HEART DISEASE IN INFANCY

HEART DISEASE IN INFANCY

James H. Moller, M.D.
Professor of Pediatrics
University of Minnesota
Minneapolis, Minnesota

William A. Neal, M.D.
Associate Professor of Pediatrics and Chairman
Section of Pediatric Cardiology
West Virginia University
Morgantown, West Virginia

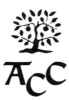

APPLETON-CENTURY-CROFTS/New York

Prentice-Hall International, Inc., London
Prentice-Hall of Australia, Pty. Ltd., Sydney
Prentice-Hall of India Private Limited, New Delhi
Prentice-Hall of Japan, Inc., Tokyo
Prentice-Hall of Southeast Asia (Pte.) Ltd., Singapore
Whitehall Books Ltd., Wellington, New Zealand

Library of Congress Cataloging in Publication Data
Moller, James H.
    Heart diseases in infancy.

    Includes index.
    1. Pediatric cardiology.   2.   Infants—Diseases.
I. Neal, William A., 1940-   joint author. II. Fuhr-
man, Bradley P., joint author.   III.   Title.   [DNLM:
1.   Heart diseases—In infancy and childhood.   WS290
M726h]
RJ421.M562   618.92′12   80-10518
ISBN 0-8385-3671-9

Cover illustration: Holly Reid
Cover design: Robert Bull

Dedicated to our children
Jim and Elizabeth Moller
and
Stephanie, Michael, Elizabeth, and James Neal

CONTENTS

ACKNOWLEDGMENTS

Contributions to books are made in various ways. Through the years, we have been fortunate to work with a number of students, residents, fellows, colleagues, and teachers who have been stimulating and knowledgeable, and our friends. It is difficult to state precisely how each person has contributed, where each thought and idea originated.

The medical students, residents, and fellows—whether in cardiology, neonatology, radiology, or cardiovascular surgery—have kept us on our toes by asking questions, sometimes simple ones, that pointed out deficiencies in our knowledge and made us search for answers, new relationships, or explanations. A special thanks should go to the pediatric cardiology fellows at the University of Minnesota who have helped train one of the authors (JHM).

A pediatric cardiologist depends heavily on his surgeons, and both authors have been fortunate to have close and friendly working and learning experiences with our cardiovascular surgeons—Dr. Neal with Dr. Herbert Warden at the University of West Virginia, and Dr. Moller with Drs. Richard Varco, Aldo Castaneda, Demetre Nicoloff, John Foker, and Robert Anderson. We have worked as colleagues in attempting to provide the best care we could for our patients.

Drs. Kurt Amplatz and Gustave Formanek, cardiovascular radiologists at the University of Minnesota, have taught us a great deal through the years. We have learned together by reviewing x-rays and attempting to solve problems presented by critically ill infants in the catheterization laboratory. Their extensive knowledge of cardiology has provided a bond and a level of understanding that has permitted our close working relationship.

Several pediatric cardiologists have been our teachers and colleagues. Dr. Paul Adams was interested in cardiac disease in infants during the 1950s and early 1960s. Unfortunately, his illness prevented him from developing fully his thoughts and knowledge, and perhaps from authoring this book. Dr. Ray Anderson is a superb clinician who taught us so much about cardiac examination and pediatric electrocardiography. We hope someday to approach the high level of clinical skills he possesses. As he nears retirement, I (JHM) begin to sense the loss of his helpful consultation as the pediatric cardiologist's cardiologist at the University of Minnesota.

Dr. Russ Lucas has provided us the opportunity to spread our wings, develop, and grow. By his piercing questions, he has prompted us to think logically and stand up for our beliefs.

Drs. Blanton Bessinger and Ed Kaplan have served as colleagues and teachers along the way.

One of our distinct pleasures has been the opportunity to work with Dr. Jesse Edwards. A great person and warm friend, he taught us not only to solve clinical problems by studying pathology, but how to organize and present material in a clear fashion. Jesse has remained interested in our activities, and we hope he will take pride in this book.

Our departmental chairmen, Dr. Gene Klingberg and Dr. John Anderson, each had faith in us and provided the opportunities and freedom to develop our careers as we saw fit.

Dr. Paul Dwan, a pioneering pediatric cardiologist in the upper Midwest, has been a friend and supporter of the activities of pediatric cardiology at the University of Minnesota. He established the Dwan Cardiovascular Learning Center, and has provided an endowed chair concerned with education in pediatric cardiology that is held by one of the authors (JHM). This support has greatly assisted the development of this text.

Linda Richter of Biomedical Graphics of the University of Minnesota worked with us in developing the illustrations and preparing the electrocardiograms and echocardiograms for photography. Keith Anderson advised us about the photographic aspects of the publication and developed techniques to best reproduce x-rays. Cheryl Lawrence helped us select appropriate echocardiograms for the book. Susan Kline and Linda Boche helped in preparing and typing the manuscript.

The person who deserves the most credit for keeping this project on the track is Mary Jo Antinozzi. She supervised the typing, proofread, checked references, pulled books, picked up artwork, but most of all, took great pride in this effort and endeavored to make certain each aspect was correct. She managed to do this with equanimity, despite many other responsibilities.

We hope you enjoy reading this book and learn as much as we have in writing it.

JHM
WAN

1 Incidence of Cardiac Malformation

In this book, we will emphasize the value of various diagnostic tools that can be used to correctly identify the underlying cardiac condition causing the signs and symptoms of an infant. In approaching diagnosis, a physician applies a wide range of knowledge, experience, and skills, which are initially learned in medical school, focused upon during residency, and expanded and widened during postresidency years. Early in a medical career, the student or resident uses knowledge as the major base on which to approach diagnosis, but with the passing years, the physician gains experience which he uses as a basis for diagnosis. Experience is invaluable in improving skills in history taking and physical examination and in interpreting electrocardiograms and chest x-rays. Experience also leads to development of diagnostic patterns that the physician can readily recognize. Experience allows the physician to weigh conflicting diagnostic information and choose the best. With experience develops intuition, an ill-defined quality that guides the physician in initiating the diagnostic process.

In this chapter, the incidence of various cardiac anomalies is discussed. Experience gained over a period of years can lead the physician to develop an idea about which cardiac conditions are common and which are rare. Information about the types of cardiac conditions that are common or rare at various ages can narrow the diagnostic possibilities as soon as the physician learns the age of the patient.

OVERALL INCIDENCE OF CONGENITAL CARDIAC MALFORMATIONS

The exact incidence of congenital cardiac malformations is difficult to determine. Table 1-1 shows the incidence of congenital cardiac malformations in several large population groups in which the population was relatively captive, so that all cases were seen either at a single center[1-7] or through a single study.[8]

TABLE 1-1

Incidence of Congenital Cardiac Malformations among Live Births

	NO. LIVE BIRTHS	NO. AFFECTED	INCIDENCE (NO. LIVE BIRTHS/1,000)
MacMahon et al.[1] (Britain) 1953	194,418	633	3.23
McIntosh et al.[2] (USA) 1954	5,628	43	7.6
Carlgren[3] (Sweden) 1959	58,105	369	6.4
Richards et al.[4] (USA) 1955	5,628	43	7.6
Kerrebijn[5] (Holland) 1966	1,817	15	8.0
Landtman[6] (Finland) 1966	1,745,419	—	8.0 (estimate)
Bound and Logan[7] (Britain) 1977	56,982	338	5.9
Mitchell et al.[8] (USA) 1966	54,765	420	7.7

A number of factors influence the reported incidence of congenital cardiac malformations. The often quoted incidence figure of 8/1,000 probably underestimates the incidence because most patients have not been followed for a long enough period to discover certain cardiac anomalies that are not recognized or present in infancy or early childhood. Examples of anomalies which may be initially recognized in later life include atrial septal defect, aortic arch anomalies, and, particularly, bicuspid aortic valve. The incidence of bicuspid valve is about 10/1,000.[9] Thus, the overall incidence of congenital cardiac malformations is at least 20/1,000.

In studying incidence, stillbirths should be excluded from the study, since the incidence of congenital cardiac malformations is higher among this group.

If the study population includes a large number of prematurely born infants, this single factor increases the incidence of congenital cardiac malformations. Both patent ductus arteriosus and ventricular septal defect are common in premature infants. Ventricular septal defect occurs three to four times as frequently in prematures[10, 11] as in full-term infants. In prematurely born infants, both a patent ductus arteriosus and a ventricular septal defect may undergo spontaneous closure, and this also can occur in full-term infants. Therefore, the age at which the population is initially screened influences the incidence of cardiac anomalies.

The incidence and relative frequency of congenital cardiac anomalies depend upon etiologic factors, such as rubella, thalidomide, or the race of the population. These factors, therefore, must be considered.

Because of the high incidence of deaths among neonates and infants with cardiac anomalies, the cardiac problems occurring in this age group deserve special attention. Landtman[6] has reported that 90 percent of deaths in children with congenital cardiac disease occur under 1 year of age, and 83 percent occur under 6 months of age. The experience of Carlgren[3] is similar, 86 percent dying by 1 year of age and 77 percent by 6 months of age.

Menashe and associates[12] studied the mortality from congenital cardiovascular disease in Oregon and found 72 percent of deaths occurred under 1 year of age and 43 percent in the neonatal period.

Feldt and associates[13] studied the incidence of congenital cardiac disease in the first year of life and indicate that approximately 43 percent of all cases were diagnosed in the first week of life, and 86 percent had a specific cardiac diagnosis established by 1 year of age. They found that 24 percent of patients died by 1 week of age and 41 percent by 1 year of age. MacMahon and co-workers[1] estimate, based on their studies in Birmingham, that about 60 percent of patients with congenital cardiac malformations die by 1 year of age.

We believe these studies overestimate the number of deaths and that the incidence is probably closer to 35 percent in the first year of life. The exact incidence also depends upon the era, particularly because of changes in operative techniques and abilities, improved recognition of affected infants, and the definition of congenital cardiac anomalies, particularly the problem of whether patent ductus arteriosus and patent foramen ovale in the first month of life should be considered congenital cardiac anomalies.

These studies indicate that most deaths from congenital cardiac disease occur in the first year of life and at least one third of children born with congenital cardiac disease die. These figures indicate the magnitude of the problem of cardiac disease in infancy, and they must be considered in relation to the continually improving diagnostic and therapeutic methods, many of which can be applied to this age group to improve survival.

FREQUENCY OF SYMPTOMATIC CONGENITAL CARDIAC ANOMALIES IN THE FIRST MONTH OF LIFE

It is difficult to obtain exact figures of the types of cardiac anomalies that lead to symptoms within the first month of life. The incidence figures vary, depending upon referral patterns, the nature of the reporting hospital, the presence of neonatal transport systems, and the degree to which physicians in the community are alert to neonatal symptoms that may indicate congenital cardiac disease. The distribution of cardiac anomalies in the first month of life can be estimated by autopsy series (Table 1-2).

Of the 10 most common cardiac conditions, 6 lesions are found predominantly in autopsies in this age group: left ventricular outflow obstruction—particularly aortic or mitral atresia, transposition of the great vessels, tetralogy of Fallot, pulmonary stenosis or atresia, coarctation of the aorta, and ventricular septal defect. Mehrizi and co-workers[14] and Rowe and Cleary [15] found that two thirds of neonatal deaths occurred in the first week of life. In Lambert's experience[16] it was 52 percent, and in our experience from 1955 to 1978[17] it was 56 percent.

Lambert and associates[16] comment that two lesions—hypoplastic left ventricle and transposition of the great vessels—were the leading causes of death in the first week of life.

In our experience, deaths in patients with tetralogy of Fallot, pulmonary

TABLE 1-2

Distribution of Cardiac Anomalies in Neonates by Percentage—Autopsy Studies

	MINNESOTA[17] 1955–1956	MINNESOTA[17] 1967–1978	JOHNS HOPKINS[14] 1927–1958	BUFFALO[16] 1949–1964	TORONTO[15] 1953–1957	GOTHENBERG[3] 1941–1950	COOPERATIVE STUDY[8]	TORONTO[18] 1965–1970	HELSINKI[19] 1947–1970
No. cases	143	211	150	165	106	81	78	111	677
Hypo LV	21	29	13	24.5	27	11.5	17	24.3	15
TGV	12	8.5	17	15	10	7	4	11.7	10
T of F	5	6	4	7	5	4	2.5	4.5	2
PS/PA	13	7.5	7	7	8	2.5	8	7	—
Coarct	5	10	16	12	13	33	13	17	11
VSD	3	2	17	2	7	15	12	4.5	14
AV	4	1	2	4	5	1	5	4	—
PDA	0.5	0.5	10	2	2	9	1	1	6
TA	2	0.5	2	2	2	0	2.5	0	2
Truncus	1	3	2	4	3	5	8	5.4	—

Abbreviations: AV, atrioventricular canal; Coarct, coarctation; Hypo LV, hypoplastic left ventricle; PDA, patent ductus arteriosus; PS/PA, pulmonary stenosis/pulmonary atresia; T of F, tetralogy of Fallot; TGV, transposition of great vessels; VSD, ventricular septal defect; —, not mentioned.

stenosis, or pulmonary atresia more commonly occurred at operation or cardiac catheterization.

The distribution of anomalies varies according to the years during which the study was carried out. For instance, with the current aggressive approach toward transposition of the great vessels, the survival rate should be improved over that of the era in which palliative and corrective procedures were unavailable. Furthermore, variations of this incidence occur if the patent ductus arteriosus accompanying the respiratory distress syndrome is included in the statistics.

Another way of determining the distribution of symptomatic cardiac disease in the first month of life is by studying the diagnosis of patients undergoing cardiac catheterization in the neonatal period, assuming that only symptomatic neonates are studied (Table 1-3).

The major cardiac conditions catheterized are transposition of the great vessels, conditions associated with hypoplastic left ventricle, coarctation of the aorta, pulmonary stenosis or pulmonary atresia, and hypoplastic right ventricle. Considering the overall frequency of ventricular septal defect, the number studied in the first month of life is small, and atrial septal defect is rare.

TABLE 1-3

Distribution of Cardiac Anomalies in First Month of Life by Percentage—Cardiac Catheterization Study

	MINNESOTA[17] <1 WEEK 1967-1976	LONDON[20] <1 WEEK 1970-1973	MINNESOTA[17] <1 MONTH 1967-1976	JOHNS HOPKINS[21] <1 MONTH 1964-1968
No. cases	177	111	344	100
Hypo LV	12	9	9	9
TGV	29	34	24	20
T of F	6	3	7	5
Coarct	8	7	12.5	9
PS/PA	8	18	5.5	5
VSD	0	1	6	11
PDA	3	0	3.5	9
Truncus	1	0	2	7
Hypo RV	5	3	3	9
AV	2	1	2	—
Single ventricle	4	4	5	—
PA with VSD single ventricle	*	I3	*	—
Misc	23	5	20	18†

* Coded under T of F.
† Includes complex cases.
Abbreviations: AV, atrioventricular canal; Coarct, coarctation; Hypo LV, hypoplastic left ventricle; Hypo RV, hypoplastic right ventricle; Misc, miscellaneous; PA, pulmonary atresia; PDA, patent ductus arteriosus; PS/PA, pulmonary stenosis/pulmonary atresia; T of F, tetralogy of Fallot; TGV, transposition of great vessels; VSD, ventricular septal defect; —, not mentioned.

Among our patients with miscellaneous conditions catheterized in the first month of life were atrial septal defect (2), corrected transposition (4), double outlet right ventricle (3), mitral insufficiency (1), mitral stenosis (2), Ebstein's malformation (8), tricuspid insufficiency (2), hypoplastic right ventricle (4), myocarditis (2), supravalvar aortic stenosis (1), absent pulmonary artery (1), pulmonary artery branch stenosis or atresia (1), interruption of the aortic arch (7), total anomalous pulmonary venous connection (8), cardiac anomalies associated with splenic anomalies (13), and arteriovenous fistula (2).

DISTRIBUTION OF CARDIAC ANOMALIES
BETWEEN 1 MONTH AND 1 YEAR

Several autopsy studies have reviewed the distribution of the congenital cardiac anomalies in infants between 1 and 12 months (Table 1-4), and four studies have studied the incidence under 1 year of age (Table 1-5). These studies show that ventricular septal defect, transposition of the great vessels, atrioventricular canal, coarctation of the aorta, and tetralogy of Fallot are the most common lesions. In the first year of life, at least one third of the deaths are related to conditions obstructing left ventricular outflow.

Infants with ventricular septal defect show a higher incidence of prematurity or die from infection or noncardiac malformations.

Other studies have presented information about distribution of cardiac anomalies catheterized in the first year (Table 1-6) and indicate that ventricu-

TABLE 1-4

Distribution of Cardiac Anomalies Between 1 and 12 Months by Percentage—Autopsy Study

	MINNESOTA[17] 1955–1966	MINNESOTA[17] 1967–1978	GOTHENBERG[3] 1941–1950	COOPERATIVE[8] STUDY	HELSINKI[19] 1947–1970
No. cases	256	125	44	50	258
VSD	11	14	11	10	13
TGV	17	10	25	10	17
Coarct	7	14	9	4	7
PDA	2	1	5	20	6
T of F	6	8	2.5	4	7.5
AV	7	7	7	4	—
PS/PA	6	4	2.5	8	—
TAPVC	8	1	2.5	—	—
AS	4	2	9	—	—
ASD	1	2	2.5	—	8
Truncus	2	5	2.5	—	10
TA	4	—	2.5	4	5

Abbreviations: AS, aortic stenosis; ASD, atrial septal defect; AV, atrioventricular canal; Coarct, coarctation; PDA, patent ductus arteriosus; PS/PA, pulmonary stenosis/pulmonary atresia; TA, tricuspid atresia; TAPVC, total anomalous pulmonary venous connection; T of F, tetralogy of Fallot; TGV, transposition of great vessels; VSD, ventricular septal defect.

TABLE 1-5

Distribution of Cardiac Anomalies Under 1 Year of Age by Percentage— Autopsy Studies

	UPPSALA[22] 1961–1970	GLASGOW[23] 1959–1962	HELSINKI[19] 1947–1970	MINNESOTA[17] 1955–1966	MINNESOTA[17] 1967–1976
No. cases	448	96	667	400	335
VSD	14	17.5	14	8	7
TGV	13	24	13	19	9
Coarct	4	15.5	10	3	6
PDA	3.6	4	6	2	0.5
EFE	1.6	8.5	5	1.5	1
T of F	5.4	—	5	5	7
Truncus	3.6	6.8	—	2	4
TA	4.2	3	4	3	<0.5
TAPVC	2.7	4	—	6	3
AV	8	—	—	6	4
PS/PA	2.9	—	—	9	6
AS	3.3	—	—	3	1
ASD	—	—	10	<1	<1
MA/AA	21.7	—	10	7	12
Combined	—	—	10	—	—

Abbreviations: AS, aortic stenosis; ASD, atrial septal defect; AV, atrioventricular canal; Coarct, coarctation; EFE, endocardial fibroelastosis; MA/AA, mitral atresia/aortic atresia; PDA, patent ductus arteriosus; PS/PA, pulmonary stenosis/pulmonary atresia; T of F, tetralogy of Fallot; TA, tricuspid atresia; TAPVC, total anomalous pulmonary venous connection; TGV, transposition of great vessels; VSD, ventricular septal defect.

TABLE 1-6

Distribution of Defects in 688 Patients Catheterized in First Year of Life at University of Minnesota, 1967–1976

CONDITION	PERCENT OF TOTAL
Ventricular septal defect	11
Transposition of great vessels	22
Coarctation of aorta	13
Patent ductus arteriosus	8
Endocardial fibroelastosis	0.5
Tetralogy of Fallot	7
Truncus arteriosus	3
Tricuspid atresia	3
Total anomalous pulmonary venous connection	2.5
Atrioventricular canal	4
Pulmonary stenosis/pulmonary atresia	4
Aortic stenosis	2.5
Atrial septal defect	2.5
Mitral atresia/aortic atresia	3
Miscellaneous	14

lar septal defect, transposition of the great vessels, coarctation of aorta, and patent ductus arteriosus account for half the cases studied. The distribution of neonates and infants seen clinically at the University of Minnesota Hospitals[24] is shown in Table 1-7. This indicates that ventricular septal defect, transposition of the great vessels, tetralogy of Fallot, coarctation of the aorta, and patent ductus arteriosus affect two thirds of all infants initially examined during the first year of life at our institution.

TABLE 1-7

Distribution of Defects in 1,368 Infants with Congenital Cardiac Disease Examined Clinically at University of Minnesota

CONDITION	NO. INFANTS	PERCENT OF TOTAL
Ventricular septal defect	337	24.6
Tetralogy of Fallot	259	17.4
Transposition of great vessels	143	10.4
Coarctation of aorta	111	8.1
Patent ductus arteriosus	109	8.0
Atrioventricular canal	78	5.7
Pulmonary stenosis/pulmonary atresia	60	4.4
Single ventricle	33	2.4
Tricuspid atresia	26	1.9
Endocardial fibroelastosis	25	1.8
Truncus arteriosus	24	1.7
Total anomalous pulmonary venous connection	20	1.5
Aortic stenosis	18	1.3
Atrial septal defect	11	0.7
Miscellaneous	134	9.0

ASSOCIATED MALFORMATIONS

Feldt and associates[13] reported associated congenital malformations in 30 percent of their patients, most commonly involving the hands, feet, and genitourinary system.

Menashe and colleagues[12] found that of infants who died with congenital cardiac anomalies, one third had associated congenital malformations. Anomalies of the gastrointestinal or genitourinary system accounted for half of the noncardiac malformations, being 25 percent each. Malformations of the central nervous system accounted for 22 percent, musculoskeletal anomalies were present in 12 percent, respiratory anomalies in 6 percent, and all other malformations comprised 10 percent. No pattern of malformations was associated with a particular congenital cardiac anomaly.

Landtman[6] studied 777 patients with cardiac anomalies at autopsy and found coexistent noncardiac congenital malformations in 353 (45 percent), but many of these were minor.[19] These malformations were most common in infants with low birth weight (53 percent) and in patients under 6 months of age (51 percent). Gastrointestinal anomalies occurred in 138 patients, musculoskeletal in 124 patients, and genitourinary in 99 patients. A higher incidence of noncardiac congenital malformations occurred in patients with combined septal defects (74 percent), patent ductus arteriosus (59 percent), and ventricular septal defect (58 percent). The incidence was low in patients with endocardial fibroelastosis or transposition of the great vessels.

Greenwood and associates[25] reviewed the data on 1,566 infants with cardiac anomalies and found that 395 (25 percent) had one or more extracardiac anomalies. Forty percent had an anomaly in one organ system, 40 percent in two organ systems, and 15 percent in three organ systems. The frequency in various systems is shown below:

System	Number	% of 1,566
Musculoskeletal	137	8.8
Specific syndromes	132	8.5
Central nervous	107	6.9
Urinary	83	5.3
Gastrointestinal	65	4.2
Respiratory	58	3.8
Endocrine	21	1.3
Immunologic-hematologic	10	<1
Reproductive	2	<1
Other	45	2.9

Interestingly, complete transposition of the great vessels, hypoplastic left ventricle, and pulmonary atresia with intact ventricular septum were associated with a lower than average number of extracardiac malformations, while more than one third of the patients with endocardial cushion defect, patent ductus arteriosus, atrial septal defect, or malposition of the heart had extracardiac anomalies. The mortality was higher in infants with associated malformations. One third of all associated malformations occurred as part of a well-recognized syndrome, such as Down's syndrome.

An interesting series of studies has reviewed the incidence and type of congenital cardiac anomalies found with particular types of major noncardiac congenital anomalies (Table 1-8). Tracheoesophageal fistula has been studied by several authors,[26-29] and probably one quarter of the patients with esophageal atresia have an associated anomaly. Ventricular septal defect, patent ductus arteriosus, coarctation of the aorta, and tetralogy of Fallot are common. There are several conditions that may be present and complicate correction—right aortic arch, aberrant subclavian artery, and persistent left superior vena cava.[26, 28] A higher mortality exists in patients with esophageal atresia and a coexistent cardiac anomaly.

Greenwood and associates[30] also studied diaphragmatic hernia, omphalocele,[31] and imperforate anus[32] and found the incidence of coexistent cardiac

TABLE 1-8

Incidence and Type of Cardiac Anomaly Associated with Major Noncardiac Malformation

NONCARDIAC MALFORMATION	REFERENCE	TOTAL NO. CASES	TOTAL NO. CHD	PERCENTAGE	TYPE OF CARDIAC ANOMALY					MORTALITY (%)	
					VSD	Coarct	T of F	ASD	Other	Without CHD	With CHD
Tracheo-esophageal fistula	26	345	96	27.8	18	2	3	11	62	26	86
Tracheo-esophageal fistula	27	326	48	14.7	17	3	6	5	17	23	79
Tracheo-esophageal fistula	28	183	48	26	—	—	—	—	—	41	96
Tracheo-esophageal fistula	29	39	16	39	3	5	0	0	8	—	—
Diaphragmatic hernia	30	48	11	23	3	1	3	1	3	27	73
Omphalocele	31	159	31 + 6	19.5	3	3	12	7	12	31	81
Imperforate anus	32	222	26 + 7	12	8	—	9	—	16	—	33

Abbreviations: ASD, atrial septal defect; CHD, congenital heart disease; Coarct, coarctation; T of F, tetralogy of Fallot; VSD, ventricular septal defect; ——, not mentioned.

anomalies to be 23 percent, 19.5 percent, and 12 percent, respectively. As in esophageal atresia, mortality was higher in those with a cardiac anomaly.

Congestive cardiac failure is rarely present at birth because most congenital cardiac malformations do not alter significantly the fetal circulation or hemodynamics. Severe valvular insufficiency, rhabdomyomas, cardiac dysrhythmias, and anemia are, however, causes which must be considered when a neonate shows cardiac failure at birth.[33-35] Other conditions, such as aortic atresia, cause problems soon after birth.

Within the first week of life, aortic atresia, transposition of the great vessels, coarctation of the aorta, and conditions associated with pulmonary valvular atresia are the most common conditions causing symptoms. In the remainder of the first month of life, these same conditions are the most common.

Conditions associated with large pulmonary blood flow, such as ventricular septal defect or patent ductus arteriosus, do not typically cause problems until 2 or 3 months of life and initially appear at this age.

It is uncommon for infants to initially develop congestive cardiac failure between 6 and 12 months of age, but myocarditis, myocardiopathies, total anomalous pulmonary venous connection, and atrioventricular canal should be considered in such infants.

SUMMARY

When approaching a neonate or an infant with an unknown form of cardiac disease, the physician must use all of the available information to reach a diagnosis. Diagnosis is a complex in which the patient's symptoms, signs, and laboratory findings are interpreted in relationship to the findings in known disease states. The task of diagnosis in any patient is considerably easier if the number of disease states that must be considered can be narrowed. Knowledge of the overall incidence of congenital cardiac malformations and the specific incidence at any given age can help the physician narrow the diagnostic possibilities for a particular child, since there will be some conditions which never or rarely occur at that age.

The age of the infant is often the first bit of data that the physician receives, and the diagnostic thought process should be initiated at and proceed from this point.

Chapters 2 through 6 present information about other methods that the physician uses in proceeding toward establishing a diagnosis.

REFERENCES

1. MacMahon B, McKeown T, Record RG: The incidence and life expectation of children with congenital heart disease. Br Heart J 15:121, 1953
2. McIntosh R, Merritt KK, Richards MR, Samuels MH, Bellows MT: The inci-

dence of congenital malformations: A study of 5,964 pregnancies. Pediatrics 14:505, 1954

3. Carlgren LE: The incidence of congenital heart disease in children born in Gothenburg 1941–1950. Br Heart J 21:40, 1959

4. Richards MR, Merritt KK, Samuels MH, Langmann AG: Congenital malformations of the cardiovascular system in a series of 6,053 infants. Pediatrics 15:12, 1955

5. Kerrebijn KF: Incidence in infants and mortality from congenital malformations of the circulatory system. Acta Paediatr Scand 55:316, 1966

6. Landtman B: The incidence of heart disease in children. Proc Assoc Eur Pediatr Cardiol 2:23, 1966

7. Bound JP, Logan WFWE: Incidence of congenital heart disease in Blackpool 1957–1971. Br Heart J 39:445, 1977

8. Mitchell SC, Korones SB, Berendes HW: Congenital heart disease in 56,109 births. Incidence and natural history. Circulation 43:323, 1971

9. Keith JD: Bicuspid aortic valve. In Keith JD, Rowe RD, Vlad P (eds): Heart Disease in Infancy and Childhood. New York, Macmillan, 1978, pp 728–735

10. Mitchell SC, Berendes HW, Clark WM Jr: The normal closure of the ventricular septum. Am Heart J 73:334, 1967

11. Hoffman JIE, Rudolph AM: The natural history of ventricular septal defect in infancy. Am J Cardiol 16:634, 1965

12. Menashe VD, Osterud HT, Griswold HE: Mortality from congenital cardiovascular disease in Oregon. Pediatrics 40:334, 1967

13. Feldt RH, Avasthey P, Yoshimasu F, Kurland LT, Titus JL: Incidence of congenital heart disease in children born to residents of Olmsted County, Minnesota, 1950–1969. Mayo Clin Proc 46:794, 1971

14. Mehrizi A, Hirsch MS, Taussig HB: Congenital heart disease in the neonatal period. Autopsy study of 170 cases. J Pediatr 65:721, 1964

15. Rowe RD, Cleary TE: Congenital cardiac malformation in the newborn period. Frequency in a children's hospital. Can Med Assoc J 83:299, 1960

16. Lambert EC, Canent RV, Hohn AR: Congenital cardiac anomalies in the newborn. A review of conditions causing death or severe distress in the first month of life. Pediatrics 37:343, 1966

17. Moller JH: Unpublished observations

18. Keith JD: Prevalence, incidence and epidemiology. In Keith JD, Rowe RD, Vlad P (eds): Heart Disease in Infancy and Childhood, New York, Macmillan, 1978, p 8

19. Landtman B: Clinical and morphological studies in congenital heart disease. A review of 777 cases. Acta Paediatr Scand 213[Suppl]:1, 1971

20. Miller GAH: Congenital heart disease in the first week of life. Br Heart J 36:1160, 1974

21. Varghese PJ, Celermajer J, Izukawa T, Haller JA, Rowe RD: Cardiac catheterization in the newborn: Experience with 100 cases. Pediatrics 44:24, 1969

22. Esscher E, Michaëlsson M, Smedby B: Cardiovascular malformation in infant deaths. 10-year clinical and epidemiological study. Br Heart J 37:824, 1975

23. Coleman EN: Serious congenital heart disease in infancy. Br Heart J 27:42, 1965

24. Eliot RS, Anderson RC, Adams P Jr, Edwards JE: Heart disease in the first year of life. In Cassels DE (ed): The Heart and Circulation in the Newborn and Infant. New York, Grune & Stratton, 1966, pp 243–254

25. Greenwood RD, Rosenthal A, Parisi L, Fyler DC, Nadas AS: Extracardiac abnormalities in infants with congenital heart disease. Pediatrics 55:485, 1975

26. David TJ, O'Callaghan SE: Cardiovascular malformations and oesophageal atresia. Br Heart J 36:559, 1974

27. Greenwood RD, Rosenthal A: Cardiovascular malformations associated with tracheoesophageal fistula and esophageal atresia. Pediatrics 57:87, 1976

28. Mellins RB, Blumenthal S: Cardiovascular anomalies and esophageal atresia. Am J Dis Child 107:160, 1964
29. Mehrizi A, Folger GM Jr, Rowe RD: Tracheoesophageal fistula associated with congenital cardiovascular malformations. Johns Hopkins Med J 118:246, 1966
30. Greenwood RD, Rosenthal A, Nadas AS: Cardiovascular abnormalities associated with congenital diaphragmatic hernia. Pediatrics 57:92, 1976
31. Greenwood RD, Rosenthal A, Nadas AS: Cardiovascular malformations associated with omphalocele. J Pediatr 85:818, 1974
32. Greenwood RD, Rosenthal A, Nadas AS: Cardiovascular malformations associated with imperforate anus. J Pediatr 86:576, 1975
33. Moller JH, Lynch RP, Edwards JE: Fetal cardiac failure resulting from congenital anomalies of the heart. J Pediatr 68:699, 1966
34. Altenburger KM, Jedziniak M, Roper WL, Hernandez J: Congenital complete heart block associated with hydrops fetalis. J Pediatr 91:618, 1977
35. Cowan RH, Waldo AL, Harris HB, Cassady G, Brans YW: Neonatal paroxysmal supraventricular tachycardia with hydrops. Pediatrics 55:428, 1975

2 History

Although data obtained from other methods may yield more diagnostic information, the history can provide important information useful in assessing the severity of the cardiac condition, in recognizing possible complications, and in identifying etiologic factors.

Knowledge about the age of onset of cardiac symptoms, particularly those related to congestive cardiac failure, yields information about the type of cardiac disease which may be present (Chap. 1). Congestive cardiac failure at birth, although rare, is caused by only a few conditions—intrauterine arrhythmias, erythroblastosis, and severe valvular insufficiencies. The onset of cardiac failure within the first week of life most commonly is related to lesions causing obstruction of blood flow from the heart, particularly aortic atresia and coarctation of the aorta. Typically, infants with conditions in which increased pulmonary blood flow places excessive volume load on the left ventricle, resulting in cardiac failure, do not have symptoms before 6 weeks of age. Examples of such conditions are ventricular septal defect, patent ductus arteriosus, or truncus arteriosus. By 6 weeks of age, the pulmonary vascular resistance has fallen sufficiently to permit the pulmonary blood flow to be large enough to cause cardiac failure.

Diagnostic information can also be obtained from knowledge of the age at which the cardiac murmur is initially heard. Significant murmurs present at birth usually result from either aortic or pulmonary stenosis. The pulmonary stenosis may be combined with a ventricular septal defect, as in tetralogy of Fallot. Murmurs related to left-to-right shunts, such as ventricular septal defect, are generally not heard until the initial postnatal visit to the physician's office.

The sex of the infant can provide diagnostic information. Complete transposition of the great vessels, coarctation of the aorta, aortic stenosis, and aortic atresia occur more commonly in males, while atrial septal defect and patent ductus arteriosus are more frequently found in females.

CYANOIS

Cyanosis is the most dramatic cardiac symptom in neonates or infants. Cyanosis is the bluish color imparted to the skin when capillaries contain more than 5 g% of reduced hemoglobin. Cyanosis may reflect a serious abnormality of oxygen transport or may be merely a normal variant. Cyanosis of the neonate has been reviewed excellently by Wiles.[1]

Cyanosis can be classified as either peripheral or central. Peripheral cyanosis (acrocyanosis) involves the extremities primarily or exclusively. Neonates often have bluish hands and feet, and normal infants may have cyanosis about the mouth when exposed to cold. Both are examples of peripheral cyanosis and are related to sluggish flow through these capillary beds. Warming or moving the extremities results in a prompt return of color to normal. Peripheral cyanosis also occurs in patients with low cardiac output, as from neonatal sepsis or adrenocortical insufficiency. Often, this is combined with cyanosis of the trunk, and the patient is initially thought to have a cyanotic form of congenital cardiac disease. This cyanosis usually improves as cardiac output is restored. In each of these examples, there is no structural abnormality of the heart, lungs, or hemoglobin to interfere with oxygen transport.

Central cyanosis regularly involves the trunk as well as the extremities and the mucous membranes and is caused by an abnormality of oxygen transport occurring from abnormalities of the heart, lungs, or hemoglobin. Cardiac anomalies can lead to cyanosis by two mechanisms. In the first, a structural abnormality is present that permits a portion of the systemic venous blood that is returning to the right side of the heart to bypass the lungs and enter the aorta. Two general forms of cardiac anomalies lead to such intracardiac right-to-left shunting: (1) the combination of an intracardiac defect and obstruction to pulmonary blood flow (e.g., tetralogy of Fallot) and (2) conditions in which both the systemic and pulmonary venous returns empty into a single chamber and are thus mixed and flow to the lungs and body (e.g., single ventricle). Central cyanosis of cardiac origin also results from abnormalities of pulmonary perfusion secondary to pulmonary edema from elevated capillary pressure, as from mitral stenosis or left ventricular failure.

In infants, particularly in the neonate, central cyanosis also commonly results from abnormalities of the respiratory tract. A congenital or acquired condition that interferes with oxygen transport from the environment to the pulmonary capillary can lead to cyanosis. This condition may occur not only in the pulmonary parenchyma but also in the respiratory passages. Choanal atresia is an example of the latter. It can lead to intense cyanosis, since neonates breathe only through their nose and, therefore, have inadequate oxygen transport. Pulmonary parenchymal diseases, such as hyaline membrane disease, pneumonitis, or atelectasis, or conditions that occupy space in the thorax and compress the lung, such as pneumothorax or diaphragmatic hernia, lead to cyanosis.

A thoracic roentgenogram is required to evaluate cyanosis and to recognize and distinguish cardiac and pulmonary causes.

Previously, it was believed that pulmonary and cardiac causes of cyanosis could be distinguished by the response to the administration of 100 percent oxygen or to crying. Unfortunately, however, there is no predictable response.

Central cyanosis rarely results from an abnormality of hemoglobin. Methemoglobinemia may be hereditary or may be acquired from ingestion of nitrate-contaminated well water or from contact with specific drugs or chemicals. Methemoglobinemia is the only form of cyanosis in which there is a normal arterial Po_2. It is caused by a reduction of elemental iron in the hemoglobin molecule and is easily treated with an oxidizing agent, such as ascorbic acid.

Among patients with cardiac disease, the age when cyanosis appears is helpful diagnostically.[2] The cyanosis in patients with complete transposition of the great vessels develops in the neonatal period. Intense cyanosis from birth suggests pulmonary or tricuspid atresia. Patients with Ebstein's malformation and an occasional patient with an atrial septal defect may show cyanosis in the neonatal period, but the cyanosis subsequently clears.

DIFFICULT FEEDING

The parent of an infant with a cardiac anomaly may complain that the child has difficulty with feeding. The history reveals that the infant is a slow eater, seems to tire on eating, and requires frequent rest. For instance, it may take 45 minutes to feed the infant only 2 ounces of milk. Often the infant is eager to feed but fatigues easily and quickly. This symptom represents dyspnea on exertion, the exertion being the act of sucking a bottle. The presence of difficult feeding usually indicates congestive cardiac failure, but it may be present in patients with severe cyanosis.

Difficult feeding must be distinguished from dysphagia—difficulty in swallowing—which may be present in an infant with a vascular ring.

DIFFICULT BREATHING

Although infants cannot describe dyspnea, difficult breathing exists and is manifested by rapid breathing, often associated with retractions and an anxious facies. This symptom may be accentuated during feeding or on other exertion but may be noticed even when the infant is asleep. Dyspnea may be associated with grunting respirations.

Difficult breathing most frequently indicates congestive cardiac failure and reflects decreased pulmonary compliance from pulmonary congestion. It can also occur in patients with severe hypoxemia.

EXCESSIVE PERSPIRATION

Parents may indicate that their infant perspires freely and easily or that the infant's head is always wet with perspiration. Heat rash may develop even in the middle of a Minnesota winter. We have observed one neonate who had numerous, 5 mm blisters of sweat over the head and upper neck. Excessive perspiration results from increased catecholamine exertion which occurs as a compensatory mechanism of congestive cardiac failure.[3]

SLOW GROWTH

Infants with congenital cardiac malformations may grow slowly, with both height and weight gain being delayed. The delay may be related to factors that caused the cardiac malformation, such as rubella, or it may be related to a syndrome, such as Down's syndrome, associated with the cardiac malformation.

Growth retardation affects weight more than height and is present in infants with either congestive cardiac failure or cyanosis.[4] The exact metabolic or physiologic mechanism for the retarded growth is unknown. Certainly, reduced caloric intake from the difficulty in feeding may be a cause. The metabolic demands are also probably increased because of the increased respiratory effort in infants with congestive cardiac failure.

RESPIRATORY INFECTIONS

In infants with cardiac malformations, respiratory infections occur frequently and tend to be severe and chronic, particularly in infants with cardiac anomalies associated with increased pulmonary blood flow. Infections frequently progress to pneumonia. It may be difficult to distinguish the symptoms of pneumonia from those of congestive cardiac failure, but usually a thoracic roentgenogram allows differentiation.

Several factors probably contribute to the frequent respiratory infections. The major bronchi may be compressed by an enlarged left atrium or by enlarged hypertensive pulmonary arteries.[5] Partial or total occlusion of the bronchi occurs, and either atelectasis or emphysema can result. In patients with increased pulmonary blood flow, the right middle or upper lobes are most frequently involved, whereas in patients with left-sided obstructive lesions or cardiomyopathy, the left lower lobe is most commonly affected. Pneumonia may develop because of atelectasis or pulmonary edema.

Respiratory problems are more frequent and severe in the first year of life and improve subsequently. Stridor or hoarse voice may be a symptom related to vascular ring.

NEUROLOGIC SYMPTOMS

Neurologic symptoms can result either from physiologic abnormalities seconary to the cardiac malformation or from coexistent developmental anomalies or syndromes.

Of the several well-known neurologic sequelae of congenital cardiac malformations, brain abscess and ruptured berry aneurysm are rare in infancy.

Cerebrovascular accidents, most frequently leading to hemiplegia, occur in infancy, but usually in those patients with a high hematocrit and a low hemoglobin value.[6]

Various types of seizures may occur in infants, particularly if they are cyanotic. These may occur as part of a tetrad spell, in which there is a sudden and often extreme decrease in arterial Po_2. Tetrad spells may be only a brief episode of unconsciousness or stiffening, or they may be associated with a grand mal convulsion. Seizures may be associated with other metabolic problems that occur in the management of an acutely ill infant or in the immediate postnatal period.

Most infants with congenital cardiac anomalies show normal mental development although those milestones depending on physical prowess may be delayed.

Developmental delay or other neurologic symptoms may occur in these children because of a coexistent condition, such as Down's syndrome, tuberous sclerosis, or others.

PAST HISTORY

In each patient, a careful history of the pregnancy should be obtained, for this may yield information to suggest an etiology of the cardiac malformation, although in general, the yield is low. An example is the association of maternal rubella in the first trimester with patent ductus arteriosus and peripheral pulmonary arterial stenosis. Maternal diabetes or ingestion of thalidomide are associated with an increased incidence of congenital cardiac disease. Whether maternal mumps infection or ingestion of sex hormonal products during pregnancy leads to cardiac malformations remains controversial. There is no evidence to indicate that parity influences the incidence of cardiac disease, nor does maternal age, other than through the recognized association with chromosomal abnormalities.

Prematurity is associated with an increased incidence of congenital cardiac malformations. A thorough family history should be obtained, since nearly every form of congenital cardiac malformation has been reported to occur in more than one member of a family. The incidence of congenital cardiac disease in the population is at least 1:135 (0.7 percent) (Chap. 1). The recurrence rate in a family is about 2 percent. The concordance of cardiac defects is about 50 percent.

REFERENCES

1. Wiles HB: Cyanosis in the new-born. Med J Aust 93:481, 1964
2. Moller JH, Anderson RC: Congenital heart disease. In Kelley VC (ed): Brennemann's Practice of Pediatrics, rev ed. Hagerstown, Md, Harper, 1969, Vol 3, p 8

3. Morgan CL, Nadas AS: Sweating and congestive heart failure. N Engl J Med 268:580, 1963
4. Linde LM, Dunn OJ, Schireson R, Rasof B: Growth in children with congenital heart disease. J Pediatr 70:413, 1967
5. Stanger P, Lucas RV Jr, Edwards JE: Anatomic factors causing respiratory distress in acyanotic congenital cardiac disease. Specific reference to bronchial obstruction. Pediatrics 43:760, 1969
6. Martelle RR, Linde LM: Cerebrovascular accidents with tetralogy of Fallot. Am J Dis Child 101:206, 1961

3 Physical Examination

Every physical examination begins with careful observation of the infant. Often, valuable clues about the infant's condition can be gathered by watching the infant while taking the history.

The general appearance of the infant may provide clues about an underlying cardiac condition. Several syndromes, most related to a chromosomal abnormality, are associated with cardiac malformations, Down's syndrome being the most widely recognized. Roughly, one third of infants with Down's syndrome have congenital cardiac malformations. Of these, one third have a ventricular septal defect, one third have endocardial cushion defect, and the remaining one third have atrial septal defect, patent ductus arteriosus, or tetralogy of Fallot.[1-3] Those with left-to-right shunt have unusually high pulmonary vascular resistance.[4] Aortic stenosis or coarctation of the aorta are rare in patients with this syndrome. The diagnosis of Down's syndrome in most neonates and infants can be made without chromosomal analysis, but such studies may be helpful in counseling the parents. Patients with Down's syndrome are delayed in growth and development. The infants are hypotonic and have characteristic facies, with a flat face, prominent epicardial folds, and a protruding tongue. Brushfield's spots in the irises, simian creases, third fontanelle, and shortened second phalanx of the little finger are usually present.

Cardiac malformations are also present in two other trisomic conditions. In 80 percent of patients with trisomy 18, cardiac malformation, usually ventricular septal defect, is present, and pulmonary hypertension coexists.[5,6] Growth and development are markedly retarded. A prominent occiput, low-set ears, and micrognathia are found. The hands show diagnostic overlapping of the index and little fingers. An umbilical hernia and rocker-bottom feet are other characteristics.

Trisomy 13 also shows cardiac malformations in about 80 percent of patients, frequently a form of dextrocardia with ventricular septal defect and pulmonary hypertension.[5,6] Central facial anomalies are common: microphthalmus, coloboma, and cleft lip and palate. Polydactyly is another frequent feature, and capillary hemangiomata are common.

Turner's syndrome, absence of a sex (X) chromosome, is associated with coarctation of the aorta in about 20 percent of cases.[7] A few other patients have systemic hypertension due to a renal abnormality. Patients with Turner's syndrome have a female phenotype. Webbing of the neck, a broad shield-shaped chest with widely spaced nipples, an increased carrying angle of the arms, low hairline, and peripheral lymphedema are other features. These patients rarely achieve 5 feet in height.

The idiopathic hypercalcemia syndrome of infancy (Williams' syndrome) is associated with congenital cardiac malformations in about one third of the patients, supravalvular aortic stenosis and peripheral arterial stenosis being the common abnormalities.[8] In infancy, serum calcium levels are elevated but usually fall to normal levels by 8 months of age. Often, by the time the cardiac disease is discovered, the serum calcium level is normal. The facies have been described as "elfin." The upper eyelids are puffy with prominent inner epicanthal folds, the nose is upturned, there is a full, prominent, cupid bow, upper lip and a broad maxilla and forehead. The voice is brassy. In infancy, hypotonia and constipation may be found.

Maternal rubella in the first trimester of pregnancy is associated with a high incidence of cardiac malformations, usually patent ductus arteriosus and/or peripheral pulmonary arterial stenosis.[9,10] The infants have microcephaly, cataracts, and deafness, and the birth weight is low. Evidence of viral infection may be found in the form of hepatosplenomegaly, jaundice, purpura, bony changes, and abnormalities of the cerebrospinal fluid.[11]

Abnormalities of the hands, either absence of the thumbs or fingerlike thumbs, have been associated with atrial septal defect and ventricular septal defect. This association is the Holt-Oram syndrome.[12,13]

The skin should be carefully observed for the presence of cyanosis, since this reflects the state of oxygenation. In the neonate, it may be difficult to determine if cyanosis is present, and often the equivocating term "dusky" is applied. A variety of factors, such as lighting, skin pigmentation, and observer experience, influence the detection of cyanosis.[14]

Neonates without known cardiac or pulmonary abnormalities but with an elevated hemoglobin and hematocrit, perhaps from umbilical cord stripping, may appear cyanotic but are actually plethoric and ruddy. Laboratory findings of elevated hemoglobin and hematocrit and a normal arterial Po_2 provide strong evidence for this situation.[15] Because of hypervolemia, these neonates may be tachypneic and have hepatomegaly. The electrocardiogram may reveal right axis deviation and right ventricular hypertrophy, and a thoracic roentgenogram may reveal cardiomegaly and prominent pulmonary vasculature, so that these infants may be confused with neonates with cardiac anomalies.

Infants of diabetic mothers also may appear cyanotic. They are plethoric, heavy infants, who are tachypneic, and they may show other features of respiratory distress. Symptoms of hypoglycemia or hypocalcemia may be present.

Normal neonates have ruddy or cyanotic hands and feet, especially when exposed to cold. Mild cyanosis of the lips may be present, especially on crying, presumably from right-to-left shunting through the foramen ovale or ductus arteriosus.

The oral mucosa is the most reliable site for determining if cyanosis is peripheral or central,[16] for although the lips may be cyanotic with peripheral cyanosis, the oral mucosa is of normal color, whereas in central cyanosis, both would be abnormal.

Cyanosis in the neonate can result from a number of causes, but in infants, it almost always results from cardiac disease. The presence of cyanosis requires careful and thorough evaluation of the patient. Often 100 percent oxygen is administered to the infant to determine if he becomes pink, the presumption being that cyanosis of pulmonary origin improves, while cyanosis of cardiac origin does not. Unfortunately, some forms of pulmonary disease do not improve, and some forms of cardiac disease, such as admixture lesions, improve considerably. In complete transposition of the great vessels, however, there is no improvement in the degree of oxygenation following administration of 100 percent oxygen.

The distribution of cyanosis should also be noted because rare cardiac anomalies are associated with differential cyanosis.[17] In patients with a reversing patent ductus arteriosus, i.e., with right-to-left shunt, the lower extremities appear cyanotic, while the upper part of the body is pink because it is perfused from the ascending aorta. Reversal of ductal flow can result from (1) elevation of pulmonary vascular resistance, as from pulmonary parenchymal disease, (2) conditions causing pulmonary venous obstruction, or (3) interruption of the aortic arch or coarctation of the aorta and distal patent ductus arteriosus. Because coarctation or interruption may coexist with ventricular septal defect, the saturation of blood in the pulmonary artery is elevated, and the difference in oxygen saturation values in the ascending and descending aorta is minimal.

Occasionally, the upper part of the body appears cyanotic, while the lower portion of the body is pink. This indicates transposition of the great vessels and interruption or coarctation of the aorta. In an occasional infant, only a single extremity is cyanotic. This form of differential cyanosis indicates obstruction to the venous return, as commonly follows a cutdown or cardiac catheterization.

Inspection of the fingertips may show them to be suffused or to have a ruddy color, indicating a mild degree of desaturation.

The neonate or infant should also be carefully evaluated to determine the presence of respiratory distress, for this is a valuable sign of cardiopulmonary disease. The respiratory rate and effort should be determined. Normally the respiration rate should be less than 45/min in a full-term infant and less than 60/min in a premature infant. Higher respiratory rates are usually abnormal and indicate cardiac or pulmonary problems. Occasionally, we have observed normal infants with higher respiratory rates, but who were breathing without difficulty. It is important to make certain the infant is in a quiet, resting state when counting the respiratory rate. Respiratory effort should also be evaluated. Infants with respiratory distress show intercostal and subcostal contractions, flaring of the alae nasae, anxious facies, and excessive perspiration.

Vital signs provide important clues to the diagnosis and severity of the cardiac condition. Blood pressure should be obtained in each neonate and infant suspected of cardiac disease, with recordings made from both arms and one leg. The same precautions should be taken in infants as in adults to obtain a reliable pressure recording. The infant should be in a quiet, resting state because excitement elevates blood pressure readings. The extremity in which the blood pressure is being taken should be at the same level as the heart, for if the extremity is lower, the reading is elevated.

The blood pressure cuff should be the proper size. A 4 to 5 cm (2 inch) cuff should be used in neonates and infants. Although a narrower cuff is available commercially, it uniformly yields falsely elevated levels. It is easier to use the forearm and lower leg than the upper arm and thigh as sites to obtain the blood pressure. In using these sites, the pressure obtained in the arms may be up to 20 mm Hg higher than that in the legs in normal infants less than 1 year of age.[18]

Several methods are available to obtain blood pressure readings. The simplest and the one we frequently use is the flush method.[19,20] In this technique, the hand or foot is gently squeezed to express blood, and the blood pressure cuff is rapidly inflated. The hand or foot now appears blanched. As the pressure in the cuff is released, the hand will suddenly flush. The pressure recording at this change in color represents the mean arterial pressure. Flush blood pressures can be obtained simultaneously from the upper and lower extremities by placing the blood pressure cuffs on both extremities and connecting them together with a Y connector (Fig. 3-1). Simultaneous blood pressure recordings show if the blood pressure is identical or lower in the legs, as in patients with coarctation of the aorta.

The blood pressure may also be obtained by the palpatory method. While the blood pressure cuff is deflating, the pressure level at which the pulse valve appears distal to the cuff is observed, and this reading approximates systolic blood pressure. Conventional auscultatory methods are used to measure blood pressure, but these are difficult procedures. More recently, blood pressure has been measured with the aid of Doppler equipment.[21,22]

The normal values for blood pressure in the neonate vary considerably with the method of delivery of the infant, the blood volume, and the presence of neonatal distress. In Table 3-1, the normal range of blood pressure is given for various ages through the first year of life.

The peripheral arterial pulses should be palpated for heart rate and character of pulse amplitude. The resting pulse rates for children in the first year of life are given in Table 3-1.

Pulses should be palpated simultaneously in one arm and one leg. They should be of equal intensity and occur synchronously. With care and gentleness, pulses can be easily palpated in the inguinal area of normal infants

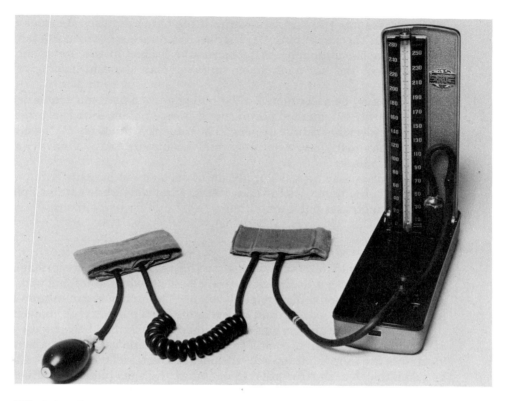

FIG. 3-1.   Apparatus for obtaining blood pressure in two extremities simultaneously.

TABLE 3-1

Normal Values of Pulse and Blood Pressure in First Year of Life

| AGE GROUP | PULSE RATE (BEATS/MIN) | | | BLOOD PRESSURE (MM HG) | |
	Lower Limits of Normal	Average	Upper Limits of Normal	Systolic	Diastolic
Premature	80	120	170	60 (50–75)	35 (30–45)
Neonate	80	120	170	75 (60–90)	45 (40–60)
1–12 Months	90	120	180	90 (75–100)	60 (50–70)

when the examiner's hands are warm. If the femoral pulses are weak or undetectable and the radial pulses are strong, coarctation of the aorta is the most likely diagnosis, although other obstructive lesions in the aorta, such as interruption of the aortic arch or supravalvular stenosis, may give similar findings.

Pulses may be accentuated or bounding in each extremity in patients with conditions with augmented aortic runoff—large patent ductus arteriosus, systemic arteriovenous fistula, or persistent truncus arteriosus. We have been impressed that many apparently normal premature infants have prominent peripheral pulses.

The pulses may be weak or absent at each site in patients with cardiovascular shock. In infants, when shock results from congestive cardiac failure, digitalization increases pulse amplitude.

THORAX

The thorax should be carefully inspected for asymmetry or precordial bulge. In the neonate, a precordial bulge is rarely present, while in infants with marked cardiomegaly, a precordial bulge develops. The upper sternum may bulge in patients with pulmonary hypertension or elevated pulmonary venous pressure.

The location of the cardiac apex should be identified because the location of the cardiac apex gives a clue to cardiac size. The cardiac apex is normally located in the fourth left intercostal space in the midclavicular line. Care must be taken to detect dextrocardia. In neonates, the apex impulse is often difficult to palpate, but there may be a heave along the left sternal border. In infancy, the precordial activity is increased in patients with large volumes of pulmonary blood flow, such as left-to-right shunts.

The precordium should be palpated for thrills, using the palm of the hand, and the suprasternal notch with a fingertip. Thrills in the latter location arise from aortic stenosis and occasionally from pulmonary stenosis. We have observed one neonate with a cerebral arteriovenous fistula with a thrill in the suprasternal notch and along the carotid arteries. Precordial thrills in the neonate are rare and, when present, usually indicate stenosis of a semilunar valve or insufficiency of an atrioventricular valve.

In infants, thrills are more common in such conditions as patent ductus arteriosus and ventricular septal defect because, with the fall in pulmonary vascular resistance, the volume of blood flow increases through the communication, leading to a louder murmur and thrill.

LUNGS

The lungs should be carefully auscultated for rales that may indicate pneumonia or left-sided cardiac failure. In the latter instance, they are dry, crackly, and indicate pulmonary edema.

HEART

Patience, care, and experience are required to gain the maximum amount of information from cardiac auscultation of the neonate and infant. Whenever possible, examine the infant when he is asleep. Despite the admonition that a physician never listens through the patient's clothing, often more is heard through the clothing of an undisturbed infant than from a crying or vigorously active, fully exposed infant. In the fearful infant near 1 year of age, it is best to examine him as he sits in his mother's lap (Fig. 3-2).

Each physician should use his personal stethoscope, rather than the one hanging at the patient's bedside that may have a bell made from a rubber nipple. Stethoscopes should have short, stout tubing and both a bell and a diaphragm. I prefer a Rappaport-Sprague stethoscope, and although it seemed expensive when initially purchased, considering the cost per patient over the past 19 years and the benefit gained from an excellent stethoscope, it has been extremely cost effective. I use the ¾ inch bell and the large diaphragm and find these satisfactory for each infant. The stethoscope, like the hand, should be warm when examining the infant.

Particularly in neonates, repeated examinations should be carried out, for, often, to the frustration of the cardiologist, auscultatory findings may vary because of physiologic changes occurring in the developing neonate.

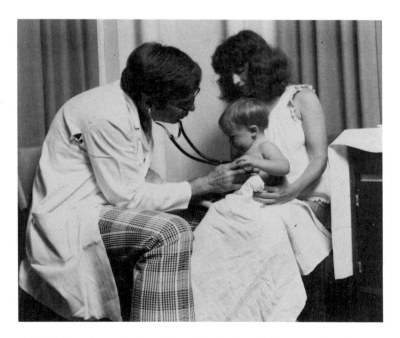

FIG. 3-2. Auscultation of an older infant sitting in mother's lap.

Heart Sounds

It is very helpful in understanding cardiac sounds and in locating murmurs within the cardiac cycle to correlate their location with the electrical and mechanical events of the heart as they are depicted in the modifications of the diagram of the classic works of Wiggers (Fig. 3-3).

The *first heart sound* is caused principally by the closure of the mitral and tricuspid valves at the onset of ventricular systole. Although mitral valve closure precedes tricuspid valve closure, they occur nearly simultaneously, so in most infants the first heart sound is single. The only exception we can recall of

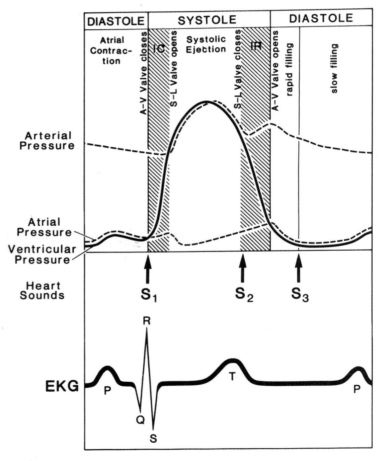

FIG. 3-3. Modification of Wiggers' diagram relating the electrocardiogram, intracardiac pressures, and location of cardiac sounds. IC, isovolumetric contraction; IR, isovolumetric relaxation; S₁, first heart sound; S₂, second heart sound; S₃, third heart sound.

a distinct split of the first heart sound has been in infants with Ebstein's malformation of the tricuspid valve. Usually the first heart sound is heard best at the cardiac apex, representing closure of the mitral valve.

The first heart sound is accentuated in several conditions:

1. Increased blood flow across an atrioventricular valve. In patients with increased flow across the mitral valve, as in patent ductus arteriosus, ventricular septal defect, or mitral insufficiency, the first heart sound at the apex is accentuated. In atrial septal defect and total anomalous pulmonary venous connection, the first heart sound along the lower left sternal border (tricuspid valve) is accentuated. We have found this to be a valuable clue in recognizing atrial shunts in infants.
2. Stenosis of an atrioventricular valve, particularly of the mitral valve. The accentuation in this instance is related to the pressure difference across the mitral valve at the end of diastole. As systole begins, the ventricular pressure must rise to a higher level before the mitral valve closes. Thus, the valve is closed at a higher pressure, and the sound is louder. Although we have observed this in older children with congenital mitral stenosis, we have not recognized it among patients with mitral stenosis in the first year of life.
3. Short PR interval, since ventricular contraction occurs soon after atrial contraction and at a time when the valves are widely opened.
4. Conditions with increased cardiac output, such as fever, arteriovenous fistula, or anemia. The loud first heart sound is related to the increased volume of flow across the atrioventricular valve and the shortened period of diastole. The atrioventricular valve leaflets are more widely open and close forcibly because of increased myocardial contractility.

The intensity of the first heart sound can be decreased by:

1. Prolonged atrioventricular conduction. Following atrial contraction, if a longer period exists before ventricular contraction occurs, the atrioventricular valve leaflets tend to drift toward a closed position, so that when systole occurs the length of excursion is slight.
2. Myocardial disease. In patients with myocarditis or other conditions decreasing myocardial contractility, the first heart sound may be soft. The first heart sound may be soft during congestive cardiac failure and increase in intensity following digitalization.

The details of the *second heart sound* provide valuable diagnostic clues. The second heart sound occurs from asynchronous closure of the semilunar valves. The pulmonary closure follows the aortic closure because right ventricular ejection takes longer than left ventricular ejection. Normally, the second heart sound has two components, and the occurrence of two heart sounds is called *splitting*. The degree of splitting varies in normal infants. With inspiration, a greater volume of blood returns to the right side of the heart and right ventricular ejection is longer, so the degree of splitting is wider. With expiration, the reverse occurs, and the degree of splitting narrows.

The components of the second heart sound are heard best in the second and third left intercostal spaces.

In neonates or infants, because of tachycardia, it may be difficult to hear splitting of the second heart sound. It is worthwhile to auscultate an infant on several occasions to make certain that splitting is present.

If only a single second heart sound is heard, an abnormality of the semilunar valves is present. There may be only one valve, as in persistent truncus arteriosus, or one of the valves may be stenotic or atretic. Pulmonary atresia, severe pulmonary stenosis, or tetralogy of Fallot are associated with a single second heart sound (the aortic component), while aortic atresia or aortic stenosis is also associated with a single second heart sound (the pulmonic component).

Wide splitting of the second heart sound occurs in conditions that prolong right ventricular ejection:

1. Conditions, such as in atrial septal defect or total anomalous pulmonary venous connection in which the right ventricle ejects a larger volume than normal, are associated with a widely split second heart sound. In anomalies with an atrial communication, the second heart sound does not vary with respiration. This is termed *fixed splitting* of the second heart sound and indicates an atrial communication.
2. Obstruction to right ventricular outflow, as occurs in pulmonary stenosis or tetralogy of Fallot, is associated with wide splitting because pulmonary valve closure is delayed.
3. In complete right bundle-branch block, right ventricular depolarization and right ventricular systole are delayed, so that the pulmonary component occurs later than normal.

In neonates or infants with tachycardia, if the second heart sound is easily heard to split, wide splitting is most likely present.

The intensity of either component of the second heart sound may be accentuated because of elevation of pressure in the respective great vessel. Although the aortic component of the second heart sound may be accentuated in infants with elevated pressure in the ascending aorta, this is rarely recognized. An accentuated pulmonic component is frequently heard and indicates pulmonary hypertension which coexists with many forms of congenital cardiac malformations.

In patients with transposition of the great vessels, particularly with l-transposition, the second heart sound is loud and single, since the aorta is located anteriorly and close to the anterior chest wall, while the pulmonary trunk is distant.

A *third heart sound* may occur at the transition between the rapid and slow filling phases of diastole. This is a normal finding in healthy children.

Third heart sounds also occur in infants with increased blood flow across an atrioventricular valve, as in left-to-right shunt or mitral or tricuspid insufficiency. In such infants, the third heart sound may initiate a middiastolic murmur. In patients with congestive cardiac failure and tachycardia, the third heart sound may be accentuated and be called a "gallop."

A *fourth heart sound* is abnormal and occurs at the time of atrial contraction. When left ventricular compliance is decreased because of left ventricular hypertrophy, from whatever cause, or because of intrinsic myocardial disease, such as myocarditis or myocardiopathy, a fourth heart sound may be heard. We have rarely heard this sound in infants, probably because tachycardia is nearly always present.

Ejection clicks may be present in certain conditions and are always abnormal, except in the first 24 hours of life.[23] Systolic ejection clicks indicate enlargement of a great vessel, either aorta or pulmonary artery. Occurring most frequently from poststenotic dilatation, systolic ejection clicks can develop in other conditions that cause great vessel dilatation. This sound occurs as the semilunar valve opens and, therefore, marks the transition from the isovolumetric contraction period to the ejection phase of systole.

Characteristics of the click allow distinction between those arising from the aorta and those arising from the pulmonary artery. Aortic systolic ejection clicks are heard best at the cardiac apex and are often heard well over the lower left back. They are louder when the patient is reclining and vary little with phases of respiration. In contrast, pulmonary systolic ejection clicks are heard better in the pulmonary area. They vary with respiration and are louder when the patient is upright.

Aortic ejection clicks in infants occur most frequently in truncus arteriosus, severe tetralogy of Fallot, and aortic stenosis, while pulmonary systolic ejection clicks usually indicate pulmonary stenosis and, less frequently, pulmonary hypertension.

Murmurs

If a murmur is present, several characteristics should be noted: location in the cardiac cycle, location on the thorax, loudness, radiation of the murmur, and pitch.

LOCATION IN THE CARDIAC CYCLE.   Systolic murmurs are classified as either ejection or pansystolic. *Ejection systolic murmurs* occur during the ejection phase of systole and occur after the period of isovolumetric contraction. Therefore, a short period of time occurs between the first heart sound and the onset of the murmur.

Ejection murmurs occur from turbulence of blood flow as it leaves the heart. Turbulence may develop from anatomic narrowing, such as aortic or pulmonary valvular stenosis, or from subvalvular stenosis, as from the infundibular stenosis in tetralogy of Fallot. Ejection systolic murmurs also develop in patients who have increased volumes of blood flow across normal semilunar valves. The latter occurs in patients with atrial septal defect or total anomalous pulmonary venous connection in which the right ventricle ejects large volumes across the right ventricular outflow area and causes an ejection murmur. The murmurs are softer in the latter circumstance than in patients with obstruction.

The other systolic murmur is *pansystolic,* occurring throughout systole and beginning with the first heart sound. It, therefore, includes the isovolumetric contraction period. Only three anatomic conditions are associated with a pansystolic murmur: mitral insufficiency, tricuspid insufficiency, and ventricular septal defect. In each of these conditions, blood flows within the heart from the onset of systole. In the first two conditions, the higher ventricular pressure communicates with the atrium, and in the ventricular septal defect, the ventricles are in communication throughout systole.

In neonates, a pansystolic murmur almost invariably indicates atrioventricular valvular insufficiency, since at this age, elevated pulmonary vascular resistance limits flow through a ventricular septal defect. The murmurs of atrioventricular valvular insufficiency, particularly of the mitral valve, are high-pitched and frequently described as "blowing" because of high pressure differences across the valve.

Diastolic murmurs are classified—early, mid, or late—depending upon their location in the cardiac cycle.

Early diastolic murmurs immediately follow the second heart sound and occupy the period of isovolumetric relaxation and occur from semilunar valvular insufficiency. Blood flows from the higher pressure great vessel into the lower diastolic pressure in the ventricle.

Early diastolic murmurs are uncommon in neonates or infants, occurring in such rare conditions as absent pulmonary valve, which is frequently associated with tetralogy of Fallot, or from ruptured sinus of Valsalva aneurysm, which leads to aortic regurgitation. These murmurs are usually high-pitched and decrescendo.

Middiastolic murmurs commonly follow a third heart sound and occupy the slow-filling phase of diastole. They are low-pitched and indicate an increased volume of blood flow across a normal atrioventricular valve. When the volume of flow across an atrioventricular valve exceeds twice normal, a middiastolic murmur is heard. Left-to-right shunts at the ventricular or great vessel level (i.e., ventricular septal defect or patent ductus arteriosus) and mitral insufficiency are among the conditions in which these murmurs may be heard. When present, they indicate at least a moderate increase in blood flow. Middiastolic murmurs can also occur from increased flow across the tricuspid valve in patients with atrial septal defect or total anomalous pulmonary venous connection.

Late diastolic murmurs, also called protodiastolic or presystolic, are associated with organic atrioventricular valvular stenosis, almost always mitral stenosis. These are crescendo, reaching a peak before the first heart sound, since the pressure gradient across the valve increases in diastole, particularly with atrial contraction.

In infants with isolated mitral stenosis, the late diastolic murmur may be the only murmur present and can be erroneously interpreted as being systolic in timing merely because isolated diastolic murmurs are rare, while systolic murmurs are so common.

Continuous murmurs, i.e., murmurs beginning in systole and continuing into diastole, indicate a communication between the aorta or one of its branches and the pulmonary artery or a right-sided cardiac chamber. The classic continuous murmur is that of patent ductus arteriosus. This murmur may occur in infants with an isolated patent ductus arteriosus or in infants with pulmonary stenosis or atresia, with or without a ventricular communication, in which a patent ductus supplies blood to the lungs.

In cyanotic infants, a continuous murmur may be found in those with severe pulmonary stenosis or pulmonary atresia and in whom the major portion of pulmonary blood flow is through bronchial collateral vessels. These murmurs may be found more diffusely over the chest than in patients with patent ductus arteriosus and may have a hollow characteristic.

Continuous murmurs also occur in patients with arteriovenous fistulae. In neonates, arteriovenous fistulae may be located intracranially (aneurysm of the great vein of Galen), between the subclavian artery and vein, within the liver (hemangiomatosis of the liver), or as coronary arteriovenous fistulae. While the last anatomic form does not result in cardiac failure in the neonatal period, other arteriovenous fistulae can. In infants with cardiac failure, auscultation over the head or abdomen may be rewarded by the discovery of a continuous murmur.

A continuous murmur can also occur diffusely over the chest or be localized over a single pulmonary segment in patients with pulmonary arteriovenous fistulae. These fistulae may be solitary or multiple and may lead to cyanosis.

Peripheral primary arterial stenosis is a rare cause of a continuous murmur. We have heard of an infant with peripheral pulmonary arterial stenosis coexisting with ventricular septal defect and large left-to-right shunt. In this infant, the greatly increased pulmonary blood flow apparently led to a pressure gradient across the stenotic area throughout the cardiac cycle.

LOCATION ON THE THORAX.   Useful diagnostic information can be gained by describing the location upon the thorax where the murmur has its loudest intensity. There are four general auscultatory areas: aortic, pulmonary, tricuspid, and mitral. Murmurs originating from the left ventricular outflow area are heard best along the midleft sternal border and beneath the right clavicle (aortic area), while those from the right ventricular outflow area are present along the upper left sternal border (pulmonary area). The murmur of patent ductus arteriosus is also heard best in the pulmonary area.

The tricuspid area describes a location along the lower left sternal border. Murmurs originating from the tricuspid valve increase on inspiration. The

34   HEART DISEASE IN INFANCY

murmur of ventricular septal defect is also heard best in this area. The mitral area describes that location about the cardiac apex. As indicated previously, localization of a murmur to the head or abdomen has rather specific meaning.

LOUDNESS OF THE MURMUR.   The loudness of the murmur is described by expressing its intensity in terms of a fraction—e.g., 1/6, 2/6—in which the numerator represents the loudness in the patient and the denominator represents the loudest murmur on the scale. Intensity of murmurs does not necessarily correlate with the severity of the condition, for there are conditions, such as tetralogy of Fallot, in which the murmur has an inverse relation—the more severe the stenosis, the softer the murmur.

The intensity of the murmur may also vary as the hemodynamic status of the patient changes. A very soft murmur, present when the patient has a reduced cardiac output from cardiac failure, may become louder as cardiac output increases following digitalization.

RADIATION OF THE MURMUR.   In the description of a murmur, both the site of maximal intensity and the direction of its radiation provide useful diagnostic information. The murmurs of aortic stenosis radiate into the carotid arteries, and those from pulmonary stenosis radiate to the left upper back, since the jet of blood is primarily into the left pulmonary artery.

In patients with complete transposition of the great vessels and pulmonary stenosis, the murmur may be heard best on the right side of the back. Murmurs of mitral regurgitation radiate forward to the left axilla.

Patients with peripheral pulmonary arterial stenosis have systolic murmurs heard well throughout the chest, particularly in the axillae.

As these facts indicate, the back should be carefully auscultated for radiation of the murmur or for the presence of a murmur when one is not heard anteriorly. Coarctation of the aorta is one condition where the murmur may be louder or heard exclusively over the back. We have also heard soft systolic murmurs in the left paraspinal area of neonates with hypoplastic left heart syndrome.

PITCH.   The frequency of the murmur should be described. High-pitched murmurs usually occur when there is turbulence from a high pressure to a low pressure area, such as in mitral insufficiency or aortic insufficiency. Murmurs from pulmonary or tricuspid insufficiency usually have a lower frequency than similar murmurs on the left side of the heart. Low-pitched murmurs occur from flow across low pressure areas.

Unique Auscultatory Findings in Normal Neonates

Studies in the early neonatal period have shown several distinctive characteristics that must be considered when auscultating neonates. A study of newborns by Braudo and Rowe[23] is perhaps the most extensive. They found that the first heart sound was loud at birth and decreased in loudness during the first 48 hours of life. They heard two components of the first heart sound in this age group, the second component being particularly loud in the tricuspid area and varying with respiration. In many neonates, systolic ejection click may be heard as well along the left sternal border. Craige and Harned[24] found a 93 percent incidence of this sound early in life.

Craige and Harned[24] and also Braudo and Rowe[23] noted that the second heart sound was single at birth, presumably because of the elevated pulmonary vascular resistance. The second heart sound was split by 4 hours of age in 50 percent of neonates, and by 2 days it was split in all neonates. The degree of splitting seemed to increase with age. Third and fourth heart sounds were not heard.

In the study by Braudo and Rowe,[23] four types of murmurs were found in normal neonates:

1. *Ejection systolic murmurs.* These were grade 1/6 to 2/6 ejection systolic murmurs heard in the pulmonary area and were present in 56 percent of patients studied, developing within the first day and lasting to 6 days. They were described as vibratory and were heard best with the bell of the stethoscope.
2. *Continuous murmurs.* These were also of grade 1/6 to 2/6, heard best with the bell and located in the pulmonary area. Fourteen percent of the patients manifested this murmur, which was heard by 8 hours of age.
3. *Crescendo systolic murmurs.* Several neonates who initially had a continuous murmur subsequently had a crescendo systolic murmur in the pulmonary area.
4. *Early systolic murmurs.* These murmurs occurred in 4 percent of babies and started with the first heart sound. These murmurs were louder (grade 3/6 to 4/6), had a blowing characteristic, and were heard along the lower left sternal border, but they were transmitted throughout the chest.

Burnard[25] also studied both normal and dyspneic newborns and premature infants. He described a continuous and a crescendo murmur, both of which he considered related to blood flow through a patent ductus arteriosus. In 37 percent of normal newborns, such a murmur was present, and it lasted a short time. The incidence was higher in prematures, neonates with asphyxia, and those with higher temperatures.

Although a continuous murmur due to a patent ductus arteriosus has been described in normal newborns,[23,26] this is usually transient, being detectable for less than 12 hours. Clarkson and Orgill,[27] in a prospective study of 100 prematurely born infants, found the continuous murmur persisted in 18, disappeared between the ages of 3 and 29 weeks, and indicated delayed closure of the ductus arteriosus.

Walsh,[28] in studying normal premature infants over a period of time, found that in 80 percent, a functional systolic murmur was heard at some time during the first 18 months of life, most frequently at 3 months of age. These murmurs were short and humming, varied with respiration, and located between the lower left sternal border and the apex. The incidence of murmurs was also greater in those with lower hemoglobin values. Hallidie-Smith[29] also found a high incidence of functional murmurs in infancy. Other authors,[30-32] however, have described a much lower incidence of functional murmurs in the neonatal period or infancy.

In the neonate, significant systolic murmurs appearing at or within hours of birth almost always result from either pulmonary stenosis or aortic stenosis. Small ventricular septal defect may result in a murmur before the patient is discharged from the hospital. Usually, in patients with a large ventricular septal defect or with similar hemodynamic conditions, such as persistent truncus arteriosus, a murmur is not heard until the first postnatal examination, because the elevated pulmonary vascular resistance in the neonatal period tends to limit the volume of pulmonary blood flow. Atrial septal defect is usually not recognized in the first year of life, presumably because the murmur is soft and the decreased right ventricular compliance limits the left-to-right shunt early in life.

ABDOMEN

In every infant, the abdomen should be gently palpated to determine the hepatic size: normally in infants it may be palpated as far as 3 cm below the right costal margin in the midclavicular line. If the hepatic edge is palpated below this level, hepatomegaly may be present. At times, however, the liver may be displaced inferiorly by overexpansion of the lungs. Therefore, in every infant suspected of having hepatomegaly, the upper edge of the liver should be percussed, and this is usually in the fifth right intercostal space in the midclavicular line. Hepatic size is a variable indicator of congestive cardiac failure, and its size may change quickly, corresponding to changes in the status of the patient.

The tip of the spleen may be palpable in many infants. Splenomegaly is infrequently the result of congestive cardiac failure.

The physician should be alert to the possibility of abdominal situs inversus.

PERIPHERAL EDEMA

At birth, clinical evidence of edema may be found in many neonates, but this usually disappears within 48 hours, although it may persist longer in prematures. Edema is generally dependent.

Other causes of edema at birth or in the neonatal period include fetal hydrops, lymphedema, and the nonpitting edema associated with Turner's syndrome. Cardiac causes are uncommon, but they include paroxysmal tachycardia. Urinary tract obstruction and hepatic cirrhosis are other causes of an uncommon symptom.

Edema occurring after the neonatal period is abnormal and develops from several causes, including cardiac failure. The edema is usually dependent and evident as puffy eyelids or by impression of clothes on the skin. Rarely is there pitting edema of the extremities. Renal diseases and exudative enteropathy are other causes, as is the feeding of formulas with high solute concentration to premature infants.

REFERENCES

1. Cullum L, Liebman J: The association of congenital heart disease with Down's syndrome (mongolism). Am J Cardiol 24:354, 1969
2. Tandon R, Edwards JE: Cardiac malformations associated with Down's syndrome (clinicopathologic correlations). Circulation 47:1349, 1971
3. Laursen HB: Congenital heart disease in Down's syndrome. Br Heart J 38:32, 1976
4. Chi TL, Krovetz J: The pulmonary vascular bed in children with Down syndrome. J Pediatr 86:533, 1975
5. Taylor AI: Autosomal trisomy syndrome. A detailed study of 27 cases of Edwards syndrome and 27 cases of Patau's syndrome. J Med Genet 5:227, 1968
6. Smith DW: The No. 18 trisomy and D_1 trisomy syndromes. Pediatr Clin North Am 10:389, 1963
7. Nora JJ, Torres FG, Sinha AK, McNamara DG: Characteristic cardiovascular anomalies of XO Turner syndrome, XX and XY phenotype and XO/XX Turner mosaic. Am J Cardiol 25:639, 1970
8. Jones KL, Smith DW: The Williams elfin facies syndrome. A new perspective. J Pediatr 86:718, 1975
9. Rowe RD: Cardiovascular lesions in rubella. J Pediatr 68:147, 1966 (Letter to the Editor)
10. Hastreiter AR, Joorbchi B, Pujatti G, et al.: Cardiovascular lesions asociated with congenital rubella. J Pediatr 71:59, 1967
11. Cooper LZ, Krugman S: Diagnosis and management: Congenital rubella. Pediatrics 37:335, 1966
12. Holt M, Oram S: Familial heart disease with skeletal malformations. Br Heart J 22:236, 1900
13. Silverman ME, Copeland AJ, Hurst JW: The Holt-Oram syndrome: The long and the short of it. Am J Cardiol 25:11, 1970
14. Mitnick S: Cyanosis. Am J Dis Child 99:88, 1960
15. Gatti RA, Muster AJ, Cole RB, Paul MH: Neonatal polycythemia with transient cyanosis and cardiorespiratory abnormalities. J Pediatr 69:1063, 1966
16. Goldman HI, Maralit A, Sun S, Lanzkowsky P: Neonatal cyanosis and arterial oxygen saturations. J Pediatr 82:319, 1973
17. Chesler E, Moller JH, Edwards JE: Anatomic basis for delivery of right ventricular blood into localized segments of the systemic arterial system. Relation to differential cyanosis. Am J Cardiol 21:72, 1968
18. Moss AJ, Adams FH: Problems of Blood Pressure in Childhood. Springfield, Ill, Thomas, 1962
19. Goldring D, Wohltmann H: Flush method for blood pressure determinations in newborn infants. J Pediatr 40:285, 1952
20 Virnig NL, Reynolds JW: Reliability of flush blood pressure measurements in the sick newborn infant. J Pediatr 84:594, 1974
21. McLaughlin GW, Kirby RR, Kemmerer WT, deLemos RA: Indirect measurement of blood pressure in infants utilizing Doppler ultrasound. J Pediatr 79:300, 1971

22. Black IFS, Kotrapu N, Massie H: Application of Doppler ultrasound to blood pressure measurement in small infants. J Pediatr 81:932, 1972

23. Braudo M, Rowe RD: Auscultation of the heart—early neonatal period. Am J Dis Child 101:67, 1961

24. Craige E, Harned HS Jr: Phonocardiographic and electrocardiographic studies in normal newborn infants. Am Heart J 65:180, 1963

25. Burnard ED: The cardiac murmur in relation to symptoms in the newborn. Br Med J 1:134, 1959

26. Burnard ED: A murmur from the ductus arteriosus in the newborn baby. Br Med J 1:806, 1958

27. Clarkson PM, Orgill AA: Continuous murmurs in infants of low birth weight. J Pediatr 84:208, 1974

28. Walsh SZ: The incidence of murmurs in healthy premature infants during the first 18 months of life. J Pediatr 62:480, 1963

29. Hallidie-Smith KA: Some auscultatory and phonocardiographic findings observed in early infancy. Br Med J 1:756, 1960

30. Lyon R, Rauch LW, Stirling JW: Heart murmurs in newborn infants. J Pediatr 16:310, 1940

31. Taylor W: The incidence and significance of systolic cardiac murmurs in infants. Arch Dis Child 28:52, 1953

32. Richards MR, Merritt KK, Samuels MH, Langemann AG: Frequency and significance of cardiac murmurs in the first years of life. Pediatrics 15:169, 1955

4 Electrocardiography

ELECTROCARDIOGRAM

Electrocardiography is one of the major noninvasive diagnostic methods for cardiac conditions of neonates and infants. It provides helpful information for the diagnosis and management of cardiac, pulmonary, and other problems of infancy.

The electrocardiogram yields information about abnormal hemodynamic loads placed upon cardiac chambers. The electrocardiogram reflects more accurately than does the thoracic roentgenogram right atrial, right ventricular, or left ventricular hypertrophy or enlargement, while the thoracic roentgenogram is a better indicator of left atrial enlargement. Often the electrocardiographic patterns are not diagnostic of the underlying cardiac condition but reflect chamber hypertrophy or enlargement that develops in response to the anomaly—e.g., a pattern of right ventricular hypertrophy may be present in several conditions, such as pulmonary stenosis, tetralogy of Fallot, or complete transposition of the great vessels. In these situations, the electrocardiogram reflects the anatomic change, but there may be no other electrocardiographic changes that allow these conditions to be distinguished.

On the other hand, certain cardiac conditions present an electrocardiographic pattern that is highly diagnostic of the underlying condition. Examples of unique electrocardiographic patterns include those present in infants with anomalous left coronary artery, glycogen storage disease, tricuspid atresia, or endocardial cushion defect. In these instances, the electrocardiogram provides a major diagnostic clue.

Once a cardiac condition has been diagnosed, the electrocardiogram can be used to assess its severity. QRS changes and ventricular hypertrophy are particularly helpful. Severe degrees of ventricular hypertrophy are associated with abnormalities of ventricular repolarization, i.e., ST and T wave changes, indicating ventricular strain.

The electrocardiogram is the principal diagnostic tool in identifying and diagnosing cardiac dysrhythmias.

The electrocardiogram can be used to recognize and evaluate electrolyte abnormalities. Electrocardiographic changes of hyperkalemia are well known, but the electrocardiogram can aid in the diagnosis of hypokalemia and disorders of calcium metabolism as well.

During the first year of life, profound electrocardiographic changes, particularly of the QRS complex, occur. In interpretation of the electrocardiogram of infants, these age-related changes and the wide range of normal must be considered.

The electrocardiographic variations taking place in the first year of life reflect the normal physiologic and anatomic developmental circulatory changes. During fetal life and in the neonatal period, major changes take place in the circulation. Because of differences in vascular resistances in fetal life, left ventricular (LV) weight exceeds right ventricular (RV) weight until about the thirtieth gestational week, after which right ventricular weight exceeds left ventricular weight. At birth (40 weeks gestation), the right ventricular:left ventricular weight ratio is 1.3:1. Because right ventricular weight exceeds left ventricular weight, the QRS axis is directed toward the right, tall R waves are present in right precordial leads, and deep S waves are found in the left precordial leads. This pattern, which is normal for a neonate, would be interpreted as right axis deviation and right ventricular hypertrophy in older children.

Following birth, as pulmonary vascular resistance falls, right ventricular afterload is decreased, and the thickness of the right ventricular wall slowly decreases, although right ventricular weight slowly increases. At birth, the immediate fall in pulmonary vascular resistance increases pulmonary blood flow and pulmonary venous return to the left atrium and left ventricle. Furthermore, the separation from the placenta increases systemic vascular resistance immediately. In response to these two changes, left ventricular weight increases at a faster rate than the right ventricular weight, and by 1 month of age, the left ventricle weighs more. This weight differential favoring the left ventricle continues to increase over a period of months and years during infancy and childhood. The QRS complex of the electrocardiogram, as a consequence, assumes a more adult pattern.

The rate of transition of the QRS axis and precordial QRS pattern varies among neonates. If the fall of pulmonary vascular resistance is delayed, as from neonatal pulmonary parenchymal disease, the thickness of the right ventricle is maintained, and transition is delayed. In prematurely born infants, however, the transition toward an adult pattern is accelerated because the right ventricular:left ventricular weight ratio is less than in full-term infants.

Although the major electrocardiographic changes during the first year of life occur in the QRS complex, age-related changes of heart rate, P waves, and T waves are also found and will be further discussed.

ELECTROCARDIOGRAM OF FULL-TERM INFANTS (Fig. 4-1)

Heart Rate

The average heart rate during the first week of life is 130 beats/min, with a minimum of 85/min and a maximum near 190/min. The heart rate is deter-

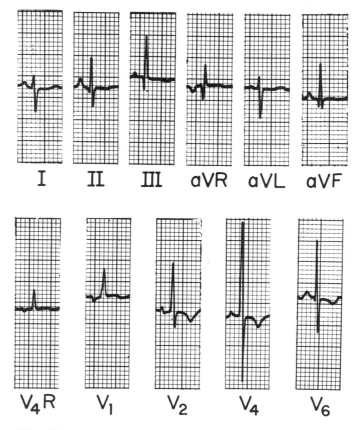

I   II   III   aVR   aVL   aVF

V₄R   V₁   V₂   V₄   V₆

FIG. 4-1. Electrocardiogram of full-term infant aged 2 days. T waves inverted in left precordial leads.

mined by the activity of the child, increasing during crying or activity and decreasing during sleep. There is a gradual increase in heart rate during the first week of life.[1, 2]

The average heart rate increases until 1 month of age and then gradually decreases throughout childhood. Sinus rates of 200 beats/min can be observed in normal infants.

Rhythm

A sinus mechanism is present in virtually all full-term infants. Sinus arrhythmia has been considered an uncommon rhythm in neonates, perhaps because they were stimulated merely by having an electrocardiogram recorded. A study by Morgan and Guntheroth,[3] however, showed that when neonates are continuously monitored, all show sinus arrhythmia, although none have nodal escape or rates below 70/min. These authors also commented that with feeding or crying, the cardiac rate accelerates over a short period of time.

TABLE 4-1

Normal Values of Electrocardiogram of Prematures, Neonates, and Infants*

AGE	QRS AXIS (DEGREES)	QRS DURATION (SEC)	LEAD V$_1$		
			R Wave (mm)	S Wave (mm)	R/RS V$_1$ (%)
0–24 hr	70–205 (137)	0.05–0.10 (0.065)	16 (6–27)	10 (0–25)	60 (25–100)
1–7 days	75–185 (125)	0.04–0.08 (0.056)	17 (4–30)	10 (0–20)	60 (35–100)
8–30 days	30–190 (108)	0.04–0.07 (0.055)	13 (3–24)	7 (0–18)	65 (35–100)
1–3 mo	25–125 (75)	0.05–0.08 (0.062)	10 (2–20)	7 (0–18)	65 (35–100)
3–6 mo	20–120 (65)	0.05–0.08 (0.069)	10 (2–20)	7 (2–12)	60 (35–85)
6–12 mo	10–115 (65)	0.04–0.08 (0.065)	10 (2–20)	8 (2–15)	55 (35–85)

* Range of normal and mean value.

P Wave

The P wave duration is variable and ranges from 0.04 to 0.066 sec,[2] and 0.04 to 0.08 sec.[4] The mean value is 0.05 to 0.06 sec. In neonates following stripping of the umbilical cord, the duration (0.082 sec) is longer than in neonates with early clamping of the cord (0.06 sec).[5] By 1 year of age, P wave duration is between 0.06 and 0.08 sec.

At birth, the P wave axis in the frontal plane is +60°, decreases to +54° by 1 week of age, and gradually decreases further to +50°. In the horizontal plane,[6] P wave axis is also about +50° during the first month of life and then moves more posteriorly.

The maximum amplitude of the P wave, which is best observed in lead II, gradually increases during the first week of life but does not exceed 3.0 mm in height. In the horizontal plane, the maximum P wave deflection in the first week of life is directed toward either lead V$_1$ or lead V$_2$. The P wave in lead V$_1$ is biphasic in 80 percent of infants in the first 8 hours of life, and this incidence decreases to 30 percent by the end of the first week.

PR Interval

The PR interval, measured in lead II, has a mean value of 0.10 sec and ranges from 0.07 to 0.13 sec. At birth, the mean value decreases slightly in the first week of life.[4, 7] The PR interval is longer in infants following stripping of the umbilical cord, and this prolongation requires 4 to 5 days to reach a level comparable to neonates with early clamping of the umbilical cord.

Throughout the remainder of the first year of life, the mean PR interval gradually increases to 0.12 sec and rarely exceeds 0.15 sec. The minimum value is 0.07 sec.

QRS Complex (Table 4-1)

The QRS interval has been studied by several authors.[2, 4, 8, 9] Soon after birth, the mean values of QRS duration range from 0.055 to 0.065 sec. The mean

TABLE 4-1 (*cont.*)

LEAD V_6			T WAVE			
R Wave (mm)	S Wave (mm)	R/RS V_6 (%)	V_1	V_2	V_4	V_6
4 (0–12)	4 (0–12)	50 (0–100)	+ or −	+ or −	+ or −	+ or −
6 (0–16)	3 (0–12)	65 (20–100)	−	+ or −	+ or −	+
8 (0–20)	2 (0–9)	75 (30–100)	−	+ or −	+ or −	+
9 (2–16)	2 (0–6)	80 (60–100)	−	+ or −	+ or −	+
10 (2–16)	1 (0–5)	85 (60–100)	−	+ or −	+ or −	+
12 (3–20)	1 (0–3)	85 (70–100)	−	+ or −	+ or −	+

value for QRS interval decreases to 0.045 to 0.055 sec in the first weeks of life and then increases gradually during the first year of life to 0.055 to 0.065 sec. In normal infants, the QRS duration rarely exceeds 0.08 sec.

The QRS axis undergoes a major change in the first year of life because of hemodynamic alterations and resultant anatomic changes occurring during this period. In the first week of life, the mean frontal QRS axis is 135°,[2, 7, 8] with a range of +60° to +180°. Following the first week of life, rapid change occurs in the QRS axis. By 1 month of age, the mean value is +100°, by 2 to 3 months of age +75°, and after 6 months of age +65°.

In the horizontal plane, the QRS axis of neonates is directed toward the right, being reported around +160° by one author[7] and +*130*° by another.[2] It decreases to +110° during the first week of life,[2] remains stable during the remainder of the first month, and then gradually shifts toward the normal adult value of −10°. It is difficult to determine accurately the QRS axis in the horizontal plane.

The amplitude of various QRS components vary considerably between individual infants and with age. We have been impressed by the low voltage, particularly in the frontal plane, of the QRS complex of many neonates.

Q waves rarely occur (13 percent)[4] in the left precordial leads or lead I of neonates, but Q waves develop in these leads with age. A Q wave is frequently present in lead III of neonates. Q waves in lead V_4R are uncommon[2, 4, 10] but are considered a normal variant.

In the right precordial leads of neonates, the R/S ratio usually exceeds 1.0, and shows an R wave (34 percent), Rs pattern (61 percent), or RS pattern (5 percent).[4] Notching of the R wave may be present. In neonates, the amplitude of the R and S waves varies considerably, and the normal values are given in Table 4-1. With age, in lead V_1, the height of the R wave gradually decreases.

Whereas Q waves in lead V_6 are uncommon at birth, most neonates show a Q wave in this lead by 1 week of age.[10] With age, the height of the R wave increases, the S wave decreases, and R/S increases remarkably. At birth, the R/S in lead V_6 is more than 1 in half of the neonates. Although the S wave may be deep at birth, by 1 month of age, it usually is less than 5 mm.

T Wave

Changes of T waves have been studied by many authors.[1, 2, 4, 11-13] The T wave axis has been most extensively studied by Hait and Gasul.[13] At birth (0 to 5 min), the T wave axis ranges from −90° to +60° (mean +7°) in the frontal plane. By 2 to 4 hours of age, the T wave axis ranges from +60° to +210° (mean +115°). During the remainder of the first week of life, the T wave returns toward the left and lies between −45° and +90° (mean +9°) at 3 days, and between 0 and +60° (mean +25°) at the end of 1 week of age. By 3 months of age, the mean T wave axis becomes +60° and remains at this point throughout the remainder of the first year of life.

It is more difficult to identify and to describe precisely the T wave axis in the horizontal plane. The following description approximates the change in T wave axis during infancy: at birth (0 to 5 min), the T wave axis is between 0° and +90° (mean +60°). By 2 to 4 hours, the T wave axis lies between +90° and +175° (mean +132°). At 3 days, it returns toward the left and is between +90° and −90° (mean −10°), and at 7 days, it is between 0° and −60° (mean −28°). During the remainder of the first year of life, the T wave axis gradually and slightly becomes more anteriorly directed.

The marked changes in the T wave axis during the first week of life have profound effects on the appearance of the T waves, particularly in the precordial leads. The T waves are usually upright in the right precordial leads in the first hours following birth. By the end of the first day of life, half of neonates have an upright T wave in lead V_1, but by 1 week, the T wave is inverted in lead V_1 and remains inverted throughout the first year of life. The upright T wave in the right precordial leads at birth is believed related to the elevated right ventricular systolic pressure and the sudden increase in the left ventricular volume. Other factors are discussed by Stern and Lind.[12]

The left precordial leads may show reciprocal changes of T waves. In lead V_6, the T wave is upright at birth and may become flattened or inverted hours following birth. The T wave becomes upright by 3 days of age and remains positive throughout childhood.

In studying neonates, Emmanouilides and co-workers[14] showed that the pulmonary arterial pressure was higher in those with an upright T wave in lead V_1 than in those with a negative T wave. Further, they found that most neonates with inverted T waves in lead V_6 were less than 10 hours of age and had a left-to-right shunt through the ductus arteriosus.

Changes of T wave amplitude also occur which are partially explained by shifts of T wave axis. The T waves frequently show low voltage during the first week of life and gradually increase in amplitude during the first year of life. The increase of T wave amplitude coincides with the age-related increase of QRS voltage, since a rough relationship exists between QRS and T wave amplitude.

QT Interval

The QT interval decreases during the first week of life. At birth, the QT interval is between 0.28 and 0.30 sec,[2, 4, 9] decreases to 0.24 sec by 3 weeks, and gradually increases to 0.27 sec by 1 year of age. Ziegler[15] considered 0.30 sec the maximum value of the QT interval between 1 week and 3 years of age.

The QT interval may be corrected for heart rate (QTc), and although conflicting information has been described,[2, 7, 9] the QTc should be between 0.40 and 0.44 sec. Walsh[5] reported a higher QTc in neonates with either late clamping or stripping of the umbilical cord, compared with those with early clamping of the umbilical cord.

ELECTROCARDIOGRAM OF POSTMATURE INFANTS

Ackerman and co-workers[16] studied the electrocardiograms of 40 postmature and 6 dysmature term infants and found that most electrocardiographic measurements were similar to those of normal term infants, except for a high R/S ratio, in leads V_3R, V_4R, or V_1. This variation occurred more commonly in the dysmature infants than in normal-appearing postmature infants.

EFFECT OF UMBILICAL CORD CLAMPING ON THE ELECTROCARDIOGRAM

Walsh[5] compared the electrocardiographic findings of 31 neonates following early clamping of the umbilical cord to those of 6 neonates following vigorous stripping of the umbilical cord. In the neonates following vigorous stripping, the PR interval, P wave duration, and QT interval were longer. In the group of 6 neonates, the P wave amplitude was greater, the R/S ratios in both leads V_1 and V_6 were lower, and inversion of the T wave in lead V_1 was delayed. The considerable increase of blood volume present in the 6 neonates following vigorous stripping caused the electrocardiographic differences.

ELECTROCARDIOGRAM OF PREMATURE INFANTS (Fig. 4-2)

Using continuous tape recordings, Morgan and co-workers[17] studied the cardiac rhythm of 20 prematurely born infants. In each infant, sinus rhythm was the principal rhythm, although sinus arrhythmia was also observed. Eight of the premature infants showed episodes of sinus bradycardia, and five others showed marked sinus bradycardia (<50 beats/min) associated with nodal escape. The marked bradycardia occurred during sleep and occasionally with defecation. An occasional ectopic atrial impulse was found. A subsequent study[18] confirmed the dysrhythmias and noted that the incidence of dysrhythmia decreased as the infant grew and matured. The frequent dysrhythmias occur because of immaturity of the autonomic nervous system.

P Wave

The P wave duration is shorter in premature than in full-term infants at similar ages.[19] Reports describing the amplitude of the P waves of premature infants vary. Hubsher[20] found that P waves were occasionally 3 mm in amplitude. Le-

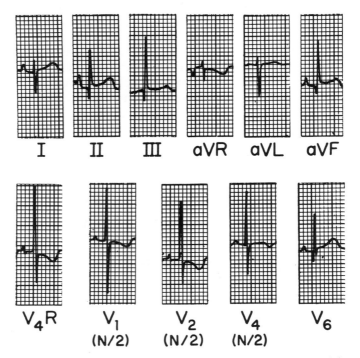

FIG. 4-2. Electrocardiogram of premature infant, weight 1,500 g. N/2, half-standardization.

vine and Griffiths[21] state that P waves are usually of low amplitude (1 mm), while Costa et al.[6] found no difference from full-term infants. Sreenivasan et al.[19] found that the P amplitude was greater during the first week of life than during the remainder of the first 2 months of life.

The P wave axis in the frontal plane is directed slightly more leftward and superiorly than in the full-term infants, being 38° in the first 24 hours and ranging between 44° and 51° for the remainder of the first year of life.[19]

PR Interval

The mean PR value for premature infants is 0.10 to 0.11 sec and changes little during the first year of life.

QRS Complex

In premature infants, the QRS duration is 0.04 sec[19, 22, 23] and remains stable for the first few months of life and then increases to 0.05 sec by the end of the first year of life. In premature infants, the QRS axis in the frontal plane is directed more toward the left than in the comparable aged full-term infants.[15] There is, however, a wide range of QRS axis.[19, 21, 22]

The QRS amplitudes are generally lower in premature than in full-term infants,[6, 19, 21] perhaps because of the smaller ventricular mass. This difference of QRS amplitude may persist for the first few months of life. Therefore, the voltage criteria for QRS amplitudes used to interpret the electrocardiogram of full-term infants cannot be applied to premature infants.

When compared to those of full-term infants, the precordial leads indicate less right ventricular dominance. With growth, the QRS pattern changes towards an adult-type pattern more rapidly than in full-term infants.

At birth the R/S ratio in lead V_1 may be less than 1. With age, the R/S ratio in this lead increases until at least 6 weeks of age rather than decreases.[6, 20, 21] The initial increase in R/S ratio is accounted primarily by an increase of R wave amplitude. Premature infants often have a tall R wave in lead V_6.

ST Segment

ST segment changes are present commonly in premature infants.[6, 22, 24] The ST segment may be scooped out and depressed in the right precordial leads. ST elevation may be present in the standard leads. The origin of the ST segment changes is unknown but is perhaps related to either hypoxia or electrolyte imbalance.

T Wave

T wave amplitudes are lower in premature infants than in full-term infants.[19] During the first day of life, there is a lower incidence of positive T waves in the right precordial leads.[6, 20, 21] The incidence of positive T waves in lead V_1 is also less in neonates with smaller birth weight. The difference in incidence of upright T waves in lead V_1 is the only major recognized difference among the electrocardiograms of premature infants of different weights. The T wave is always positive in lead V_6.

QT Interval

The QT interval is 0.28 to 0.30 sec at birth and decreases with age (0.24 to 0.26 sec). The interval then gradually increases until 1 year of age (0.26 to 0.28 sec). The QTc, early in life, is 0.44 sec.[20, 21]

CRITERIA FOR DIAGNOSING ELECTROCARDIOGRAPHIC ABNORMALITIES

In the previous sections, the ranges of normal values for electrocardiograms of normal and premature infants have been described. This information was provided as a standard for comparison to electrocardiograms of patients with abnormalities. The electrocardiogram of neonates and infants is difficult to interpret because of the normal changes that occur during the first year of life and the wide range of normal changes. In the neonatal period particularly, difficulty is encountered in distinguishing right ventricular hypertrophy from the normal neonatal pattern.

P Waves

The P waves should be interpreted for axis, amplitude, and duration. The normal P wave axis has been described. If the P wave axis is abnormal, there may be junctional rhythm, and atrial depolarization occurs from an ectopic site. Frequently with junctional rhythm, the PR interval is short. The P wave axis may also be abnormal in patients with malposition of the heart. Infants with polysplenia tend to have left axis P waves, whereas infants with asplenia tend to have P waves directed slightly to the right. Some patients with atrial septal defect also have P waves directed leftward (0 to $-30°$), and controversy exists whether these are associated with a sinus venosus type defect.

The P wave amplitude should not exceed 3 mm. Right atrial enlargement is diagnosed when P waves exceed this value. In right atrial enlargement, the P waves are also peaked and pointed.

If the P wave is greater than 0.08 sec, left atrial enlargement is present, particularly if the P wave is broad and notched. Left atrial enlargement can also be recognized by a prominent, wide, negative component of a diphasic P wave in leads V_1 or V_4R.

PR Interval

The PR interval reflects transmission through the atrioventricular node. When shorter than normal, either a junctional rhythm or preexcitation (Wolff-Parkinson-White syndrome) is present.

Prolongation of the PR interval usually is acquired and occurs with various conditions, such as digitalis administration, fever, and myocarditis. It is also a frequent component of the electrocardiographic pattern of endocardial cushion defect.

QRS Complex

In each electrocardiogram, the QRS axis is calculated. When the value is greater than the upper limit of normal for any age (Table 4-1), right axis deviation is present and indicates the presence of right ventricular hypertrophy.

Left axis deviation is diagnosed when the axis is less than the smallest value of the normal QRS axis range. Left axis deviation is rarely associated with left ventricular hypertrophy. In infancy, left axis deviation is often associated with an intraventricular conduction abnormality, the classic example being endocardial cushion defect. Tricuspid atresia is also associated frequently with left axis deviation, but the reason for this is not clear. Other causes of left axis deviation in infancy include single ventricle, pulmonary valvular dysplasia, and myocardiopathy.

If the QRS axis is located between $+210°$ and $+270°$ ($-90°$ and $-150°$), either marked right axis deviation or marked left axis deviation is present. Any of the conditions associated with left axis deviation can be included in causes of QRS axis in this sector.

The normal values of QRS duration are given (Table 4-1). If the QRS duration is prolonged, an intraventricular conduction abnormality, such as bundle-branch block, is present. While in older patients, 0.11 sec is the upper limit beyond, in neonates and infants we consider 0.08 sec the upper limits of normal. We have seen neonates with a QRS complex of 0.09 sec and a pattern of complete right bundle-branch block, in whom over a period of observation, the QRS complex gradually increased to 0.12 sec and still showed an rSR′ complex in lead V_1. Ebstein's malformation and right ventriculotomy are the most frequent causes of complete right bundle-branch block in infants. Left bundle-branch block is rare but may be found in infants with cardiomyopathy or in an occasional infant with anomalous origin of the left coronary artery.

The QRS amplitude and the configuration are used primarily to diagnose ventricular hypertrophy.[25]

Right ventricular hypertrophy is diagnosed when:

1. R wave voltage in lead V_1 is greater than normal, or
2. S wave voltage in lead V_6 is greater than normal, or
3. qR pattern is present in lead V_1, or
4. The T wave is upright in lead V_1 after 3 or 4 days, provided the T wave is upright in the left precordial leads, also.

Left ventricular hypertrophy is diagnosed when:

1. R wave voltage in lead V_6 is greater than normal (generally about 20 mm), or
2. S wave voltage in lead V_1 is greater than normal (generally about 20 mm), or
3. R/RS ratio in lead V_1 is less than normal.

Combined ventricular hypertrophy:

1. Any sign of right ventricular hypertrophy and any sign of left ventricular hypertrophy
2. Large (>70 mm), equiphasic RS complexes in midprecordial leads
3. Pattern of right ventricular hypertrophy, plus 2 mm Q in lead V_6 or negative T wave in lead V_6
4. Pattern of left ventricular hypertrophy, plus a large R or R′ in lead V_1

ST Segment

In normal infants, the ST segment may be elevated 1 mm in the standard leads and 2 mm in the midprecordial leads. Depression of the ST segment greater than 1 mm is abnormal. Digitalis is the most common cause of ST segment depression but does not indicate toxicity (Fig. 4-3).

T Wave

If the T wave is located outside the normal sector, an abnormality of ventricular repolarization is present which needs to be interpreted in relation to the QRS complex. If the QRS complex is normal in duration, amplitude, and configuration, the T wave changes are related most likely to a primary repolarization abnormality such as occurs in myocarditis, pericarditis, or electrolyte abnormalities. If, however, the QRS complex is abnormal, the T wave changes are most likely secondary to abnormal ventricular depolarization. Frequently, when the T wave axis is abnormal, it is directed away from the QRS axis and

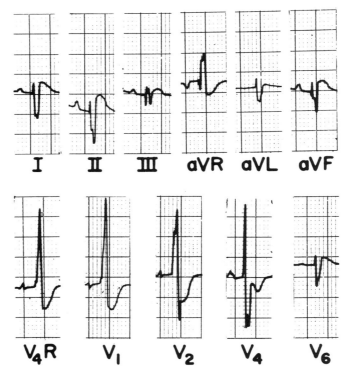

FIG. 4-3.   Electrocardiogram showing ST segment changes caused by digitalis. In infants, ST segment depression often occurs in right precordial leads.

the QRS-T angle is widened. The T wave abnormality may also be associated with ST segment changes. When there is evidence of ventricular hypertrophy, ST segment depression, and wide QRS-T angle, the combination is considered to represent ventricular strain, i.e., severe ventricular hypertrophy.

The T waves should be about one fifth the height of the QRS complex. Tall T waves may indicate hyperkalemia, especially if they are symmetrical. T wave changes roughly correlate with serum potassium levels. Small amplitude T waves may reflect low amplitude QRS complexes or hypokalemia. Hypokalemia, however, shows progressive depression of the ST segment and the presence of a U wave.

QTc Interval

Analysis of the QTc interval can yield information about serum calcium levels. Hypocalcemia is associated with prolongation of the QTc level (Fig. 4-4), whereas hypercalcemia shortens the QTc interval, as does digitalis (Fig. 4-5).

Q-oTc Interval

The interval from the beginning of the Q wave to the onset of the T wave (Q-oTc) has been used to screen for hypocalcemia. Two reports[26, 27] have shown correlations between this electrocardiographic interval with both the total and the ionized serum calcium values of healthy full-term and premature infants. If the Q-oTc is prolonged (greater than 0.19 sec in full-term babies, and 0.20 sec in premature infants), hypocalcemia is usually present. Giacoia and Wagner[27] indicated a poor correlation between Q-oTc and calcium levels in critically ill premature infants because of the effects of catecholamines and cardiac sympathetic nervous system on the duration of ventricular repolarization.

RECORDING OF AN ELECTROCARDIOGRAM IN INFANTS

With care, patience, diligence, and experience, high-quality electrocardiographic tracings can be obtained in neonates and infants. Special precautions include the use of small electrodes (2 by 3 cm), narrow electrode straps, and a 1.5 cm diameter chest piece. We do not use suction to hold the chest piece in place because of the tendency to cause petechiae in neonates. In all infants, we record lead V_4R, but often in prematures and neonates, we omit leads V_3 and V_5. Generally, we use a nonabrasive electrode jelly.

It is easy to introduce artifacts into the electrocardiographic tracings of infants, and aside from the well-recognized patterns associated with reversal of the leads, other artifacts can be produced easily in this age group.

A common artifact is caused by the infant's muscular movements (Fig. 4-6). This is shown by a pattern of fine, high-frequency deflections, frequently observed best in the limb leads as the infant moves an extremity. Another type of artifact is related to respiration, presumably from movement of the thorax (Fig.

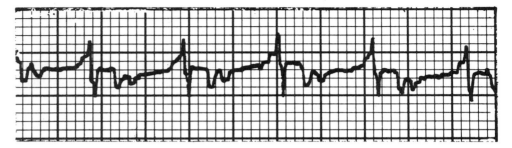

FIG. 4-4. Electrocardiographic tracing of prolonged QT interval (0.3 sec) in a 1-month-old infant with DiGeorge syndrome and tetralogy of Fallot.

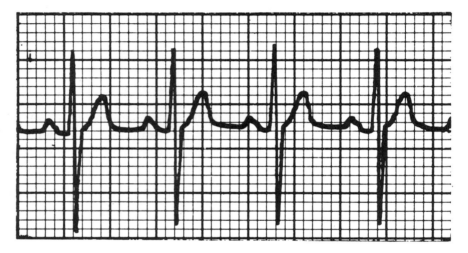

FIG. 4-5. Electrocardiographic tracing of short QT interval (0.2 sec) in a 2-week-old infant receiving a digitalis preparation.

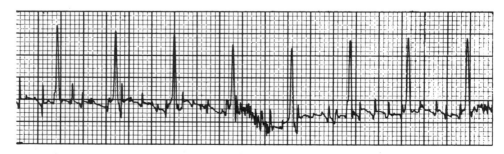

FIG. 4-6. Electrocardiographic tracing of artifact of muscular movement.

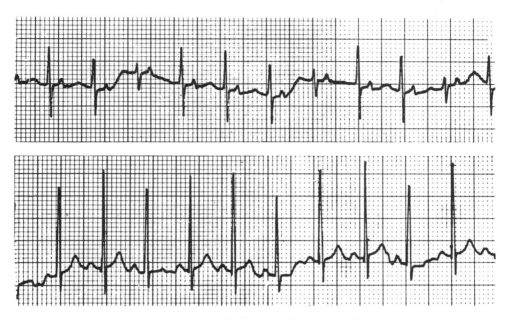

FIG. 4-7. Lead V₁ (upper) and lead V₅ (lower) of electrocardiogram show variation in QRS amplitude secondary to respiration.

4-7). The lateral precordial leads may show large deflections of the ST and T wave away from the baseline, and the heart rate often occurs as a multiple of this deflection.

Sometimes in an effort to minimize the infant's movements, the nurse restrains his arms. This produces a subtle, but at other times very confusing, artifact, in which the electrocardiogram of the restraining individual is superimposed upon the patient's electrocardiogram. This artifact is usually best seen in the limb leads (Fig. 4-8).

Babies hiccup frequently. Hiccups are recorded on the electrocardiogram as large complexes with the appearance of P waves, which occur sporadically and independently of QRS complexes (Fig. 4-9).

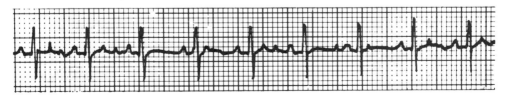

FIG. 4-8. Electrocardiographic tracing of artifact caused by person restraining infant. Lead I, small electrocardiographic complexes superimposed on tracing of patient.

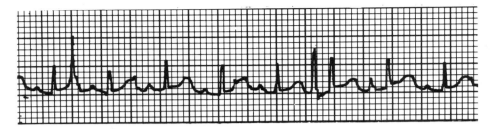

FIG. 4-9.   Electrocardiographic tracing of artifact caused by hiccups. The two large spike complexes were caused by hiccups.

Another common artifact results from smearing of the electrode paste across the anterior chest. Consequently, the entire area covered by the electrode paste acts as a common electrode. No matter where the electrode is placed along the course of the paste, the electrocardiographic pattern appears similar and represents a composite of the voltages underlying the entire area under the smeared paste.

HIS BUNDLE ELECTROCARDIOGRAM

Two studies[28, 29] have dealt extensively with His bundle recordings in children and include information from several infants. The study by Abella and co-workers[29] indicates that, for children, the average values, range, and cycle-to-cycle variability of the intervals represent a certain proportion of the PR interval, the PH representing 77 percent of PR, PA 23 percent, AH 56 percent, and HV 25 percent. The normal values and ranges for the first year are shown in Table 4-2.

VECTORCARDIOGRAM

The vectorcardiographic changes that occur with age and the patterns in various cardiac anomalies parallel the changes found in scalar electrocardiograms. Although several vectorcardiographic systems are available, the Frank[30–32] and Schmitt SVEC III systems have been most widely used in infants. Examples of vectorcardiograms of normal infants are shown in Figure 4-10.

Frontal Plane

In the first month of life, the initial QRS vectors may be directed into each of the four quadrants, but after that age, in three fourths of infants, the initial vectors are directed rightward and superiorly. Rarely, the direction is inferiorly and leftward. The direction of the terminal QRS vectors shows a similar pattern.

The mean QRS axis of the vectorcardiogram parallels the QRS axis of the

TABLE 4-2

AV Conduction Intervals Measured by His Electrocardiography in Children

AGE	CONDUCTION INTERVALS (MSEC)				
	PR	PH	PA	AH	HV
1 day	75–125 (100)*	53–98 (75)	13–31 (22)	32–74 (53)	15–35 (25)
2 weeks	71–119 (95)	50–93 (71)	13–29 (21)	30–71 (50)	14–33 (24)
1 mo	80–133 (106)	56–104 (80)	14–33 (23)	34–79 (56)	16–37 (27)
3 mo	85–142 (113)	60–110 (85)	15–35 (25)	36–84 (80)	17–40 (28)
6 mo	88–147 (118)	62–115 (88)	16–36 (25)	37–87 (62)	18–41 (29)
12 mo	92–153 (122)	64–119 (92)	16–38 (27)	39–91 (65)	18–43 (31)
24 mo	95–161 (128)	67–125 (96)	17–40 (28)	41–95 (68)	19–45 (32)
3 yr	99–165 (132)	69–129 (99)	17–41 (29)	42–98 (70)	20–46 (33)
5 yr	103–171 (137)	72–133 (103)	18–42 (30)	44–101 (73)	21–48 (34)
8 yr	109–182 (145)	76–142 (109)	19–45 (32)	46–108 (77)	22–51 (36)
12 yr	115–191 (153)	80–149 (115)	20–47 (34)	49–113 (81)	23–53 (38)
15 yr	118–196 (157)	82–153 (117)	21–48 (35)	50–116 (83)	24–55 (39)
18 yr	119–198 (159)	83–155 (119)	21–49 (35)	51–118 (84)	24–56 (40)

* Figures in parentheses indicate average values.
From Abella et al.: Am J Cardiol 30:876, 1972.

scalar electrocardiogram and shows a wide range during the first month of life. After 1 month of age, the mean QRS axis is directed leftward and inferiorly (mean, +70°) and then moves slightly more leftward (+45°) with age.

In 90 percent of infants, the QRS loop is inscribed in a clockwise direction in the frontal plane, and the remaining infants show either a figure-of-eight or counterclockwise rotation. In our experience, these latter two patterns of rotation occur more commonly in patients with more leftward direction of the QRS axis.

Horizontal Plane

The horizontal plane shows dramatic changes in the QRS vector loop. The initial QRS vector is directed anteriorly and rightward and shifts more toward the right after the age of 3 months. The terminal QRS forces are directed posteriorly and rightward (about +240°) throughout the first year of life. The mean QRS axis may be directed in a wide range until 1 month of age. Following this age, the mean QRS axis is directed anteriorly and leftward and becomes progressively more leftward with age, moving from a mean value of +41° at 2 months of age to +15° at 12 months of age. The T wave axis shows a wide scatter under 30 hours of age and then becomes directed leftward and slightly posterior. With age, the QRS loop progressively changes from a clockwise rotation, which is directed anteriorly and rightward, to a loop, which is counterclockwise in rotation and directed leftward. In this progression, the loop passes through a transition of a figure-of-eight pattern, which initially crosses in front of the E

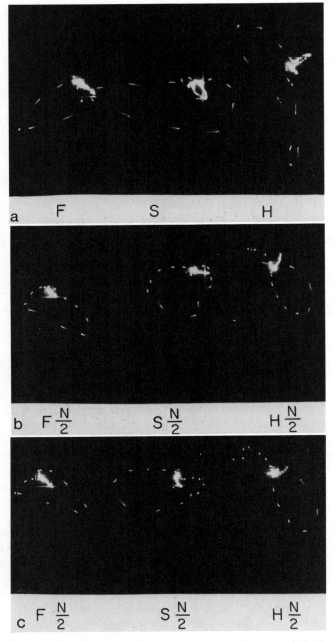

FIG. 4-10. Vectorcardiograms of normal infants, Schmitt SVEC III system. **a.** Six days. **b.** Six months. **c.** Fourteen months. In frontal plane (F), QRS loop initially directed inferiorly and rightward, subsequently leftward and inferiorly. In horizontal plane (H), QRS loop initially clockwise rotation toward right. Subsequently, loop forms a figure-of-eight contour, predominantly oriented toward left. Sagittal plane (S) is recorded as left sagittal. N/2, half-standardization.

point and then behind the E point. This sequence toward a counterclockwise loop reflects the progressive increase in left ventricular electrical forces.

The vectorcardiogram can be interpreted by a computer, utilizing multifactorial analysis to recognize abnormalities, particularly of the QRS complex. These techniques combine voltage and directional data of various points in three-dimensional space. The bedside interpretation of abnormalities, however, can be made generally by comparing the pattern recorded in a patient to that expected in the normal. The frontal plane usually gives information about the QRS axis and discordance of the QRS and the T waves, and this information can be combined with the appearance of the horizontal plane.

The horizontal plane is particularly useful in recognizing ventricular hypertrophy and other QRS patterns, such as complete right bundle-branch block, or that associated with anterolateral myocardial infarction, as in anomalous left coronary artery.

Patterns of right ventricular hypertrophy can be recognized by change in the QRS loop of the horizontal plane. Right ventricular hypertrophy is recognized by persistence of the neonatal QRS loop pattern and a clockwise rotation, being directed anteriorly and rightward. After 1 month of age, it is rare for a normal infant to have an entirely clockwise loop in the horizontal plane. Signs of severe right ventricular hypertrophy include direction of the initial QRS vectors anteriorly and leftward, the T wave being directed more posteriorly than normal, and a wide QRS-T angle.

Left ventricular hypertrophy is indicated by an accelerated progression of the QRS forces leftward and in a counterclockwise direction. At any age, when major QRS forces are accentuated and directed posteriorly and leftward, left ventricular hypertrophy should be diagnosed. Severe left ventricular hypertrophy is also indicated by the T wave being directed anteriorly and rightward, therefore yielding a wide QRS-T angle.

Biventricular hypertrophy may be manifested by either of two patterns which show large QRS voltages, particularly in the horizontal plane. In one pattern, the QRS loop is directed predominantly in an anteroposterior direction, with the anterior voltage being approximately equal to the posterior voltage. In the other pattern, as occurs in patients with a large ventricular septal defect, the loop shows large voltages laterally as well as anteriorly and posteriorly. The midportion of the QRS loop is directed leftward, while the terminal portion of the QRS loop is enlarged and directed posteriorly and rightward.

CARDIAC DYSRHYTHMIAS

Cardiac dysrhythmias occur more commonly in the first week of life than later in infancy.[33] Several factors account for this tendency: (1) the major physiologic changes that occur in the transition from fetal to adult circulation and the number of metabolic, pharmacologic, and disease alterations that occur during this period and that can affect the cardiac conduction system, (2) the altered autonomic control in neonates in which cholinergic influences predominate and sympathetic innervation develop, and (3) the continued postnatal development of the cardiac conduction system.

Dysrhythmias in infants and children[34, 35] and neonates[36] have been the subject of excellent reviews.

SINUS RHYTHM

Three variations of sinus rhythm may be observed in neonates and infants.

Sinus Arrhythmia

This is a phasic variation of the heart rate which may occur with respiration, increasing on inspiration and slowing on expiration, or which may be unassociated with respiration. Although it was previously considered uncommon in the first year of life, studies by Morgan et al.[3, 17] and Valimaki[37] have shown that sinus arrhythmia occurs frequently in both healthy and sick prematures and in full-term infants.[38] In fact, the presence of a relatively fixed cardiac rhythm may indicate cerebral dysfunction.

Sinus Tachycardia

Sinus tachycardia is diagnosed when a sinus rate exceeds the upper range of normal (Fig. 4-11). It may reach a value of 200 or 220 beats/min, although an instance of sinus tachycardia of 260 beats/min[37] has been described. In the neonate or young infant, a variety of stimuli, such as crying, feeding, or disturbance from procedures, can lead to sinus tachycardia which persists as long as 1 hour.[37]

In any infant with sinus tachycardia, an underlying cause, such as congestive cardiac failure, shock, anemia, fever, or pulmonary disease, should be sought.

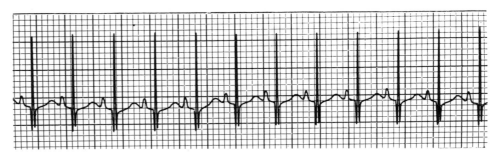

FIG. 4-11. Electrocardiographic tracing of sinus tachycardia. Lead II, heart rate 210/min.

Sinus Bradycardia

Sinus bradycardia is a sinus rhythm with a rate below the lower limit of normal. It may be associated with junctional escape beats. Sinus bradycardia occurs in both premature and full-term neonates. Various events, such as defecation, hiccups,[37] and nasopharyngeal stimulation,[39] can cause sinus bradycardia in neonates and are perhaps heightened because of cholinergic predominance of this age group. Bradycardic episodes may be associated with apnea. Although most episodes of bradycardia are brief, prolonged episodes may require treatment.

Not infrequently, the pediatrician is called to the nursery or neonatal intensive care unit to evaluate a neonate with occasional or frequent episodes of bradycardia. The most common cause of transient slowing of the heart rate is junctional rhythm, with a rate of approximately 80 beats/min. This phenomenon usually is of no significance and is most likely related to relative immaturity of the anatomic nervous system and increased vagal tone. Treatment is unnecessary, since these infants seem to be completely unaffected by short periods of mild bradycardia. Persistent junctional rhythm is uncommon and is encountered most frequently in asplenia syndrome.

Premature babies, especially those of less than 34 weeks gestation, may have bradycardia secondary to prolonged periods of apnea. Recurrent episodes of apnea leading to bradycardia require continuous monitoring of the infant and treatment. Aminophylline in a dose of 3 mg/kg every 8 to 12 hours is currently recommended for symptomatic apnea. Though apnea and bradycardia after the second day of life are expected in very small premature infants, causes such as sepsis, necrotizing enterocolitis, and patent ductus arteriosus should be investigated.

SUPRAVENTRICULAR OR VENTRICULAR PREMATURE CONTRACTIONS

If continuous monitoring is carried out, premature contractions may be observed in nearly one fourth of healthy premature or full-term neonates, but the incidence actually observed in a newborn nursery is considerably less. Supraventricular extrasystoles occur more frequently than do ventricular extrasystoles.[33, 40]

Supraventricular premature beats show an early occurring P wave with an abnormal contour (Fig. 4-12). The P waves may precede, follow, or coincide with the QRS complex. Usually the QRS complex shows a normal contour, but when widened, differentiation from a premature ventricular contraction may be difficult. Supraventricular premature beats are followed by an incomplete compensatory pause.

Ventricular premature contractions show a wide, abnormal QRS complex and a tall T wave, which often is directed opposite the QRS complex (Fig. 4-13). There is a compensatory pause.

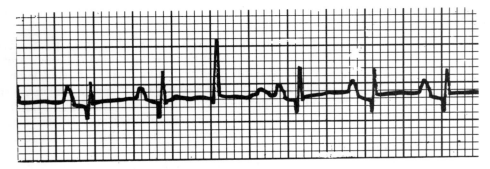

FIG. 4-12. Electrocardiographic tracing of a single junctional premature contraction. Lead II, normal neonate.

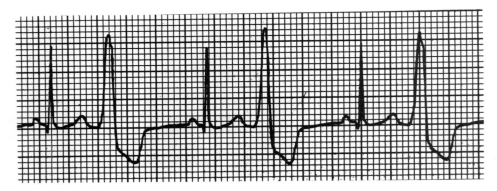

FIG. 4-13. Electrocardiogram of ventricular premature contraction occurring every other beat. Lead II.

The prognosis for each of these premature contractions is excellent, providing there is no underlying abnormality. Premature supraventricular contractions indicate a more benign condition than do premature ventricular contractions. Premature contractions may occur during cardiac catheterization, cardiac operation, metabolic abnormalities, or various neonatal diseases of infancy.

No therapy is required, except for correction of associated condition.

WOLFF-PARKINSON-WHITE SYNDROME

Wolff-Parkinson-White (preexcitation) syndrome occurs more commonly in neonates than in older infants or children, and in many instances it is transient and disappears.[41, 42] Wolff and associates[41] and Massing and associates[43] suggest that atrioventricular bypass fibers may be present at birth. The activity through the bypass fibers is enhanced by the predominant cholinergic activity and the reduced adrenergic activity of the neonate. With maturation of the heart and adrenergic activity, these bypass fibers become quiescent. It occurs more commonly in males than females (3:2 ratio).

The Wolff-Parkinson-White syndrome is characterized by (1) short PR interval, (2) widened QRS complex, and (3) delta wave (Fig. 4-14). The delta wave represents the preexcitation of ventricular myocardium. It may be difficult to recognize the Wolff-Parkinson-White syndrome in neonates because electrocardiographic intervals are shorter than in older children.

Wolff-Parkinson-White may be merely an asymptomatic electrocardiographic abnormality or may lead to paroxysmal supraventricular tachycardia (66 percent[44] to 90 percent of infants[42, 45]). During the episode of tachycardia, the QRS complex may be narrow or widened. Episodes of paroxysmal supraventricular tachycardia occur more commonly in early infancy[42, 44, 46] and may lead to congestive cardiac failure.

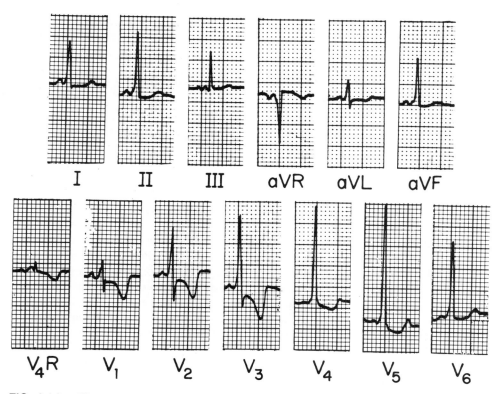

FIG. 4-14.   Electrocardiogram of Wolff-Parkinson-White syndrome in a neonate. PR interval of 0.07 seconds. Delta wave seen well in leads II, aVF, V$_5$, and V$_6$. QRS duration of 0.08 sec.

The Wolff-Parkinson-White syndrome has been classed into two types: type A—with large R waves in the right precordium, suggesting that the anomalous pathway involves the left bundle of His and the left side of the heart; type B—with large negative deflections in the right precordium, suggesting that the right bundle of His is involved. In a review by Bhandhusavee and associates[42] of Wolff-Parkinson-White syndrome, among 25 neonates without congenital cardiac disease, 85 percent had type A, and 23 of these 25 had paroxysmal atrial tachycardia. In nearly half of these 25, the Wolff-Parkinson-White syndrome disappeared with time. In 10 cases with congenital cardiac disease, most had type B Wolff-Parkinson-White syndrome, and 30 percent had paroxysmal atrial tachycardia. Swiderski and colleagues[46] found that type B Wolff-Parkinson-White syndrome was present in 19 of their 20 patients with cardiac anomalies, and half of these had episodes of paroxysmal supraventricular tachycardia. Although Ebstein's malformation is frequently associated with Wolff-Parkinson-White syndrome, central nervous system disorders and cardiomyopathies have also been associated with this electrocardiographic abnormality.[46, 47]

Digitalization is indicated for the occurrence of paroxysmal supraventricular tachycardia and is very successful in converting the dysrhythmia to a sinus rhythm and in preventing recurrence of the tachycardia.[44] The digitalis therapy should be continued until 1 year of age and then discontinued. Following discontinuance of therapy, in 85 percent of patients[44] paroxysmal tachycardia does not recur.

PAROXYSMAL SUPRAVENTRICULAR TACHYCARDIA

Paroxysmal supraventricular tachycardia is the most commonly occurring dysrhythmia in neonates. It is a rapid (250 to 320 beats/min) rhythm, originating in either the atria or junctional region. Differentiation between atrial and junctional tachycardia is difficult. The QRS complex usually shows a normal configuration but may be widened. Typically, the rhythm is remarkably regular and the RR interval is constant. Depending upon the origin of the tachycardia and the cardiac rate, the P waves may be inapparent or precede or follow the QRS complex (Fig. 4-15). ST segment depression occurs in patients with prolonged tachycardia and persists a few days following conversion. P waves may appear enlarged following conversion and take longer to become normal. When the rate is slower, it may be difficult to distinguish paroxysmal supraventricular tachycardia from sinus tachycardia. Usually there is one to one atrial to ventricular conduction, but occasionally there may be a block (Fig. 4-16).

Paroxysmal supraventricular tachycardia may originate from either an ectopic pacemaker or from a reentry phenomenon. In about 10 percent of infants, Wolff-Parkinson-White syndrome is found, although Lundberg[48] reported a 49 percent incidence, and Andersen et al.[49] reported a 46 percent incidence. It is perhaps due to persistent atrioventricular muscle bridges and Mahaim fibers.[43]

Paroxysmal supraventricular tachycardia occurs most frequently in males

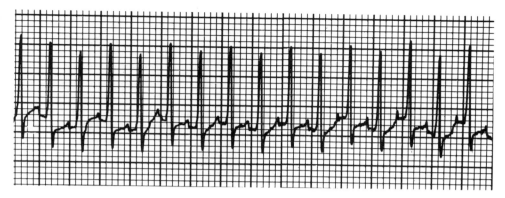

FIG. 4-15. Electrocardiographic tracing of paroxysmal supraventricular tachycardia. Heart rate, 300/min. Each P wave followed by a QRS complex.

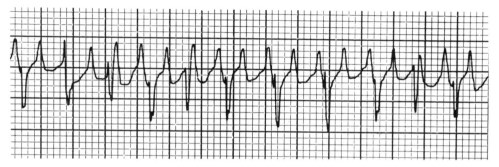

FIG. 4-16. Electrocardiographic tracing of paroxysmal supraventricular tachycardia with variable block. Atrial rate, 370 beats/min; ventricular rate, 200 beats/min.

less than 4 months of age. Rarely, it develops in utero[50] and causes fetal hydrops.[51, 52] Generally, the infant presents with symptoms related to the tachycardia, but it may be recognized initially during routine examination of an asymptomatic infant. Nadas and his colleagues[53] indicated that the age of the child and duration of the tachycardia were the two factors influencing the development of symptoms. Seventy-five percent of their infants were under 4 months of age, and the majority of these had developed congestive cardiac failure.

These authors describe clearly the clinical picture:

The majority of patients, especially the group of young infants with idiopathic paroxysmal tachycardia, were very ill patients. The color was often ashen grey. The skin was cold and wet with perspiration. They were restless and irritable. Respirations were rapid and labored. Often a hacking cough was present. The abdomen was distended.[53]

The clinical picture resembles severe pneumonia or sepsis, but the excessively rapid cardiac rate leads to the diagnosis of paroxysmal supraventricular tachycardia.[53] Soft systolic murmurs may be present,[53, 54] as may cardiomegaly and pulmonary congestion. These roentgenographic findings decrease markedly in the 36 hours following conversion to sinus rhythm and reach normal in 2 weeks if there is no underlying cardiac problem.

In early infancy, there is a male (3:2) predominance,[49, 53, 55] whereas in the latter half of infancy, the male to female ratio is equal. The age of onset was the first month of life for 18 of 30 infants. Although in most infants, paroxysmal supraventricular tachycardia is considered idiopathic, it has been associated with a variety of cardiac anomalies.[49, 56] Myocarditis, myocardiopathy, and Ebstein's malformation are the most common conditions associated with this rhythm disturbance. Saccular aneurysms of the atria were described in a patient with paroxysmal supraventricular tachycardia. When the aneurysms were resected, sinus rhythm persisted.[57]

Individual neonates have been described with paroxysmal supraventricular tachycardia occurring during a course of theophylline therapy[58] or complicating thyrotoxicosis.[59]

Therapy should be initiated with parenterally administered digoxin. The usual digitalizing doses and frequency of administration should be followed. If the infant is acutely ill, two thirds or three fourths of the digitalizing dose should be given initially, and digitalization should be completed within 4 to 8 hours, depending upon the severity of illness. If paroxysmal supraventricular tachycardia persists, another one fourth of the digitalizing dose should be given. Diuretics and oxygen are often indicated as well. Propranolol, 0.1 mg/kg, can be given slowly intravenously if paroxysmal supraventricular tachycardia fails to convert to digitalization. In our experience, in 95 percent of neonates and infants, conversion occurs during digitalization. We have never seen vagal stimulation cause conversion. Ocular compression should never be used, for it can cause retinal detachment. In a critically ill infant, DC conversion with 10 watts should be given before digitalization.

The prognosis for paroxysmal supraventricular tachycardia of infancy is excellent, particularly in neonates and in those without cardiac disease.[49, 53] Nadas and colleagues[53] reported that 22 percent of infants less than 4 months of age had a recurrence after 1 year, but, in our experience, this is a high rate. If paroxysmal supraventricular tachycardia initially developed after 4 months of age, 83 percent had recurrences.[53]

Lundberg[48] followed 47 individuals with paroxysmal supraventricular tachycardia in infancy for periods of 10 to 26 years. The recurrence rate dropped from 55 percent in the first year to 17 percent for ages up to 10 years and 23 percent during adolescent years. In another long-term study, recurrence was found in 25 percent, more commonly in individuals with Wolff-Parkinson-White syndrome.[49]

ATRIAL FLUTTER

Atrial flutter is a rare dysrhythmia occurring in the neonatal period or infancy which resembles paroxysmal supraventricular tachycardia in many respects.

In atrial flutter, the atrial rate ranges between 320 and 480 beats/min, with the average being over 400 beats/min. Characteristically, atrial activity is evident as sawtoothed flutter waves (Fig. 4-17). Depending upon atrioventricular conduction, the ventricular response is variable. Second degree atrioventricular block is usually present, permitting conduction either at a fixed rate, leading to 2:1, 3:1, or 4:1 block and regular RR intervals, or less frequently, at variable rates and irregular RR intervals. The ventricular rate ranges from 60 to 240 beats/min.[60]

Many individual infants with atrial flutter have been reported and summarized in two reviews.[61, 62] A more recent report of eight cases[63] adds additional experience and knowledge.

Atrial flutter can cause signs and symptoms similar to paroxysmal supraventricular tachycardia and lead to congestive cardiac failure. The neonate may be asymptomatic because the degree of atrioventricular block leads to a slow ventricular rate.[62, 63] The dysrhythmia may be recognized prior to birth, as in 11 of the 24 neonates we classified as congenital atrial flutter,[62] and it has been associated with congestive cardiac failure in utero and with fetal hydrops.

We grouped atrial flutter occurring in the first year of life into two categories[62] and believe this classification has value in establishing response to treatment and prognosis:

	Congenital	*Paroxysmal*
Frequency	More common	Less common
Age onset	Before or soon after birth	After third week of life
Tolerance	Good	Poor
Duration	Continuous	Paroxysmal
Spontaneous conversion	Occasional	Rare
Response to digitalization	Good	Poor
Prognosis	Usually good	Appears poor

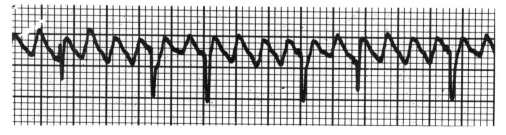

FIG. 4-17.   Electrocardiographic tracing from a neonate with atrial flutter and variable block. Atrial activity evident as sawtoothed wave form at a rate of 400 beats/min; ventricular rate, 120/min.

As in paroxysmal supraventricular tachycardia, atrial flutter occurs more commonly in males (3:1),[62] and this is much more striking after 1 week of age. Prognosis is not as favorable as it is with paroxysmal supraventricular tachycardia: 11 of the 36 reported neonates with atrial flutter died, and deaths occurred more frequently in neonates with coexistent cardiac anomalies or when atrial flutter alternated with atrial fibrillation.

Following digitalization, atrial flutter converts less frequently than paroxysmal supraventricular tachycardia, but digitalis affects atrioventricular nodal conduction and slows the ventricular rate. If conversion with digitalis is unsuccessful or if the neonate is acutely ill, cardioversion should be used. Atrial flutter usually converts using a remarkably low energy level.[63, 64] In most patients, follow-up examination is normal, even though cardiac anomalies are often suspected initially because of the severity of cardiac symptoms and the cardiomegaly.

ATRIAL FIBRILLATION

Atrial fibrillation is a rare dysrhythmia in neonates and infants[65-69] and may be associated with atrial flutter.[61, 62] Atrial fibrillation is recognized by a wavy or undulating baseline and irregular ventricular complexes (Fig. 4-18). It often causes congestive cardiac failure. Digitalization results in reduction of ventricular rate, but conversion to sinus rhythm is rare. The rhythm may convert spontaneously,[68] but if it does not, quinidine, procainamide, or cardioversion may be used. We indicated[62] that the prognosis was poor for infants with atrial fibrillation, but Radford and Izukawa[65] report that prognosis is good, for they had one neonate and three infants in whom atrial fibrillation was transient, and each patient survived.

VENTRICULAR TACHYCARDIA

Ventricular tachycardia, a rare dysrhythmia of neonates and infants, has serious consequences of reduced cardiac output, which may be profound, and of progression to ventricular fibrillation.[70-73]

In ventricular tachycardia, the QRS complexes are wide and tall. The T waves, which are also tall, are directed opposite to the QRS complex (Figs. 4-19 and 4-20). The ventricular rate may reach 270 beats/min. It may be difficult to distinguish ventricular tachycardia from junctional or paroxysmal supraventricular tachycardia with aberrant ventricular conduction, but the following electrocardiographic features are useful in identifying ventricular tachycardia: (1) premature ventricular contractions with similar contour occurring prior to or following ventricular tachycardia, (2) presence of fusion or capture beats, (3) P waves appearing independently of the QRS complex, (4) irregular ventricular rate, (5) varying QRS configuration, and (6) slower rate than paroxysmal supraventricular tachycardia.

Ventricular tachycardia can develop at the time of cardiac operation, dur-

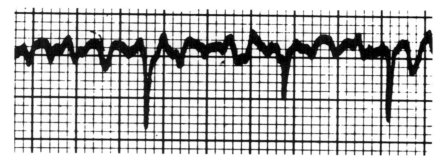

FIG. 4-18. Electrocardiographic tracing of a neonate with atrial fibrillation. Irregular atrial rate and contour. Ventricular complexes also irregular in frequency and contour.

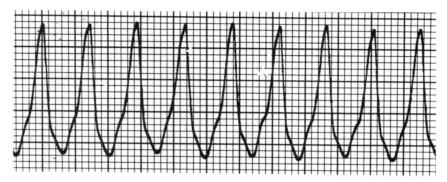

FIG. 4-19. Electrocardiographic tracing of ventricular tachycardia. Rate, 206 beats/min.

ing cardiac catheterization, with severe metabolic abnormalities, or with digitalis toxicity. Myocardial abnormalities, such as myocarditis,[74] myocardiopathy,[71] or cardiac tumor,[75] may be the etiologic factors, but often, ventricular tachycardia occurs without identifiable cause.[34, 76]

In infancy, ventricular tachycardia may present, with failure to thrive, congestive cardiac failure,[34] syncope, or shock. The natural history is largely unknown because it depends upon the presence of underlying conditions. Of 57 infants and children with idiopathic ventricular tachycardia reviewed by Hernandez and associates,[76] 16 (28 percent) have died.

Treatment of ventricular tachycardia is often difficult and may require the use of various medications, often in combination and, at times, in very large doses. Still, recurrences are frequent.

The initial treatment should be intravenous lidocaine or, if the condition is critical, cardioversion.[77] Cardioversion with 10 watts may convert the ventricular tachycardia in infants. Diphenylhydantoin may be beneficial in infants with ventricular tachycardia from digitalis toxicity. In infants, procainamide, quini-

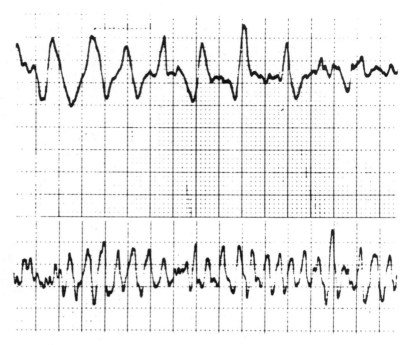

FIG. 4-20. Electrocardiographic tracing of ventricular fibrillation and tachycardia in neonate without evident cardiac disease.

dine, and propranolol have also been used with variable degrees of success. One striking feature of ventricular tachycardia in infancy is the large doses of medication needed to terminate episodes of the disorder. Sanchez and associates[73] used 3,000 mg procainamide per day in an 8 kg, 10-month-old infant and obtained a blood level of 33 μg/ml. Mortimer and associates[74] used 6,000 mg/24 hours in an 11 kg, 14-month-old infant and obtained a blood level of 26 μg/ml. Gelband and associates[78] used 3,600 mg procainamide per day in an 18-month-old, 10 kg child and obtained a blood level of 9 μg/ml. Despite these large doses and their use over a long period of time, toxic effects were minimal.

Treatment has to be individualized, depending upon the seriousness of the infant's condition, the response to therapy, and the presence of an underlying condition.

In each patient, an echocardiogram should be obtained, and angiograms should be performed in each ventricle to identify underlying cardiac conditions, particularly cardiac tumors. Tumors can be resected successfully and the tachycardia terminated.[75]

Hernandez and colleagues[76] find procainamide and propranolol are the most effective combination in children and suggest that Holter monitoring is helpful in assessing the therapeutic response.

spatial vectorcardiogram during the first week of life. Am J Cardiol 12:482, 1963

5. Walsh SZ: Early clamping versus stripping of the cord: Comparative study of the electrocardiogram in the neonatal period. Br Heart J 31:122, 1969

6. Costa AF, Faul BC, Ledbetter MK, Oalmon MC: The electrocardiogram in the premature infant. Am Heart J 67:4, 1964

7. Craige E, Harned HS Jr: Phonocardiographic and electrocardiographic studies in normal newborn infants. Am Heart J 65:180, 1963

8. Michaëlsson M: Electrocardiographic studies in the healthy newborn. Acta Paediatr Scand 48 [Suppl 117]:108, 1959

9. Walsh SZ: Electrocardiographic intervals during the first week of life. Am Heart J 66:36, 1963

10. Walsh SZ: The electrocardiogram during the first week of life. Br Heart J 25:784, 1963

11. Walsh SZ: The S-T segment and T wave during the first week of life. Br Heart J 26:679, 1964

12. Stern L, Lind J: Neonatal T wave patterns. Acta Paediatr Scand 49:329, 1960

13. Hait G, Gasul BM: The evolution and significance of T wave changes in the normal newborn during the first seven days of life. Am J Cardiol 12:494, 1963

14. Emmanouilides GC, Moss AJ, Adams FH: The electrocardiogram in normal newborn infants: Correlation with hemodynamic observations. J Pediatr 67:578, 1965

15. Ziegler RF: Electrocardiographic Studies in Normal Infants and Children. Springfield, Ill, Thomas, 1951

16. Ackerman BD, Sperling DR, O'Loughlin BJ: Electrocardiographic observations in postmature infants. J Pediatr 76:399, 1970

17. Morgan BC, Bloom RS, Guntheroth WG: Cardiac arrhythmias in premature infants. Pediatrics 35:658, 1965

18. Church SC, Morgan BC, Oliver TK Jr, Guntheroth WG: Cardiac arrhythmias in premature infants: An indication of autonomic immaturity? J Pediatr 71:542, 1967

19. Sreenivasan VV, Fisher BJ, Liebman J, Downs TD: Longitudinal study of the standard electrocardiogram in the healthy premature infant during the first year of life. Am J Cardiol 31:57, 1973

20. Hubsher JA: The electrocardiogram of the premature infant. Am Heart J 61:467, 1961

21. Levine OR, Griffiths SP: Electrocardiographic findings in healthy premature infants. Pediatrics 30:361, 1962

22. Walsh SZ: Evolution of the electrocardiogram of healthy premature infants during the first year of life. Acta Paediatr Scand 38[Suppl 145]:1, 1963

23. Walsh SZ: Comparative study of electrocardiograms of healthy premature and full-term infants of similar weight. Am Heart J 68:183, 1964

24. Wenger NK, Watkins WL, Hurst JW: A preliminary study of the electrocardiogram of the normal premature infant. Am Heart J 62:304, 1961

25. Hastreiter AR, Abella JB: The electrocardiogram in the newborn period. II. The infant with disease. J Pediatr 78:346, 1971

26. Colletti RB, Pan MW, Smith EWP, Genel M: Detection of hypocalcemia in susceptible neonates. The Q-oTc interval. N Engl J Med 290:931, 1974

27. Giacoia GP, Wagner HR: Q-oTc interval and blood calcium levels in newborn infants. Pediatrics 61:877, 1978

28. Roberts NK, Olley PM: His bundle recordings in children with normal hearts and congenital heart disease. Circulation 45:295, 1972

29. Abella JB, Teixeira OHP, Misra KP, Hastreiter AR: Changes of atrioventricular conduction with age in infants and children. Am J Cardiol 30:876, 1972

30. Namin EP, Miller RA: The normal electrocardiogram and vectorcardiogram in

children. In Cassels DE, Ziegler RF (eds): Electrocardiography in Infants and Children. New York, Grune & Stratton, 1966, pp 99–108
31. Namin EP, Arcilla RA, D'Cruz IA, Gasul BM: Evolution of the Frank vectorcardiogram in normal infants. Am J Cardiol 13:757, 1964
32. Liebman J: The normal electrocardiogram in newborns and infants (a critical review). In Cassels DE, Ziegler RF (eds): Electrocardiography in Infants and Children. New York, Grune & Stratton, 1966, pp 79–98

Cardiac Dysrhythmias

33. Ferrer PL, Gelband H, Garcia OL, Tamer DM, Jesse MJ: Occurrence of arrhythmias during the newborn period. Clin Res 25[Abstr]:64A, 1977
34. Ehlers KH: Supraventricular and ventricular dysrhythmias in infants and children. Cardiovasc Clin 4:59, 1972
35. Paul MH: Cardiac arrhythmias in infants. and children. Prog Cardiovasc Dis 9:136, 1966
36. Ferrer PL: Arrhythmias in the neonate. In Roberts NK, Gelband H (eds): Cardiac Arrhythmias in the Neonate, Infant and Child. New York, Appleton-Century-Crofts, 1977, pp 265–316
37. Valimaki I: Postnatal alterations of cardiac rhythm. Clin Pediatr 9:652, 1970
38. Landtman B: Heart arrhythmias in children. Acta Paediatr Scand 34[Suppl 1]:1, 1947
39. Cordero L Jr, Hon EH: Neonatal bradycardia following nasopharyngeal stimulation. J Pediatr 78:441, 1971

Supraventricular or Ventricular Contractions

40. Valimaki I: Heart-rate variation in full-term newborn infants. I. Use of a small, special-purpose computer. Biol Neonate 18:129, 1971

Wolff-Parkinson-White Syndrome

41. Wolff GS, Han J, Curran J: Wolff-Parkinson-White syndrome in the neonate. Am J Cardiol 41:559, 1978
42. Bhandhusavee RV, Walters LR, Noonan JA: Wolff-Parkinson-White in the neonate: 9 cases including 2 with intrauterine defects. Am J Cardiol 29[Abstr]:253, 1972
43. Massing GK, Liebman J, James TN: Cardiac conduction pathways in the infant and child. Cardiovasc Clin 4:28, 1972
44. Giardina ACV, Ehlers KH, Engle MA: Wolff-Parkinson-White syndrome in infants and children. A long-term follow-up study. Br Heart J 34:839, 1972
45. Mantakas ME, McCue CM, Miller WW: Natural history of Wolff-Parkinson-White syndrome discovered in infancy. Am J Cardiol 41:1097, 1978
46. Swiderki J, Lees MH, Nadas AS: The Wolff-Parkinson-White syndrome in infancy and childhood. Br Heart J 24:561, 1962
47. Schiebler GL, Adams P Jr, Anderson RC: The Wolff-Parkinson-White syndrome in infants and children. A review and a report of 28 cases. Pediatrics 24:585, 1959

Paroxysmal Supraventricular Tachycardia

48. Lundberg A: Paroxysmal tachycardia in infancy: Follow-up study of 47 subjects ranging in age from 10 to 26 years. Pediatrics 51:26, 1973
49. Andersen ED, Jacobsen JR, Sandøe E, Videbaek J, Wennevold A: Paroxysmal tachycardia in infancy and childhood. I. Paroxysmal supraventricular tachycardia. Acta Paediatr Scand 62:341, 1973

50. Wilburne M, Mack EG: Paroxysmal tachycardia in the newborn with onset in utero. JAMA 154:1337, 1954
51. Cowan RH, Waldo AL, Harris HB, Cassady G, Brans YW: Neonatal paroxysmal supraventricular tachycardia with hydrops. Pediatrics 55:428, 1975
52. Silber DL, Durnin RE: Intrauterine atrial tachycardia. Associated with massive edema in a newborn. Am J Dis Child 117:722, 1969
53. Nadas AS, Daeschner CW, Roth A, Blumenthal SL: Paroxysmal tachycardia in infants and children. Study of 41 cases. Pediatrics 9:167, 1952
54. Simcha A, Bonham-Carter RE: Paroxysmal atrial tachycardia in infants and children. Lancet 1:832, 1971
55. Klint RB, Hernandez A, Goldring D, Behrer RM: Paroxysmal supraventricular tachycardia (PST) in infants and children. Clin Pediatr 11:475, 1972
56. Apley J, Corner BD, Gibson TC: Paroxysmal tachycardia in infancy. Arch Dis Child 30:517, 1955
57. Varghese PJ, Simon AL, Rosenquist GC, et al: Multiple saccular congenital aneurysms of the atria causing persistent atrial tachyarrhythmia in an infant. Report of a case successfully treated by surgery. Pediatrics 44:429, 1969
58. Loughnan PM, McNamara JM: Paroxysmal supraventricular tachycardia during theophylline therapy in a premature infant. J Pediatr 92:1016, 1978
59. Riopel DA, Mullins CE: Congenital thyrotoxicosis with paroxysmal atrial tachycardia. Pediatrics 50:140, 1972

Atrial Flutter

60. McDonagh BJ: Congenital atrial flutter. Arch Dis Child 43:731, 1968
61. Rodriguez-Coronel A, Sueblingvong V, Hastreiter AR: Clinical forms of atrial flutter in infancy. J Pediatr 73:69, 1968
62. Moller JH, Davachi F, Anderson RC: Atrial flutter in infancy. J Pediatr 75:643, 1969
63. Rowland TW, Mathew R, Chameides L, Keane JF: Idiopathic atrial flutter in infancy: A review of eight cases. Pediatrics 61:52, 1978
64. Hassenrück A, Chojnacki B, Barker HJ: Cardioversion of auricular flutter in a newborn infant. Am J Cardiol 15:726, 1965

Atrial Fibrillation

65. Radford DJ, Izukawa T: Atrial fibrillation in children. Pediatrics 59:250, 1977
66. Hung W, Walsh BJ: Congenital auricular fibrillation in a newborn infant with endocardial fibroelastosis. Report of a case with necropsy. J Pediatr 61:65, 1962
67. Edeiken J, Rugel SJ: Auricular fibrillation in infancy. Report of a case with fleeting paroxysms. J Pediatr 28:471, 1946
68. Goldbloom A, Segall HN: Progress report on a case of auricular fibrillation demonstrated in infant of three months. Can Med Assoc J 55:501, 1946
69. Zaldivar N, Gelband H, Tamer D, Garcia O: Atrial fibrillation in infancy. J Pediatr 83:821, 1973

Ventricular Tachycardia

70. Palaganas MC Jr, Fay JE, Delahaye DJ: Paroxysmal ventricular tachycardia in childhood. Report of a case and review of the literature. J Pediatr 67:784, 1965
71. Videbaek J, Andersen ED, Jacobsen JR, Sandøe E, Wennevold A: Paroxsymal tachycardia in infancy and childhood. II. Paroxysmal ventricular tachycardia and fibrillation. Acta Paediatr Scand 62:349, 1973
72. Rosenbaum FF, Johnston FD, Keller AP: Paroxysmal ventricular tachycardia in childhood. Am J Dis Child 64:1030, 1942

73. Sanchez J, Christie K, Cumming GR: Treatment of ventricular tachycardia in an infant. Can Med Assoc J 107:136, 1972
74. Mortimer EA Jr, Rakita L: Ventricular tachycardia in childhood controlled with large doses of procainamide. N Engl J Med 262:615, 1970
75. Engle MA, Ebert PA, Redo SF: Recurrent ventricular tachycardia due to resectable cardiac tumor. Report of two cases in two-year-olds in heart failure. Circulation 50:1052, 1974
76. Hernandez A, Strauss A, Kleiger RE, Goldring D: Idiopathic paroxysmal ventricular tachycardia in infants and children. J Pediatr 86:182, 1975
77. Canent RV Jr, Spach MS, Morris JJ Jr, London WL: Recurrent ventricular tachycardia in an infant—use of high voltage DC shock therapy in management. Pediatrics 33:926, 1964
78. Gelband H, Steeg CN, Bigger JT Jr: Use of massive doses of procainamide in the treatment of ventricular tachycardia in infancy. Pediatrics 48:110, 1971

Atrioventricular Block

79. Griffin JH: Neonatal hypocalcemia and complete heart block. Am J Dis Child 110:672, 1965
80. Michaëlsson M, Engle MA: Congenital complete heart block: An international study of the natural history. Cardiovasc Clin 4:85, 1972
81. Crittenden IH, Latta H, Ticinovich DA: Familial congenital heart block. Am J Dis Child 108:104, 1964
82. McCue CM, Mantakas ME, Tingelstad JB, Ruddy S: Congenital heart block in newborns of mothers with connective tissue disease. Circulation 56:82, 1977
83. Anderson RH, Wenick ACG, Losekoot TG, Becker AE: Congenitally complete heart block. Developmental aspects. Circulation 56:90, 1977
84. Lev M: The pathology of complete atrioventricular block. Prog Cardiovasc Dis 6:317, 1964
85. James TN: Cardiac conduction system: Fetal and postnatal development. Am J Cardiol 25:213, 1970
86. Carter JB, Blieden LC, Edwards JE: Congenital heart block. Anatomic correlations and review of the literature. Arch Pathol 97:51, 1974
87. Hofschire PJ, Nicoloff DM, Moller JH: Postoperative complete heart block in 64 children. Treated with and without cardiac pacing. Am J Cardiol 39:559, 1977

5 Radiology

Each of the major noninvasive diagnostic techniques provides unique information about the cardiovascular system. Thoracic roentgenography yields three important types of diagnostic information:

1. Pulmonary vascularity. Thoracic roentgenography is the only noninvasive diagnostic method that can assess the pulmonary vasculature. Knowledge of the status of the pulmonary vasculature is one of the two major pieces of clinical information used in this book to develop a classification of congenital cardiac malformations and serves as an initial and major clue to quickly focus on the differential diagnosis.
2. Cardiac and specific chamber size. Although overall cardiac size can be assessed on physical examination by location of the cardiac apex, the thoracic roentgenogram more accurately demonstrates cardiac size. It can also provide information about the size of the great vessels. Cardiac chamber enlargement can be evaluated by thoracic roentgenography, echocardiography, and electrocardiography, and each technique has certain limitations.
3. Cardiac contour. Certain cardiac contours are very diagnostic and provide an important clue, but in many infants, the cardiac contour is not diagnostically specific. As in any thoracic roentgenogram, bony and soft tissue structures should be evaluated for unrelated conditions and the occasional instance in which they may provide information relative to the cardiac diagnosis.

Together with history, physical examination, electrocardiography, and echocardiography, thoracic roentgenography is one of the five major initial methods in cardiac diagnosis and in evaluating the status of the patient subsequently.

Meticulous care must be taken to obtain high-quality thoracic roentgenograms. Analysis of films of low quality or those carelessly taken can yield unreliable and misleading information, particularly about the pulmonary vasculature and cardiac contour.

Neonates and infants should be restrained on a board, the arms extended above the head, the head in the midline, and the back flat against the board. The infant should be placed so that the roentgenographic beam passes through the midthorax. Because of the rapid heart and respiratory rates, short time exposures should be used.

In infants, particularly neonates, certain features of the thoracic roentgenogram deserve special mention because they are different from those present in roentgenograms of older children and often reflect transitional changes in the circulation.

Fluoroscopy is rarely indicated in the evaluation of cardiac disease in neonates and infants. The details of the heart and vessels are less clearly seen, and the amount of x-ray exposure is greater than with thoracic roentgenograms.

NORMAL ROENTGENOGRAM

Thymus

In neonates and infants, the borders of the cardiac silhouette are frequently obscured by the thymus, this being particularly true for the supracardiac structures. In this age group, the thymus blends with the cardiac silhouette, forming a cardiothymic contour.

The thymus changes considerably in size and contour during the first week of life. Although there is a great variation in the weight of the thymus at any age, it averages 10 to 15 g at birth, decreases to half this size by 2 weeks of age, and then increases to about 20 to 25 g by 6 months. The thymus is principally a supracardiac structure, but the large venous channels, superior vena cava, innominate and subclavian veins undoubtedly contribute to the enlarged supracardiac shadow.[1] The thymic shadow may have distinctive characteristics (Fig. 5-1). There may be a notch at the junction of the thymus with the cardiac border, which may be prominent enough to yield a sail sign. The thymus may also have a wavy border caused by pressure from the ribs (Fig. 5-2). In infants, the thymus may extend down nearly to the diaphragm and cover both cardiac borders and may suggest right atrial or left ventricular enlargement. It covers both the aorta and the pulmonary artery, making it virtually impossible to evaluate these structures in many infants. On lateral views, the thymus is an anterior and superior structure.

The thymic shadow fluctuates and is widened in a recumbent patient, during expiration, or with increased intraabdominal pressure, but these changes may also be related to variation in patterns of venous return.

With stress, as from severe hypoxemia, the thymus involutes, making evaluation of the cardiac size and contour more reliable. In fact, it has been suggested that if difficulty is encountered in distinguishing the configuration of the heart and thymus, small doses of corticosteroids will shrink the thymus. However, this is rarely necessary. Following relief of the stress, the thymus regrows (Fig. 5-3).

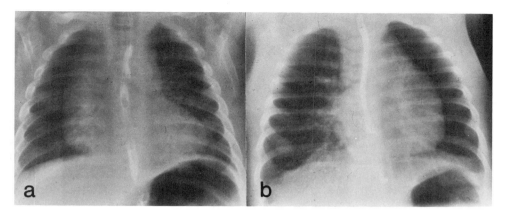

FIG. 5-1. Thoracic roentgenogram, posteroanterior view, in two normal infants. **a.** Prominent right lobe of thymus. **b.** Prominent left lobe of thymus.

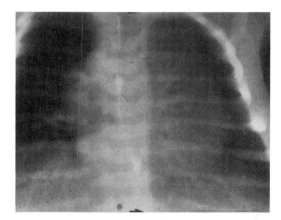

FIG. 5-2. Thoracic roentgenogram, posteroanterior view. Prominent left lobe of thymus, lateral margin of thymus wavy from impression of ribs.

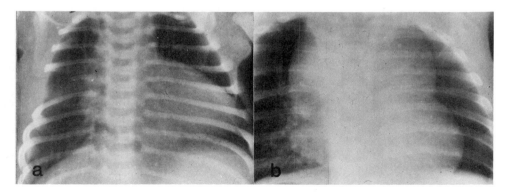

FIG. 5-3. Thoracic roentgenogram, posteroanterior view, of infant with single ventricle, transposition of great vessels, and pulmonary stenosis. **a.** Aged 3 months, immediately following Waterston anastomosis for severe hypoxemia. **b.** Aged 9 months when infant showed mild cyanosis. Marked regrowth of thymus.

The thymic shadow is characteristically absent in patients with complete transposition of the great vessels, so that the superior mediastinum is narrow. In our experience, symptomatic infants with tetralogy of Fallot often do not have a visible thymus.

In a study of 1,020 thoracic roentgenograms of newborns, Tausend and Stern[2] found that in half, there was not prominence of either lobe of the thymus. There was unilateral prominence in another one third of the patients, much more frequently on the right. In the remaining newborns, there was bilateral prominence, but to a greater degree on the right. They found no patients in whom the trachea was compressed or displaced by the thymus.

Heart

In the neonate, the cardiac shadow appears broad, primarily because the heart is anatomically more transverse and the thoracic cage is relatively short. During infancy, the heart becomes more vertical. The heart in the neonate is also more globular, and with age, its borders become more distinct.[3]

The heart, particularly the right side, is not as well defined as in older patients.[4] Following birth, the right cardiac border is large because of the right atrial prominence at this age. The left cardiac border shows left ventricular convexity, but a distinct pulmonary artery and aorta may not be able to be differentiated, perhaps because of the thymus.

A number of factors affect the cardiac size in the neonatal period. Valsalva maneuvers decrease cardiac size and Müller effect increases it, and the phases of respiration also cause changes[5] (Fig. 5-4).

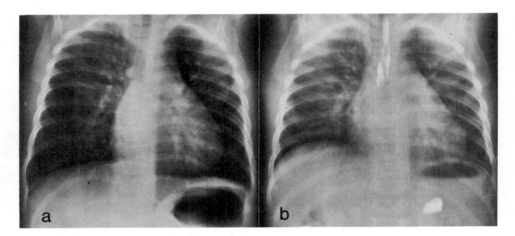

FIG. 5-4.   Effect of depth of respiration upon cardiac size. Posteroanterior views of thoracic roentgenograms of the same patient taken on the same day. **a.** Full inspiration. **b.** Incomplete inspiration. Cardiac size larger in **b.**

The heart decreases in size from 15 minutes to 4 hours of age and then shows further decrease by 24 hours and has a larger volume with delayed clamping of the umbilical cord. The minimum heart volume, as calculated radiographically, is reached at 4 days of age and is reduced 25 percent from the volume at birth.[6]

The cardiothoracic ratio should be less than 0.60 in neonates beyond 24 hours of age and 0.55 in infants.

Lungs

In a study, Nadelhaft and Ellis[4] reviewed thoracic roentgenograms of 1,000 normal neonates in the first 4 days of life. In 95 percent, they found patterns they considered normal: radiolucent lung fields without prominent pulmonary markings, focal areas of increased density, mild generalized increased density, or fine, coarse, or mixed markings. In the other 5 percent, although the lungs appeared abnormal, the patients were asymptomatic. The roentgenographic findings included generalized increased pulmonary markings or densities, either nodular or diffuse, or local areas of increased pulmonary density.

ABNORMAL ROENTGENOGRAM

The thoracic roentgenogram should be assessed for three features: pulmonary vascularity, cardiac or chamber size, and cardiac contour.

Pulmonary Vascularity

Five patterns of pulmonary vascularity can be recognized (Fig. 5-5).

1. Normal pulmonary vascular markings indicate normal blood flow (Fig. 5-5a). The right hilus is evident, but the left hilus is usually hidden behind the pulmonary trunk. The vessels gradually taper toward the periphery of the lungs.
2. Increased pulmonary arterial markings indicate increased pulmonary blood flow (Fig. 5-5b). The hilar markings are enlarged, and enlarged pulmonary markings are present in the middle third of the lungs.
3. Decreased pulmonary vascular markings reflect decreased volume of pulmonary blood flow (Fig. 5-5c). The lungs appear dark, the hila appear small, and the peripheral vessels appear stringy.
4. Increased pulmonary venous markings indicate obstruction to pulmonary venous flow (Fig. 5-5d). The hila may be prominent and hazy. There is a relative increase in the upper lobe markings. The lung fields are diffuse and hazy, and there may be Kerley's B lines.
5. Bronchial arterial patterns occur in cyanotic patients, with obstruction to pulmonary blood flow, and the pulmonary arteries are supplied through bronchial collaterals. Distinct hilar vessels are not present, but enlarged vessels may be observed at other sites.

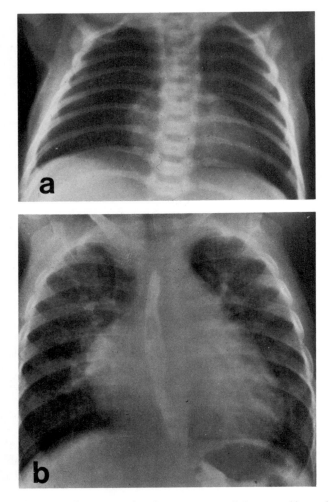

FIG. 5-5. Patterns of pulmonary vasculature. **a.** Normal pulmonary arterial. **b.** Increased

In neonates and infants, pulmonary parenchymal disorders may complicate cardiac disease. The lung fields must be carefully reviewed to identify pulmonary abnormalities. Pneumonia occurs more commonly in infants with cardiac conditions associated with increased pulmonary blood flow than in infants without cardiac disease, but the reason is unknown. Lobar abnormalities, such as atelectasis, emphysema, or pneumonia, also occur among patients with congenital cardiac malformations because of compression of the bronchi (Fig. 5-6).

Primary pulmonary disorders in neonates lead to symptoms that mimic

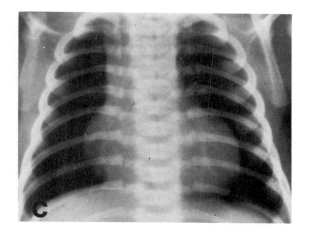

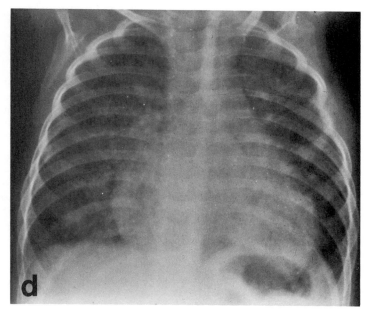

FIG. 5-5 (*cont.*).   c. Decreased pulmonary arterial. **d.** Increased pulmonary venous.

cardiac disease, particularly cardiac conditions that cause pulmonary venous obstruction. Respiratory distress syndrome causes the greatest confusion, since these neonates have tachypnea, tachycardia, cyanosis, and hepatomegaly at times, and often increased cardiac size. The lung fields show stippling and, frequently, air bronchograms. The latter feature should serve to distinguish respiratory distress syndrome from pulmonary venous obstruction, but the roent-

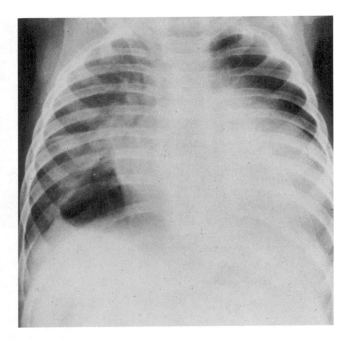

FIG. 5-6. Thoracic roentgenogram, posteroanterior view, of anomalous left coronary artery in 3-month-old infant. Massive cardiomegaly. Left lower lobe and right middle lobe atelectasis.

genographic features may be indistinguishable. Although a history of prematurity or maternal diabetes may direct the diagnosis toward respiratory distress syndrome, the features are sufficiently similar that further cardiac studies, such as cardiac catheterization, may be required to exclude a correctable cardiac lesion.

Cardiac Size

Various factors affect the size of the cardiac silhouette. Cardiac size reflects the volume of blood in the heart and not hypertrophy of the myocardium. Any cause, such as an insufficient cardiac valve or left-to-right shunt, that places extra volume of blood in a cardiac chamber leads to cardiac enlargement. Although in almost all instances, enlargement of the cardiac silhouette is caused by cardiac enlargement, pericardial effusion must always be considered. The cardiac contour has been described as "water bottle" shaped, since on an upright film the cardiac shadow above the diaphragm bulges. Distinct contours, such as the pulmonary artery segment, may be missing. If pericardial effusion is suspected, more detailed studies are indicated, such as echocardiography or intravenous CO_2 injection. Fluoroscopy shows poor or absent cardiac contractions, but this is not sufficiently diagnostic to exclude conditions such as myocarditis.

Chamber Size

Although four views of the heart with barium swallow are often ordered in the investigation of an infant with cardiac disease, usually the principal information is obtained from the posteroanterior and lateral projections. The left atrium is the cardiac chamber that is best assessed by the thoracic roentgenogram. Left atrial enlargement causes posterior displacement of the barium-filled esophagus (Fig. 5-7). The finding of left atrial enlargement is very important in the differential diagnosis and ongoing evaluation of many patients with cardiac malformations because it provides important anatomic and hemodynamic information. The other three cardiac chambers are much less easily evaluated, particularly in infants, because the heart is more transverse and may be distorted by the cardiac malformation. On roentgenogram, it is impossible to separate left from right ventricular enlargement because even in oblique views, only the borders of the ventricle are evaluated. The electrocardiogram gives a better indication of right atrial, right ventricular, and left ventricular enlargement.

The posteroanterior view also allows assessment of the size of the aorta and pulmonary artery, although in young infants these may be obscured by the thymus. Aortic enlargement is seen best on posteroanterior view of the thorax and also on the left anterior oblique views as a prominent bulge along the upper right cardiac border. Pulmonary arterial enlargement is seen as a prominence of this segment along the left cardiac border. Its enlargement can occur from increased pulmonary arterial pressure, increased pulmonary blood flow, or poststenotic dilatation from valvular pulmonary stenosis.

In the AP view, the presence of a right aortic arch should be looked for (Fig. 5-8). The lateral view provides (1) information about left atrial enlargement, (2) information about possible vascular ring—because of displacement of the esophagus from behind, (3) evaluation of pulmonary parenchyma, and (4) information about pectus excavatum (lateral view of sternum), which may compress the heart, causing an increased transverse diameter of the heart that might be falsely interpreted as cardiomegaly.

Cardiac Contour

There are several cardiac contours that are diagnostic and are present in many infants with that particular cardiac condition:

1. Complete transposition of the great vessels—egg-shaped heart, egg on its side, or apple on a string, indicating a round-shaped heart and a narrow mediastinum (Fig. 5-9a).
2. Tetralogy of Fallot—boot-shaped heart. The cardiac size is normal, cardiac

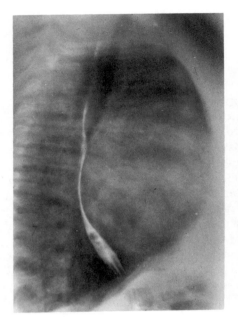

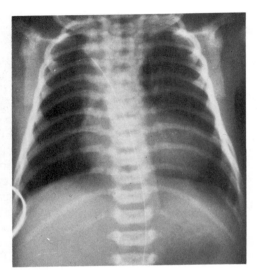

FIG. 5-7. Thoracic roentgenogram, lateral view with barium swallow. Posterior displacement of esophagus indicates left atrial enlargement.

FIG. 5-8. Thoracic roentgenogram, anteroposterior view. Umbilical arterial catheter in right aortic arch of neonate with tetralogy of Fallot.

apex is tilted upward, pulmonary arterial segment is concave, and aorta is prominent (Fig. 5-9b).

3. Total anomalous pulmonary venous connection to a left superior vena cava—snowman or figure-of-eight heart (Fig. 5-9c). The supracardiac portion of the cardiac silhouette is prominent because of the enlarged venous structures. This contributes to the upper portion and the heart to the lower portion of the snowman.

4. Congenitally corrected transposition—the left cardiac border is smooth and shows no distinct pulmonary arterial segment since the left cardiac border is composed only of the aorta and the ventricle (Fig. 5-9d).

5. Conditions associated with a hypoplastic right ventricle—show absence of the pulmonary arterial segment and a broad prominent left cardiac border (Fig. 5-9e).

6. Cardiomyopathy or left-sided obstructive lesion—show cardiomegaly and a left ventricular contour with the cardiac apex displaced laterally and downward (Fig. 5-9f).

7. Ebstein's malformation of tricuspid valve—greatly enlarged heart and decreased pulmonary vascular markings (Fig. 5-9g).

8. Endocardial cushion defect—shows cardiomegaly out of proportion to in-

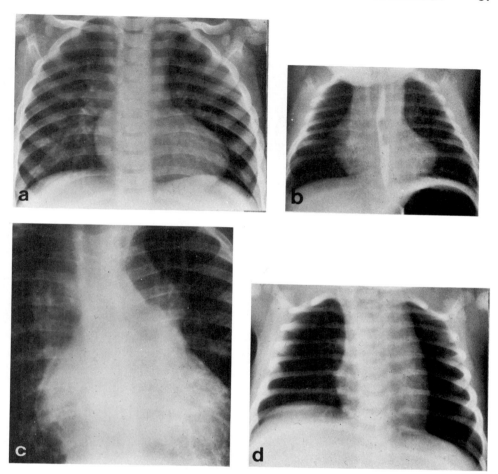

FIG. 5-9.   Thoracic roentgenograms of specific contours, posteroanterior view. **a.** Complete transposition of great vessels. Egg-on-side contour. Concave pulmonary arterial segment. Increased pulmonary vasculature. **b.** Tetralogy of Fallot. Normal size, upturned apex. Concave pulmonary arterial segment. Right aortic arch. **c.** Total anomalous pulmonary venous connection to left superior vena cava. Snowman or figure-of-eight heart. **d.** Congenitally corrected transposition of great vessels. Coexistent ventricular septal defect and pulmonary stenosis. Normal sized heart. Diminished pulmonary arterial markings. Left cardiac contour smooth and shows no distinct pulmonary arterial segment.

     crease in pulmonary arterial markings (Fig. 5-9h).

  9. Pericardial effusion—shows an enlarged cardiac silhouette without recognizable cardiac contours (Fig. 5-9i).

10. Aortic atresia—this condition is the leading cause of cardiomegaly in the first week of life. Pulmonary vasculature shows a mixture of increased pulmonary arterial and venous markings (Fig. 5-9j).

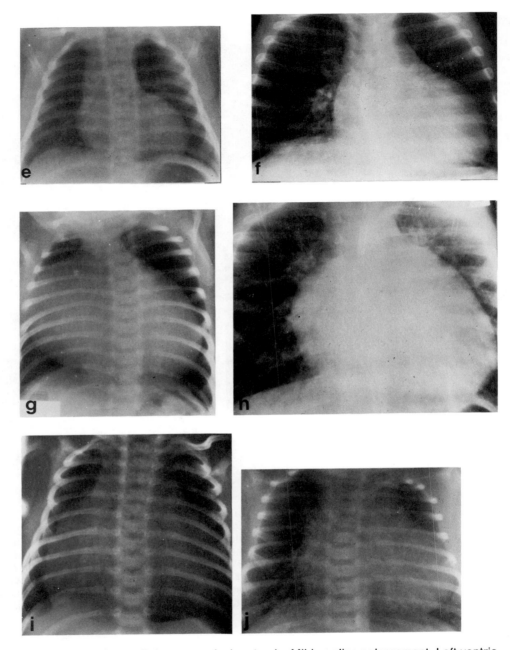

Fig. 5-9. (cont.).   e. Pulmonary valvular atresia. Mild cardiac enlargement. Left ventricular contour. Decreased pulmonary arterial vasculature. **f.** Endocardial fibroelastosis. Massive cardiomegaly. Normal pulmonary vascular markings. Left ventricular contour. **g.** Ebstein's malformation of tricuspid valve. Massive cardiomegaly. Prominent right cardiac border. Diminished pulmonary vasculature. **h.** Endocardial cushion defect. Massive cardiomegaly out of proportion to increased pulmonary arterial markings. **i.** Pericardial effusion. Massive cardiomegaly. Water-bottle contour. **j.** Aortic atresia. Massive cardiomegaly. Mixed pulmonary arterial and venous markings.

In three conditions—vascular ring, origin of left pulmonary artery from right pulmonary artery (vascular sling), and malposition of the heart—thoracic roentgenograms provide major and important diagnostic clues.

VASCULAR RING

Normally, no blood vessel passes behind the esophagus. When on lateral view of a barium swallow, the esophagus in the upper thoracic area is displaced anteriorly by a circumscribed round structure, a vascular ring should be suspected.

Anatomy

Vascular abnormalities of the aortic arch and its branches have various forms. Using a scheme of an embryologic double aortic arch, Stewart and colleagues[7] have explained the various anomalies on the basis of abnormal regression or persistence of fetal vascular structures.

The four most commonly occurring anomalies in which a vascular structure passes retroesophageally are (1) double aortic arch, (2) right aortic arch with aberrant left subclavian artery and left ligamentum arteriosus, (3) right aortic arch with mirror image branching and left ligamentum arteriosus, and (4) left aortic arch and aberrant right subclavian artery. In the first three, a true vascular ring is present in that the trachea and esophagus are surrounded by vascular structures. In the fourth, the ring is incomplete, except in the rare instance in which the right-sided ductus is present. Congenital cardiac anomalies may coexist with each of these vascular anomalies.[8]

Clinical Features

Symptoms can occur and are related to tracheal and esophageal compression. Usually, respiratory symptoms predominate.[9, 10] Dysphagia may occasionally be present, particularly with solid foods. Many infants are, however, slow feeders because of dyspnea. Stridor, hoarseness, wheezing, episodes of choking, coughing, and cyanosis may be present. Parents complain that their child has noisy breathing and a barky cough.

Physical examination may reveal no abnormalities or may reveal rhonchi and intercostal retractions. Noisy respirations may improve by extending the neck. The age of onset and severity of symptoms vary. Most patients with double aortic arch are symptomatic, while most patients with retroesophageal subclavian artery, particularly the right, are asymptomatic.

Thoracic Roentgenogram

A simple thoracic roentgenogram without barium swallow does not show the vascular ring, but a right aortic arch may be recognized on the view. Posteroanterior and lateral views of a barium swallow are helpful in identifying the presence of a vascular ring and giving information about its anatomic form.

In a double aortic arch, an indentation is found on each side of the esophagus in the PA view as well as the one present posteriorly (Fig. 5-10). Right aortic arch with mirror image branching and left ligamentous ductus yields a similar pattern.

In patients with right aortic arch and aberrant left subclavian artery, the right aortic arch is seen, and the indentation of the esophagus is angulated upward toward the left shoulder. The opposite picture is found with left aortic arch and aberrant right subclavian artery.

Bronchoscopy is not indicated in these patients and carries greater risk than in a child without a vascular anomaly. In symptomatic patients, we have usually carried out aortography before operation to identify the aortic arch and major brachiocephalic vessels. Aortography may not clearly identify all the relationships and does not negate the necessity of careful dissection and identification of vascular structures at the time of operation.

Treatment

Only symptomatic patients with vascular ring should be surgically treated. Most patients with double aortic arch require operation. Only an occasional patient with right aortic arch and aberrant left subclavian artery and, rarely, a patient with left aortic arch and aberrant right subclavian artery require surgery. Operation is carried out through a left thoracotomy.[9, 10] In double aortic arch, the left arch is usually smaller and is divided at the time of operation. In patients with right aortic arch and aberrant left subclavian artery, the left

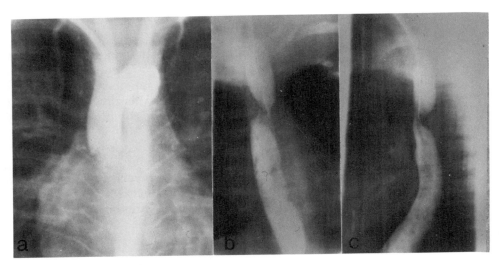

FIG. 5-10.   Double left aortic arch. **a.** Aortogram, anteroposterior view. Barium swallow. **b.** Anteroposterior view. **c.** Lateral view. Shows indentation on both lateral sides and posteriorly.

ductus arteriosus is divided, and the area about the trachea and esophagus is dissected free. It is unnecessary to relocate the subclavian on the aortic arch.

During and following operation, the area of the narrowed trachea must not be traumatized as from an endotracheal tube. The respiratory symptoms of stridor, hoarseness, or noisy breathing gradually improve in a month or so.

PULMONARY ARTERIAL SLING

Pulmonary arterial sling has been the subject of three recent reviews.[11-13] In this condition, the left pulmonary artery arises from the right pulmonary artery and passes over the right main stem bronchus and then between the trachea and esophagus on its course to the left hilus. The left pulmonary artery compresses the trachea or right main stem bronchus and causes respiratory symptoms. Other abnormalities of the tracheobronchial tree may coexist, and, in our experience, a bronchus suis has been present. A variety of congenital cardiac anomalies may coexist.

The symptoms of respiratory obstruction—stridor and wheezing—appear by 1 month of age. Symptoms may be continuously present or caused by or exacerbated by respiratory infections.

Thoracic roentgenograms are diagnostic. On the lateral view, a mass is present between the trachea and esophagus at the level of the carina and represents the left pulmonary artery (Fig. 5-11). This appearance is not found in other conditions or from other types of abnormal blood vessels, such as vascular ring or bronchial collaterals. The anteroposterior view may show hyperaeration of the right lung.

Pulmonary arteriography is not necessary to make the diagnosis, since the roentgenogram is characteristic, and, in fact, the anomaly may be difficult to demonstrate angiographically.

Bronchoscopy and bronchography should be performed to define abnormalities of the tracheobronchial tree so that appropriate care may be given postoperatively.

The mortality either with or without operation is 50 percent. If the condition is diagnosed, operation should be performed to divide the left pulmonary artery from the right pulmonary artery and anastomose it to the pulmonary trunk. The major postoperative complications are respiratory, since the deformed tracheobronchial tree does not return immediately to normal, and symptoms may persist from a few days to months. Postoperatively, in many infants, the left pulmonary artery becomes occluded by scarring or thrombosis at the anastomotic site.

CARDIAC MALPOSITION

The heart may be malpositioned in either the right or left hemithorax. Recognition of the exact form of malposition can give diagnostic information about coexisting cardiac malformations. We will use one classification of cardiac mal-

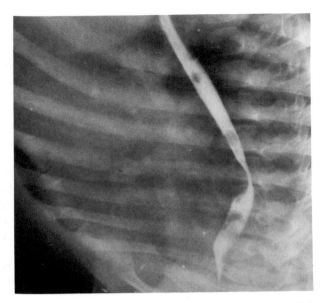

FIG. 5-11. Thoracic roentgenogram, lateral view. Pulmonary arterial sling. Circumscribed round indentation in anterior wall of upper esophagus. Trachea displaced anteriorly.

position which has been clinically helpful and uses terms similar to those used by Lev and associates[14] and by Grant.[15]

In almost all individuals, certain relationships exist between organs, and these are important in understanding cardiac malpositions. The inferior vena cava, major lobe of the liver, and anatomic right atrium lie on one side of the body, while on the opposite side lie the stomach, descending aorta at the diaphragm, and anatomic left atrium. Perhaps of all structures, the inferior vena cava at the level of the diaphragm is most important, for it serves to position the right atrium in relationship to the viscera. Occasionally, these relationships do not exist, and in such cases, as will be discussed subsequently, abnormalities of the spleen are common, and there is frequently abnormal placement of the inferior vena cava.

In situs solitus, the inferior vena cava, major hepatic lobe, and right atrium lie on the right side of the body, while the descending aorta, stomach, and left atrium are on the left side (Fig. 5-12). Other familiar features of situs solitus are a trilobed lung on the right, a bilobed lung on the left, and a spleen on the left. In situs inversus, the relationships are opposite (Fig. 5-12). The major hepatic lobe, inferior vena cava, and anatomic right atrium are on the left side of the body, and the stomach, descending aorta, and anatomic left atrium are on the right. The left lung is trilobed, the right lung is bilobed, and the spleen is on the left. In either situs solitus or situs inversus, the cardiac apex may be in the left hemithorax (levocardia) or right hemithorax (dextrocardia).

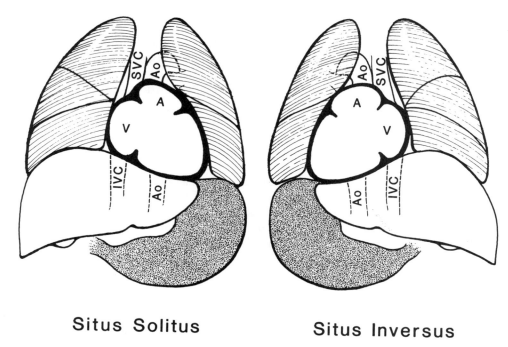

FIG. 5-12.   Diagrams of anatomic relationships in (left) situs solitus and (right) situs inversus. Inferior vena cava (IVC), systemic venous atrium (V), and liver are on one side, while aorta (Ao), pulmonary venous atrium (A), and stomach are on the opposite side. SVC, superior vena cava.

DEXTROCARDIA

Dextrocardia is a general term indicating that the heart is located in the right hemithorax, regardless of the exact anatomic details. There are several anatomic forms of dextrocardia.[14, 16–18]

Situs Inversus Heart

This has also been called "mirror-image dextrocardia." The anatomic relationships of the body are those of situs inversus. The exact incidence of this condition probably lies between 1:5,000 and 1:10,000. A genetic factor is occasionally involved, since it occurs frequently in siblings. In about 15 percent, it may be associated with bronchiectasis and sinusitis (Kartagener's syndrome). The incidence of cardiac anomalies in situs inversus heart is unknown but is overestimated by necropsy studies. The incidence is probably about 3 to 5 percent. If a cardiac anomaly coexists, it is usually complex, including transposition of the great vessels, double outlet right ventricle, or endocardial cushion defect. The ventricles may be either normally related or inverted.[17, 19] This form can usually be recognized by inversion of P and T waves in lead I of the electrocardiogram, and the cardiac silhouette appears the opposite of normal.

Dextroposition of Situs Solitus

We use this term to indicate the situation wherein the heart is located in the right hemithorax because of extrinsic factors, such as hypoplasia of the right lung, agenesis of the right lung, or eventration of the left hemidiaphragm. Although the heart is displaced into the right hemithorax, the cardiac apex points toward the left (Fig. 5-13).

Cardiac anomalies are common and include ventricular septal defect, atrial septal defect, and anomalies of pulmonary venous connection. Pulmonary hypertension frequently coexists because of the hypoplastic pulmonary arterial tree in the right lung.

The thorax is asymmetrical, with the right hemithorax being smaller than the left. This may be observed on physical examination and is accompanied by decreased excursion of the ribs on the right side. The thoracic roentgenogram shows the diminished volume of the right hemithorax and right lung.

Scimitar syndrome[20] is a particular type of dextroposition of the heart. In this syndrome, one or more of the right pulmonary veins enter the inferior vena cava, either immediately above or below the diaphragm. The anomalously coursing right pulmonary veins form a slightly curved shadow in the right lung, similar to a scimitar (a Turkish sword) (Fig. 5-14). Scimitar syndrome is associated with a variable degree of hypoplasia of the right lung, leading to dextro-

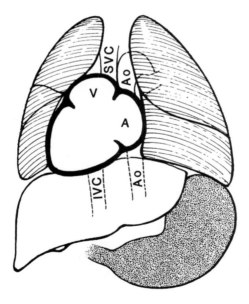

Dextroposition

FIG. 5-13.   Diagram of anatomic relationship of dextroposition of situs solitus heart displaced into right hemithorax because of hypoplastic right lung. A, pulmonary venous atrium; Ao, aorta; IVC, inferior vena cava; SVC superior vena cava; V, systemic venous atrium.

position of the heart. There may be anomalous arterial blood supply from the descending aorta. Cardiac anomalies, such as ventricular septal defect, patent ductus arteriosus, and tetralogy of Fallot, are common.

Dextroversion of the Heart

In dextroversion of the heart, situs solitus is present and atrial relationships are normal, but the cardiac apex is directed toward the right (Figs. 5-15 and 5-16). Dextroversion of the heart may be associated with inverted ventricles, noninverted ventricles, or a single ventricle.

INVERTED VENTRICLES.   In over half of the infants with dextroversion, the ventricles are inverted.[17, 19] The right atrium, receiving the vena cava, empties across a mitral valve into a morphologic left ventricle, while the left atrium empties into morphologic right ventricles across the tricuspid valve. The morphologic right ventricle has an infundibulum from which the aorta arises, while posteriorly the pulmonary trunk arises from the left ventricle. Thus, the relationship of the ventricles and great vessels is like that of congenitally corrected transposition of the great vessels. With inverted ventricles, ventricular septal defect, pulmonary stenosis, AV valve insufficiency, or double outlet right ventricle may coexist.

This malposition can be suspected by the findings present in infants with congenitally corrected transposition of the great vessels: loud single second heart sound and abnormality of initial depolarization of the QRS complex, so that the leads over the right chest show a q wave and initial R wave in left precordial leads. The P waves are normally upright in lead I.

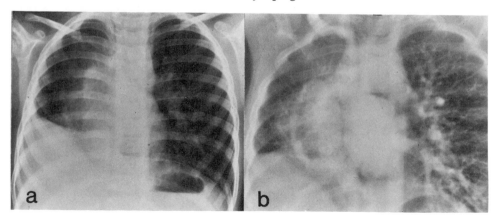

FIG. 5-14.   Dextroposition of situs solitus, scimitar syndrome. **a.** Thoracic roentgenogram, posteroanterior view. Cardiac silhouette predominantly in right hemithorax. Right hemidiaphragm elevated. Scimitar shadow in right thorax. **b.** Angiocardiogram, anteroposterior view. Scimitar vein visualized in right lung.

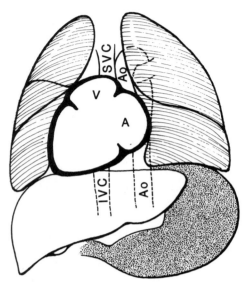

Dextroversion

FIG. 5-15. Diagram of anatomic relationships of dextroversion of situs solitus. A, pulmonary venous atrium; Ao, aorta; IVC, inferior vena cava; SVC, superior vena cava; V, systemic venous atrium.

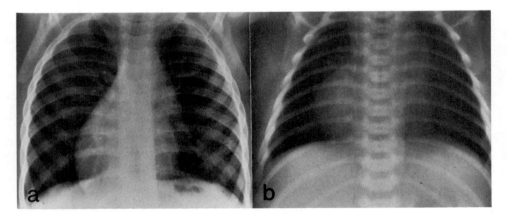

FIG. 5-16. **a** and **b.** Dextroversion of situs solitus. Two infants with corrected transposition of great vessels, ventricular septal defect, and pulmonary stenosis. Cardiac apex directed toward right. Left aortic arch. Pulmonary vasculature diminished.

NONINVERTED VENTRICLES. In the infants with noninverted ventricles, the atria and ventricles are correctly related. The great vessels may be normally related or show a pattern of complete transposition of the great vessels.

One form of dextroversion and noninverted ventricles is associated with a left ventricular diverticulum,[21, 22] which projects through a defect in the ante-

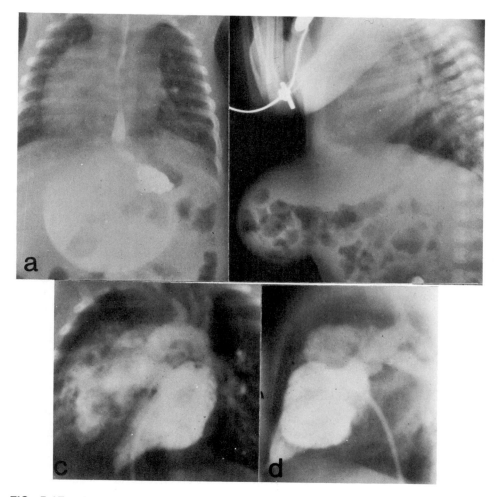

FIG. 5-17. Dextroversion of heart. Situs solitus. Thoracic roentgenogram. **a.** Posteroanterior view. **b.** Lateral view. Cardiac silhouette predominantly in right hemithorax. Pulmonary vasculature accentuated. Large epigastric hernia. Left ventriculogram. **c.** Anteroposterior projection. **d.** Lateral projection. Concordant ventricles. Origin of both great vessels from right ventricle. Diverticulum of left ventricle passing anteriorly and inferiorly.

rior diaphragm (Fig. 5-17). There is a ventral hernia above the umbilicus, and the diverticulum appears as a pulsatile mass in the hernia. The sternum may also be short.

In our opinion, this particular form should not be corrected in infancy. Repair should be delayed until childhood. It is difficult to demark clearly the origin of the diverticulum, and the defect in the upper abdominal wall may be difficult to repair.

SINGLE VENTRICLE. In a few cases of dextroversion, a single ventricle may be found and, as expected, has a high frequency of coexistent transposition of the great vessels. Pulmonary stenosis is common.

LEVOCARDIA

The heart may also be malpositioned in the left chest, but this occurs rarely.

Levoposition

In a rare patient with situs solitus, the left lung may be hypoplastic and the normally positioned heart displaced further into the hemithorax (Fig. 5-18). When levoposition is associated with cardiac anomalies with increased pulmonary blood flow, pulmonary hypertension is present.

Levoversion

Levoversion of the heart can occur in patients with situs inversus, yielding a pattern of left-sided cardiac apex but a body configuration of situs inversus (Fig. 5-18). Almost always, the heart shows inverted venticles and transposition of the great vessels, yielding a pattern of corrected transposition of the great vessels. Coexistent cardiac malformations, as in corrected transposition of the great vessels, are present.

SPLENIC ABNORMALITIES

As indicated previously, there are certain rules of body configuration which indicate that the liver, anatomic right atrium, and inferior vena cava lie on one side of the body, and that the stomach and anatomic left atrium lie on the opposite side. As has been shown, this pattern of visceroatrial concordance holds true whether there is situs inversus or situs solitus and whether the heart is located in the right or left hemithorax.

In a few infants, however, this pattern is not followed. Such infants almost always have abnormalities of the spleen, and it is difficult or impossible to determine visceral situs. As a result, they are considered to have situs ambiguous. The other remarkable feature of patients with situs ambiguous is the tendency for symmetry of organ development, unlike the asymmetrical organ development (e.g., the lungs) found in individuals with situs solitus or situs inversus. Because of the abnormality of the spleen, patients with situs ambiguous are classified according to the splenic abnormality—either asplenia or polysplenia.

Asplenia Syndrome

In patients with asplenia, there is abnormal visceral organ development, with a tendency for symmetrical organ development of normally asymmetrical organs. The lungs, for example, are an important indication of symmetry, since

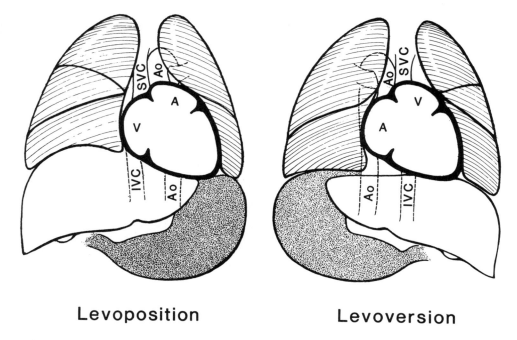

Levoposition   **Levoversion**

FIG. 5-18.   Diagrams of anatomic relationships of (left) levoposition of situs solitus and (right) levoversion of situs inversus. A, pulmonary venous atrium; Ao, aorta; IVC, inferior vena cava; SVC, superior vena cava; V, systemic venous atrium.

the left lung resembles its right-sided counterpart by having three lobes and an epiarterial bronchus.

The liver tends to be symmetrical. The left lobe is enlarged and similar in size to the right lobe. Because of these features of the lungs and liver, the name *bilateral right-sidedness* has been given to the asplenia syndrome.

Abnormalities of mesentric attachment of the bowel are common,[23] and the bowel shows either nonrotation or reverse rotation of the midgut loop. This leads frequently to the entire small intestine's being located on one side of the abdomen and the entire colon on the opposite side, with the cecum and various portions of the ascending colon not being positioned retroperitoneally (Fig. 5-19). Bowel obstruction may occur.

Cardiac anomalies may be present in each portion of the heart. Bilateral superior vena cavae occur in two thirds of the cases. If a single superior vena cava exists, it may be present on either the left or the right side. The inferior vena cava may be present on either the left or right side but almost always lies on the same side of the abdomen as the aorta, as opposed to the normal, where these two major vessels are on opposite sides of the spine[24] (Fig. 5-20). We have not observed this particular feature in any condition other than asplenia.

The atria resemble one another, and, in fact, bilateral sinoatrial nodal tissue has been reported in asplenia.[25] The atrial septum is almost totally absent,

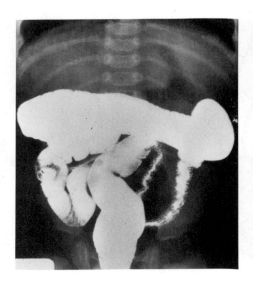

FIG. 5-19. Asplenia syndrome. Barium enema shows malrotation of bowel.

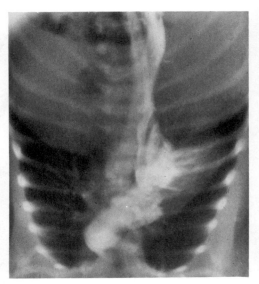

FIG. 5-20. Inferior venacavogram, antero-posterior view, of asplenia syndrome in a 2-week-old infant. Contrast material passes in inferior vena cava to right of spine. Ventricle and aorta opacified. Left aortic arch, but abdominal aorta to right of spine.

and only a thin band of tissue extends from the midportion of the posterior to the anterior atrial walls. The lower part of the atrial defect is continuous, with a defect in the ventricular septum forming a complete atrioventricular canal. This may be associated with a common ventricle. Some variation of an endo-cardial cushion defect is nearly always present.

Transposition of the great vessels and pulmonary stenosis or atresia each occur in about three fourths of the patients.

Total anomalous pulmonary venous connection is frequently present and may connect to any of the usual sites. The frequent association of total anomalous pulmonary venous connection supports the fact that each atria has features of a right atrium. If each atria is developmentally a right atrium, no analagen for the common pulmonary vein is present. Thus, the pulmonary veins are not incorporated into the heart, and embryonic connecting vessels persist.

The infants present with severe cyanosis, but congestive cardiac failure is not a feature.

The asplenia syndrome is suspected from the thoracic roentgenogram. The cardiac apex may be directed toward the right or left, and the pulmonary vascularity is diminished. The liver is symmetrical,[26] and the stomach may be in the midline (Fig. 5-21). The electrocardiogram shows P wave axis direction inferiorly and rightward.[27]

The other clinical and laboratory features reflect the coexistent cardiac condition. The presence of Howell-Jolly bodies on a peripheral blood smear is diagnostic of splenic agenesis, except in the neonatal period, when they may be found in neonates with a normal spleen.

Making a diagnosis of asplenia is extremely helpful, since the coexistent cardiac conditions are so predictable. Ninety percent of the patients die in the first year of life, and even the creation of an aorticopulmonary shunt has not improved longevity. The prognosis is gloomy, since their cardiac anomalies are not correctable, and even with palliative operation, the outlook is bleak. Because of the absence of the spleen and the possible increased incidence of pneumococcal infections, we believe prophylactic penicillin should be given.

Polysplenia

In the polysplenia syndrome, two or more splenic masses are present. This situation is distinct from accessory spleen, in which there is a large, normal-appearing spleen and a small additional spleen. In polysplenia, each lung shows two lobes and hyperarterial bronchi, and, therefore, the term *bilateral left-*

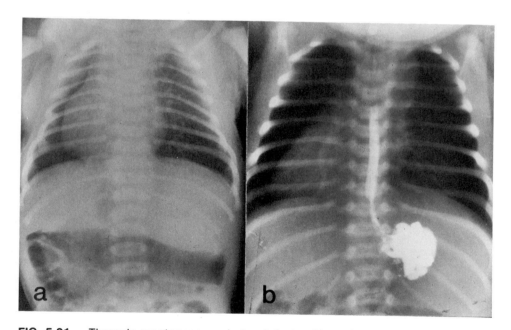

FIG. 5-21. Thoracic roentgenogram in two infants with asplenia syndrome. **a.** Dextrocardia. Characteristic horizontal lower margin of liver. **b.** Dextrocardia. Midline stomach. Horizontal liver. Diminished pulmonary vascular markings.

sidedness has been applied. Symmetry of the liver occurs, but much less frequently than in asplenia. Abnormalities of the gastrointestinal tract, similar to those in asplenia, are always present.

Cardiac anomalies are present and less complicated than in asplenia and are associated usually with increased pulmonary blood flow.

Abnormalities of the superior and inferior vena cavae occur. In half of patients, bilateral superior vena cavae are present. Interruption of the inferior vena cava (infrahepatic absence) with azygos continuation is present in 90 percent of patients. The inferior vena caval blood flows into the azygos system, which connects to the superior vena cava (Fig. 5-22). Connection can occur to either superior vena cava or the coronary sinus.

Anomalous pulmonary venous connection is common. Total anomalous pulmonary venous connection may occur directly to the right atrium. Partial anomalous pulmonary venous connection occurs in half the patients and in a unique form, in which the right pulmonary veins connect directly to the right atrium and the left pulmonary veins directly to the left atrium. Authors[17, 28] have considered this type of anomalous pulmonary venous connection to support the concept that each atrium resembles a left atrium. Defects in the atrial septum, such as ostium primum, ostium secundum, or single atrium, are common.

Supportive evidence of atrial symmetry includes each atrial appendage showing smooth walls and absence of the septum secundum.

Ventricular septal defects can occur and may be associated with origin of both great vessels from the right ventricle. Transposition of the great vessels and pulmonary stenosis rarely occur.

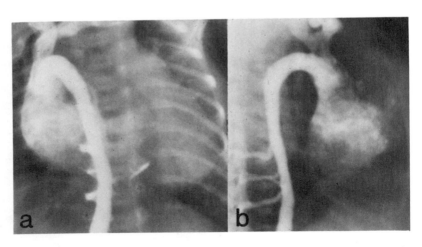

FIG. 5-22.   Inferior venacavogram of 1-month-old infant with polysplenia syndrome. **a.** Anteroposterior view. **b.** Lateral view. Infrahepatic interruption of inferior vena cava with azygous continuation to right superior vena cava.

Patients with polysplenia are acyanotic or show minimal cyanosis. Congestive cardiac failure may develop because of the increased pulmonary blood flow or mitral insufficiency present as part of an endocardial cushion defect. The physical findings are those of a left-to-right shunt, although the presence of the heart in the right chest should lead one to suspect polysplenia.

The thoracic roentgenogram gives important clues. If there is interruption of the inferior vena cava, the azygos vein is large and forms a prominent bulge on the cardiac border. Polysplenia can also be suspected if the relationship and contour of the heart do not fit with the location of the liver and stomach. The electrocardiogram commonly shows leftward (−30° to −60°) P waves.

Recognition of the polysplenic state helps in understanding the associated cardiac conditions. The discovery of an interrupted inferior vena cava is diagnostic of this condition. Howell-Jolly bodies do not occur.

Some authors[17, 29] have indicated that heavily penetrated thoracic roentgenograms will demonstrate the bronchi and show their symmetry, but we have not found this helpful. Occasionally, we have been able to observe symmetry of the pulmonary arteries on lateral views of pulmonary angiograms.

Authors[30, 31] have indicated the value of radioisotopic scanning techniques to demonstrate the abnormal hepatic contour and splenic state, although we believe that the diagnosis of asplenia and polysplenia can be made on the basis of thoracic roentgenogram and observations at angiography.

In approaching a thoracic roentgenogram of a patient with malposition of the heart:

1. Review the thoracic cage and lung fields to determine if there is an extrinsic factor influencing cardiac position.
2. Identify situs by locating the major lobe of the liver and the stomach bubble—these should be on opposite sides of the abdomen. If these two organs are not in this relative position, a splenic anomaly is likely to be present.
3. Determine if dextroversion or levoversion is present by combining evidence of situs and the location of the cardiac apex.

ROENTGEN LOCALIZATION OF CATHETERS

Many neonates with cardiac disease are managed with the assistance of catheters inserted through either the umbilical arteries or the umbilical vein into the aorta or the inferior vena cava, respectively,[32] and these catheters may be used for angiography.[33]

In the lateral projection, arterial catheters follow a course that is initially inferior and caudal and then posterior along the anterior edge of the spine. It lies to the left side of the spine. At times, it is passed into the thoracic aorta. Placement into the ascending aorta may be achieved, but frequently it passes through a patent ductus arteriosus into the pulmonary trunk (Fig. 5-23). Since the ductus arteriosus normally passes inferiorly from the aorta superiorly to the pulmonary artery, the course into the pulmonary artery forms an arch, as it

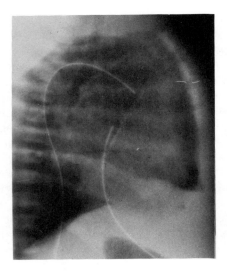

FIG. 5-23. Thoracic roentgenogram, lateral view, of neonate with two catheters in place. Umbilical arterial catheter (arrow) passes through patent ductus arteriosus into pulmonary trunk. Umbilical venous catheter passed into right atrium.

would into the ascending aorta. The course, however, forms a broad arch, rather than the more acute arch of the aorta.

The umbilical venous course on lateral films passes along the anterior abdominal wall and then along the inferior hepatic border through the ductus venosus into the inferior vena cava, which crosses the diaphragm about midway between the anterior and posterior chest wall. The catheter in an AP view is located to the right of the spine. It may be advanced into the heart. If it remains to the right of the spine, it is located in the right atrium. If the tip of the catheter is directed to the left of the spine, it most likely is located in the left atrium or the right ventricle.

If it forms a hook below the diaphragm, it most likely is wedged in the liver, having passed into the inferior vena cava and then back into the hepatic vein.

REFERENCES

Normal Roentgenogram

1. Burnard ED, James LS: The cardiac silhouette in newborn infants: A cinematographic study of the normal range. Pediatrics 27:713, 1961
2. Tausend ME, Stern WZ: Thymic patterns in the newborn. Am J Roentgenol Radium Ther Nucl Med 95:125, 1965
3. Lind J: Heart volume in normal infants. A roentgenological study. Chapter 2. Heart size estimations in infants. Acta Radiol 82[Suppl]:34, 1950
4. Nadelhaft R, Ellis K: Roentgen appearances of the lungs in 1,000 apparently normal full term newborn infants. Am J Roentgenol Radium Ther Nucl Med 78:440, 1957

5. Burnard ED, James LS: Radiographic heart size in apparently healthy newborn infants: Clinical and biochemical correlations. Pediatrics 27:726, 1961
6. Kjellberg SR, Rudhe U, Zetterström R: Heart volume variations in the neonatal period. 1. Normal infants. Acta Radiol 42:173, 1954

Vascular Ring

7. Stewart JR, Kincaid OW, Edwards JE: An Atlas of Vascular Rings and Related Malformations of the Aortic Arch System. Springfield, Ill, Thomas, 1964
8. Edwards JE: Malformations of the aortic arch system manifested as "vascular rings." Lab Invest 2:56, 1953
9. Wychulis AR, Kincaid OW, Weidman WH, Danielson GK: Congenital vascular ring: Surgical considerations and results of operation. Mayo Clin Proc 46:182, 1971
10. Arciniegas E, Hakimi M, Hertzler JH, Farooki ZQ, Green EW: Surgical management of congenital vascular rings. J Thorac Cardiovasc Surg 77:721, 1979

Pulmonary Arterial Sling

11. Grover FL, Norton JB Jr, Webb GE, Trinkle JK: Pulmonary sling. Case report and collective review. J Thorac Cardiovasc Surg 69:295, 1975
12. Sade RM, Rosenthal A, Fellows K, Castaneda AR: Pulmonary artery sling. J Thorac Cardiovasc Surg 69:333, 1975
13. Koopot R, Nikaidoh H, Idriss FS: Surgical management of anomalous left pulmonary artery causing tracheobronchial obstruction. Pulmonary artery sling. J Thorac Cardiovasc Surg 69:239, 1975

Cardiac Malposition

14. Lev M, Liberthson RR, Eckner FAO, Arcilla RA: Pathologic anatomy of dextrocardia and its clinical implications. Circulation 37:979, 1968
15. Grant RP: The syndrome of dextroversion of the heart. Circulation 18:25, 1958
16. Arcilla RA, Gasul BM: Congenital dextrocardia. Clinical, angiocardiographic, and autopsy studies on 50 patients. J Pediatr 58:39, 58:251, 1961
17. Stanger P, Rudolph AM, Edwards JE: Cardiac malpositions. An overview based on study of sixty-five necropsy specimens. Circulation 56:159, 1977
18. Elliott LP, Jue KL, Amplatz K: A roentgen classification of cardiac malpositions. Radiology 1:17, 1966
19. Squarcia U, Ritter DG, Kincaid OW: Dextrocardia: Angiocardiographic study and classification. Am J Cardiol 32:965, 1973
20. Neill CA, Ferencz C, Sabiston DC, Sheldon H: The familial occurrence of hypoplastic right lung with systemic arterial supply and venous drainage: "scimitar syndrome." Johns Hopkins Med J 107:1, 1960
21. Edgett JW Jr, Nelson WP, Hall RJ, Fishback ME, Jahnke EJ: Diverticulum of the heart. Part of the syndrome of congenital cardiac and midline thoracic and abdominal defects. Am J Cardiol 24:580, 1969
22. Symbas PN, Ware RE: A syndrome of defects of the thoracoabdominal wall, diaphragm, pericardium, and heart. One-stage surgical repair and analysis of the syndrome. J Thorac Cardiovasc Surg 65:914, 1973
23. Moller JH, Amplatz K, Wolfson J: Malrotation of the bowel in patients with congenital heart disease associated with splenic anomalies. Radiology 99:393, 1971
24. Elliott LP, Cramer GG, Amplatz K: The anomalous relationship of the inferior vena cava and abdominal aorta as a specific angiocardiographic sign of asplenia. Radiology 87:859, 1966

25. Van Mierop LHS, Patterson PR, Reynolds RW: Two cases of congenital asplenia with isomersion of the cardiac atria and the sinoatrial nodes. Am J Cardiol 13:407, 1964

26. Lucas RV Jr, Neufeld HN, Lester RG, Edwards JE: The symmetrical liver as a roentgen sign of asplenia. Circulation 25:973, 1962

27. Blieden LC, Moller JH: Analysis of the P wave in congenital cardiac malformations associated with splenic anomalies. Am Heart J 85:439, 1973

28. Van Mierop LHS, Gessner I, Schiebler GL: Asplenia and polysplenia syndromes. Birth Defects 8:74, 1972

29. Van Mierop LHS, Eisen S, Schiebler GL: The radiographic appearance of the tracheobronchial tree as an indicator of visceral situs. Am J Cardiol 26:432, 1970

30. Freedom RM, Treves S: Splenic scintigraphy and radionuclide venography in the heterotaxy syndrome. Radiology 107:381, 1973

31. Shah KD, Neill CA, Wagner HN Jr, Taussig HB: Radioisotope scanning of the liver and spleen in dextrocardia and in situs inversus with levocardia. Circulation 29:231, 1964

Roentgen Localization of Catheters

32. Baker DH, Berdon WE, James LS: Proper localization of umbilical arterial and venous catheters by lateral roentgenograms. Pediatrics 43:34, 1969

33. Emmanouilides GC, Hoy RC: Transumbilical aortography and selective arteriography in newborn infants. Pediatrics 39:337, 1967

6

Other Diagnostic Studies

Although there are a variety of diagnostic studies that might be used to assist in the diagnosis and management of cardiac problems and their complications in neonates and infants, in this chapter three major diagnostic studies are presented: echocardiography, radioisotopic techniques, and measurement of hemoglobin and hematocrit.

ECHOCARDIOGRAPHY

ROLE OF ECHOCARDIOGRAPHY

Echocardiography has become increasingly useful in the diagnosis of congenital cardiac anomalies.[1-5] Though it is doubtful that diagnostic ultrasound will completely replace cardiac catheterization, application of this technique to infants and children with suspected cardiac disease may obviate the need for cardiac catheterization in certain instances and can reduce the need for frequent serial catheterizations in others. At the very least, the clinician is armed with more information about the structure and function of the heart before cardiac catheterization.

The biologic safety of pulsed ultrasound has not been fully determined, but it is unlikely that the amount of acoustical energy used in the standard echocardiographic study causes tissue damage.[6, 7] The procedure is noninvasive, and application of the physical principle of acoustical impedance yields information not readily obtainable by other means. For example, blood and cardiac valves cannot be differentiated radiographically because of their similar x-ray density, but they can be differentiated by ultrasound. These and other advantages account for the increasing popularity of echocardiography in recent years.

There are, however, disadvantages of echocardiography. In contrast to the electrocardiogram, a high-quality echocardiogram is relatively difficult to obtain and requires the time-consuming attention of an experienced technician or physician. Furthermore, standardization of technique is inherently difficult. Despite these drawbacks, the echocardiogram parallels the electrocardiogram and thoracic roentgenogram in providing information to the clinician managing an infant with cardiac disease.

PHYSICAL PRINCIPLES

Echocardiographic instruments both transmit and receive ultrasonic energy through ultrasound transducers made of ceramic material which change dimension when voltage is applied (piezoelectric effect). Each second, a thousand or more pulses of electrical energy are converted by the transducer to sound-producing vibrations. Sound waves are propagated during only 0.1 percent of the cycle. The remaining 99.9 percent of the time, the transducer receives or listens for reflected echoes of ultrasound. The energy from the returning sound waves distorts the transducer crystal, and this is converted into an electrical signal which is displayed on an oscilloscope. The magnitude of the signal recorded is directly proportional to the intensity of the echo.

The velocity of sound depends upon the medium through which it passes. Through cardiac tissue, sound travels at approximately 1,540 m/sec. By knowing the time elapsed from emission of sound until the reflected sound returns, the distance penetrated by the reflected sound waves can be calculated. This information can be used to determine intracardiac dimensions.

By the use of acoustical impedance, various structures of the heart can be identified and differentiated. When sound waves strike an interface between tissues of different density, some waves are reflected from this surface. Other sound waves pass through the new medium until they strike a deeper interface of two tissues, again causing some reflection. Since the angle of reflection equals the angle of incidence, only those ultrasound waves which strike an interface in nearly perpendicular fashion are received by the small transducer head.

Resolution of the ultrasound image is a function of the wavelength, and this is inversely proportional to frequency of the sound. Frequencies used in diagnostic ultrasound range between 2.25 MHz (million cycles per second) and 7.50 MHz. High-frequency transducer crystals allow greater resolution but less penetrability. Thus, whereas 5.0 and 7.5 MHz transducers are most suitable for echocardiographic studies in infants, echocardiograms in adults are usually performed with 2.25 MHz transducers.

TECHNIQUE

We will not describe the operation of the controls of various echocardiographic devices or describe optimal transducer position and angulation for detection of various cardiac structures. The interested reader is referred to echocardiography texts[8-11] for more complete discussions of methods. However, the general approach to ultrasound study of the infant is pertinent to this discussion.

The usual practice of obtaining the echocardiogram in the noninvasive diagnostic laboratory is not always feasible when evaluating critically ill infants. It is frequently necessary to perform this study using portable apparatus in the intensive care unit or on the ward. Adequate space for the echocardiographic device and technician, usually to the right of the incubator or radiant warmer, is a prerequisite for a satisfactory study. The operator should assume a comfortable sitting position with the transducer held lightly on the infant's chest (Fig. 6-1).

The echocardiogram consists of images obtained from a reflected surface perpendicular to the plane of the ultrasound beam. Several modes of display are possible, but the most useful (M-mode echocardiography) records dots on photosensitive paper moving perpendicular to the dots.

A complete echocardiographic study of a normal infant consists of a single-dimension image of each cardiac valve, both ventricles, the left atrium, both great vessels, the intraventricular septum, anterior and posterior walls of the heart, and the pericardium. To obtain a complete study, it is necessary to direct the ultrasound beam at various angles through the heart so that the desired structures are transected. Usually, the echocardiographer begins by placing the

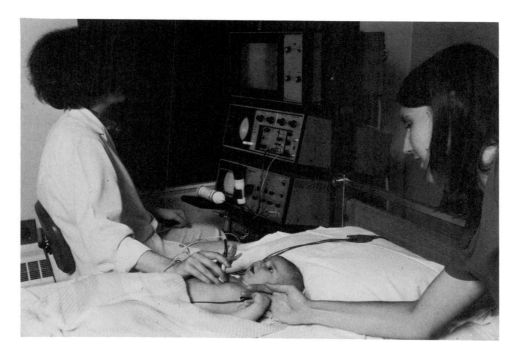

FIG. 6-1.   Recording of echocardiogram in an infant.

transducer nearly perpendicular to the fourth left intercostal space along the left sternal border and directs the ultrasound beam through the anterior leaflet of the mitral valve. The mitral valve can be easily identified on the oscilloscope. By slowly angulating the transducer cephalad and slightly to the right (medially), a sweep can be recorded from the anterior leaflet of the mitral valve to the posterior wall of the aorta (Figs. 6-2 and 6-3). On this sweep, the interventricular septum is found in continuity with the anterior wall of the aorta. The pulmonary artery is visualized by placing the transducer in the second or third left intercostal space and angulating it to the left (laterally). Similar minor variations in transducer position allow imaging of other intracardiac structures.

Movement of the infant hampers the study, and offering a pacifier or bottle may be helpful. Echocardiographic examination of the infant is facilitated by the relative lack of ossification of the thorax, thus the echo window is larger than in the older child or adult.

EVALUATION

As with data obtained from cardiac catheterization, analysis of the infant echocardiogram is best approached from two perspectives: anatomic and functional. The former involves scrutiny of the record for structural relationships and dimensions, whereas the functional perspective assesses hemodynamics, such as presence of a shunt, pulmonary vascular resistance, or ventricular performance.

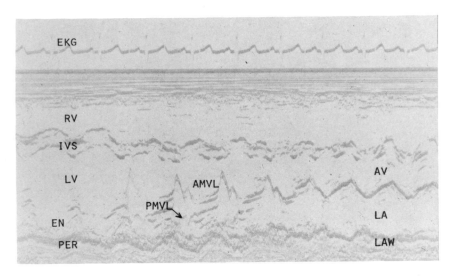

FIG. 6-2. Echocardiographic tracing recorded as transducer sweeps from left ventricle (LV) to aorta, visualizing aortic valve (AV). EKG, electrocardiogram; RV, right ventricular cavity; IVS, interventricular septum; EN, endocardium; PER, pericardium; AMVL, anterior mitral valve leaflet; PMVL, posterior mitral valve leaflet; LA, left atrium; LAW, left atrial wall.

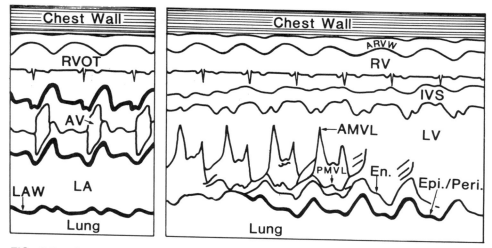

FIG. 6-3. Drawing of an echocardiographic tracing of a newborn. For abbreviations, see Figure 6-2. RVOT, right ventricular outflow tract; Epi, epicardium.

ANATOMIC PERSPECTIVE

Solinger and co-workers[12] have proposed an innovative deductive approach to analysis of the infant with suspected congenital cardiac malformation. Visceral-atrial situs is determined by the chest roentgenogram (Chap. 5). Then, by echocardiography, great vessel and atrioventricular valve relationships are analyzed according to the pathologic nomenclature of Van Praagh.[13] This sophisticated approach maximizes the available information one can obtain from the echogram. The ability to accurately differentiate one valve from another may be difficult, however, and does not necessarily imply an unsatisfactory study. It is nearly always possible to determine the presence and size of each cardiac valve, each great vessel, each ventricle, and the intraventricular septum. Various cardiac structures can be measured and compared to normal values (Tables 6-1, 6-2, and 6-3). This information alone is extremely helpful. Inability to visualize one or more of these structures by ultrasound implies its absence (atresia). In certain circumstances, the echocardiogram is diagnostic of the underlying cardiac condition.

HYPOPLASTIC LEFT HEART SYNDROME

Atresia or severe stenosis of the aortic valve and hypoplasia of the left ventricle produce a characteristic clinical picture of profound shock, inadequate tissue perfusion, weak arterial pulses, and pulmonary edema. Hypoplastic left heart syndrome remains one of the few congenital cardiac lesions for which no palliative or corrective operative procedure exists. Infrequently, cardiac catheterization is needed to make the diagnosis, since a carefully performed echocardiographic study demonstrates very diminutive or absent left ventricle

TABLE 6-1

Selected Echocardiographic Values for Normal Prematures

WEIGHT (GM)	LEFT ATRIAL DIAMETER (CM) RANGE AND MEAN	LEFT VENTRICULAR INTERNAL DIAMETER (CM) RANGE AND MEAN
600–900	0.5–0.7 (0.60)	0.9–1.2 (1.07)
901–1,200	0.5–0.8 (0.65)	0.9–1.3 (1.08)
1,201–1,500	0.5–0.9 (0.69)	1.0–1.3 (1.18)
1,501–1,800	0.6–1.0 (0.79)	1.2–1.5 (1.37)
1,801–2,200	0.7–1.1 (0.88)	1.1–1.6 (1.39)

From Meyer: Pediatric Echocardiography, 1977. Courtesy of Lea & Febiger.

TABLE 6-2

Echocardiographic Values for Normal Newborn Infants

	MEYER AND KAPLAN[14]	SOLINGER ET AL.[3]	HAGAN ET AL.[15]	GODMAN ET AL.[2]
Number studied	50	240	200	50
Weight (kg)	2.3–4.9 (3.2)	2.27–4.54	2.7–4.5 (3.4)	1.9–4.3 (3.2)
Ao (mm)	7–12 (10)	9–14	8–12 (10)	8–11 (10)
LAD (mm)	6–13 (9)	7–14	5–10 (7)	4–10 (6)
LVD (mm)	12–20 (16)	16–24	12–23	12–20 (16)
RVD (mm)	10–17 (13)	11–22	8–19 (14)	10–17 (14)
Septal thickness (mm)	—	2–5	2–4 (3)	—
LVW thickness (mm)	—	2–5	2–4 (3)	—
RVW thickness (mm)	—	1–4	2–5 (3)	—
PA (mm)	—	11–16	9–13 (11)	9–13 (11)

Abbreviations: Ao, aortic root; LAD, left atrial dimension; LVD, left ventricular end-diastolic internal dimension from left septal surface to LV endocardium; RVD, right ventricular dimension measured in diastole from the epicardial to right septal surface; LVW, left ventricular wall thickness, measured in end-diastole; RVW, right ventricular wall thickness, measured in end-diastole; PA, pulmonic root, measured in end-diastole.

and mitral valve.[14, 15] The ascending aorta is narrow, and the aortic valve echoes are absent or abnormal (see Fig. 13-15).

HYPOPLASTIC RIGHT HEART SYNDROME

Pulmonary atresia and tricuspid atresia are often associated with hypoplastic right ventricle, and rarely, isolated hypoplasia of the right ventricle is found.

TABLE 6-3

Normal Echocardiographic Values for Children of Various Ages

	1 WEEK TO 3 MONTHS	4 MONTHS TO 12 MONTHS	1 YEAR TO 2 YEARS
Number of subjects	24	15	23
Weight (kg)	4.80	7.77	10.86
	(1.55)	(1.80)	(2.15)
Height (cm)	57.20	69.98	81.90
	(4.80)	(3.98)	(6.60)
RVD	1.00	1.12	1.12
	(0.19)	(0.18)	(0.22)
LVD	1.86	2.28	2.82
	(0.31)	(0.36)	(0.26)
Ao	1.01	1.21	1.38
	(0.15)	(0.14)	(0.15)
LAD	1.30	1.59	1.82
	(0.27)	(0.33)	(0.30)
Septum	0.36	0.38	0.47
	(0.06)	(0.08)	(0.09)
LVW	0.34	0.38	0.45
	(0.08)	(0.08)	(0.09)
PA	1.20	1.25	1.41
	(0.20)	(0.09)	(0.33)
RVOT	1.04	1.19	1.21
	(0.24)	(0.32)	(0.22)

From Meyer: Pediatric Echocardiography, 1977. Courtesy of Lea & Febiger.
Weight is in kg; all other measurements are in cm. Numbers in parentheses are ± 2 standard deviations from the mean.
Abbreviations: RVD, right ventricular dimension measured in diastole from the epicardial to right septal surface; LVD, left ventricular end-diastolic internal dimension from left septal surface to LV endocardium; Ao, aortic root; LAD, left atrial dimension, both Ao and LAD measured in end-systole; Septum, septal thickness; LVW, left ventricular wall thickness, measured in end-diastole; PA, pulmonic root; and RVOT, right ventricular outflow tract, PA and RVOT measured in end-systole.

In echocardiograms of such patients, the tricuspid valve echo is absent, the anterior wall of the right ventricle is markedly thickened, and the right ventricle is rudimentary (see Figs. 12-9 and 12-15). This pattern is diagnostic of tricuspid atresia. Similarly, failure to record the pulmonary valve in the presence of a very small right ventricle strongly suggests pulmonary atresia. Occasionally, the tricuspid valve, the right ventricle, and the pulmonary valve, though present, are quite diminutive, characteristic of isolated hypoplasia of the right ventricle.[14]

CARDIAC TUMORS

Intracavitary tumors of the heart can be detected by ultrasound. The first reported echocardiographic demonstration of a right ventricular tumor in a neonate was a 1-day-old female with a rhabdomyoma studied at the University of Minnesota.[16] In this neonate, a continuous stream of dense echoes was detected between the anterior right ventricular wall and the ventricular septum. An example of a cardiac tumor is seen in Figure 6-4.

PERICARDIAL EFFUSION

A large cardiac silhouette on a thoracic roentgenogram should suggest the possibility of pericardial effusion.[17] An echo-free space throughout the cardiac cycle between the posterior epicardium and the pericardium is diagnostic of pericardial effusion.[18] An echocardiogram obtained from a 1-year-old child with massive pericardial effusion and tamponade demonstrates an anterior, fluid-filled, echo-free space (Fig. 6–5). Effusions are more frequently recorded when they are large. Serial echograms are often obtained to determine whether reaccumulation has occurred.

OTHER CARDIAC CONDITIONS

Only those cardiac conditions in infancy which can be most readily diagnosed by single plane echocardiography have been discussed. The echocardiogram, though not as diagnostic in other conditions, can be useful. For example, the presence of a ventricular septum differentiates a large ventricular septal defect

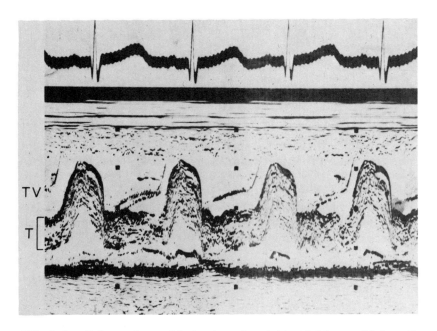

FIG. 6-4.   Echocardiographic tracing of a right atrial tumor (T) in a 2-month-old infant. The tumor, shown by a dense band of echoes, prolapses through the tricuspid valve (TV) during diastole.

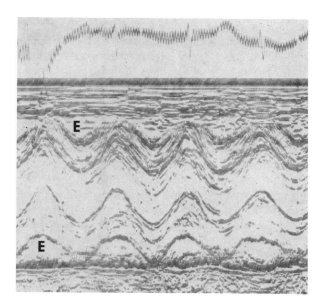

FIG. 6-5.   Pericordial effusion in 1-year-old infant. Echo-free spaces anteriorly and posteriorly (E) indicate pericardial effusion.

from single ventricle.[15] Failure to record echoes from the pulmonary valve and the presence of an overriding aorta suggest pulmonary atresia with a ventricular septal defect, severe tetralogy of Fallot, double-outlet right ventricle, or truncus arteriosus.[19-21] An increased ratio of septal to posterobasal free wall thickening (1.8 to 2.6) is present in idiopathic hypertrophic subaortic stenosis.[22] A very skilled echocardiographer may reliably diagnose transposition of the great vessels by combining knowledge of the transducer position necessary to record the pulmonary valve with systolic time intervals to differentiate one semilunar valve from the other.[12, 23, 24]

One must caution, however, against overreliance on a single diagnostic tool. For instance, the skilled clinician usually knows with a high degree of accuracy whether the patient has transposition of the great vessels before an echo study is performed. If the infant is severely hypoxic and acidotic, the echocardiogram should be bypassed and the diagnosis quickly substantiated by cardiac catheterization and a balloon atrial septostomy should be performed.

FUNCTIONAL PERSPECTIVE

Echocardiography is equally useful as a noninvasive means of studying hemodynamic changes and cardiac performance. In most patients with congenital cardiac malformations, cardiac catheterization is eventually performed, and this establishes the anatomic relationships and confirms the diagnosis. Often, while the anatomic details are unlikely to change, hemodynamics change over a period of time. Periodic echograms can provide reliable information about hemodynamics, particularly the state of the pulmonary vascular bed and ventricular performance. Serial cardiac catheterizations to assess hemodynamics may, therefore, be avoided in some infants.

PULMONARY VASCULAR RESISTANCE

Right ventricular performance and pulmonary vascular resistance can be assessed from simultaneous recording of pulmonary valve motion and of the electrocardiogram. It may be impossible to record adequately the opening and closing of the pulmonary valve, but the posterior cusp motion is often visualized. Echocardiograms of the pulmonary valve in older children and adults characteristically show straightening of the diastolic configuration of the pulmonary cusp echoes, and the "a" wave which is produced by right atrial systole disappears.[25] Hirschfeld and associates[26] correlated pulmonary arterial diastolic pressure, a reflection of pulmonary vascular resistance, with the ratio of right ventricular preejection period (RPEP) to right ventricular ejection time (RVET). Right ventricular preejection period is measured from the q wave of the electrocardiogram to opening of the pulmonary valve, and right ventricular ejection time is the interval between opening and closure of the pulmonary valve. When the ratio of RPEP/RVET is less than 0.3, the pulmonary arterial diastolic pressure is less than 20 mm Hg. A RPEP/RVET ratio between 0.31 and 0.34 indicates borderline pulmonary hypertension, and a ratio greater than 0.34 is strong evidence of increased pulmonary vascular resistance.

VOLUME OVERLOAD OF THE RIGHT VENTRICLE

Cardiac conditions, such as atrial septal defect, tricuspid insufficiency, and pulmonary insufficiency, cause increased right ventricular diastolic volume. Volume overload of the right ventricle, especially when secondary to an atrial septal defect, is associated with paradoxical (anterior) septal motion during systole.[27, 28] This echocardiographic phenomenon is caused by right ventricular dilatation in the absence of significant left ventricular dilatation.[29] In a normal individual, the intraventricular septum moves anteriorly at the end of diastole and moves posteriorly during systole. With a volume-overloaded right ventricle, the interventricular septum is displaced posteriorly, and the superior portion of the septum moves anteriorly (and paradoxically) during systole.[30]

VOLUME OVERLOAD OF THE LEFT VENTRICLE

Any condition which places an increased volume on the left ventricle and/or left atrium can be estimated by measurement of the left ventricular and left atrial internal dimensions.[31] In infancy, cardiac conditions with left-to-right shunts, such as ventricular septal defect or patent ductus arteriosus, are the most common causes of left atrial and left ventricular dilatation. The ratio of left atrial to aortic dimension (LA/Ao) has been used to estimate the volume of left-to-right shunt.[32] An LA/Ao ratio less than 0.9 is normal, whereas a value greater than 1.2 indicates that the left atrium is enlarged. This measurement is of greatest use when measured serially in an individual patient, especially in a premature infant with patent ductus arteriosus whose left atrial dimension rapidly increases as congestive cardiac failure develops.

VENTRICULAR PERFORMANCE

Echocardiographic evaluation of cardiac performance has been succinctly reviewed by Feigenbaum.[33] Considerable progress has been made since Edler's observation[6] that the free wall of the left ventricle moved about 1 cm anteriorly during ventricular systole. Recent investigators have applied diagnostic ultrasound to the study of ventricular function in infants and children.[34, 35] At the present time, there are several useful quantitative techniques for assessing ventricular contractility.

Systolic Time Intervals

Both preejection period (PEP) and ejection time (ET) can be measured for either the left or the right ventricle and are usually combined as a ratio. The ratio is not affected by heart rate, age, or sex but is influenced by preload, afterload, ionotropic state of the myocardium, and intraventricular conduction.[36] Preejection period is measured from the onset of the q wave of the electrocardiogram to the opening of the semilunar valve, and ejection time is measured from the opening to the closure of the semilunar valve. An increased PEP/ET indicates either increased great vessel pressure or congestive cardiac failure. A decrease in PEP/ET indicates that contractility of the heart is enhanced. The normal value of PEP/ET for the left ventricle is 0.35 (range 0.30 to 0.39) and for the right ventricle is 0.24 (range 0.16 to 0.30).[26]

Isovolumetric Contraction Period

The isovolumetric contraction period (IVT), a component of the preejection period, is the interval between atrioventricular valvular closure and semilunar valvular opening. The isovolumetric contraction period is influenced by heart rate, age, stroke volume, and myocardial contractility. A value of isovolumetric contraction greater than 40 msec indicates myocardial disease regardless of the age of the child.

Mean Circumferential Fiber Shortening (V_{cf})

$$\text{Mean } V_{cf} = \frac{\text{LVID}_d - \text{LVID}_s}{\text{LVID}_d \times \text{ET}}$$

$LVID_d$ = left ventricular internal diameter in diastole; $LVID_s$ = left ventricular internal diameter in systole.

The mean circumferential fiber shortening is an index of ejection similar to ejection fraction (EF) and defines basal contractility.[36] In the presence of mitral insufficiency, V_{cf} detects depressed function more readily than ejection fraction, since ejection fraction is falsely elevated because of reduced afterload.[37] Sahn and co-workers[34] have established values for normal newborns (1.51 ± 0.04 circ/sec) and for infants in congestive cardiac failure (1.8 ± 0.06 circ/sec).

Shortening Fraction (SF)

Shortening fraction is the index of contractility easiest to derive and one of the most valid. It is expressed as a percentage of internal diameter shortening and calculated as follows:

$$SF = \frac{LVID_d - LVID_s}{LVID_d} \times 100$$

Left ventricular internal dimension in diastole is measured at the time of the q wave of the electrocardiogram, and left ventricular internal dimension in systole is measured when the ventricular chamber is of minimal size.[38] Shortening fraction is more appealing than ejection fraction because it is a direct measurement and not a value derived from uncertain volume formulae.

These measurements permit an evaluation of ventricular performance, and when combined with the ability of the echogram to determine major anatomic features, they make echocardiography an invaluable diagnostic tool for evaluation of the infant with suspected cardiac disease.

CROSS-SECTIONAL (REAL-TIME) ECHOCARDIOGRAPHY

This chapter has dealt primarily with M-mode echocardiography because of its wide availability and applicability to infants and children with cardiac disease. Recently two-dimensional (real-time) diagnostic ultrasound has emerged as a highly sophisticated diagnostic method for evaluation of cardiac structure and function.

Real-time ultrasound imaging of the heart was developed a decade ago.[39-42] Sahn and co-workers[43] deserve the major credit for successfully applying this technique to infants and children and demonstrating its usefulness. Several real-time ultrasonic techniques have been developed and include multielement linear array systems, mechanical sector scanners, and phased-array systems utilizing electronic steering of the ultrasound beam. The latter method has gained increasing popularity in recent years.

In the phased-array system, a stationary transducer produces an 80° pie-shaped image of the beating heart at a rate of 30 frame/sec. These real-time images are recorded on videotape for playback and review. Single frames may be photographed with a Polaroid camera. Using this technique, cross-sectional views of the heart in its long and short axes can be recorded by placing the transducer in several different positions on the chest: parasternal, apical, and subxiphoid. Great vessel orientation is observed by placing the transducer in the suprasternal notch.

Cross-sectional echocardiography allows more precise determination of spatial relationships within the heart and of great vessel orientation than do single crystal techniques. Therefore, it is particularly useful in infants with congenital heart disease because of the complexity of the anatomy in many such infants. Details about the performance and analysis of real-time, wide-angle, two-dimensional echocardiography are available to the reader in an excellent review by Tajik and associates.[44]

RADIOISOTOPIC TECHNIQUES

Although radioactive tracers have been used for many years in studying the cardiovascular system, development of gamma scintillation cameras and radio-isotopes with short half-lives made this a more applicable technique, which yields a variety of information. Portable cameras have been developed so that radioisotopic studies can now be performed in neonatal nurseries and on the wards. Despite the possibility of studying the heart with a relatively noninvasive method, radioisotopic study of the heart has not been more widely used because:

1. Echocardiography has progressed to the point where it can provide detailed information about the structure of the heart in many neonates or infants with congenital cardiac malformations.
2. The information obtained is often insufficient to reach decisions about operation.
3. In a specific pediatric application, the separation of pulmonary and cardiac causes of cyanosis, the distinction could not be easily resolved.

Despite these limitations, there may be applications of this technique to answer specific clinical questions.

TECHNIQUE

Technetium-99m in a dose of about 200 microcuries/kg is given intravenously, as rapidly as possible and as a bolus. A gamma scintillation camera views the heart and lungs for 25 to 30 sec. Polaroid pictures of the scintillation screen are made at frequent intervals and subsequently viewed. Data are also collected by an on-line computer for both qualitative and quantitative analysis.

In neonates and infants, there are three possible uses of scintillation scanning techniques:

Evaluation of the Cyanotic Neonate

Because of the risk of cardiac catheterization in neonates and the common problem of distinguishing cardiac and pulmonary origins of cyanosis, it was hoped that nuclear angiocardiography could resolve these clinical problems. Unfortunately, in neonates with pulmonary parenchymal disease, such as respiratory distress syndrome, pulmonary vascular resistance may be elevated and associated with right-to-left shunting through a patent foramen ovale or patent ductus arteriosus. Therefore, radioactive material appears rapidly in the left atrium, left ventricle, or aorta, as in some cyanotic forms of cardiac disease.

Several types of congenital cardiac malformations, however, do yield characteristic scintillation scanning pictures:[45-47]

1. *l*-Transposition
2. *d*-Transposition
3. Truncus arteriosus
4. Pulmonary atresia with intact ventricular septum
5. Aortic atresia
6. Total anomalous pulmonary venous connection (infradiaphragmatic type)
7. Ebstein's malformation
8. Position of inferior vena cavae in malpositions of the heart

In most of these situations, more detailed information is needed to make decisions about management.

In cyanotic patients, the amount of right-to-left shunt can be quantitated by comparing the amount of radioactivity within the body to that in the lungs.[48, 49]

Quantitation of Left-to-right Shunt

When analyzing the stored data, a window of radioactivity over an area of interest of the heart or lungs can be selected and a time-activity curve generated from the window. A curve obtained from a section of the right lung can be analyzed for left-to-right shunt. The time-activity recorded resembles curves obtained using Cardio-Green dye during cardiac catheterization. As with Cardio-Green dye curves, if a left-to-right shunt is present, a secondary peak or plateau is recorded after the primary curve and reflects the volume of left-to-right shunt. The time-activity curves can be quantitated for size of the left-to-right shunt.[45, 47, 48] Serial studies may be helpful in estimating changes of pulmonary vascular resistance in patients with large left-to-right shunt.

Evaluation of Operative Results

There are perhaps three uses of scintillation scanning techniques in postoperative evaluation: (1) patients with residual murmur in whom the scan might be used to detect and quantify residual shunt, (2) patients in whom major intracardiac baffling, as in Mustard procedure,[47] conduit (e.g., Fontan), or Rastelli-like procedure, has been performed, and (3) evaluation of extracardiac shunt. A simple method to evaluate patency of an aorticopulmonary shunt or to determine distribution of blood flow through the shunt would be extremely helpful in many situations. Radionuclide scanning is useful in infants whose cardiac anomalies have either pulmonary atresia or severe stenosis, so that the volume of blood passing through the operatively created shunt represents most or all of the pulmonary blood flow. However, in most infants the pulmonary circulation also receives blood directly from the right ventricle. In the latter instance, analysis is complicated, for the appearance of radioactivity in both lungs does not exclude an occluded shunt.

The amount of radioactivity reaching the lung on the side of the operatively created shunt is determined by the size of the shunt, the amount of right-to-left shunt, and the distribution of blood reaching the pulmonary arteries from the ventricle. Because several factors influence the amount of radioactivity, it is difficult to determine the precise status of the pulmonary vasculature and the shunt. The use of preoperative scans and then serial determinations following the placement of the shunt can provide better insight into the meaning of postoperative changes.[49]

HEMOGLOBIN AND HEMATOCRIT

In infants with cardiac disease, hemoglobin and hematocrit values should be measured periodically during the first year of life, particularly if cyanosis is present, because oxygen is carried almost entirely on hemoglobin, and the total amount of oxygen carried at any given level of hemoglobin saturation, or Po_2, varies with the hemoglobin level.

The level of hemoglobin has important effects on infants with congenital cardiac anomalies:

1. In patients with cyanotic congenital cardiac disease and hypoxemia, polycythemia develops and hemoglobin increases. Therefore, the oxygen-carrying capacity increases, but since the hemoglobin is only partially saturated, the total amount of oxygen being transported is often the same as in a noncyanotic patient.
2. In patients with a low hemoglobin value, as from anemia, the total amount of oxygen delivered to tissue is compensated by an increased cardiac output.

Iron deficiency anemia can develop in normal infants because of the limited absorption of iron by the intestine in early infancy, limited dietary intake, and increased demand for iron because of growth. In infants with congenital cardiac disease, intake of iron may be limited because of feeding habits, such as easy fatigability, and the requirement for iron may be accentuated in infants with cyanotic congenital cardiac disease.

A low hemoglobin level can have profound effects. For instance, the development of anemia in an infant with a compensated ventricular septal defect may increase cardiac output sufficiently to lead to congestive cardiac failure. Or, in infants with cyanotic congenital cardiac anomalies, limitation of hemoglobin production can limit oxygen transport and cause hypoxic syndromes.

Therefore, we routinely determine hematocrit, because it reflects the stimulus for erythrocyte production, whereas the hemoglobin value is partially determined by adequate amounts of iron and other substances for hemoglobin formation.

In our experience, many infants with cyanotic congenital cardiac anomalies have iron deficiency even when their hemoglobin value is in the normal range. In such patients, the hematocrit is elevated, so the hemoglobin is low in relation to the hematocrit value. When such patients are treated with iron, the hemoglobin rises to a value appropriate to the hematocrit. We believe that it is not necessary to measure serum iron or erythrocyte count but that decisions can be made solely on hemoglobin and hematocrit values.

REFERENCES

Echocardiography and Functional Perspective

1. Sahn DJ, Allen HD, Goldberg SJ, Solinger R, Meyer RA: Pediatric echocardiography: A review of its clinical utility. J Pediatr 87:335, 1975
2. Godman MJ, Tham P, Kidd BSL: Echocardiography in the evaluation of the cyanotic newborn infant. Br Heart J 36:154, 1974
3. Solinger R, Elbl F, Minhas K: Echocardiography: Its role in the severely ill infant. Pediatrics 57:543, 1976
4. Hagler DJ: The utilization of echocardiography in the differential diagnosis of cyanosis in the neonate. Mayo Clin Proc 51:143, 1976
5. Meyer RA: Echocardiography in congenital heart disease. Cardiovasc Clin 6:226, 1975
6. Edler I, Gustafson A, Karletors T, Christensson B: Ultrasound cardiography. Acta Med Scand 370[Suppl]:67, 1961
7. Ziskin MC: Survey of patient exposure to diagnostic ultrasound. In Reid JM, Sikov MR (eds): Workshop Proceedings of Interactions of Ultrasound and Biologic Tissues. DHEW Publication no. (FDA) 73-8008, Washington, DC, 1972
8. Feigenbaum H: Echocardiography, 2nd ed. Philadelphia, Lea & Febiger, 1976
9. Gramiak R, Waag RC: Cardiac Ultrasound. St. Louis, Mosby, 1975
10. Goldberg SJ, Allen HD, Sahn DJ: Pediatric and Adolescent Echocardiography. Chicago, Year Book, 1975
11. Meyer RA: Pediatric Echocardiography. Philadelphia, Lea & Febiger, 1977
12. Solinger R, Elbl F, Minhas K: Deductive echocardiographic analysis in infants with congenital heart disease. Circulation 50:1072, 1974
13. Van Praagh R: Malposition of the heart. In Moss AJ, Adams FH (eds): Heart Disease in Infants, Children and Adolescents. Baltimore, Williams & Wilkins, 1968, pp 602–636
14. Meyer RA, Kaplan S: Echocardiography in the diagnosis of hypoplasia of the left or right ventricles in the neonate. Circulation 46:55, 1972
15. Hagan AD, Deely WJ, Sahn D, Friedman WF: Echocardiographic criteria for normal newborn infants. Circulation 48:1221, 1973
16. Allen HD, Blieden LC, Stone FM, Bessinger FB Jr, Lucas RV Jr: Echocardio-

graphic demonstration of a right ventricular tumor in a neonate. J Pediatr 84:854, 1974

17. Pieroni DR, Park SC, Holbrook PR, Houghton PB: Echocardiographic diagnosis of septic pericarditis in infancy. J Pediatr 82:689, 1973
18. Horowitz MS, Schultz CS, Stinson EB, Harrison DC, Popp RL: Sensitivity and specificity of echocardiographic diagnosis of pericardial effusion. Circulation 50:239, 1974
19. French JW, Popp R: Variability of echocardiographic discontinuity in double outlet right ventricle and truncus arteriosus. Circulation 51:848, 1975
20. Chung KJ, Alexson CG, Manning JA, Gramiak R: Echocardiography in truncus arteriosus: The value of pulmonic valve detection. Circulation 48:281, 1973
21. Assad-Morell JL, Seward JB, Tajik AJ, Hagler DJ, Giuliani ER: Echo-phono-cardiographic and contrast studies in conditions associated with systemic arterial trunk overriding the ventricular septum. Circulation 53:663, 1976
22. Maron BJ, Edwards JE, Henry WL, et al.: Asymmetric special hypertrophy (ASH) in infancy. Circulation 50:809, 1974
23. Dillon JC, Feigenbaum H, Konecke LL, et al.: Echocardiographic manifestations of d-transposition of the great vessels. Am J Cardiol 32:74, 1973
24. Gramiak R, Chung KJ, Nanda N, Manning J: Echocardiographic diagnosis of transposition of the great vessels. Radiology 106:187, 1973
25. Nanda NC, Gramiak R, Robinson TI, Shaw PM: Echocardiographic evaluation of pulmonary hypertension. Circulation 50:575, 1974
26. Hirschfeld S, Meyer R, Schwartz DC, Korfhagen J, Kaplan S: The echocardiographic assessment of pulmonary artery pressure and pulmonary vascular resistance. Circulation 52:642, 1975
27. Diamond MA, Dillon JC, Haine CL, Chang S, Feigenbaum H: Echocardiographic features of atrial septal defect. Circulation 43:129, 1971
28. Asad-Morell JL, Tajik AJ, Giuliani ER: Echocardiographic analysis of the ventricular septum. Prog Cardiovasc Dis 17:219, 1974
29. Pearlman AS, Clark CE, Henry WL, et al.: Determinants of ventricular septal motion. Influence of relative right and left ventricular size. Circulation 54:83, 1976
30. Neal WA, Moller JH, Lucas RV Jr, Anderson RC: Operative repair of atrial septal defect without cardiac catheterization. J Pediatr 86:189, 1975
31. Baylen BG, Meyer RA, Kaplan S, Ringenburg WE, Korfhagen J: The critically ill premature infant with patent ductus arteriosus and pulmonary disease—an echocardiographic assessment. J Pediatr 86:423, 1975
32. Silverman NH, Lewis AB, Heymann MA, Rudolph AM: Echocardiographic assessment of ductus arteriosus shunt in premature infants. Circulation 50:821, 1974
33. Feigenbaum H: Echocardiographic examination of the left ventricle (Editorial). Circulation 51:1, 1975
34. Sahn DJ, Deely WJ, Hagan AD, Friedman WF: Echocardiographic assessment of left ventricular performance in normal newborns. Circulation 49:232, 1974
35. Kaye HH, Tynan M, Hunter S: Validity of echocardiographic estimates of left ventricular size and performance in infants and children. Br Heart J 37:371, 1975
36. Braunwald E, Ross J Jr, Sonnenblick EH: Mechanism of Contraction of the Normal and Failing Heart, 2nd ed. Boston, Little, Brown, 1976
37. Eckberg DL, Gault JH, Bonchard RL, Karliner JS, Ross J Jr: Mechanisms of left ventricular contraction in chronic severe mitral regurgitation. Circulation 47:1252, 1973
38. Belenkie I, Nutter DO, Clark DW, McCraw DB, Raizner AE: Assessment of left ventricular dimension and function by echocardiography. Am J Cardiol 31:755, 1973
39. Åsherg A: Ultrasonic cinematography of the living heart. Ultrasonics 6:113, 1967
40. Ebina T, Oka S, Tanaka M, et al.: The ultrasono-tomography for the heart and great vessels in living human subjects by means of the ultrasonic reflection technique. Jpn Heart J 8:331, 1967

41. Somer JG: Electronic sector scanning for ultrasonic diagnosis. Ultrasonics 6:153, 1968
42. Bom N, Lancée CT, Honkoop J, Hugenholtz PG: Ultrasonic viewer for cross-sectional analyses of moving cardiac structures. Biomed Eng 6:500, 1971
43. Sahn DJ, Terry R, O'Rourke R, Leopold G, Friedman WF: Multiple crystal cross-sectional echocardiography in the diagnosis of cyanotic congenital heart disease. Circulation 50:230, 1974
44. Tajik AJ, Seward JB, Hagler DJ, Mair DD, Lie JT: Two-dimensional real-time ultrasonic imaging of the heart and great vessels. Technique, image orientation, structure identification, and validation. Mayo Clin Proc 53:271, 1978

Radioisotopic Techniques

45. Hagan AD, Friedman WF, Ashburn WL, Alazraki N: Further applications of scintillation scanning technics to the diagnosis and management of infants and children with congenital heart disease. Circulation 45:858, 1972
46. Wesselhoeft H, Hurley PJ, Wagner HN Jr, Rowe RD: Nuclear angiocardiography in the diagnosis of congenital heart disease in infants. Circulation 45:77, 1972
47. Treves S, Collins-Nakai RL: Radioactive tracers in congenital heart disease. Am J Cardiol 38:711, 1976
48. Stocker FP, Kinser J, Weber JW, Rösler H: Pediatric radiocardioangiography. Shunt diagnosis. Circulation 47:819, 1973
49. Gates GF: Radionuclide Scanning in Cyanotic Heart Disease. Springfield, Ill, Thomas, 1974, p 18

7 Cardiac Catheterization and Angiocardiography

Although there has been extensive development of cardiac diagnostic techniques which do not require insertion of catheters, these have not supplemented cardiac catheterization in most instances. Cardiac catheterization remains a key in the diagnostic process for neonates and infants because it provides anatomic and hemodynamic information which other diagnostic methods cannot. The noninvasive diagnostic methods—history, physical examination, electrocardiography, thoracic roentgenography, echocardiography, and radionucleotide studies—provide important data that allow the clinician to establish a diagnosis or, at least, a differential diagnosis and to estimate the severity of a condition. But often such clinical assessment of a patient is inadequate to make decisions regarding management and prognosis. Thus, cardiac catheterization plays a role. Cardiac catheterization is not undertaken without careful clinical and laboratory evaluation by the previously described methods and is only undertaken to answer specific questions. It is rarely necessary for catheterization to be performed to determine the diagnosis. The physician should enter the catheterization laboratory with a diagnosis or differential diagnosis and a plan for the systematic approach to catheterization. The attitude should be that cardiac catheterization confirms a diagnosis and not that catheterization establishes a diagnosis.

In considering any diagnostic or therapeutic maneuver, a physician must consider the risk and the benefit, and the same principle should be applied to cardiac catheterization in neonates and infants. In a critically ill neonate, the risk of cardiac catheterization is higher than in older children, but the benefits of demonstrating an operatively treatable condition are also great. The physician recommends catheterization because the possible benefits exceed the risks.

INDICATIONS FOR CATHETERIZATION

Cardiac catheterization is performed in neonates and infants when the symptoms and/or signs indicate that operative or other extensive therapeutic procedures may be indicated.

Cyanosis

Any neonate or infant with cyanosis of cardiac origin should be catheterized. Many instances of cardiac cyanosis present initially during the neonatal period. In these neonates, cardiac catheterization should be performed as an emergency procedure, since severe cyanosis at this age results either from inadequate mixing, as in transposition of the great vessels, and is benefited by creating an atrial septal defect, or from inadequate pulmonary blood flow, as in conditions in tetralogy of Fallot, in which an aorticopulmonary shunt or infusion of prostaglandin E_1 is beneficial. Precise diagnosis is necessary for proper management.

Because hypoxemia in neonates can progress rapidly and lead to acidosis and disseminated intravascular coagulation, the study of cyanotic neonates is expedited. Following a thorough but quick diagnostic evaluation, cardiac catheterization is undertaken immediately. In cyanotic neonates, an unsatisfactory outcome occurs more commonly from delay rather than from prompt and expeditious catheterization.

In infants in whom cyanosis has appeared more slowly, catheterization is not performed as an emergency procedure, but such infants are admitted and catheterized within a day or two.

Occasionally, in neonates with cyanosis and respiratory distress, distinction of a pulmonary from a cardiac cause of the cyanosis may be difficult. The cardiac cause in the differential diagnosis may be a condition associated with pulmonary venous obstruction. Despite careful observation and frequently repeated laboratory studies, cardiac catheterization may be required to establish a diagnosis. In such instances, even if a cardiac lesion is not found, catheterization is warranted because of the possibility of identifying a correctable cardiac lesion.

Congestive Cardiac Failure

All neonates with congenital cardiac anomalies who develop congestive cardiac failure should be studied after their condition has been stabilized. If during digitalization, the condition deteriorates further, study should be undertaken without waiting for full digitalization. An exception is a premature infant with typical clinical findings of a patent ductus arteriosus in whom catheterization is not indicated before operation. Obvious causes of congestive cardiac failure, such as myocarditis, anemia, or paroxysmal atrial tachycardia, do not require study.

Most infants who develop congestive cardiac failure should be catheterized to define the anatomy of the underlying malformation and to assess its severity. Catheterization provides information needed to make decisions regarding further management, to provide prognosis, and to define the clinical course. Cardiac catheterization is not needed in the occasional infant who improves promptly following digitalization and in whom the diagnosis and the hemodynamic features of the associated cardiac condition are obvious.

Asymptomatic Infant

Asymptomatic neonates and infants with findings of a congenital cardiac malformation do not require cardiac catheterization routinely as soon as the presence of cardiac disease is discovered. Usually the clinical and laboratory features are sufficient to allow the physician to make a diagnosis with a high degree of certainty and to safely follow the infant into childhood. In a few infants, the clinical or laboratory findings indicate that the condition is very severe, as in aortic stenosis or pulmonary stenosis, where the electrocardiogram shows severe ventricular hypertrophy and strain. Cardiac catheterization is indicated in these instances. Cardiac catheterization is also indicated in an asymptomatic infant whose clinical and laboratory findings are typical of a particular condition, such as anomalous left coronary artery, which may deteriorate. An asymptomatic infant with clinical findings that suggest progression of the condition, such as development of pulmonary vascular disease, should be studied.

Preoperative Evaluation

In preparation for cardiac operation, cardiac catheterization should be performed in any infant not previously studied. The only exception is typical patent ductus arteriosus. Some infants need to be catheterized prior to operation if the condition is known to change with age or if there is specific information that the surgeon requires preoperatively.

Evaluation of the Results of Operation

Cardiac catheterization is occasionally used in infancy, but much more commonly in childhood, to evaluate the results of an operation or therapeutic procedure, particularly if the postoperative course has not been as expected. In infancy, evaluation of the results of a previous Rashkind or Blalock-Hanlon procedure or an aorticopulmonary shunt is the most common indication.

REQUIREMENTS AND PRECAUTIONS

The requirements for cardiac catheterization are designed to (1) provide the optimum diagnostic information, (2) reduce the incidence and severity of complications, and (3) maintain the infant's homeostasis.

The requirements for a cardiac catheterization laboratory were outlined by the Report of the Inter-Society Commission for Heart Disease Resources.[1] Subsequently, federal guidelines were developed which further defined requirements for cardiac catheterization units. The latter indicate that a laboratory must study 150 children per year. Both of these documents were developed to establish and maintain high standards of cardiac care.

Several requirements are absolutely necessary for optimum cardiac care of neonates and infants. Cardiac catheterization of neonates and infants should be undertaken only at centers with facilities to provide the necessary medical and surgical treatment. Cardiac surgeons must be available for acute situations, but, more importantly, the cardiologists and surgeons dealing with a patient must have ongoing communication, for this process establishes concepts of care and diagnostic approaches. For instance, individual surgeons may desire particular types of diagnostic information prior to operation which must be considered by the cardiologist when evaluating the patient. The continuing dialogue between cardiologists and surgeons can provide peer review and review of management and results, and can mobilize resources for proper care.

Only hospitals with a sufficient volume of patients, well-trained professional staff, and necessary equipment should undertake the care of neonates and infants with congenital cardiac disease.

The number of staff and type of equipment differs among institutions. In this section, we discuss what we consider the optimal requirements, and in each instance these equal or exceed those in the report of the Inter-Society Commission.[1]

Staff

The cardiac catheterization laboratory and its staff should be available 24 hours a day. If this is not possible, an institution cannot provide adequate care for neonates and infants with congenital cardiac malformations. It seems the sickest infants often must be catheterized on weekends or nights, and they deserve the best staff and facilities for management and diagnosis. We inform our cardiac surgeons when an infant is being catheterized and of the suspected diagnosis, so that if an emergency arises in the laboratory or if an operation is required, they are prepared.

Personnel

Two physicians should be present during the cardiac catheterization—one performing the study, the other monitoring the patient, treating complications, and assisting in other ways. In addition, there should be (1) a radiographic technician to operate the radiographic equipment and develop angiographic studies, (2) a technician to record pressures and perform blood gas analysis, and (3) a nurse with knowledge of cardiac catheterization procedures to monitor and care for infants and assist in cardiopulmonary resuscitation. Exactly who performs these tasks is immaterial, but the tasks need to be performed by properly trained individuals.

Whenever possible, when we catheterize neonates, the nurse caring for a neonate on the intensive care unit accompanies the child to the catheterization laboratory and can monitor the neonate, relieving others to assist the physician or perform other duties. We routinely have a radiologist in attendance during the procedure to help make decisions regarding angiocardiographic techniques and to interpret the films.

A physician and nurse accompany the sick neonate to and from the catheterization laboratory.

Equipment

In the study of the sick neonate or infant, catheterization should be performed as quickly as possible. With proper training, delegation of responsibilities, and skill, each step can be performed expeditiously. In the catheterization of most neonates and many infants, the most important information is usually obtained by angiography. Catheterization laboratories should have the capability of both biplane cineangiography and biplane rapid film changer. While biplane cutfilms provide better information about anatomic detail, they require a minimum of 10 minutes before the films can be viewed, and in most laboratories the room must be darkened to remove the films, making it difficult to observe the infant during this period.

Biplane cineangiographic equipment should be combined with biplane videorecorders so that the angiogram can be immediately replayed. This saves valuable time and makes it possible to reach rapid decisions about the diagnosis and additional procedures which may be required.

Biplane image intensifiers allow the possibility of biplane fluoroscopy to aid manipulation of the catheter. Most cardiologists have been trained to use the anteroposterior view for fluoroscopy, but during manipulation of the catheter, there are situations when viewing both planes simultaneously is helpful.

The radiographic equipment in a properly equipped laboratory should include:

1. Biplane image intensifiers and biplane cameras
2. TV system for each image intensifier
3. Vidoesystem for each image intensifier
4. Biplane rapid film changer

Physiologic Recording and Monitoring Equipment

The laboratory should have at least two fluid-filled pressure transducers and a cuvette oximeter prepared for each catheterization. A multiple channel recorder is used so that an electrocardiogram, pressures, and other functions can be recorded simultaneously and at speeds of 100 mm/sec. The recorder is attached to an oscilloscope so that the patient can be continuously monitored. The oscilloscope is placed adjacent to the fluoroscope screen so that the physician can simultaneously observe fluoroscopy, electrocardiogram, pressure, and other functions.

Equipment to Measure Oxygen

Equipment is needed to measure oxygen. Blood oxygen saturation can be measured spectrophotometrically, using either transmission or reflective oximetry. We use the former, although many workers use reflective oximetry, drawing less than 0.25 ml of blood per sample. This blood is not returned to the patient. This procedure has the advantage of being faster than transmission oximetry.

During catheterization, we draw small (1 ml) blood samples for determination of pH, P_{CO_2}, and P_{O_2} from sites with high oxygen saturation and with low oxygen saturation. With the use of a monogram, the oxygen saturations can be calculated, and these values help to standardize the spectrophotometric oximetry values. In neonates and infants, we do not measure oxygen using the Van Slyke method because of the volume of blood required to make this determination. By determining the hemoglobin and oxygen saturation, the oxygen content can be calculated:

Oxygen content = Hb × 1.34 × % O_2 saturation

Blood samples for pH, P_{O_2}, and P_{CO_2} should be drawn at other times during the cardiac catheterization if the infant's condition is unstable. In neonates and infants with cyanosis or congestive cardiac failure, we draw a blood sample for blood gas analysis, as an initial step of the cardiac catheterization, either from a previously placed umbilical arterial catheter or from the catheter as soon as it has been inserted and is located within the heart.

The patient's rate of oxygen consumption can be measured during the catheterization, and cardiac output can be calculated by the Fick principle.

Techniques have been described for the measurement of oxygen consumption by a flow-through method.[2-4] The head and shoulders of the infant are placed in a plastic hood, and the space around the neck is closed loosely by plastic. A pump is attached to the hood, and room air is drawn through the box at a rate of five times the infant's minute volume. The exhaust is analyzed to determine the difference in oxygen content between inspired and expired air. We collect the expired air in a chain-driven Tissot spirometer and analyze the expired air by the Sholander method. The flow-through method was established because it is impossible to use a mouthpiece in infants and because of the need to measure oxygen consumption in order to calculate accurate cardiac output. Many centers estimate oxygen consumption from established tables or equations, but studies[3,4] indicate a wide variation of oxygen consumption: in 20 percent of patients, the measured oxygen consumption differed from the assumed value by at least 20 percent. A number of variables, such as sedation, temperature, and activity level,[3,5] affect the measured oxygen consumption.

Emergency Equipment

Equipment must be available to manage emergencies. The catheterization laboratory should have an oxygen supply. A DC defibrillator with pediatric size paddle must be available. Pacemaker units and small pacemaker catheter units should be available for the conversion of atrial tachycardia or for infants who develop and are symptomatic from heart block or bradycardia.

Suction equipment, Ambu bag, appropriately sized face masks, laryngoscope, and variously sized endotracheal tubes are needed for resuscitation and ventilation.

Appropriate pharmacologic agents must be available in the laboratory to treat arrhythmias and other emergencies.

CATHETERIZATION PROCEDURE

The catheterization procedure must be discussed with the parents and the relative risks and benefits explained. In most instances, the indications for the procedure are fairly obvious to the parents because most neonates and infants undergoing cardiac catheterization are symptomatic. Parents of neonates must be told that the risks are higher in this age group than at any other time in life. Following discussion and explanation, written permission must be obtained.

The initial preparation of the neonate for cardiac catheterization can be accomplished on the station prior to transfer to the catheterization laboratory. If the neonate is in an isolette or warmer, he can be restrained to a padded board with elastic bandages, and electrocardiographic leads can be placed. The arms are restrained over the head, the body restrained by bandages over the upper pelvis and abdomen, and the legs restrained by bandages from the feet to above the knee. The legs should be slightly abducted and externally rotated.

We do not administer premedication to any neonate or infant, but we do restrict oral intake for 4 hours prior to the study.

Monitoring

During the procedure, we make the following measurements, generally every 15 min.

TEMPERATURE.   We place a rectal thermistor to measure the infant's temperature, since neonates and small infants may become hypothermic during cardiac catheterization.[6] Efforts to maintain the infant's temperature are carried out. When catheterizing neonates, we dial the thermostat of the catheterization laboratory up so that the ambient temperature reaches 80F. We perform the cutdown on a hooded warmer, and once the catheter has been inserted into the vein, the infant is transferred to the catheterization table.

We apply a heating pad to the chest and place a blanket about the infant's head. By frequent monitoring of the temperature, the infant's temperature can be maintained.

PULSE RATE AND RHYTHM.   An electrocardiographic trace must be continuously observed on an oscilloscope. It is helpful to have interchangeable electrocardiographic electrodes on the neonatal intensive care unit and catheterization laboratory, so the leads can be merely plugged in when the infant arrives in the laboratory. The electrodes are placed on the extremities, rather than on the trunk where they might interfere with fluoroscopy or angiography.

One individual, in our case the recording technician, must constantly observe the oscilloscope and call out ectopic beats or changes in cardiac rate.

RESPIRATION.   Respiratory rate and effort must be monitored frequently. Respiration can easily be neglected because each of the other functions is monitored by a device. During catheterization, respirations may become depressed, occurring much more frequently in neonates than in older infants. Should this respiratory depression occur, the infant is intubated and placed on a respirator. Recently, many of our infants have been placed on a respirator prior to catheterization, for we believe this technique maintains respiratory rate, controls oxygen consumption, and eases respiratory effort. The patient's metabolic rate is thereby reduced. The respirator improves pulmonary edema if it is present.

INTRAVASCULAR PRESSURE.   In many neonates, an umbilical arterial catheter is placed and connected to a pressure transducer. Arterial pressure can be monitored provided a coarctation is not present. The blood pressure may be measured either by cuff or a Doppler unit.

Throughout the catheterization procedure, intracardiac pressures are monitored as the catheter tip is manipulated, and these pressures provide a valuable guide to the patient's hemodynamic status.

pH, P_{CO_2}, AND P_{O_2}.   In a sick neonate, we obtain these values initially and repeat them depending upon the patient's status and after each angiographic injection. In infants, the frequency of determination of pH, P_{CO_2}, and P_{O_2} depends upon the underlying cardiac defect, catheterization complications, and duration of procedure. If an umbilical arterial catheter is in place, blood can be withdrawn from this site.

Although we prefer to measure blood gases from the arterial side of the circulation, this is not always possible, and measurements of venous pH, P_{O_2}, and P_{CO_2}, particularly if they are performed serially, permit the physician to recognize and treat abnormalities. On the venous side of the circulation, the pH is slightly lower (0.5 units) and P_{CO_2} slightly higher (5 torr). pH, P_{CO_2}, and P_{O_2} are monitored to detect hypercapnia (from respiratory depression), acidosis (either respiratory or metabolic), and hypoxemia. When disturbances occur, the underlying cause is sought, and appropriate treatment is given. Metabolic disturbances are treated by respirator support and administration of bicarbonate or oxygen.

BLOOD LOSS.   Prior to cardiac catheterization, we type and crossmatch each infant for whole blood. The volume of blood loss from the catheterization site and from blood sampling is carefully monitored. If blood loss is excessive, a transfusion is given.

FLUID.   The volumes of intravenous fluid administered and of contrast material injected are accurately recorded. Fluid is used to flush catheters and cuvettes and is administered through peripheral intravenous sites or umbilical catheters. The volume must be carefully monitored. We use a constant infusion pump to control volume infused through umbilical catheters.

The amount of contrast material used for test injections and for angiograms is also recorded. Following injection, we always clear the catheter of contrast material by withdrawal until blood flows.

BLOOD CHEMISTRIES.   Prior to catheterization of neonates, we obtain serum electrolytes and blood glucose and, if necessary, make repeat determinations made during the catheterization.

Approach

Depending upon the questions to be answered by cardiac catheterization in neonates and infants, one of three sites is generally used. The inguinal area is the most frequent catheterization site. In neonates, the umbilical vessels provide a potential site to insert the catheter, whereas in particular situations, the antecubital fossa is used.

While we perform cutdowns for most catheterizations in neonates and infants, other workers prefer the percutaneous method.

INGUINAL AREA.   In our laboratory, over 90 percent of catheterizations in neonates and infants are performed in the inguinal area. The veins are larger in the inguinal area than in the arm, and this approach makes it easier to pass the catheter into the left side of the heart through the foramen ovale or atrial septal defect and to identify left-sided cardiac anomalies.

Unless an aortogram is to be performed, the inguinal approach is used to reach most intracardiac sites. Some have considered interruption of inferior vena cava with azygous continuation a contraindication for the inguinal approach, but in most of these infants, it is possible to advance the catheter into the ventricle for an angiogram. This ventriculogram usually provides sufficient information for reaching decisions regarding the patient.

The inguinal approach has an advantage in cyanotic conditions, since injection of contrast medium into the right side of the heart usually visualizes the site of the right-to-left shunt. Usually, the catheter can be passed into the aorta if a ventricular communication is present. Occasionally, passing the catheter into the pulmonary artery is difficult from the inguinal approach, but this can usually be accomplished with balloon catheters.

It is preferable to use the right inguinal area, since it may be difficult to pass the catheter through the left iliac vein into the inferior vena cava because the catheter may pass repeatedly into a lumbar vein. The torque of the catheter from the left leg is not as favorable for manipulating the catheter within the heart.

Two approaches have been used for introducing the catheter in the inguinal area.

INGUINAL CUTDOWN. After cleaning and draping the inguinal area, 0.5 percent Xylocaine is injected. A 2 cm incision is made 0.5 cm below and parallel to the inguinal crease, starting from the point of the femoral arterial pulse and extending medially. The saphenous vein is located by blunt dissection. The saphenous vein courses on the medial side of a lymph node before it joins the saphenous bulb. Once the skin is incised, damp rather than dry sponges are used, because they are less traumatic to vessels. Several small veins enter the saphenous vein or saphenous bulb. If a small vein is the first vessel identified, it can be followed toward the saphenous vein. The saphenous vein courses in an obtuse angle to the femoral vein. In infants, the vein appears white and has a thicker wall than a deep vein.

Once the saphenous vein has been identified by blunt dissection, the saphenous vein is mobilized up to the saphenous bulb. If the saphenous vein is small or if a balloon atrial septostomy is anticipated, the femoral vein is also isolated. By blunt dissection through the cribriform fascia, the femoral vein is located in the femoral triangle. The femoral vein lies posteriorly and medially to the femoral artery. Usually, the femoral vein can be isolated without disturbing the femoral artery. The femoral vein can be isolated at either of two locations:

1. The common femoral vein: a 2 cm section of the common femoral vein is isolated above and below the saphenous bulb. Care must be taken in isolating the distal end of the femoral vein because profundal branches join the posterior aspect of the femoral vein. If excessive traction is exerted on the femoral vein, a profundal branch can be evulsed and extensive hemorrhage occur.
2. Superficial femoral vein: a segment distal to insertion of the profundal branch.

In order to maintain hemostasis once the vein is isolated, place gut sutures proximally and distally to the site where the vein is to be opened and make certain that tributaries entering this section of vein are also looped or tied.

In handling veins, gentleness must be used to avoid venospasm or tearing of the vein. Gentle traction is placed proximally and distally, and the vein is opened. I prefer using a curved iris scissors to open the vein, making a cut on the upper surface of the vein, at an angle of about 45° with the long axis of the vein.

Occasionally, the incision is made at a confluence of veins, giving a larger site for catheter insertion. A single blade of a curved iris forceps is inserted into the vein, and the vein wall is lifted. The catheter tip is inserted into the vein. Other workers use a catheter introducer. When inserting the catheter, the distal end of the vein is retracted. There is no traction placed on the proximal end, since the tie will occlude the vein, making it impossible to advance the catheter.

The catheter must be inserted in the direction of the vein. If the catheter passes freely, it is inserted several centimeters. At this point, the distal end of the vein is ligated, a single knot is made in the proximal tie, and this is pulled tightly around the vein and catheter. The proximal tie ensures hemostasis but allows easy movement of the catheter.

If the saphenous vein is small and inadequate to accept a catheter, the femoral vein should be isolated for catheterization.

Hemostasis must exist before the catheter is further manipulated. It is not wise to continue the procedure trying to maintain hemostasis by applying intermittent or continuous pressure with a sponge. If there is bleeding or oozing and the catheterization continues, excessive blood loss can occur easily, particularly when the room is darkened and attention is focused on fluoroscopy screens, pressure monitors, and oscilloscopes. Having made certain hemostasis exists, the physician can turn his attention to other aspects of the procedure.

In infants in whom balloon atrial septostomy is expected, some cardiologists make the incision above the inguinal ligament and use the external iliac vein.

We rarely use the femoral artery in neonates and infants because, usually, the left side of the heart can be approached in other ways. Because, in infancy, the femoral arteries are very small, it is difficult to maintain the patency following cutdown.

PERCUTANEOUS METHOD.   The percutaneous method of cardiac catheterization was introduced more than 25 years ago by Seldinger,[7] and was first extensively applied to children by Lurie and associates.[8] Although it has gained wide popularity and has largely replaced the cutdown technique, only recently has it been applied to a large number of neonates and infants.[9-13]

The percutaneous method has the following advantages: a lower incidence of infection, the possibility of inserting a larger catheter, not interfering with venous return by ligation, a lower incidence of interference with arterial flow if an artery is used, less time required, easy exchanging of catheters, and ability to use veins repeatedly.

The technique has been further described by Takahashi and Kirkpatrick,[14,15] and recommendation has been made for the type of catheter, guidewire, and introducer for infants. Gay[13] described the successful use of the percutaneous technique in 20 infants weighing less than 4.2 kg. Neches and colleagues[12] reported a large experience with the percutaneous sheath technique, including 33 infants under 1 year of age and 114 children weighing less than 10 kg. Carter et al.[11] reported a series of neonates weighing less than 4.5 kg and described a 77 percent success rate for left-sided cardiac catheterization and a 41 percent success rate for right-sided cardiac catheterization. Subsequently, Sunderlund and colleagues[9] described an experience with the percutaneous sheath technique in 195 infants weighing less than 5 kg, of whom 133 were neonates, and indicated doing a Rashkind procedure by this method. They report success rates of 85 percent for the right side of the heart and 91 percent and 95 percent success rates for left-sided catheterization in infants and neonates, respectively.

The percutaneous technique has been described for neonates and infants.[9-14] The inguinal area is prepared, local anesthesia is given, and the femoral artery is palpated. The type, length, and gauge of the needle to be inserted vary among institutions. The needle is inserted through the skin below the inguinal ligament, medial to the arterial pulse, and parallel to the artery at an angle of 30° to 45° from the skin. Once blood flows freely, the flexible tip of a guidewire is passed through the needle. If it does not pass easily, the needle is manipulated slightly either by withdrawing it slightly or by depressing the hub of the needle, without forcing the guidewire. Once the guidewire is freely in the vein, the needle is removed and the guidewire is left in the vein. With a No. 11 scalpel blade, a small nick is made at the site where the wire penetrates the skin. At this point, two techniques can be used. In one, a dilator is passed over the wire and advanced with a rotating motion through the subcutaneous tissues into the vein. The dilator is then withdrawn, and an end-hole catheter is advanced over the guidewire into the vein. The other technique, which is becoming more popular, involves passing a dilator and sheath over the guidewire into the vein. The guide and dilator are then removed from the vein, leaving a thin-walled sheath in the vein. Different types of catheters can then be advanced through the sheath into the vein. Upon completion of the study, the catheter is removed. The sheath is allowed to bleed briefly and then is withdrawn. Pressure is applied for 5 to 10 min. to obtain hemostasis.

Femoral arterial catheterization is carried out in a similar fashion, inserting the needle over and parallel to the femoral arterial pulse.

In the experience of Sunderlund and colleagues,[9] following femoral arterial catheterization, all neonates and infants had normal skin temperature, color, and capillary filling in the involved leg within 48 hours, although 15 percent of patients under 5 kg and 20 percent of patients between 5 and 10 kg had reduced or absent arterial pulses after 48 hours. The long-term effects of the decreased arterial pulse are unknown, although Boros and associates[16] studied 14 children 4 years following demonstration of umbilical arterial catheter thrombus formation and found no difference in femoral or tibial lengths, leg length, or pulse pressure difference. Carter and colleagues[11] described diminished arterial pulse in 3 of 97 catheterized neonates at the time of hospital discharge but indicated that pulses usually return to normal within 24 hours of the arterial catheterization.

UMBILICAL ARTERY AND VEIN.   In the neonate, catheterization through the umbilical artery or vein has several advantages: the method is quick, since time-consuming cutdown is not required, the vessels are large and can be ligated without ill effect, and two arteries and one vein are present at a single site.

The umbilical artery can usually be catheterized during the first 3 days of life and the umbilical vein up to 7 to 10 days, but the likelihood of being able to pass the ductus venosus decreases with age.[17]

Several authors[17-19] have described a technique for using the umbilicus as a site for catheterization. The umbilicus is cleaned and draped, and the cord is cut at a level above the skin. One or two silk sutures can be placed in the umbilicus to help in traction. The arteries are white, located together, and show a smaller lumen than the thin-walled vein, which has an elliptical orifice.

The arterial orifice can be gently opened by an iris forceps and any thrombus removed. Usually, a polyethylene catheter is inserted. It is important to remember that the umbilical arteries are branches from the iliac arteries, and, therefore, the catheter must be passed inferiorly to the iliac arteries and then into the aorta. The catheter can be advanced into the aortic arch and ascending aorta in many neonates who do not have an obstructive lesion in the aortic arch. The physician must be alert to its passage through the ductus arteriosus into the pulmonary trunk.

Aortography through umbilical arterial catheterization is very helpful in identifying aortic obstructions, particularly aortic atresia, where a characteristic picture is demonstrated. Coarctation of the aorta and interruption of the aortic arch may also be suspected or diagnosed. Information about the aortic arch may be insufficient, however, to make decisions regarding operation.

In neonates, the presence of an umbilical arterial catheter can be very useful in monitoring pH, Po_2, Pco_2, and blood pressure during this procedure. If a catheter has been placed prior to arrival at the catheterization laboratory, it should be replaced under sterile conditions before being manipulated for aortography.

Upon removal of the catheter, the artery usually seals, but a pursestring suture may be necessary for hemostasis.

By umbilical venous catheterization, the right and left atrium can be catheterized, but less frequently the ventricles, and rarely the pulmonary artery. Either a polyethylene catheter or a standard cardiac catheter is inserted into the umbilical vein. It is directed superiorly and passes through the ductus venosus into the inferior vena cava. Gentle manipulation is used, and the catheter course is carefully observed because the catheter tip may enter the portal venous system. Because of its slightly tortuous course, it is difficult to manipulate the catheter tip once it is within the heart. One of the major drawbacks to umbilical venous catheterization is closure of the ductus venosus. Linde et al.[17] found that the ductus venosus was patent in 61 percent of neonates less than 6 days of age. Even during a single study, the ductus venosus may close, making it impossible to replace a catheter. If a catheter cannot be easily advanced into the heart from the umbilical vein, the inguinal area should be prepared and the procedure performed from that site. Silk pursestring sutures are placed in the umbilical venous wall, and as the catheter is withdrawn, the sutures are pulled closed.

The umbilical venous approach can be used for pressure and oximetry determinations, angiography, and performance of balloon atrial septostomy. Newfeld and associates[20] described successful balloon atrial septostomy in 16 neonates under 4 days of age but indicated an inability to pass the catheter through the ductus venosus in 5 other neonates.

Porter and associates[10] were able to catheterize each cardiac chamber using the umbilical venous approach but with more difficulty than was encountered using the inguinal approach. It is easier and less traumatic to catheterize various chambers with a balloon-tipped catheter. Porter's experience[10] is similar to ours in encountering difficulties during balloon atrial septostomy, frequently necessitating a change to the inguinal site.

BRACHIAL APPROACH.   Although arteries are small in the antecubital fossa, we have sometimes performed cutdowns on the brachial artery. We prefer to use the brachial artery rather than the femoral artery because the potential long-term effects of arterial occlusion are less in the arm than in the leg.

Performance of a retrograde aortogram from left brachial arterial cutdown may provide important diagnostic information more quickly and safely than will cardiac catheterization. We use it in neonates or infants with congestive cardiac failure and clinical findings suggestive of isolated coarctation of the aorta, in symptomatic infants in whom a patent ductus arteriosus is suspected but cannot be diagnosed by clinical means, or in an occasional infant with an abnormality of the great vessels, such as vascular ring or interruption of the aortic arch, in which information is needed about the precise origin of brachiocephalic vessels.

We have used the right brachial artery to pass a catheter into the aorta for angiography in anomalous left coronary arterial or aorticopulmonary communications in which the anatomic features have not been clearly demonstrated by other means. In an occasional patient with aortic stenosis, left ventricular cardiomyopathy, or mitral insufficiency, we have used this approach to obtain hemodynamic information and to visualize the left ventricle, aortic, and mitral valves.

In performing this cutdown, we restrain the arm on a board, with the forearm extended, externally rotated, and the palm up. This position facilitates isolation of the brachial artery beneath the biceps. Following injection with 0.5 percent Xylocaine into the skin and deeper tissues, a short incision is made 1 cm above the antecubital crease, starting over the brachial arterial pulse and extending medially. Blunt dissection is carried out through the subcutaneous tissue. The radiating fibers of the lacertus fibrosus sweep from the biceps tendon to the medial epicondyle. By dissecting either through these fibers or immediately superior to this fascia, one can approach the undersurface of the biceps muscle and tendon. The brachial artery is accompanied by two thin-walled veins, the venae comitantes, and the median nerve, which lies adjacent and medial to the artery.

A 1 to 2 cm section of artery is dissected free. Either a gut suture or a short length of sterile rubber band can be placed above and below the site at which the artery is to be opened. With an iris scissor, a transverse opening is made on the top surface of the artery. A small polyethylene catheter is inserted distally into the artery, and 0.5 to 1 ml of heparin solution is injected.

If only an aortogram is to be performed, a No. 16 or No. 18 Robb-Steinberg cannula is inserted into the artery, and the proximal tie is narrowed around the artery to hold the cannula in place. If a catheter is to be inserted, the technique is similar to inserting a venous catheter. Either a No. 4 or No. 5F catheter can be inserted. Tension on the distal tie generally stops the bleeding from the distal artery, and proximally the artery constricts about the catheter and leads to hemostasis.

Following completion of the study, the catheter or cannula are removed. A fine polyethylene catheter is advanced proximally, and a small amount of heparin solution is injected. The arteriotomy is closed with interrupted 6-0 to 7-0 Tevdek sutures. Previously, in neonates and small infants, we have ligated the artery proximally and distally and had no complications, but we believe it is preferable to attempt to establish continuity. If the pulse is absent at the completion of the study, we do not explore the artery.

Technique

The cardiac catheterization of neonates and infants should be carried out expeditiously, for many are critically ill and may require emergency operation. During catheterization, their condition may deteriorate further because of the time and stress involved.

Two factors are important to expedite the catheterization. First, the physician must be well trained and experienced in the technical aspects of catheterization, and the supporting nursing, laboratory, and radiologic staff must be skilled and have clearly defined responsibilities. Each new supporting staff member must be fully trained. Second, the physician must be knowledgeable about the patient and his clinical and laboratory findings and have discussed the patient's problems. Based on this knowledge prior to entering the laboratory, the goals of the study should be clearly established, the needed information outlined, and methods of accomplishing the goals defined.

During a cardiac catheterization, the physician must maintain flexibility and be able to alter the course of the catheterization if the findings so indicate. For example, if the catheter is passed to a site which is difficult to reach or which was not meant to be catheterized at this time, take the opportunity to obtain all the information you can before moving on—you may not get another chance! The physician must quickly recognize when findings vary from those anticipated and make adjustments in the plan of the catheterization.

Every catheterization is associated with risk, and steps must be taken to monitor the patient and to minimize complications. The physician must be experienced, so that during the procedure he can weigh the risk in this particular patient of proceeding further or following a particular course. The physician must recognize when problems are developing and must be able to recognize and treat serious complications.

In catheterization, we feel it is important to have two methods of proving the existence of a shunt. For instance, the presence of an increase in oxygen saturation at the ventricular level on right-sided cardiac catheterization, while highly probable of a ventricular septal defect, should be verified by angiography or passage of a catheter through the defect.

Catheters

Many different catheters are available, and each laboratory or physician may have particular ones which they use most frequently. There are three basic types of catheters:

SIDE HOLES AND CLOSED END.   The NIH angiocatheter is an example of this type of catheter with closed tip and multiple side holes. This is the catheter we most frequently use in neonates and infants. There are two disadvantages of this catheter. First, a wedge pressure cannot be recorded, but usually in neonates and infants it is possible to pass the catheter into the left atrium and measure pressure. Therefore, in most instances it is not necessary to record the wedge pressure. Second, this catheter cannot be advanced over a guidewire, but if a sheath is used in the percutaneous method, this is not a problem. In most diagnostic situations in neonates and infants, angiography plays an important role, so that using this catheter allows one to be prepared to perform an injection if one reaches a particular site. With multiple holes, it is easy to withdraw blood. Pressure can be recorded, and although the presence of several holes over the length of a centimeter at the tip of the catheter might interfere with recording of transvalvular gradients, in our experience, this has rarely caused confusion in the analysis of pressure recordings.

END-HOLE CATHETERS.   Catheters with end holes may also have side holes. The Goodale-Lubin is an example of a catheter with both an end hole and side holes. We use it to measure pulmonary arterial wedge pressure or when the catheter is advanced over a guidewire to reach unusual sites. It should not be used for angiography, but it is satisfactory for pressure recording and blood withdrawal.

FLOW-DIRECTED CATHETERS.   Flow-directed catheters have been welcomed by pediatric cardiologists because their use has made it easier to reach certain sites, such as the pulmonary artery in transposition of the great vessels or the pulmonary arteries in a patient with an aorticopulmonary shunt.[21]

Flow-directed catheters may have either two or three lumens, one lumen being connected to the balloon. The number and location of the holes vary. A single hole may be located distal to the balloon, as in the Swan-Ganz catheter, and this hole is used to measure the pulmonary arterial wedge pressure. The holes may be located proximally (Behrman angio, Swan-Ganz angio catheters),[22] and these may be used for blood sampling, pressure recording, and angiography. While using these catheters, the pressure recordings may be damped or easily become damped.

CO_2, not air, is used to inflate the balloon because, should the balloon break, CO_2 is easily absorbed from the circulation, while air is not. Therefore, a CO_2 embolus which might pass to the brain in an infant with a right-to-left shunt would be rapidly absorbed.

SPECIAL CATHETERS. A variety of types of catheters has been developed for particular uses to answer particular questions arising in the catheterization laboratory.

1. Electrode catheter—used to measure intracardiac electrical potentials, or detect ascorbic acid or H^+ if either of these is used as an indicator
2. Thermistor—used to measure cardiac output by thermodilution method
3. Catheter-tip transducer—a microtransducer is mounted in the catheter to obtain high-fidelity pressure recording

CATHETERS FOR THERAPEUTIC USE. The most widely used therapeutic catheter is a balloon atrial septostomy catheter, which may have either one or two lumens. It is used to create an atrial septal defect, most often in infants with complete transposition of the great vessels. Catheters have been developed for closure of atrial septal defect or a patent ductus arteriosus. A blade atrial septostomy catheter has been developed but has had limited use.

SIZE OF THE CATHETER. In most infants the vessels are large enough that a No. 5F catheter can be inserted, and in older infants a No. 6F can be used. These catheters are usually large enough for satisfactory injection of contrast material, particularly if they are short (50 cm). Occasionally, only a No. 4F can be inserted. These are unsatisfactory for angiography but do permit measurement of pressures and oxygen saturations.

Procedure

The catheter is connected to a manifold through a stiff-walled connecting tube, so that adequate frequency response is maintained. Care needs to be exercised throughout the procedure to guard against inadvertently injecting air bubbles into the patient. The techniques of catheter manipulation are familiar to experienced cardiologists and have been described, so we will mention only a few points which we believe will help reduce risk and speed the procedure. Whenever advancing the catheter, advance to a point and then withdraw slightly to avoid wedging the catheter tip in a vein. It may be difficult to withdraw the catheter tip from a wedged peripheral vein. When advancing the catheter in the inferior vena cava, follow its course by fluoroscopy because it is easy to advance it into renal or hepatic veins.

Catheter manipulation should be gentle and by probing, not stabbing, motions. The tip of the catheter responds best to rotation if the catheter is gripped close to the site of entry of the catheter through the skin, rather than at a distance. The catheter should not be rotated unless it is being withdrawn or advanced.

The heart of a neonate or infant can inadvertently be perforated by the catheter tip. Perforation of the heart can occur easily at three sites—right atrial appendage, left atrial appendage, and right ventricular outflow area. Care must be taken in maneuvering catheters in these areas to recognize the catheter position in these sites and not advance the catheter with force. Avoid wedging or jamming the catheter at any site.

During the manipulation of the catheter within the heart, we continuously monitor pressure through the catheter, because these data, combined with fluoroscopic visualization of the catheter, inform the physician of the location of the catheter tip.

In catheterizing from the inguinal area and attempting to obtain information about particular cardiac anomalies of infants, data may be needed from the pulmonary artery, aorta, or left ventricle. Particular techniques are needed to successfully catheterize these structures.

Although flow-directed catheters make it easier to reach these sites, the cardiologist should know techniques using other catheters. To enter the pulmonary artery, the catheter is passed in a gentle curve into the midright ventricle with the tip pointed toward the lateral wall. The catheter tip is then rotated clockwise, directing the catheter tip superiorly and gently advancing. To enter the aorta through a ventricular septal defect, start with the catheter tip pointed laterally and withdraw slightly toward the spine and turn clockwise, directing the catheter tip upward and medially toward the spine. Do not force the catheter, because this maneuver has been associated with cardiac perforation. To enter the left ventricle from the left atrium, the maneuver that has helped us most frequently is advancing the catheter tip to the superior aspect of the left atrium, forming a curve, which is rotated into the left ventricle. Another method is to advance the catheter into the right upper pulmonary vein, and on withdrawal of the catheter, when it reaches the left atrium, to turn it clockwise rapidly, sharply, and inferiorly, with the tip slightly lateral to the spine.

When the catheter is initially advanced into the heart from the inferior vena cava, it usually passes to one of three sites, superior vena cava, left atrium, or right ventricle. From each of these sites, collection of data can commence: from the superior vena cava—an oximetry series through the atrium, from the left atrium—entry into the left ventricle, pressure and oximetry from left to right atrium to evaluate patency of the atrial septum, from the right ventricle—measurement of pressure and then advance into a great vessel.

Oximetry series are usually performed during cardiac catheterization. Optimally, at least two samples should be withdrawn from different locations of each chamber and as many samples obtained within as short a period of time as possible. To expedite oximetry series, the catheter should be advanced to a distal point, such as a pulmonary artery or the superior vena cava, and samples obtained as the catheter is successively withdrawn to each site. Only after it has been withdrawn to the most distal site (such as inferior vena cava) should it be advanced to other sites (such as left atrium) not in the withdrawal course. If a shunt is present, the oximetry series should be repeated to improve the accuracy of estimating the volume of shunt.

Phasic and mean pressures should be recorded in each great artery, atria, or pulmonary vein entered, and phasic pressures should be recorded from each ventricle. The attenuation must be selected so that pressure recording is as large as possible on the calibrated scale. Phasic pressures should be recorded on withdrawal across the cardiac valves. When withdrawing across an atrioventricular valve, a low attenuation should be used to more accurately measure the end-diastolic pressure and detect a diastolic gradient.

CATHETERIZATION DATA AND INTERPRETATION

Four types of information can be gathered at cardiac catheterization: catheter course, oxygen data, pressures, and angiography. The information derived from these sources is used to establish a diagnosis, estimate the severity of the condition, and assess the effect of the condition on myocardial function. In infants, the emphasis is placed on the first two purposes.

Catheter Course

The course the catheter takes through the vena cava, cardiac chambers, or great vessels may in itself be diagnostic. A variety of characteristic catheter courses have been described and were summarized by Taketa and associates.[23] The catheter course can verify the presence of a defect (such as ventricular septal defect or patent ductus arteriosus), demonstrate abnormal venous structures (such as persistent superior vena cava), and outline an abnormal position of a great vessel (such as the aorta in corrected transposition of the great vessels). An abnormal catheter course may, therefore, either make a diagnosis or verify one established by other means.

Oxygen Data

Oximetry data are used to diagnose cardiac conditions associated with a shunt and can be used either alone or with other data to assess the severity of the condition, as in determining the magnitude of the shunt or calculating the cardiac output, using the Fick principle.

As blood flows from the vena cava through the right side of the heart, mixing becomes more uniform. The superior vena caval oxygen saturation is normally around 70 percent. An oxygen saturation value considerably higher than 70 percent suggests partial or total anomalous pulmonary venous connection to superior vena cava or one of its tributaries, an arteriovenous fistula emptying into superior vena cava or tributary, or a high cardiac output, as from anxiety.

An abnormally low oxygen saturation indicates low cardiac output or a cyanotic form of congenital cardiac disease.

Oxygen saturation of blood in the inferior vena cava is variable because this vein receives blood from various sources, renal venous blood having an oxygen saturation of at least 80 percent and hepatic venous blood with 65 percent, and reflux of right atrial blood. Because of this variability, it is difficult to obtain a blood sample truly representing inferior vena caval flow. In calculating the magnitude of shunt at the atrial level, we use only the superior vena caval saturation for the calculation. Inferior vena caval oxygen saturation is higher than that of the superior vena cava, about 75 percent. If the saturation is lower than that of the superior vena cava, a reversing patent ductus arteriosus is present.

The right atrium receives vena caval and coronary sinus blood. The latter, which may represent 10 percent of the cardiac output, has an oxygen saturation of 30 percent, unless there is persistence of left superior vena cava or anomalous pulmonary venous connection to the coronary sinus. Considering the various venous returns to the right atrium, the best site at which to obtain a sample representative of the right atrium is at the midright atrium lateral wall. Because of the wide variation of oxygen saturation of blood entering the right atrium, a greater increase in oxygen saturation must be found between superior vena cava and right atrium than at the right ventricular or pulmonary arterial level to diagnose a left-to-right shunt. With repeated series of oxygen sampling, a smaller increase is needed to diagnose a left-to-right atrial shunt. An increase greater than 1.5 vol% of oxygen between superior vena cava and right atrium is significant. Other investigators have indicated significance if there is an increase in oxygen saturation of 10 percent if one series is performed and 7 percent if two series are performed.[24]

In neonates and infants, an increase in oxygen saturation in the right atrium results from isolated atrial septal defect, atrial septal defect related to a left-sided cardiac condition, endocardial cushion defect, anomalous pulmonary venous connection to right atrium or coronary sinus, left ventricular-right atrial communication, or ventricular septal defect with tricuspid insufficiency.

There may be a slight (usually less than 3 percent) increase in oxygen saturation between the right atrium and right ventricle, and there is normally little variation among oximetry samples in the right ventricle. An increase of 1 vol% or 7 percent on one or 5 percent on two oximetry series is considered significant of a left-to-right shunt at the ventricular level. Isolated ventricular septal defect is the most common cause, but other conditions associated with a ventricular septal defect and single ventricle may show this finding.

The saturations between the right ventricle and pulmonary artery are the same within the errors of the measurement technique. The presence of a left-to-right shunt at the pulmonary arterial level is diagnosed if there is a 0.5 vol% or 5 percent or 3 percent oxygen saturation increase from right ventricle to pulmonary artery on one or two series, respectively. Patent ductus arteriosus and aorticopulmonary window are the major conditions with left-to-right shunts at the pulmonary artery in the first year of life. Since the patent ductus arteriosus connects to the left pulmonary artery, saturated blood flows preferentially into the left lung, and, therefore, an increase in oxygen saturation is detected in the left pulmonary artery.

Occasionally, the presence of the defect or oximetry values reflecting its true magnitude may be recognized by the oximetry samples in the chamber immediately beyond the shunt—thus, an atrial septal defect may be found by an increase at the right ventricular level or a supracristal ventricular septal defect may be detected by increased oxygen saturation in the pulmonary artery.

The oxygen saturation of the pulmonary veins should be 96 percent and Po_2 should be 90 to 100 torr. In neonates and infants being catheterized from the inguinal area, pulmonary veins can usually be catheterized. In patients with pneumonia or atelectasis, a lower value of oxygen saturation is obtained from the vein draining the involved lobe. With sedation or hypoventilation, pulmonary venous Po_2 and O_2 saturation are reduced from each lobe and associated with elevated Pco_2. Infants with a large volume of pulmonary blood flow may have slightly reduced pulmonary venous oxygen saturation, and those with congestive cardiac failure or pulmonary edema may have even larger reductions.

If blood from a systemic artery is desaturated, the pulmonary veins should also be sampled to make certain the hypoxemia is unrelated to pulmonary disease.

A 5 percent decrease in oxygen saturation between the pulmonary veins and the aorta is needed to diagnose a right-to-left shunt. At the atrial level, a right-to-left shunt could occur through an atrial septal defect or foramen ovale, associated with a variety of conditions. A shunt at the ventricular level occurs with ventricular septal defect and pulmonary stenosis or pulmonary vascular disease, or with a single ventricle. A shunt at the aortic level occurs with truncus arteriosus or tetralogy of Fallot.

There are occasions when the aortic and pulmonary arterial oxygen saturations are identical, indicating an admixture lesion, such as total anomalous pulmonary venous connection, single atrium, single ventricle, truncus arteriosus, tricuspid atresia, pulmonary atresia, mitral atresia, or tetralogy of Fallot with pulmonary atresia.

In neonates, the ductus arteriosus may shunt right to left. Therefore, descending aortic oxygen saturation is lower than the ascending aortic oxygen saturation. A right-to-left ductal shunt can be detected by comparing right brachial arterial blood to samples drawn from the descending aorta or its tributaries.

Oximetry data can be used to calculate a number of variables about the circulation, especially when combined with information about the oxygen consumption. As indicated previously, the oxygen consumption can be measured in infants and used to calculate the cardiac output by the Fick principle. If the oxygen consumption is not measured, it can be assumed to be 120 to 130 $ml/mm/M^2$ in neonates or 150 to 160 $ml/mm/M^2$ for infants.[24] It is preferable to measure the oxygen consumption:

$$CO = \frac{V_{O_2}}{A\text{-}V_{O_2}\ Diff}$$

$$Qp = \frac{V_{O_2}}{PV\text{-}PA_{O_2}\ Diff}$$

$$Qs = \frac{V_{O_2}}{AO\text{-}MV_{O_2}\ Diff}$$

$$Qp/Qs = \frac{AO\text{-}MV_{O_2}\ Diff}{PV\text{-}PA_{O_2}\ Diff}$$

$$\text{L-R shunt }(\%) = \frac{PA\text{-}MV}{SA\text{-}MV} \times 100$$

$$\text{R-L shunt }(\%) = \frac{PV\text{-}SA}{SA\text{-}MV} \times 100$$

CO = cardiac output; V_{O_2} = oxygen consumption; A-V_{O_2} Diff = arteriovenous oxygen difference (in vol %); Qs = systemic blood flow; Qp = pulmonary blood flow; *AO* = aorta; MV = mixed venous; PV = pulmonary venous; PA = pulmonary arterial; SA = systemic artery; L-R shunt = left-to-right shunt; R-L shunt = right-to-left shunt.

There are a number of considerations and precautions about calculated blood flows by the Fick principle and these are discussed in a number of other texts.

Pressure

Pressure data are used to diagnose obstructive lesions, such as aortic or pulmonary stenosis, or to assess the severity of a condition, as the level of pulmonary arterial pressure in patients with left-to-right shunt.

RIGHT ATRIAL PRESSURE.   The mean right atrial pressure of neonates and infants is lower than in older children and is frequently 0 to 2 mm Hg, even in the presence of congestive cardiac failure. The a wave is the predominant wave form and is usually 5 to 7 mm Hg in amplitude.

The a wave and mean right atrial pressure are elevated in patients with obstruction to the tricuspid valve, decreased right ventricular compliance, or pericardial tamponade. The v wave is prominent in patients with tricuspid insufficiency.

RIGHT VENTRICULAR PRESSURE.   In normal infants, the right ventricular systolic pressure reflects pulmonary arterial systolic pressure. It is equal to left ventricular systolic pressure at birth and declines rapidly in the first week as pulmonary vascular resistance falls postnatally and reaches adult levels (25 mm Hg) by 1 week of age.[25]

Right ventricular systolic pressure is increased if there is obstruction to pulmonary blood flow from either pulmonary stenosis or increased pulmonary vascular resistance, in the presence of a large communication between the ventricles or great vessels, or from greatly increased pulmonary blood flow. In patients with obstruction to pulmonary blood flow coexisting with a ventricular septal defect, the right ventricular pressure contour shows a plateau-topped curve, while with an intact septum, it has a pointed, peaked contour.

PULMONARY ARTERIAL PRESSURE.   The pulmonary arterial pressure in normal neonates undergoes considerable change. Emmanouilides and co-workers[26] studied normal neonates and found a gradual decrease in pulmonary arterial pressures in the first 3 days of life, with the most abrupt decline occurring in the first 24 hours. The status of the ductus arteriosus, the degree of hypoxia, and the amount of placental transfusion affect the level and rate of decline of pulmonary arterial pressure. Under 1 hour of age, mean pulmonary arterial pressure equals or exceeds mean aortic pressure. Under 10 hours of age, the pulmonary arterial pressure equals 70 to 76/16 to 40 mm Hg, with mean values from 26 to 52 mm Hg. After 10 hours, systolic pressure gradually declines, and diastolic pressure falls abruptly. By 36 hours of age, the pressure is 32 to 40/10 to 22 mm Hg, with a mean of 20 to 31 mm Hg, and it reaches normal by 3 days. Krovetz and Goldbloom[27] found that after 1 week of age, the ratio of mean pulmonary arterial to mean systolic arterial pressure remains constant.

Pulmonary arterial pressure can be elevated because of increased resistance to blood flow through the lungs or increased volume of pulmonary blood flow. Increased resistance can occur at either a precapillary or postcapillary level. The pulmonary arterioles may narrow because of pulmonary vascular disease or pulmonary parenchymal disease. Any condition causing obstruction to blood flow into the left ventricle or left atrium, such as mitral stenosis or cor triatriatum, can also elevate pulmonary arterial pressure. In conditions with increased pulmonary resistance, the pulmonary pulse pressure is narrow (about 35 percent of peak systolic pressure).

Pulmonary hypertension also occurs in large communication at the ventricular or great vessel level with an increased pulmonary blood flow, but the pulse pressure is wide (at least 50 percent of peak pressure). The pulse pressure is also widened proximal to peripheral pulmonary arterial stenosis or in pulmonary valvular insufficiency.

Danilowicz and associates[28] found that a small (10 to 15 mm Hg) systolic pressure difference between the main pulmonary artery and branch pulmonary arteries in normal neonates subsequently disappeared. The gradient is presumably related to the acute angle of origin of the pulmonary arteries from the pulmonary trunk in infancy and subsequently disappears.

LEFT ATRIAL PRESSURE.   In the left atrium, the v wave is the predominant wave form, and although the left atrial pressure is higher than the right atrial pressure, the mean value is normally lower in infants than older children. We consider a mean pressure of 13 mm Hg as upper limits of normal, but usually it is less than 7 mm Hg.

In patients with large left-to-right shunts occurring distal to the mitral valve, the atrial pressures are elevated, particularly the v wave. In patients with obstruction to left ventricular filling, as from mitral stenosis or decreased left ventricular compliance, atrial pressures, particularly the a wave, are increased. The a wave may be the dominant wave form in patients with right-to-left atrial shunt, as in tricuspid atresia or total anomalous pulmonary venous connection.

The left atrial pressure is low and equal to the right atrial pressure in patients with a large atrial communication, but the presence of equal atrial pressures does not in itself indicate an atrial communication.

LEFT VENTRICULAR PRESSURE.   Peak left ventricular pressure in normal neonates ranges between 65 and 80 mm Hg and is slightly lower in premature infants. By 1 year of age, it is usually 90 to 100 mm Hg.

Left ventricular systolic pressure is increased in conditions with obstruction to left ventricular outflow, such as aortic stenosis, coarctation of the aorta, or systemic hypertension.

AORTIC PRESSURE.   Aortic pressures gradually increase in the first year of life, and the pulse pressure is usually 35 percent of the systolic pressure level. A wide pulse pressure is found in conditions with aortic runoff, such as patent ductus arteriosus, aorticopulmonary window, systemic arteriovenous fistula, truncus arteriosus, aortic insufficiency, or high output states. A narrow pulse pressure is found in aortic stenosis or low cardiac output.

Calculations

Pressure data can be combined with information about cardiac output to calculate vascular resistance according to the relationship:

Resistance = Pressure/Flow.

This can be calculated:

$$SVR = \frac{\overline{AO} - \overline{RA}}{SBF}$$

$$PAR = \frac{\overline{PA} - \overline{LA}}{PBF}$$

SVR = systemic vascular resistance; PAR = pulmonary arterial resistance; SBF = systemic blood flow; PBF = pulmonary blood flow; $\overline{AO}$ = mean aortic pressure; $\overline{\mathrm{RA}}$ = mean right atrial pressure; $\overline{\mathrm{PA}}$ = mean pulmonary arterial pressure; $\overline{\mathrm{LA}}$ = mean left atrial pressure.

Both the pulmonary and systemic vascular resistances are elevated at birth and subsequently fall. Although there are arguments against it, we have found it useful to express resistance on the basis of body surface area in terms of mm Hg/l/min/m^2, also called resistance units. On this basis, systemic vascular resistance is 10 to 12 units in infants and rises to 14 to 18 units in older children. In contrast, pulmonary vascular resistance is 8 to 10 units at birth and falls to less than 3 units by 8 weeks of age.

The area of a stenotic valvular orifice can be calculated, using pressure and flow data, by the formula developed by Gorlin and Gorlin. We have rarely used these formulae in infants because of inaccuracies in calculating flow from assumed oxygen consumption. Most infants with stenotic valves catheterized in the first year of life have obviously severe stenosis, and such calculations are not required.

ANGIOGRAPHY

The principal use of angiography is to establish a diagnosis. Of all the data derived from catheterization, angiography provides the greatest amount of information about the heart of symptomatic neonates. It is also used to determine ventricular and atrial volumes, providing details about the severity of many conditions and their effect upon the myocardium.

Many of the specific indications and the details of angiography, such as projection and choice of x-ray technique, are discussed later in relation to specific cardiac malformations. Although there are many specific indications, there are two general indications for specific types of angiography. A right ventriculogram should be performed in any patient whose right ventricular systolic pressure is at systemic levels, and an aortogram should be performed to exclude a patent ductus arteriosus in any patient whose aortic and pulmonary arterial pressures are equal.

Before making any injection, the site of injection should be identified by recording the pressure and obtaining an oxygen saturation. In addition, a test injection of contrast medium should be made by rapidly injecting by hand a small amount of contrast material to verify the position of the catheter. It is important that the catheter tip is not wedged into the wall of a chamber and that the contrast material can flow freely from the catheter.

For optimal visualization, the contrast material should be injected as rapidly as possible. The size and length of the catheter are the major determinants of the speed at which the injection can be made. In neonates, we use a No. 5F NIH angiocatheter, 50 cm long, and find it gives us very satisfactory angiography. In infants, we often use a No. 6F NIH angiocatheter.

In infants, Hypaque and Renografin are the contrast media commonly used. These contrast media contain high concentrations of sodium, combined with iodine (iothalanat). Because of the myocardial depressive effects of high sodium concentrations, contrast media currently combine both methylglucanine and sodium-iodine salts. Methylglucanine, however, has a higher viscosity than sodium iodine, so that most contrast media have equal portions of sodium and methylglucanine salts. For neonates and infants, 50 to 60 percent concentrations of these contrast media are used. The contrast media should be warmed to body temperature to reduce viscosity.

The amount of contrast medium given per injection and the total amount given to any infant during a catheterization vary. When injecting into an enlarged chamber or in the presence of a large left-to-right shunt, 1.5 to 2 ml/kg is used instead of the usual 1 mg/kg. For aortography, slightly less is needed unless there is a large aortic flow, as in patent ductus arteriosus or truncus arteriosus. The total amount of contrast material injected should probably not exceed 4 ml/kg, with a smaller limit in infants with severe congestive cardiac failure or in premature infants. Occasionally, when this limit has been reached, the diagnosis may still not be clear. The physician must then consider the infant's condition, the interval over which the contrast material has been given, and how critical it is to establish an immediate diagnosis. We have exceeded 4 ml/kg when the urine output has been satisfactory, the contrast injections have been made over a period of a couple of hours, the patient (usually a neonate) is critically ill, and immediate decisions need to be made about further management.

The angiogram may be recorded by cine technique or by using a rapid film changer. The cine technique is faster, since it usually does not require moving the patient, and the results can be viewed almost immediately on video recorder. Cine technique is very useful, particularly in assessing valvular insufficiency and when critical events are occurring at a rapid rate. Cineangiography can be used to study the volumes of cardiac chambers. The technique and normal values have been reported.[29-31] The film changer shows anatomic detail and is preferred in many infants because the cardiac malformations may be complicated. Since anatomic detail is often needed to clearly diagnose the condition, individual frames of angiograms obtained on the film changer can be studied. There are several disadvantages to the film changer. The patient must be moved to the film changer, during which the catheter tip may be dislodged to a less favorable or a more hazardous position. In addition, the films must be removed in the dark, and they are not available for viewing for at least 15 min.

Newer angiographic techniques involve angling and rotating the patient in various projections to better visualize certain anatomic relationships.[32-34] These projections can clarify, for instance, mitral valve-semilunar valve relationships, abnormalities of left ventricular outflow tract, details of endocardial cushion defects, and anatomy of the bifurcation of the pulmonary arteries.

Angiograms can be performed through umbilical arterial catheters, which are usually made of polyethylene. Polyethylene catheters were not designed primarily for angiography. They cannot withstand high injection pressures, may have only end holes, and are not stiff. Because of the end hole and the flexibility, the catheter tip can recoil during the injection. We had one instance of aortic laceration occurring as the catheter straightened following the recoil. Therefore, we use a polyethylene catheter and inject at low pressure, but we prefer to use polyethylene feeding tubes that have an occluded end.

COMPLICATIONS

Complications can occur during cardiac catheterization directly from the procedure or from a problem arising from the stress placed on an acutely ill infant.

In 1968, a cooperative study on cardiac catheterization was reported.[35] This multicenter study included the experience with cardiac catheterization in 1,161 neonates and infants. Of these, 105 had complications, the rate being higher (15 percent) in infants less than 2 months of age. The death rate of catheterization in neonates (<30 days) was 20/325 (6.2 percent) and in infants between 1 and 2 months 9/155 (5.8 percent). Among 681 infants between 2 and 12 months of age, 9 (1.2 percent) died. Deaths occurred most frequently from perforation of the heart, cardiac arrhythmia, or from deterioration in the catheterization laboratory or, subsequently, on the ward. Deterioration occurred most often in the critically ill and those with inoperable conditions, although at times no explanation was found. This extensive study described many individual complications, and most of these will be discussed in this chapter.

Subsequent to the cooperative study, Stanger and associates[36] reported a 3-year experience with 1,160 catheterizations in children, 439 of the children being under 1 year of age. These authors, who had been involved in the cooperative study, modified their catheterization procedures according to the findings of that study and reported a lower rate of complications. There were 2 deaths among 218 neonates and 1 death among 221 infants. In this excellent study, the incidence of major complications was similar to the cooperative study, but many of the complications could be treated with relatively simple methods.

The authors believe that the improved mortality and morbidity were related to (1) prompt recognition and treatment of metabolic abnormalities, such as acidosis, hypoglycemia, and hypocalcemia, and the judicious use of oxygen; (2) changes in volume and type of contrast material; and (3) the development of flow-directed catheters, which reduce the incidence of cardiac perforation and shorten the duration of catheterization.

Perforation of the Heart

Cardiac chambers or great vessels can be perforated by the catheter tip,[36-42] particularly when stiff catheters are used. Perforation occurs most often through (1) the left atrial appendage when attempting to pass the catheter into the left ventricle, (2) the right ventricle when attempting to pass the catheter into the aorta through a ventricular septal defect, and (3) the right atrial appendage in attempts to enter the left atrium.

Perforation of the heart must be suspected when (1) the catheter course is abnormal, (2) systemic or ventricular pressure drops suddenly, (3) blood cannot be withdrawn from the catheter, or (4) the patient's status changes.

If perforation of the heart is believed to occur, the catheter tip should not be withdrawn from its location. Attempts should be made to withdraw blood from the catheter. If the tip of the catheter is within a cardiac chamber, blood can be withdrawn. If none is obtained, the catheter is either clotted, or the tip is within the pericardium. One milliliter of contrast material should be injected slowly through the catheter to verify the position. If it is in the pericardium, the contrast material should be withdrawn from the pericardial sac, since it is hyperosmotic, and the volume of fluid in the pericardial sac could be increased.

It has been recommended that when either atrium has been perforated, a thoracotomy should be performed, the catheter removed, and the perforation closed. If a perforation occurs, regardless of the site, our policy has been to call the cardiovascular surgeon and have him available in the catheterization laboratory. Whole blood is ordered and made available in the laboratory, and a means to monitor systemic pressure is established. If there is distress, the infant is intubated, and an intravenous solution of isoproterenol and a pericardiocentesis tray are prepared. The catheter tip is withdrawn into the heart, and pressure is monitored. The catheter can be used as an intravenous line.

Pressures and pulse rate are monitored, the cardiac silhouette is fluoroscoped periodically, and the infant is observed. If there is deterioration, blood and isoproterenol are infused, and pericardiocentesis is performed. Even with an atrial perforation, we have not had to perform more than one pericardiocentesis in an individual patient.

Perforation can be prevented by flow-directed catheters, knowledge of the anatomy, and gentleness during manipulation of the catheter.

Intramyocardial or transmyocardial injection of contrast material is potentially a serious complication. This complication occurs most frequently in the trabeculated ventricles in patients with complicated anatomy or when the catheter course is complicated, such as an interrupted inferior vena cava, or with right ventriculography. The chances of myocardial injection on right ventriculography are less when the catheter tip is withdrawn into the right ventricle from a great vessel, rather than merely advanced into the right ventricle.

Intramyocardial injection of contrast material can be minimized by performing angiograms through catheters with occluded ends or with flow-directed catheters. In the latter, since the holes are proximal to the balloon, they cannot be wedged into the ventricular wall. A test injection of contrast material should always be made prior to angiography to verify the position of the catheter tip and to make certain that contrast material flows freely. An occasional PVC before a ventriculogram is preferable to a perfectly quiet tracing, for the former indicates the catheter tip is free within the ventricle, whereas in the latter it may be wedged.

Intramyocardial injection can cause widening of the QRS complex and ST and T wave changes. Occasionally, ventricular arrhythmias, hypotension, or low cardiac output may develop and must be treated promptly. Usually, the myocardial stain of contrast material disappears within 15 min. Krovetz and associates[25] showed histologic changes of myocardial necrosis, hemorrhage, and subsequent scarring following angiocardiography.

Vascular Complications

Arterial complications occurring from various arterial routes of catheterization were discussed earlier in this chapter, and the general problems of arterial complications, methods of prevention, and techniques for the closure of arteriotomies are discussed well by Stanger and associates.[36]

In 688 catheterizations of neonates and infants, we have had 3 instances where the femoral vein or one of its major tributaries tore and 13 instances where the saphenous vein tore. This number can be reduced by careful dissection, good exposure, isolating a long segment of vein, and gentle handling of the vein during insertion of the catheter.

Hemorrhage can occur from tearing a vein, but otherwise blood loss should be minimal during the procedure. Excessive blood loss is the responsibility of the physician and can easily be and must be prevented by the physician. When catheterizing a vein, the distal end and any tributaries should be ligated and a simple knot placed around the proximal end of the vein once the catheter has been inserted. Even with the proximal tie about the catheter and vein, the catheter can be manipulated easily, and bleeding does not occur. If oozing or bleeding develops, the catheterization should be momentarily stopped and the source of the bleeding identified.

Blood loss may also occur while catheters are being exchanged, particularly if the infant is crying, thereby elevating venous pressure. A pacifier or sugar nipple will quiet the baby during this critical time.

Wound Infections

Wound infections rarely occur from cutdown procedures in the arm but can occur in the inguinal area, perhaps because of the moisture in this area. Following the cutdown, the wound should be thoroughly flushed and the subcutaneous tissues closed by gut sutures. This eliminates a dead space and approximates the skin so that it will not be closed under tension.

Arrhythmias

Stanger and associates,[36] in their review, found 59 instances of arrhythmias among 439 procedures in neonates and infants, an incidence which was higher than that found in older children.

Arrhythmias, usually isolated premature atrial or ventricular beats, occur in virtually all patients undergoing cardiac catheterization and result from manipulation of the catheter. Most arrhythmias lead to no serious problem and stop when the catheter is withdrawn from the heart.

Paroxysmal atrial tachycardia can develop as the catheter is being manipulated in an atrium, particularly when trying to form a loop. In the experience of Stanger et al.,[36] it occurred in nearly 6 percent of the infants undergoing study. They comment on its frequent occurrence in infants with complete transposition of the great vessels or Ebstein's malformation, and this has been our experience also. Atrial flutter occurs less frequently but does occur in infants with enlarged atria, particularly Ebstein's malformation.

When paroxysmal atrial tachycardia or atrial flutter develops, the catheter tip should be withdrawn to the vena cava. If it persists, the catheter tip should be advanced into the ventricle to produce a PVC. This maneuver often converts the rhythm. Most episodes of paroxysmal atrial tachycardia revert within 10 min. If it persists, attempts at vagal stimulation should be applied but, in our experience, are rarely effective.

Cyanotic patients become more hypoxemic during these episodes, and patients with poor myocardial effusion or obstructive valvular lesions may have markedly reduced cardiac output. In these patients or those with persistent tachycardia, cardioversion is needed.

Ventricular premature contractions, bigeminy, or short episodes of ventricular tachycardia can develop during manipulation in the ventricle but usually revert to sinus rhythm upon withdrawal of the catheter. Ventricular fibrillation can develop, particularly in sick neonates, and should be treated promptly with cardioversion. Occasionally, with manipulation of the catheter tip into the outflow area, a pattern of right bundle-branch block can develop. This is usually transient.

Heart block can develop but usually reverts spontaneously. We have never had to use a pacemaker to treat this complication.

Sinus bradycardia occurs, particularly in neonates, and has serious effects. When sinus bradycardia develops, pH and Po_2 should be measured promptly, oxygen should be administered, and the catheter should be withdrawn from the heart. The bradycardia may be transient, but if it is persistent, intravenous atropine should be given, and respiratory support may be needed. If bradycardia recurs, atropine should be given, and acid-base balance, temperature, and oxygenation should be checked because bradycardia often indicates a complicating factor.

Hypoxic Episodes

In neonates or infants with cyanotic cardiac anomalies associated with diminished pulmonary blood flow, hypoxic spells can occur during catheterization, particularly if an arrhythmia occurs, acidosis develops, or blood loss is excessive. Adequate hydration, monitoring, minimal blood loss, and expeditious catheterization help prevent this complication. In neonates with pulmonary atresia, Prostaglandin E_1 infusion during the study can maintain ductal patency and maintain systemic arterial oxygen saturation above the level which leads to acidosis and its complications.

Obstruction of Orifice

Paul and Rudolph[43] report the complication of obstruction of the pulmonary valve by the catheter. In infants, if the right ventricular pressure is suprasystemic, we do not attempt to pass the catheter into the pulmonary artery because of the potential of developing this complication. The additional information is unnecessary for the diagnosis, and arrhythmias can occur during such maneuvers. This complication is recognized by increasing cyanosis, bradycardia, and restlessness.

Acidosis

Acidosis can develop from a number of different factors during cardiac catheterization: hypothermia, sedation, hypoxemia, low cardiac output, and pulmonary complications. Since infants have limited renal and pulmonary compensatory mechanisms, the infant should be carefully observed for development of acidosis. If acidosis develops, it should be promptly treated, and underlying causes should be sought and corrected. In one study, 91 percent of infants had uncompensated acidosis at completion of catheterization, and the degree was more pronounced in young cyanotic infants with pulmonary congestion.[44] Angiography contributes to acidosis, since it adds organic anions to the circulation and abruptly reduces pH.[45]

Renal Complications

Renal medullary necrosis,[46,47] renal venous thrombosis,[47] and renal tubular changes have been found in infants following angiography. Gruskin and associates[46] studied the urine of infants less than 3 months of age following angiography. Eight of 30 developed hematuria, which lasted as long as 28 hours, and each received more than 3 ml/kg of contrast material. The renal abnormalities are perhaps related to decreased oxygen delivery to the medulla and to osmotic diuresis. Renal changes are more likely to occur in patients with hypoxemia, dehydration, low cardiac output, or in newborns who normally have reduced renal function. Renal complications can be minimized by limiting the amount of contrast material and maintaining adequate fluid intake and urine output. Spacing contrast injections over a period of time and fluoroscopy of the bladder to observe if contrast material is being excreted are preventive steps if the physician cannot limit the total amount of contrast material injected.

Temperature

As indicated, the temperature of neonates or infants must be carefully monitored. In severely ill neonates, hypothermia may develop, but with warming pads and increased environmental temperature, the frequency and severity of hypothermia can be reduced. Hyperthermia is another complication and occurred in 36 percent of infants and children studied by Gilladoga and associates.[48] Hyperthermia is usually transient, generally less than 39C, and appears related to the number of angiograms. Bacteremia is rarely a cause. Observation is required, and, generally, the temperature returns to normal within 4 hours of catheterization. If it persists, the infant should be investigated for sources of fever.

BALLOON ATRIOSEPTOSTOMY

Although there are complications, such as balloon embolization,[49] inability to deflate the balloon,[50] intraabdominal hemorrhage,[51] atrial perforation,[52] and avulsion of the inferior vena cava, with improved catheters, experience, care to follow the procedures, and observance of the precautions outlined by Rashkind,[53] balloon atrial septostomy can be performed with little morbidity. We have had no important complications in over 6 years. It is necessary to make certain that no air bubbles are injected into the balloon, to slowly inflate the balloon so as not to damage the pulmonary vein, to carefully observe the catheter course so that it is not across the AV valve, and to make certain not to pull the catheter into the inferior vena cava.

REFERENCES

1. Markowitz M, Weidman WH, McNamara DG: Standards for a cardiac catheterization laboratory. A guide for cardiologists and for institutions sponsoring cardiac catheterization laboratories. Circulation 42:557, 1970
2. Wessel HU, Rorem D, Muster AJ, Acevedo RE, Paul MH: Continuous determination of oxygen uptake in sedated infants and children during cardiac catheterization. Am J Cardiol 24:376, 1969
3. Fixler DE, Carrell T, Browne R, Willis K, Miller WW: Oxygen consumption in infants and children during cardiac catheterization under different sedation regimens. Circulation 50:788, 1974
4. Lister G, Hoffman JIE, Rudolph AM: Oxygen uptake in infants and children: A simple method for measurement. Pediatrics 53:656, 1974
5. Baum D, Brown AC, Church SC: Effect of sedation on oxygen consumption of children undergoing cardiac catheterization. Pediatrics 39:891, 1967
6. Baum D, Mullins G: Core temperature in infants undergoing cardiac catheterization. Pediatrics 36:88, 1965
7. Seldinger SI: Catheter replacement of the needle in percutaneous arteriography. A new technique. Acta Radiol 39:368, 1953
8. Lurie PR, Armer RM, Klatte EC: Percutaneous guidewire catheterization—diagnosis and therapy. Am J Dis Child 106:189, 1963

9. Sunderland CO, Nichols GM, Henken DP, et al.: Percutaneous cardiac catheterization and atrial balloon septostomy in pediatrics. J Pediatr 89:584, 1976
10. Porter CJ, Gillette PC, Mullins CE, McNamara DG: Cardiac catheterization in the neonate. A comparison of three techniques. J Pediatr 93:97, 1978
11. Carter GA, Girod DA, Hurwitz RA: Percutaneous cardiac catheterization of the neonate. Pediatrics 55:662, 1975
12. Neches WH, Mullins CE, Williams RL, Vargo TA, McNamara DG: Percutaneous sheath cardiac catheterization. Am J Cardiol 30:378, 1972
13. Gay JH: Cardiac catheterization in small infants: The percutaneous approach. Am J Cardiol 36:493, 1975
14. Takahashi M, Petry EL, Lurie PR, Kirkpatrick SE, Stanton RE: Percutaneous heart catheterization in infants and children. I. Catheter placement and manipulation with guide wires. Circulation 42:1037, 1970
15. Kirkpatrick SE, Takahashi M, Petry EL, Stanton RE, Lurie PR: Percutaneous heart catheterization in infants and children. II. Prospective study of results and complications in 127 consecutive cases. Circulation 42:1049, 1970
16. Boros SJ, Nystrom JF, Thompson TR, Reynolds JW, Williams HJ: Leg growth following umbilical artery catheter-associated thrombus formation. A 4-year follow-up. J Pediatr 87:973, 1975
17. Linde LM, Higashino SM, Berman G, Sapin SO, Emmanouilides GC: Umbilical vessel cardiac catheterization and angiocardiography. Circulation 34:984, 1966
18. Sapin SO, Linde LM, Emmanouilides GC: Umbilical vessel angiocardiography in the newborn infant. Pediatrics 31:946, 1963
19. Emmanouilides GC, Hoy RC: Transumbilical aortography and selective arteriography in newborn infants. Pediatrics 39:337, 1967
20. Newfeld EA, Purcell C, Paul MH, Cole RB, Muster AJ: Transumbilical balloon atrial septostomy in 16 infants with transposition of the great arteries. Pediatrics 54:495, 1974
21. Stanger P, Heymann MA, Hoffman JIE, Rudolph AM: Use of the Swan-Ganz catheter in cardiac catheterization on infants and children. Am Heart J 83:749, 1972
22. Swan HJC, Ganz W, Forrester J, et al.: Catheterization of the heart in man with use of a flow-directed balloon-tipped catheter. N Engl J Med 283:447, 1970
23. Taketa RM, Sahn DJ, Simon AL, Pappelbaum SJ, Friedman WF: Catheter position in congenital cardiac malformations. Circulation 51:749, 1975
24. Rudolph AM: Congenital Diseases of the Heart. Chicago, Year Book, 1974, p 120
25. Krovetz LJ, Shanklin DR, Schiebler GL: Serious and fatal complications of catheterization and angiocardiography in infants and children. Am Heart J 76:39, 1968
26. Emmanouilides GC, Moss AJ, Duffie ER Jr, Adams FH: Pulmonary arterial pressure changes in human newborn infants from birth to 3 days of age. J Pediatr 65:327, 1964
27. Krovetz LJ, Goldbloom S: Normal standards for cardiovascular data. II. Pressure and vascular resistances. Johns Hopkins Med J 130:187, 1972
28. Danilowicz D, Rudolph AM, Hoffman JIE, Heymann MA: Physiologic pressure differences between main and branch pulmonary arteries in infants. Circulation 45:410, 1972
29. Graham TP Jr, Jarmakani JM, Canent RV Jr, Morrow MN: Left heart volume estimation in infancy and childhood. Re-evaluation of methodology and normal values. Circulation 43:895, 1971
30. Graham TP Jr, Jarmakani JM, Atwood GF, Canent RV Jr: Right ventricular volume determinations in children. Normal values and observations with volume or pressure overload. Circulation 47:144, 1973
31. Graham TP Jr, Atwood GF, Faulkner SL, Nelson JH: Right atrial volume mea-

surements from biplane cineangiocardiography. Methodology, normal values, and alterations with pressure or volume overload. Circulation 49:709, 1974

32. Fellows KE, Keane JF, Freed MD: Angled views in cineangiocardiography of congenital heart disease. Circulation 56:485, 1977

33. Bargeron LM Jr, Elliott LP, Soto B, Bream PR, Curry GC: Axial cineangiography in congenital heart disease. Section I. Concept, technical and anatomic considerations. Circulation 56:1075, 1977

34. Elliott LP, Bargeron LM Jr, Bream PR, Soto B, Curry GC: Axial cineangiography in congenital heart disease. Section II. Specific lesions. Circulation 56:1084, 1977

35. Braunwald E, Swan HJC (eds): Monograph 20: Cooperative study on cardiac catheterization. Circulation 37–38[Suppl III]:1, 1968

36. Stanger P, Heymann MA, Tarnoff H, Hoffman JIE, Rudolph AM: Complications of cardiac catheterization of neonates, infants, and children. A three-year study. Circulation 50:595, 1974

37. Kazenelson G, Rowe RD, Bender HW, Haller JA Jr: Nonfatal accidental atrial perforation during cardiac catheterization in the newborn. J Pediatr 69:127, 1966

38. Lawton RL, Rossi NP, Funk DC: Intracardiac perforation. Arch Surg 98:213, 1969

39. Lurie PR, Grajo MZ: Accidental cardiac puncture during right heart catheterization. Pediatrics 29:283, 1962

40. Pocock WA, Barlow JB, Berezowski A: Perforation of the heart during cardioangiography. Case report of a six month old infant. Am J Cardiol 11:819, 1963

41. Gengos DC, Celermajer JM, Morgan WW Jr: A simplified method of internal cardiac compression and open pericardial drainage in the infant. J Pediatr 72:543, 1968

42. Gorlin R: Perforations and other cardiac complications. Monograph 20: Cooperative study on cardiac catheterization. Circulation 37–38[Suppl III]:36, 1968

43. Paul MH, Rudolph AM: Pulmonary valve obstruction during cardiac catheterization. Circulation 18:53, 1958

44. Srouji MH, Rashkind WJ: The effect of cardiac catheterization on the acid-base status of infants with congenital heart disease. J Pediatr 75:943, 1969

45. Lichtman MA, Murphy MS, Whitbeck AA, Pogal M, Lipchik EO: Acidification of plasma by the red cell due to radiographic contrast materials. Circulation 52:943, 1975

46. Gruskin AB, Oetliker OH, Wolfish NM, et al.: Effects of angiography on renal function and histology in infants and piglets. J Pediatr 76:41, 1970

47. Gilbert EF, Khoury GH, Hogan GR, Jones B: Hemorrhagic renal necrosis in infancy: Relationship to radiopaque compounds J Pediatr 76:49, 1970

48. Gilladoga AC, Levin AR, Deely WJ, Engle M: Cardiac catheterization and febrile episodes. Pediatrics 80:215, 1972

49. Vogel JHK: Balloon embolization during atrial septostomy. Circulation 42:155, 1970

50. Ellison RC, Plauth WH Jr, Gazzaniga AB, Fyler DC: Inability to deflate catheter balloon: A complication of balloon atrial septostomy. J Pediatr 76:604, 1970

51. Ehmke DA, Durnin RE, Lauer RM: Intra-abdominal hemorrhage complicating a balloon atrial septostomy for transposition of the great arteries. Pediatrics 45:289, 1970

52. Venables AW: Balloon atrial septostomy in complete transposition of great arteries in infancy. Br Heart J 32:61, 1970

53. Rashkind WJ: The complications of balloon atrioseptostomy. J Pediatr 76:649, 1970

8 Hemodynamics and Classification of Cardiac Anomalies

This chapter summarizes some of the information about the fetal and transitional circulation that has been excellently reviewed by Dawes[1] and Rudolph.[2,3] Because the pulmonary arterial system shows such major changes in the neonatal and early infancy periods and because these changes have important effects on the circulation of many congenital anomalies, pulmonary vascular resistance is discussed. Finally, a classification of congenital cardiac disease is presented.

FETAL CIRCULATION

The structure and function of the fetal circulation differ in many ways from the adult circulation. In the fetus, blood is oxygenated in the placenta and returns to the heart through the umbilical vein (Fig. 8-1). Part of the blood passes through the liver, preferentially flowing to the left lobe, while the fetal portal venous blood flows preferentially to the right lobe. A variable amount bypasses the liver through the ductus venosus and mixes with the small amount of blood returning from the lower extremities in the inferior vena cava.

The total inferior vena caval flow, representing umbilical venous, portal venous, and inferior vena caval flow, is 65 to 75 percent of total venous return to the heart. Inferior vena caval flow is preferentially shunted through the foramen ovale into the left atrium because of the position of the crista dividens of the atrial septum. The foramen ovale can really be considered to face the inferior vena cava and to open off the inferior vena cava.

The blood from the head and upper extremities returns in the superior vena cava and accounts for 25 percent of venous return to the heart. Various studies have indicated that only a minute quantity of superior vena caval blood crosses the atrial septum, but most of the blood joins the remaining inferior vena caval flow and coronary sinus blood to enter the right ventricle.

Right ventricular blood is ejected into the pulmonary artery, but only a small amount of right ventricular output flows through the lungs. Most flows through the ductus arteriosus to the descending aorta, with a large amount

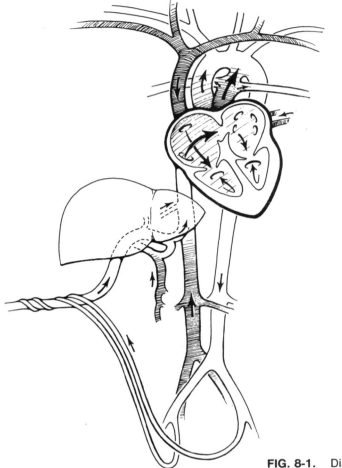

FIG. 8-1.   Diagram of fetal circulation.

passing through the umbilical arteries to the placenta. Only a small amount flows to the abdominal organs and lower extremities.

Pulmonary venous return represents only about 10 percent of venous return to the heart. The left ventricle receives predominantly inferior vena caval blood and also the small volume of pulmonary venous blood. Since it receives blood predominantly from the placenta, the left ventricular oxygen saturation is higher than the right ventricular saturation. Left ventricular output flows to the head and upper extremities, and a small amount passes through the aortic isthmus into the descending aorta.

The division of blood flow in the right atrium leads to blood with a higher oxygen saturation being delivered to the coronary arteries and brain, and that with a lower saturation being delivered to the placenta.

The pathways of fetal blood flow are principally governed by the relative resistances of the pulmonary and systemic circulations. In the fetus, pulmonary resistance is elevated primarily because of the low oxygen environment of the fetus. This relatively hypoxic state causes pulmonary vasoconstriction. Only a minor portion of the elevated pulmonary vascular resistance can be accounted for by the unexpanded state of the lungs in utero. In the fetus, systemic vascular resistance is decreased because the placenta is a low-resistance organ.

Unlike the adult circulation in which the ventricles and their respective circulations are in series, the two sides of the heart and systemic and pulmonary circulations in the fetus are in parallel. Therefore, distribution of blood flow is considered as a percentage of combined ventricular output (Table 8-1).

CHANGES IN CIRCULATION AT BIRTH

At birth, abrupt changes occur in the circulation that are followed by more gradual changes in the next few hours. Finally, the circulation approaches adult circulation in several weeks. The most dramatic events relate to the neonatal changes in pulmonary and systemic vascular resistances.

Systemic resistance increases abruptly with the separation of the infant from the placenta. The placenta has been a low-resistance organ and has received 40 to 50 percent of the combined ventricular output. The elimination of the placenta from the circulation doubles the systemic vascular resistance. Elimination of the placenta also markedly reduces inferior vena caval blood flow. With respiration, oxygen saturation improves, and this relieves the hypoxic pulmonary vasoconstriction, causing a prompt fall in pulmonary vascular resistance and an increase in volume of pulmonary blood flow. Thus the volume of pulmonary venous return increases. This increase, coupled with a decrease in inferior vena caval blood flow, causes functional closure of the foramen ovale.

TABLE 8-1

Distribution of Blood Flow in Fetus*

SITE	FLOW (%)	SATURATION (%)
Right ventricle	66	55
Ductus	59	55
Pulmonary artery	7	55
Descending aorta	69	60
Left ventricle	34	65
Aortic isthmus	10	65
Inferior vena cava	69	70
Superior vena cava	21	40
Foramen ovale	27	—
Placenta	40–50	—

* Flow expressed in percentage of combined left and right ventricular outputs; percentage of oxygen saturation from various sites given.

Flow through the ductus arteriosus remains right to left for periods up to 1 hour after birth, but as pulmonary vascular resistance falls, flow through the ductus becomes bidirectional and, subsequently, left to right. Usually the ductus arteriosus closes by 18 hours of age. Increased oxygen saturation is the major factor causing closure of the muscular ductus arteriosus. The role of vasoactive substances, such as bradykinin and prostaglandins, in normal closure of the ductus needs further exploration.

Following these immediate changes, the circulation undergoes more gradual evolution during the first week of life. The ductus venosus closes between 3 and 7 days of age, but the mechanism of its closure is unknown. The foramen ovale is closed, and gradually the valve of the foramen ovale seals to the atrial septum. This process takes months or years, and in 25 percent of adults, a valvular competent foramen ovale may persist. Conditions causing an increased atrial pressure, either right or left, may open the foramen ovale, allowing a shunt. In full-term infants, the ductus arteriosus, following its constriction, is anatomically closed by thrombosis and then fibrosis, the process usually being complete by 2 weeks of age. The process is delayed in premature infants or in some infants with conditions associated with hypoxemia.

The other major change occurs in the pulmonary circulation. With the increase in oxygen levels, the pulmonary vascular resistance falls dramatically, and following closure of the ductus arteriosus, right ventricular and pulmonary arterial systolic pressures fall in a parallel manner. Pulmonary blood flow increases. The immediate fall is related principally to release of hypoxic vasoconstriction and partially to expansion of the lungs. Following these immediate events, there is a more gradual decrease in pulmonary vascular resistance, related to thinning of the media of the small pulmonary arteries. This process, which continues until about 2 months of age, probably occurs in response to the fall in pulmonary arterial pressure. The other effect, lowering pulmonary vascular resistance during this time and continuing into childhood, is the continual growth of the lung and further branching of bronchioles and associated arteries and veins as new alveolar units are formed, leading to a greater cross-sectional area of the pulmonary arterial bed.

PULMONARY VASCULATURE

There are two conflicting views about the development of small pulmonary arteries in utero. Wagenvoort and associates[4] showed that medial thickness, measured as a percent of external diameter of an artery, remained constant (between 14 and 17 percent) in the late fetal life and decreased postnatally. These authors, however, also determined an index of medial surface area by relating arterial media to parenchyma and showed that this index gradually increased during fetal life and fell postnatally.

Naeye[5] also studied fetal arterial changes. He found an increase in smooth muscle in both systemic and pulmonary arterioles during fetal life and also found that the relative muscular mass in the pulmonary circuit slightly exceeded that in the systemic circuit. Following birth, systemic arterial muscle mass increased, while pulmonary arterial muscle mass decreased. He compared the area of medial muscle to the area of the media and found that this ratio doubled during fetal life and showed a 40 percent decrease in the first 2 weeks of life. He assumed these changes were due to increase in medial muscle mass in the fetus and to decrease in postnatal life.

More information is required to understand the prenatal changes of pulmonary vasculature, although the experience with premature infants with persistence of patent ductus arteriosus who develop congestive cardiac failure soon after birth suggests that perhaps the media is not as fully developed and that the arteries attain adult characteristics sooner than in a full-term infant.

Because of the amount of smooth muscle in the small arteries in the lungs of neonates and infants, these vessels are considerably more reactive to pharmacologic agents and hypoxemia. Although in the normal neonate the pulmonary arterial musculature regresses markedly by 2 months, even at this age the vessels remain reactive. If elevated pulmonary arterial pressure is present because of a large ventricular septal defect or pulmonary parenchymal disease and resultant hypoxemia, the thickened medial musculature persists. If the factors causing elevated pressure are corrected, the pulmonary arteries mature, and pulmonary vascular resistance falls.

The hypoxic stimulus to pulmonary vasoconstriction is accentuated in the presence of acidosis.[6] Figure 8-2 shows that with hypoxia, the pulmonary vas-

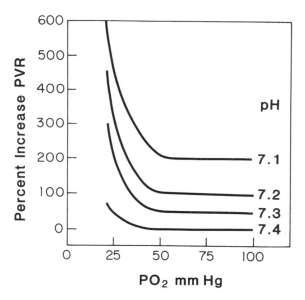

FIG. 8-2. Relationship between P_{O_2} and pulmonary vascular resistance (PVR). (From Rudolph and Yuan: J Clin Invest 45:399, 1966)

cular resistance rises, but the rate of rise and the values obtained are considerably higher when acidosis coexists.

In neonates or young infants with pulmonary or cardiac disease, hypoxemia and acidosis not infrequently develop. These factors, combined with a vasoreactive pulmonary arterial tree, can profoundly alter the circulation, particularly if there is a communication at the ventricular or ductal level. This accounts for the development of a reversing ductus arteriosus in many neonates with respiratory distress syndrome.

Chronic hypoxemia can maintain the pulmonary vasculature and be a factor in patients living at higher altitudes, such as the Colorado Rockies, by preventing full maturation of the lungs even in normal individuals. In infants with large communications at the ventricular or great vessel level, the pulmonary vascular resistance may be elevated. This limits pulmonary blood flow but is associated with earlier development of intimal and fibrotic changes of pulmonary vascular disease.

VENTRICULAR ANATOMY

Ventricular shape and wall thickness reflect the pressures to which ventricles are submitted. An example is the left ventricular hypertrophy that develops in patients with aortic stenosis. In the fetal circulation, right ventricular pressure is elevated secondary to the high level of pulmonary vascular resistance. As the fetus grows and pulmonary vascular resistance increases, the thickness of the right ventricular wall equals that of the left ventricular wall, and right ventricular weight exceeds left ventricular weight. The shape of the fetal right ventricle resembles that of the left ventricle in being round and conical. As pulmonary vascular resistance and right ventricular systolic pressure fall postnatally, the right ventricular free wall thins, so that by 1 month of age, right and left ventricular weights are equal, following which left ventricular weight increases considerably faster than that of the right ventricle. The right ventricle in this process assumes a crescent or bellowslike shape, as in the adult. The left ventricular wall becomes thicker because of rising systemic vascular resistance at birth and subsequent rise in aortic pressure.

If a congenital cardiac anomaly is present that maintains right ventricular systolic pressure, such as in infants with tetralogy of Fallot or transposition of the great vessels, right ventricular weight, wall thickness, and shape are maintained. Thickness of the ventricular wall affects ventricular compliance. A thicker wall decreases compliance and impedes ventricular filling.

The shape of the ventricles is probably important in determining their response to different types of overload. The left ventricle generally can accommodate increased pressure load better than it can increased volume. LaPlace's law helps to understand the relationship between anatomy and function, but it is an oversimplification:

$$T = Pr$$
T = tension; P = pressure; r = radius.

LaPlace's law indicates that in a cylindrical object, a certain level of tension must be developed in the wall to maintain that pressure-volume relationship.

In the left ventricle, pressure is high, and the radius is small. If left ventricular systolic pressure increases since the radius is small, only small changes in tension would be needed to maintain the pressure-volume relationship. In contrast, an increase in volume increases considerably the small radius, and when multiplied by the relatively high level of pressure, larger changes in tension would be required to maintain this pressure-volume relationship. The same could be considered true for the neonatal right ventricle, but in the older individual with a thinned right ventricular wall and crescent shape, the response to pressure and volume is different from that of the left ventricle. In the normal right ventricle, the resting right ventricular systolic pressure is low, and the radius of the free wall of the right ventricle is large. Thus, the right ventricle responds well to increased volume loads, since the radius is already large, and relatively small increases would be required to handle the extra volume. In contrast, increased right ventricular systolic pressure, when added to relatively low resting value and multiplied by the large radius, would require large changes of tension.

Perhaps this explanation helps in understanding why patients with an increased volume of blood in the left ventricle may develop congestive cardiac failure, while an increased volume in the right ventricle is relatively well tolerated unless the pressure is also elevated.

Generally, increased pressure loads in the right ventricle that have been present since birth are well tolerated, but certain major increases in right ventricular systolic pressure, as in pulmonary stenosis, can cause congestive cardiac failure in the first year of life.

Friedman and co-workers[7] have studied myocardial function in the fetus and found important differences from the adult. At any given fiber length, fetal myocardium developed less tension, perhaps helping to understand the inability of ventricles to respond to increased pressure loads. Perhaps this limitation of contractility is related to delayed development of sympathetic innervation of the neonatal heart, which Friedman et al.[7] found in rabbits, but, as yet, information is unavailable about the rate of development in humans.

Friedman et al.[7] also observed that at any myocardial segment length, the resting tension was higher in the fetus than in the adult. This would decrease ventricular compliance. The compliance does change rapidly in the first 2 weeks of life.

CLASSIFICATION OF CONGENITAL CARDIAC DISEASE

Congenital cardiac anomalies can be classified in various ways, but in this text, we have chosen to divide them according to two clinical features: the presence or absence of cyanosis and the status of the pulmonary vasculature as observed on a thoracic roentgenogram.

This classification is harder to apply to neonates than it is to infants or children because of difficulties in assessing the presence and origin of cyanosis. As indicated in Chapters 2 and 3, cyanosis can result from a number of noncardiac causes, such as inadequate peripheral perfusion or pulmonary conditions. Even neonates or infants with cardiac lesions that do not cause a right-to-left shunting of blood may have cyanosis of pulmonary origin, as from pulmonary edema or pulmonary parenchymal complications, such as pneumonia or atelectasis. The presence of pulmonary factors leading to cyanosis in a neonate or infant can usually be recognized either by the response to treatment of congestive cardiac failure or by the appearance of the thoracic roentgenogram.

In some neonates and infants, the cardiac condition may not be severe, and the degree of right-to-left shunt may be slight. Such mild degrees of hypoxemia are not evident clinically as cyanosis but are recognized only on measurement of arterial Po_2 or determination of hemoglobin and hematocrit values.

The status of pulmonary blood flow and vasculature is assessed by a review of the thoracic roentgenogram, as discussed in Chapter 5. In our classification, four states of pulmonary vascular markings will be described: normal, increased pulmonary blood flow, decreased pulmonary blood flow, and increased pulmonary venous markings. Combining these features of cyanosis/acyanosis and pulmonary vasculature, eight divisions could be made, but, in fact, only six are hemodynamically possible.

Acyanotic and Normal Pulmonary Blood Flow

In this group of conditions, discussed fully in Chapter 10, there is no shunting of blood either left to right or right to left. Thus, the pulmonary vasculature is normal, and the patient appears acyanotic. Two types of conditions give this combination.

OBSTRUCTION TO BLOOD FLOW THROUGH THE HEART.   Conditions causing obstruction to blood flow from the left side of the heart fall in this category. Some infants with pulmonary stenosis are acyanotic and have normal pulmonary blood flow, but in most neonates and infants with obstruction at either the tricuspid or pulmonary valve level, a right-to-left shunt is present at the atrial level, so cyanosis or arterial desaturation is present. Patients with conditions obstructing blood flow through the left atrium and adjacent structures, such as mitral stenosis, usually show a pattern of venous obstruction. These are discussed in Chapter 13.

MYOCARDIAL DISEASE.   A variety of diseases can affect the myocardium primarily and lead to symptoms in infancy. The pulmonary vasculature most often is normal but may show increased pulmonary venous markings, which often improve with treatment. Myocardial disease must also be considered in the differential diagnosis of increased pulmonary venous obstruction.

Acyanotic and Increased Pulmonary Blood Flow

This group of conditions, discussed more fully in Chapter 9, includes those associated with a left-to-right shunt which may occur at the atrial, ventricular, or great vessel level. The cardiac anomaly may occur by itself or coexist with such conditions as coarctation or myocarditis (Chap. 10), or such conditions as mitral stenosis (Chap. 13), which when present may increase the magnitude of the shunt.

Cyanosis and Increased Pulmonary Blood Flow

Several congenital cardiac anomalies cause both a right-to-left shunt, leading to cyanosis, and a left-to-right shunt, leading to the appearance of increased pulmonary arterial markings on thoracic roentgenogram (Chap. 11). In each condition there is a cardiac chamber allowing mixing of the systemic and pulmonary venous returns. Thus, these conditions have been called "admixture lesions."

Cyanosis and Decreased Pulmonary Blood Flow

This category of congenital cardiac conditions (Chap. 12) is associated with a right-to-left shunt. In each anomaly, an obstruction to pulmonary blood flow usually at either the pulmonary or tricuspid level coexists with an intracardiac anomaly. As a result, the volume of pulmonary blood flow is reduced, and a portion of systemic venous return is shunted into the aorta. The form and site of the obstruction varies, and the shunt can occur at either the atrial or ventricular level.

Acyanotic and Increased Pulmonary Venous Markings

The conditions associated with increased pulmonary venous markings are presented in Chapter 13. In each, pulmonary venous return is obstructed, and pulmonary edema can develop and lead to cyanosis, but this usually clears or improves significantly with treatment. There is a variety of anomalies involving the left ventricle, mitral valve, left atrium, or pulmonary veins in which the cardiac septae are intact, and, therefore, cyanosis is absent.

Cyanosis and Increased Pulmonary Venous Markings

In certain congenital cardiac anomalies, obstruction to pulmonary venous return coexists with a communication between the right and left sides of the heart, and through this communication, a right-to-left shunt can occur. An example of this pattern is total anomalous pulmonary venous connection with obstruction. These conditions are also discussed in Chapter 13.

Despite the variety of congenital cardiac anomalies, four basic hemodynamic principles govern the flow of blood and cardiac response, regardless of the anatomic nature of the anomaly. These concepts allow understanding of the similarities between conditions and many of the clinical and laboratory findings.

COMMUNICATION AT THE VENTRICULAR OR GREAT VESSEL LEVEL. In any cardiac anomaly in which the ventricles (as in ventricular septal defect or tetralogy of Fallot) or great vessels (as in patent ductus arteriosus or truncus arteriosus) are in communication, flow through the communication is dependent upon the relative resistances to flow into the lungs and into the body. When the communication is large (about three fourths the size of the aortic orifice) and there is no stenotic lesion, such as coexistent coarctation of the aorta or pulmonary stenosis, the direction and magnitude of flow through the communication are governed by the resistances imposed by the pulmonary and systemic vascular beds. Vascular resistance is determined by the caliber of the arterioles, and, as indicated previously in this chapter, major changes occur in vascular resistances, particularly the pulmonary resistances in the neonatal period and in early infancy. This change has a profound effect on the volume of shunt because, as the pulmonary vascular resistance decreases, the pulmonary blood flow increases. In infants with a large communication, however, the pulmonary vascular resistance does not follow the normal pattern of regression of arterial media, but the regression is delayed. Therefore, the decrease in pulmonary vascular resistance is delayed and not as severe, so these infants often have mild or moderate elevation of pulmonary vascular resistance. This elevation is perhaps related to persistent elevation of pulmonary arterial pressure. Because the pulmonary resistance is elevated, the excessive pulmonary blood flow is limited to some extent.

In patients with large communications and anatomic sites of obstruction distal to the communication, such as pulmonary stenosis in tetralogy of Fallot, the obstructive lesion can act as a major resistance factor, instead of that in the more distal arteriolar bed. The resistance of the pulmonary stenosis then must be considered in relation to the systemic vascular resistance.

When the communication is small, the flow through the communication is dependent upon pressure differences across the communication and the systemic vascular resistance.

COMMUNICATION AT THE ATRIAL LEVEL. The direction and magnitude of blood flow through atrial communications are dependent upon factors influencing ventricular filling. If there is no abnormality of the atrioventricular valves, flow is determined by relative compliance of the ventricles. Ventricular compliance can be decreased by either of two factors: thickness of the ventricular wall, as from hypertrophy, and factors influencing elasticity of the ventricle, as occurs with myocardial fibrosis, myocardial storage disease, or in the normal neonate. Ventricular hypertrophy is the most important factor influencing compliance in the neonatal period or in infancy.

Since, in the neonatal period, right ventricular weight exceeds left ventricular weight, its compliance is less, and the direction of shunt would be toward the left ventricle. As pulmonary vascular resistance decreases, the right ventricle thins, and its compliance increases. The direction of shunt would change toward the right ventricle.

If either atrioventricular valve is stenotic, this can cause a major obstruction to ventricular inflow and can be more important than the compliance of that ventricle. This obstruction must be considered in relation to the compliance of the opposite ventricle.

INSUFFICIENT VALVE. The chamber or great vessel on either side of an insufficient valve dilates. Ventricular dilatation occurs, since the ventricle must maintain the normal cardiac output. Therefore, with each systole, the ventricle ejects the normal stroke volume plus an amount equal to the regurgitant volume. It does not matter whether the regurgitation occurs into the ventricle from the great vessel during diastole in the case of semilunar valve insufficiency or into the atrium during systole in the situation of atrioventricular valve deformity. The ventricle must handle the regurgitant flow.

Many of the clinical and laboratory features reflect ventricular dilatation. Depending upon the ventricular compliance, pressures in the atria and ventricles may be elevated. If the ventricle is very compliant, a large volume of blood may be accommodated with little increase in end-diastolic pressure or atrial pressure. In contrast, if ventricular compliance is reduced, as from ventricular hypertrophy or myocardial fibrosis, augmentation of ventricular volume is associated with higher levels of end-diastolic and atrial pressures. In this circumstance, venous pressure becomes elevated and may lead to symptoms, such as pulmonary edema on the left side or hepatomegaly if the right side is involved.

In the first year of life, aortic regurgitation is extremely rare. It will not be discussed in this book. Pulmonary insufficiency does occur, usually associated with tetralogy of Fallot, and is discussed in Chapter 12. Mitral insufficiency can occur in infancy either as an isolated condition or, more commonly, secondary to another cardiac lesion, such as endocardial cushion defect or congenitally corrected transposition of great vessels (Chap. 9) or conditions which cause dilatation of the left ventricle (endocardial fibroelastosis) or infarction of papillary muscles (aortic stenosis, anomalous left coronary artery) (Chap. 10). Tricuspid insufficiency can also occur as either an isolated or as a secondary condition. In almost all circumstances of tricuspid insufficiency, because of the right atrial dilatation that occurs from elevated atrial pressure and volume, the foramen ovale is stretched open, allowing a right-to-left atrial shunt. Conditions associated with tricuspid insufficiency are discussed in Chapter 12.

OBLIGATORY SHUNT Rudolph[2] introduced the concept of dependent and obligatory shunts. Dependent shunts are those in which flow is governed by such factors as resistance or compliance. In contrast, obligatory shunts occur independent of either of these factors because communication exists between a high pressure ventricle or great vessel and a low pressure area. Examples are atrioventricular canal (with shunt from left ventricle to right atrium) or systemic arteriovenous fistulae with communication between an artery and a vein. In these infants, blood shunts early in life, even with pulmonary vascular resistance. The high volume of blood flow in the presence of elevated pulmonary vascular resistance can lead to early congestive cardiac failure and to development of pulmonary vascular disease at an accelerated rate.

REFERENCES

1. Dawes GS: Foetal and Neonatal Physiology. A Comparative Study of the Changes at Birth. Chicago, Year Book, 1968, pp 79, 91, 160
2. Rudolph AM: The fetal circulation and its adjustments after birth in congenital heart disease. In Adams FH, Swan HJC, Hall VE (eds): Pathophysiology of Congenital Heart Disease. Berkeley, U. of California Press, 1970, pp 105–118
3. Rudolph AM: The changes in the circulation after birth. Their importance in congenital heart disease. Circulation 41:343, 1970
4. Wagenvoort CA, Neufeld HN, Edwards JE: The structure of the pulmonary arterial tree in fetal and early postnatal life. Lab Invest 10:751, 1961
5. Naeye RL: Arterial changes during the perinatal period. Arch Pathol 71:121, 1961
6. Rudolph AM, Yuan S: Response of the pulmonary vasculature to hypoxia and H^+ ion concentration changes. J Clin Invest 45:399, 1966
7. Friedman WF, Pool PE, Jacobowitz D, Seagren SC, Braunwald E: Sympathetic innervation of the developing rabbit heart. Biochemical and histochemical comparisons of fetal, neonatal, and adult myocardium. Circ Res 23:25, 1968

9 Acyanosis and Increased Pulmonary Blood Flow

The combination of increased pulmonary arterial markings and absence of cyanosis indicates the presence of a left-to-right shunt. The shunt can occur at the level of the pulmonary arteries, the right ventricle, the right atrium, or the systemic veins.

The conditions included in this chapter comprise at least 40 percent of the congenital cardiac anomalies present in the first year of life. The conditions can cause congestive cardiac failure, failure to thrive, frequent respiratory infections, and death but usually are first evident because of a murmur.

Because of differences in hemodynamics, the conditions will be divided into three groups, shunts at the ventricular or great vessel level, shunts at the atrial level, and systemic arteriovenous fistulous communication.

SHUNTS AT THE VENTRICULAR OR GREAT VESSEL LEVEL

Congenital cardiac anomalies in which a communication occurs between the great vessels or ventricles are presented in this chapter. These include:

1. Ventricular septal defect
2. Patent ductus arteriosus
3. Congenitally corrected transposition of the great vessels with ventricular septal defect
4. Aorticopulmonary septal defect
5. Aortic origin of the pulmonary artery

As indicated in Chapter 8, the volume of blood flow through the abnormal communication depends upon the size of the communication and the relative systemic and pulmonary vascular resistances.

In most infants symptomatic from these conditions, the communication is large, so that relative vascular resistances are the major factors influencing shunt, and pulmonary hypertension is common.

VENTRICULAR SEPTAL DEFECT

Isolated ventricular septal defect is the most common congenital cardiac anomaly. Hoffman[1] reported an incidence of 30.8 percent among neonates with cardiac malformations. This incidence represents a minimal occurrence rate of ventricular septal defect of 2 per 1,000 live births, a rate predicted by Keith et al.[2] Females account for slightly more than half (56 percent) of neonates with ventricular septal defect.[1]

The occurrence rate is much lower in older children and adults. Patients with large ventricular septal defect may die in infancy, especially when the defect is associated with other complex cardiac anomalies[3, 4] or with chromosomal anomalies.

The high spontaneous closure rate of small ventricular septal defect is a more important cause of reduction in occurrence with age. Hoffman,[1] drawing upon data from a number of sources, estimated that spontaneous closure occurred in 45 percent of children with ventricular septal defect.

It is our impression, though not documented, that most of the small defects close spontaneously by the time the child is 5 or 6 years of age. In our cardiac clinic, we follow a number of children with typical murmurs of a small ventricular septal defect and have noted that spontaneous closure of the defect is the rule rather than the exception.

DEVELOPMENTAL ANATOMY.   The heart is incompletely separated into right and left ventricles until the end of the seventh week of gestation, when closure of the intraventricular foramen occurs. In the broad sense, tissue from three sources—the right and left bulbar ridges and the right endocardial cushion—fuses with the aorticopulmonary septum and the muscular septum to complete closure of the interventricular septum.[5] Failure of fusion of these tissues results in a ventricular septal defect. The most frequent abnormality is the failure of the right-sided endocardial cushion to form the membranous interventricular septum.

Thus, the location of the interventricular septal defect can vary, and its exact anatomic position is important to the operating surgeon, for technical details of operation and prognosis vary according to its position.

In almost all infants, only one ventricular septal defect is found, although its position may vary (Fig. 9-1). Eighty percent of ventricular septal defects, because of their location, are called "membranous." These involve only a portion of the membranous septum but also part of the adjacent muscular septum. They lie beneath the right and noncoronary aortic valve cusps and beneath the septal leaflet of the tricuspid valve.

Less commonly, the defect is located above the crista supraventricularis and lies between the right and left coronary cusps. Defects may occur in the muscular interventricular septum, and frequently these are large and multiple. The least frequent ventricular septal defect is of the atrioventricular canal type.

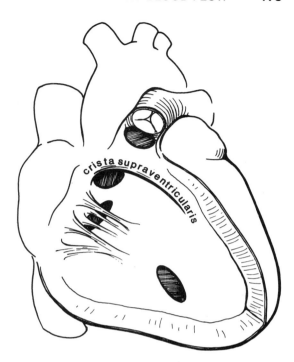

FIG. 9-1. Diagram of right ventricular aspect of interventricular septum, showing typical locations of ventricular septal defect.

HEMODYNAMICS. The effect of a ventricular septal defect depends more on its size and the status of the pulmonary vasculature than on its location. Ventricular septal defects can be broadly divided into two categories: (1) large ventricular septal defect, in which the size of the defect is similar to that of the aortic orifice, or greater than 1 cm^2/m^2, and (2) small- or moderate-sized defects, in which the defect is less than the size of the aortic orifice or less than 1 cm^2/m^2.

Large Ventricular Septal Defect

Ten percent of ventricular septal defects in infancy are large. The flow through the defect is unrestricted because the major determinant of the volume and direction of intracardiac shunting of blood is the pulmonary vascular resistance. Systolic pressure in the right ventricle and pulmonary artery is at systemic levels and equals aortic and left ventricular systolic pressure. Both great vessels are exposed to a common ventricular ejection force.[6]

In large ventricular septal defects, the level of pulmonary arterial pressure is determined by systemic pressure. Considering:

$$P = R \times F$$

the elevated pulmonary arterial pressure (P) is maintained by a combination of pulmonary vascular resistance (R) and pulmonary blood flow (F). As is well known, pulmonary vascular resistance changes with age.

Immediately after birth, pulmonary vascular resistance is elevated to near systemic level, and significant shunting of the blood through a large ventricular septal defect does not occur. As the pulmonary vascular bed matures, the degree of medial hypertrophy of arterial smooth muscle gradually diminishes, lowering pulmonary vascular resistance. The declining pulmonary vascular resistance leads to progressive increase in the volume of blood shunted left to right through the septal defect. As pulmonary blood flow exceeds three times the systemic output, the excessive volume overload upon the left ventricle leads to congestive cardiac failure. In isolated large ventricular septal defects, cardiac failure rarely occurs before 6 weeks of age.

A number of cardiopulmonary adaptive changes occur in infants with congestive cardiac failure secondary to a ventricular septal defect with large left-to-right shunt. Increased end-diastolic volume of the left ventricle (preload) augments cardiac contractility by the Frank-Starling mechanism, which is also enhanced by an increase in sympathetic stimulation. An increase in 2,3-DPG causes a rightward shift in the oxygen dissociation curve, resulting in easier release of oxygen to tissues. Development of myocardial hypertrophy provides greater muscle mass and reduces compliance of the ventricle somewhat, thereby improving performance characteristics.

The architecture of the pulmonary vascular bed in infants with a large ventricular septal defect differs from that of normal neonates and is not static. Secondary to the increased pressure and flow, the muscularity of larger arterioles (>250 mm diameter) and pulmonary venules is increased. Medial muscle tissue extends into smaller and more peripheral arteries, and the arterioles are reduced in number.[7] Eventually, obliterative intimal changes develop.[8] Each of these changes is initially protective because it limits the volume of left-to-right shunt through the ventricular septal defect. In time, the pulmonary arteriolar changes progress, intimal proliferation occurs, and pulmonary vascular resistance rises gradually and eventually exceeds systemic resistance. These changes in pulmonary vasculature are accompanied by a period of bidirectional shunting across the ventricular septal defect, followed by progressive cyanosis, and eventually death (Eisenmenger's syndrome).[9] Such progression rarely occurs in infancy.

The importance of the pulmonary vasculature as a determinant of the natural history of ventricular septal defect is well known but somewhat taken for granted today. During the early era of cardiac surgery, our knowledge of cardiopulmonary hemodynamics associated with ventricular septal defect was less well defined and understood. Dammann and Ferencz[10] and Adams and associates[11] were among the first to relate clinical findings to changes in the pulmonary vascular bed. Edwards,[12] Wagenvoort,[13] and Lucas and associates[14] more precisely defined the structural changes occurring in the lung subjected to increased flow and pressure.

The pressure-flow dynamics during each phase of the cardiac cycle in patients with ventricular septal defect have been described in detail.[15, 16] During diastole, a larger volume of blood fills the left ventricle than the right, resulting in some left-to-right spillover across the defect. Further flow of blood into the body of the right ventricle occurs during isovolumetric contraction. When the semilunar valves open, ventricular systole is characterized by rapid egress of blood to the great vessels, especially the pulmonary artery (assuming pulmonary resistance is lower than systemic). The predominant left-to-right shunting of blood occurs during early systole, the outflow tract of the right ventricle merely acting as a passive conduit during this phase of the cardiac cycle.

Small Ventricular Septal Defect

The small size of a ventricular septal defect can prevent the free transmission of left ventricular systolic pressure. Therefore, pulmonary arterial pressure is not fixed at systemic levels, as in a large ventricular septal defect. The change in pressure depends almost entirely upon the volume of pulmonary blood flow, since the pulmonary vascular resistance follows a normal or near-normal course.

Infants with a small ventricular septal defect show a wide range of hemodynamics. The defect may be so small that pressure in the right side of the heart is normal and the pulmonary system flow rate is less than 2:1. These defects may undergo spontaneous closure, and the patients are asymptomatic. In other patients with larger defects, the right-sided pressures may reach 75 percent of the left ventricle. Such patients may develop congestive cardiac failure because the shunt is large.

CLINICAL FEATURES.   The newborn with a ventricular septal defect is acyanotic and asymptomatic. When the defect is small, a short, soft systolic murmur may be audible at the mid to lower left sternal border by the third or fourth day of life. Spontaneous closure of the defect without sequelae is expected within 1 to 2 years. In such infants the murmur is always soft, squirty, and gradually disappears.

An infant with a moderate to large ventricular septal defect presents differently. In these infants, a systolic murmur is noted at the time of the postnatal visit to the physician. Then, the previously healthy infant begins to develop signs and symptoms of congestive cardiac failure during the second month of life. The initial manifestations are tiring during feeding and, subsequently, failure to gain weight normally. The parents may relate that the baby can suck only 1 to 2 ounces of formula per feeding. The infant becomes diaphoretic and tachypneic.

Physical examination shows evidence of slow growth and tachypnea. There may be a precordial bulge and displacement of the cardiac apex laterally, indicating cardiac enlargement. Precordial activity is increased, and a systolic thrill along the midleft sternal border is almost always present. A grade 3–4/6 long systolic murmur is present along the left sternal border.

Two auscultatory features indicate features of the hemodynamics. The intensity of the pulmonary second sound (P_2) reflects the level of pulmonary arterial pressure. In large defects, P_2 is accentuated and more narrowly split, reflecting the presence of pulmonary hypertension. When the left-to-right shunt is large (Qp/Qs > 2:1), a low frequency diastolic rumble is audible at the apex, due to excessive blood flow across the mitral valve. If pulmonary vascular resistance rises and pulmonary blood flow decreases, the diastolic murmur softens and disappears.

In the infants with congestive cardiac failure, hepatomegaly is found.

ELECTROCARDIOGRAM. In most infants, the electrocardiogram also reflects the hemodynamics. If a small defect is present, the electrocardiogram is normal and remains so. Among patients with large defects, a pattern of biventricular hypertrophy, left atrial enlargement, and normal frontal plane QRS axis is found.[17] The presence of left ventricular hypertrophy reflects the volume overload on the left ventricle, and right ventricular hypertrophy reflects the increased right ventricular systolic pressure (Fig. 9-2). Although left atrial enlargement may be found, it is uncommon.

In patients with a moderate-sized left-to-right shunt, the electrocardiogram shows predominant left ventricular hypertrophy.

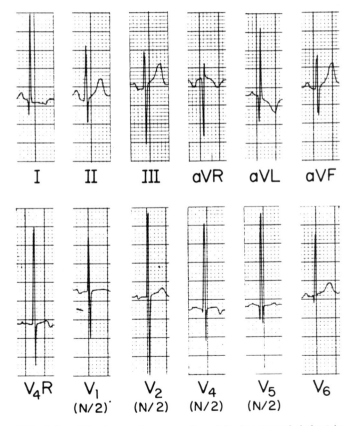

FIG. 9-2. Electrocardiogram of ventricular septal defect in 3-month-old infant in congestive cardiac failure. QRS axis is 0°. Biventricular hypertrophy. N/2, half-standardization.

Slight degrees of left axis deviation (less than −30°) may be found. We were unable to associate slight left axis deviation with any particular anatomic form of ventricular septal defect.

THORACIC ROENTGENOGRAM.   The thoracic roentgenogram may be normal in infants with a small defect. Cardiac enlargement and increased pulmonary arterial markings are present depending on the size of the shunt (Fig. 9-3a). The cardiac contour is nonspecific. Left atrial enlargement, evident by posterior displacement of the barium-filled esophagus (Fig. 9-3b), is present when pulmonary blood flow exceeds twice the systemic flow.

ECHOCARDIOGRAM.   M-mode echocardiogram is not diagnostic of the condition but can yield information about the hemodynamics. In small defects, it is normal. In infants with increased pulmonary blood flow, the diameters of both the left atrium and left ventricle are increased. With pulmonary hypertension, the right ventricle may become dilated and the right ventricular wall thickened, but the latter may be difficult to detect. Measurement of preejection period may be helpful in detecting elevated pulmonary arterial pressure.

CARDIAC CATHETERIZATION AND ANGIOCARDIOGRAM.   Cardiac catheterization is unnecessary for asymptomatic infants with ventricular septal defect. It should, however, be carried out in infants who develop congestive cardiac failure or have evidence of increasing pulmonary vascular resistance.

The purposes of cardiac catheterization are:

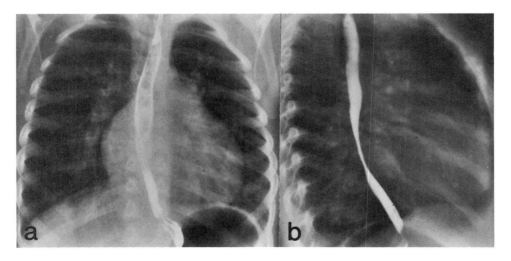

FIG. 9-3.   Thoracic roentgenogram of ventricular septal defect in 3-month-old infant. **a.** Posteroanterior view. **b.** Lateral view. Cardiomegaly. Increased pulmonary arterial markings. Left atrial enlargement.

1. To measure pulmonary arterial pressure
2. To determine the volume of pulmonary blood flow
3. To locate the position of the ventricular septal defect
4. To exclude coexistent cardiac conditions

The usual catheter approach for an infant with a ventricular septal defect is through the saphenous vein. This approach facilitates the passage of the catheter across the foramen ovale into the left side of the heart. In at least half of the patients, it is possible to pass the catheter through the ventricular septal defect into the aorta, but rarely can it be positioned in the left ventricle. The passage of the catheter into the aorta indicates the presence of the ventricular septal defect. In all likelihood, it is in the membranous septum.

Careful oximetry data should be obtained, and at least two oximetry series performed. The series should include serial sampling from the superior vena cava, through the right atrium to the inferior vena cava, to detect an additional left-to-right shunt at the atrial level, which occurs frequently, presumably through a stretched foramen ovale.

During the oximetry series, pressure data can be obtained. Oxygen consumption can be measured in the catheterization laboratory. From the pressure and oximetry data, absolute pulmonary and systemic blood flow can be easily calculated, allowing definitive quantitation of resistances of the respective vascular beds. When absolute blood flows are not measured, pulmonary resistance relative to systemic resistance (Rp/Rs) can be calculated.

Angiography plays an important role in the diagnostic evaluation of an infant with a ventricular septal defect. Left ventriculography should be performed in each infant to locate the position of the ventricular septal defect and to make certain multiple defects are not present (Fig. 9-4). The left ventricle can be approached through the foramen ovale. We prefer to use a balloon-tipped angiocatheter, for this facilitates passage of the catheter into the left ventricle and reduces the incidence of perforation of the left atrial appendage. The inflated balloon holds the catheter holes away from the left ventricular wall, thereby reducing the possibility of intramyocardial injection.

The left ventriculogram should be performed on cine film with the patient in a left anterior oblique position, so that the plane of the x-ray beam is parallel to the ventricular septum. Slight rotation of the infant from the left anterior oblique position may be necessary to properly position the septum.

Right ventriculography should be performed in anteroposterior and lateral projections to visualize the right ventricle, its outflow area, and, on pulmonary venous phase, the pulmonary veins. Aortography is also necessary in infants with pulmonary hypertension to exclude a coexistent but silent patent ductus arteriosus. These angiographic studies can demonstrate other conditions, such as coarctation of the aorta or origin of both great vessels from the right ventricle, which may coexist.

Repeat cardiac catheterization is sometimes necessary during the latter part of the first year of life to accurately assess the patient's hemodynamics.

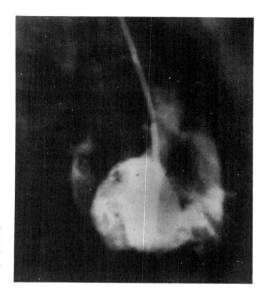

FIG. 9-4. Left ventriculogram of ventricular septal defect. Lateral view following opacification of left ventricle, right ventricle opacified through muscular ventricular septal defect.

Keith and co-workers,[18] found that, whereas less than one fourth of their patients with ventricular septal defect had small left-to-right shunts and normal pulmonary vascular resistance early in infancy, half fell within this category by the time subsequent catheterization was performed. Thus, in some children, ventricular septal defects gradually diminish in size and become hemodynamically insignificant.

MANAGEMENT.   Many patients with ventricular septal defect require no treatment in infancy and, in the long term, none other than prophylaxis for bacterial endocarditis. Since subacute bacterial endocarditis is exceedingly rare during infancy and dental procedures are unnecessary until 2 or 3 years of age at the earliest, we usually do not stress antibiotic prophylaxis until early childhood. Many defects will have spontaneously closed by then, in which case no further instruction or follow-up is necessary.

Congestive cardiac failure is usually managed quite successfully with digoxin. Some infants benefit from the addition of oral diuretic therapy and an aldosterone antagonist.[19] The addition of a peripheral vasodilator to reduce afterload in intractable congestive cardiac failure has met with little success in our patients. Following initial treatment for congestive cardiac failure, cardiac catheterization is recommended to obtain information to aid in management.

Typically, treatment of congestive cardiac failure is successful, and the infant is discharged from the hospital following cardiac catheterization. Frequent clinic visits are essential to monitor the infant's course.

Most commonly, the infant remains in chronic compensated congestive cardiac failure until near the end of the first year of life, at which time symptoms diminish and growth improves. The clinician must watch carefully for the development of significant pulmonary vascular changes. Persistence of a diastolic murmur and normal intensity of pulmonic closure are clinically reassuring, as is the transition from biventricular to a left ventricular pattern electrocardiographically. Serial echograms are useful in semiquantitating the volume of left-to-right shunt and pulmonary arterial pressure.[20]

Most children with a defect large enough to cause congestive cardiac failure during early infancy continue to have symptoms and may eventually develop irreversible pulmonary vascular disease if operation is not performed.[21] Though the majority can be followed safely for about 2 years, approximately 10 to 15 percent require operation during the first year of life because of intractable congestive cardiac failure or rapidly progressive pulmonary vascular disease.

A few infants may develop infundibular hypertrophy. This obstructs flow into the pulmonary artery and protects the pulmonary vascular bed.[22] These infants become, in effect, pink tetrads, with small, predominantly left-to-right shunts.

Aortic insufficiency secondary to prolapse of the right coronary cusp may develop.[23,24] This rare complication does not appear to be related to the size of the defect and does not occur until later in childhood.

Operation is required in some infants, and the indications vary. Decisions regarding operation in infants are not as difficult as they were previously, for operative mortality and morbidity have decreased because of more sophisticated intraoperative and postoperative management,[25] and the incidence of postoperative heart block is less than 1 percent.[26,27]

In infants who have a large defect with pulmonary blood flow at least twice the systemic blood flow and who either do not develop cardiac failure or do not respond well to digitalization, the defect should be closed, but operation can be deferred until age 18 to 24 months. This age range is chosen, since residual pulmonary hypertension is present in half of such children operated after 2 years of age,[28-31] and the operative risk is lower (less than 7 percent mortality)[32,33] than at an earlier age.

This recommendation does not imply that every patient with a large ventricular septal defect should have surgery during infancy, since in some patients the size of the defect may decrease sufficiently so that surgery is no longer necessary. This prospect must be considered against the risk of development of pulmonary vascular changes in patients in whom the defect remains large.

Some infants remain in intractable congestive cardiac failure secondary to ventricular septal defect throughout infancy. These infants may have associated cardiac lesions, such as coarctation of the aorta or multiple ventricular septal defects. Failure to thrive is marked, and operative intervention is not only advisable but lifesaving. In a few infants, congestive cardiac failure does not develop, but pulmonary vascular changes progress rapidly and may become irreversible. In either instance, an operation must be performed. Two operative choices are available.

Pulmonary arterial banding is a palliative operation that reduces the magnitude of the left-to-right shunt and protects the pulmonary vascular bed.[34] This operation is used less frequently because of the rather high incidence of complications,[35,36] the desire to avoid two operations, and the improved ability of cardiac surgeons to close ventricular septal defect in infants. Pulmonary arterial banding is indicated in a few circumstances, however. For example, we recently chose pulmonary band palliation in a 1 kg premature infant with a large ventricular septal defect and intractable congestive cardiac failure. We prefer banding in infants with large or multiple muscular ventricular septal defects.

The preferred choice if operation becomes necessary during infancy is total correction. Hypothermia has gained increasing popularity over the past several years, significantly improving the utility and safety of cardiopulmonary bypass in young infants.[37] Many centers now employ moderate core cooling maintained by low-flow circulatory perfusion rather than profound hypothermia and total circulatory arrest.

The long-term morbidity associated with total correction under hypothermia has not been completely assessed, although in several series, development and cognitive ability appear to be normal and hemodynamic repair excellent.[38,39]

Early surgical correction should be considered in a final group of children with ventricular septal defect. In an occasional child, who has tolerated a large defect throughout infancy, which becomes smaller by 2 years of age, cardiomegaly persists. The long-term outlook for such a child is unknown, but we are concerned. Often, cardiac catheterization is reassuring in terms of substantiating the presence of a small defect and normal pulmonary vascular resistance, but biventricular chamber enlargement, slight elevation of end-diastolic pressure, and the subjective impression of suboptimal ventricular contractility are found. Graham et al.[16] have data showing that children operated on for ventricular septal defect during infancy have better postoperative ventricular performance and regression of myocardial hypertrophy than do children who are corrected at an older age. Therefore, indications for operation may need cautious modification as more postoperative hemodynamic data and natural history studies become available. Our knowledge of pulmonary vascular pathophysiology in relation to ventricular septal defect is reasonably well delineated. The effects of left-to-right shunt on the myocardium are unknown.

The prognosis for an infant with an uncomplicated ventricular septal defect is good. The majority of defects are small enough to be hemodynamically insignificant, precluding the need for corrective surgery. Larger defects require surgical closure, which can usually be accomplished with acceptably low risk to the patient.

PATENT DUCTUS ARTERIOSUS

Whereas correction of most congenital cardiac lesions remains a technical challenge to the surgeon, patent ductus arteriosus has for many years been readily amenable to simple operative ligation and, thus, from a surgical point of view, is of very little interest. The perspective of the pediatric cardiologist is quite different. Perhaps no other defect presents as formidable a daily challenge. Knowledge of normal physiology of the ductus is rudimentary. Continued patency of the ductus is of concern when one is dealing with a ductus-dependent lesion, such as pulmonary atresia. Failure of the ductus arteriosus to close after birth in an infant without intrinsic cardiac disease is of nearly equal concern. In terms of numbers of patients alone, problems related to the ductus arteriosus confront the pediatric cardiologist and neonatologist far more than any other isolated cardiac defect.

In this chapter, three major clinical problems of the patent ductus arteriosus are discussed:

1. Persistent patency of the ductus arteriosus in premature infants
2. Persistence of the ductus arteriosus in the term infant
3. The ductus arteriosus in association with other congenital cardiac anomalies

As an isolated lesion or accompanying other cardiac anomalies, patent ductus arteriosus occurs in approximately 10 percent of patients with congenital heart disease.[40] The exact incidence is difficult to determine because of factors discussed in Chapter 1. The ratio of females to males with patent ductus arteriosus is 2:1 to 3:1. Familial aggregation occurs, typical of a polygenic mode of inheritance.

The incidence of patent ductus arteriosus is influenced by the frequency among premature infants.[41,42] Kitterman and co-workers [43] reported that 42 percent of premature infants weighing less than 1,750 g had evidence of patent ductus arteriosus. Seventy-six of 396 premature infants (19 percent) admitted to the newborn intensive care unit at the University of Minnesota Hospitals during a 2-year period had clinical signs of patent ductus arteriosus.[44]

The incidence of patent ductus arteriosus is inversely related to the gestational age. Babies who are small for gestational age have a lower incidence of patent ductus arteriosus than do babies who have appropriate weight for gestational age. When corrected for gestational age, the incidence of patent ductus arteriosus in infants recovering from respiratory distress syndrome is higher than in premature infants without pulmonary disease.[45] Premature infants born of mothers with prolonged rupture of fetal membranes have a lower incidence of patent ductus arteriosus, perhaps because they are less likely to develop respiratory distress syndrome.[46] A number of factors, in addition to the gestational age of the infant, determine patency of the ductus arteriosus.

Role of the Ductus Arteriosus in Utero

Embryologically, the ductus arteriosus represents persistence of the left sixth aortic arch. At birth, the ductus appears as a continuation of the pulmonary artery and may have a diameter equal to the aorta. Its important role in the fetus is to allow egress of blood pumped from the right ventricle into the pulmonary trunk to the descending aorta, thus bypassing the nonaerated lungs.

Studies carried out at the Cardiovascular Research Institute in San Francisco have substantially added to our understanding of fetal hemodynamics.[47] The combined output of the right and left ventricles of the fetal lamb is 500 ml/kg/min. The right ventricle ejects approximately two thirds of this volume via the pulmonary trunk and ductus arteriosus to the descending aorta (lower circulation); the left ventricle ejects the remaining one third to the ascending aorta (upper circulation). The two circulations are kept relatively separate by the minimal blood flow across the narrow isthmus of the aorta.

Right-to-left shunting through the ductus is favored by the low resistance placental circulation as opposed to the high resistance pulmonary vascular bed. Following birth, expansion of the lungs results in a substantial decrease in pulmonary resistance. Constriction and clamping of the umbilical arteries cause an abrupt increase in systemic vascular resistance, and flow through the ductus becomes bidirectional for about 6 hours.[48] Further decline in pulmonary vascular resistance accounts for a net left-to-right shunt in most infants 6 to 18 hours of age. Functional patency of the ductus arteriosus beyond 24 hours is considered abnormal, though anatomic closure may not be complete until several weeks following birth.[49]

Morphologic and Biochemical Mechanisms of Contraction

The ductus arteriosus possesses less elastic tissue and more circumferential smooth muscle than either the aorta or the pulmonary trunk. Ductal smooth muscle extends slightly into the wall of the pulmonary artery and elastic tissue into the wall of the aorta. Perhaps because of the relatively larger amount of smooth muscle near the pulmonary arterial end of the ductus, this is the area of initial ductal constriction.

There is a disproportionately greater amount of elastic tissue and less smooth muscle distributed near the aortic end of the ductus,[50] supporting the commonly held view that persistence of the ductus arteriosus may be related to deficient amount and distribution of smooth muscle within its wall. Gittenberger-deGroot[51] has proposed an alternative mechanism based upon histologic examination of human ductus arteriosus from premature as well as adult subjects. She postulates that the aberrant distribution of elastic material and the presence of a subendothelial elastic lamina, which interferes with intimal cushion formation, are primary anatomic defects resulting in patent ductus arteriosus. Whichever mechanism of constriction is correct, the end result is shortening and obliteration of the lumen.

Increased oxygen tension in blood is a potent stimulant of ductal smooth muscle constriction and, undoubtedly, is the major factor influencing closure of the ductus after birth.[52-54] Beyond this, we can do little more than speculate. Diminished responsiveness of the premature ductus to oxygen does not appear to be simply related to adrenergic and cholinergic receptor function, since these are well developed early in human fetal life.[55] The role of the cyclic nucleotides as ultimate mediators of smooth muscle contraction is less certain now than it was believed to be in the past, as is the importance at one time ascribed to bradykinin.[56] More recently, interest has been focused on prostaglandin biochemistry and the effects these potent vasoactive substances have on the ductus arteriosus. Heymann and Rudolph[57] have shown that in fetal lambs, PGE_1 and PGE_2 act at relatively low levels of Po_2 to preserve ductal patency. The metabolites of prostaglandin synthesis responsible for ductal smooth muscle constriction have not been positively identified as yet, though thromboxane A_2 and PGF_2 have been proposed as possible mediators.

Persistent Patency of the Ductus Arteriosus in Premature Infants

A premature infant is more likely than a term infant to develop congestive cardiac failure secondary to patent ductus arteriosus because the magnitude of the left-to-right shunt through the ductus is greater and the ability of the left ventricle to compensate for volume overload is less well developed.

The quantity of left-to-right shunt depends upon the size of the ductus and the relationship between pulmonary and systemic vascular resistances. In premature infants, a patent ductus arteriosus is invariably large and nonrestrictive. The development of resistance vessels in the lungs occurs predominantly during the third trimester of pregnancy. Thus, a 30-week gestation premature baby, for example, has not developed sufficient numbers of fourth and fifth generation pulmonary arterioles in relation to the total amount of lung parenchyma to impart enough resistance to flow to protect the volume-sensitive left side of the heart. This phenomenon of decreased pulmonary vascular resistance in prematurely born infants was initially thought to be due to incomplete development and thickening of the medial layer of the pulmonary arterioles.[58] More recent studies have demonstrated a constant ratio of medial width to external vessel diameter throughout gestation.[59]

The ability of the immature left ventricle to handle excessive volume stress is compromised by deficient contractile ability. Sarcomere development may be incomplete, and sympathetic innervation of the heart is not fully developed in the very premature infant, so that the force of contraction is decreased. The low aortic diastolic pressure in infants with patent ductus arteriosus decreases subendocardial perfusion.[60] Thus, the premature heart, inherently less capable of responding to volume overload, is further compromised in the presence of patent ductus arteriosus by inadequate coronary perfusion during diastole.

CLINICAL FEATURES. Characteristically, patent ductus arteriosus becomes evident by the development of a murmur toward the end of the first week of life. Many of these premature infants are in the early recovery stage of hyaline membrane disease and may still require ventilatory assistance. The cardiac murmur may be either systolic or continuous and tends to be loudest beneath the left clavicle. Frequently, the murmur is loud and well heard over the entire precordium, so that localization is impossible. Occasionally, the murmur appears to be most prominent along the lower left sternal border and, therefore, mimics ventricular septal defect. A separate middiastolic rumble at the apex is infrequently heard, even when the left-to-right shunt is large. The second heart sound is usually narrowly split but often is obscured by the continuous murmur. The precordium is hyperdynamic. Peripheral pulses are brisk, and one may even palpate digital or palmar pulses when a significant left-to-right shunt through the ductus exists.

Unfortunately, there are no generally accepted criteria for determining whether or not a patent ductus arteriosus is significant. A significant ductus implies that the left-to-right shunt is large enough to have caused congestive cardiac failure, and this determination may be difficult, at best.

Persistent tachycardia (heart rate > 140) is a reliable indication of congestive cardiac failure in premature infants with patent ductus arteriosus. Other causes of tachycardia, such as severe anemia, hyperthermia from an overheated isolette, hyperthyroidism, or shock, must be excluded.

Cardiomegaly, as seen on serial thoracic roentgenograms, and hepatomegaly are usually present with severe congestive cardiac failure. However, these signs are not invariably present in milder degrees of congestive cardiac failure, even though the ductus may be significant.

Tachypnea is not helpful in determining the presence of congestive cardiac failure, since most premature infants have intrinsic pulmonary disease and respiratory distress on that basis. The development of congestive cardiac failure, when other signs of a large ductus arteriosus are present, is often indicated by a change in ventilatory status, manifested by increasing respiratory rate, increased oxygen requirements, hypercarbia, or occasionally even apnea.

Additional signs and symptoms of circulatory insufficiency secondary to ductus arteriosus may include abdominal distention and ileus, decreased urine output, and metabolic acidosis. These relatively frequent complications of prematurity can result from a wide variety of causes, often incompletely understood, and should not necessarily be ascribed to patent ductus arteriosus just because a murmur is present.

Judging the significance of a patent ductus arteriosus in a given premature infant is difficult. Acceptance of criteria that are too liberal results in treatment of a patent ductus arteriosus which may not be contributing to the infant's illness and which, if left alone, would close spontaneously in time. The opposite is also true: utilization of rigid criteria for determining the presence of congestive cardiac failure may lead to failure of treatment of a symptomatic infant and adversely affect the outcome. Currently, a dogmatic approach is completely unjustified, and as is usually the case, the truth lies somewhere between these two extremes.

The clinical diagnosis of patent ductus arteriosus is not difficult and is quite reliable. Assessing its severity is not easy, and, unfortunately, there is no single diagnostic study which provides consistent objective determination of the hemodynamics and effects of a patent ductus arteriosus in a premature infant.

ELECTROCARDIOGRAM. The electrocardiogram reflects the excessive left ventricular volume overload encountered in a large patent ductus arteriosus, but the development of left ventricular hypertrophy (Fig. 9-5) comes relatively late in the course of the disease (4 to 6 weeks).[44] Interpretation of the electrocardiogram must be based upon the gestational age and chronologic age of the infant, since premature infants normally show less right ventricular preponderance than do normal term infants.[61] When a ductus with a large shunt has been present for a number of weeks, the T waves over the left precordium may become flattened or inverted and, along with increased left ventricular forces, indicate left ventricular strain. At times, only the T wave changes are seen, and the QRS voltages are normal. The T wave findings slowly reverse after closure of the ductus arteriosus.

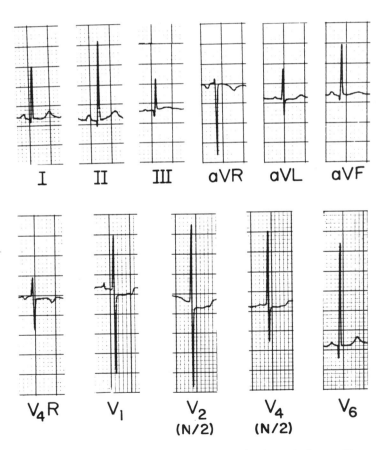

FIG. 9-5. Electrocardiogram of patent ductus arteriosus. Two-month-old, prematurely born infant in mild congestive cardiac failure. QRS axis is +45°. Left ventricular hypertrophy. N/2, half-standardization.

THORACIC ROENTGENOGRAM.   The thoracic roentgenogram, especially when evaluated serially, usually shows increasing heart size and increased pulmonary vascular markings (Fig. 9-6). Left atrial enlargement is expected and may be evident by elevation of the left main stem bronchus. While left atrial enlargement would be better evaluated using a barium swallow, it may be difficult to obtain such a study in a premature infant. If severe hyaline membrane disease is present, pulmonary vascular markings are difficult to assess, and the poorly compliant left ventricle of the premature infant may not dilate appreciably even though a large left-to-right shunt exists.

ECHOCARDIOGRAM.   The echocardiogram has been used to assess, in a semi-quantitative way, the size of a left-to-right ductal shunt,[62-64] using measurement of the left atrial and/or left ventricular internal dimension (Fig. 9-7). The ratio of the left atrial to aortic diameter has been widely used and provides a means of serially following in an infant the changes of left atrial dimension by comparing them to the unchanging aortic root diameter. Normally, the left atrial dimension equals or is slightly less than the aortic root diameter. A left atrial to aortic ratio of greater than 1.2 is abnormal and considered to indicate left atrial enlargement. Serial echograms are helpful, but therapy should not be based solely upon changes in the left atrial to aortic ratio. There are few data relating left atrial to aortic ratio or left ventricular internal dimension to the volume of left-to-right shunt. Infants with a patent ductus arteriosus and congestive cardiac failure may have normal serial echograms[65] because the left atrial dimension may increase asymmetrically and not be reflected in the plane of the echogram. Furthermore, there is an unpredictable effect of positive end expiratory pressure on left atrial filling in an infant receiving respiratory assistance.

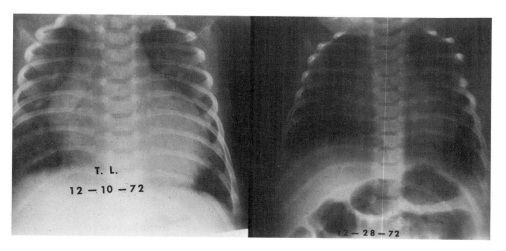

FIG. 9-6.   Thoracic roentgenogram before (left) and following (right) ligation of patent ductus arteriosus.

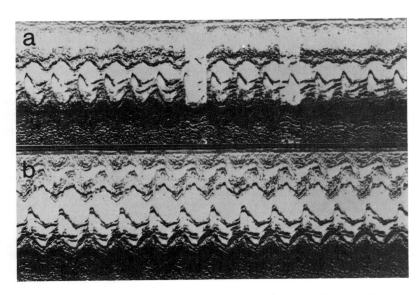

FIG. 9-7.   a and **b.** Serial echocardiograms of patent ductus arteriosus. Increase in left ventricular internal diastolic diameter (LVID$_d$) from 13 mm to 21 mm.

CARDIAC CATHETERIZATION AND ANGIOCARDIOGRAM.   Usually the diagnosis of patent ductus arteriosus is made on auscultatory findings, and further studies are unwarranted. Retrograde aortograms through an umbilical arterial catheter have been used to confirm the presence of a patent ductus arteriosus.[42] The authors cannot recommend this as a routine, since there is no way to quantitate the magnitude of the left-to-right shunt by this method, and there is a danger of causing embolization of a clot present on the tip of the catheter.[66,67] If we perform an aortogram we prefer to use an approach through the left brachial artery (Fig. 9-8).

It would be helpful if catheterization data could be obtained which would allow distinction between the respiratory symptoms caused by the ductus and those caused by the underlying pulmonary disease.

We attempted to separate infants with respiratory distress syndrome and patent ductus arteriosus who were dependent upon the respirator because of pulmonary disease from infants who require prolonged ventilatory assistance because of congestive cardiac failure.[68] We performed cardiac catheterizations to obtain data which would allow prediction of which infant would respond to ligation of the patent ductus arteriosus. We measured pulmonary function with a mass spectrophotometer and, simultaneously, intracardiac pressure and measured such shunt calculation from indocyanine green dye curves. We studied each premature infant at several ambient oxygen concentrations. No parameter measured, such as the AaCO$_2$ gradient, distinguished the infant with

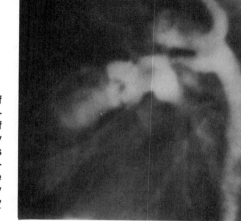

FIG. 9-8. Aortogram, lateral view, of patent ductus arteriosus in infant with rubella syndrome. Following injection of contrast material into aorta, pulmonary artery opacifies through patent ductus arteriosus. Characteristic findings of rubella syndrome are shown and include shortened pulmonary trunk, vertically oriented pulmonary valve, and pulmonary regurgitation.

heart disease from the infant with lung disease. Our purpose in recounting these negative data is to underscore that there is no consistent, reliable means of objectively predicting which premature infant is going to respond to closure of the ductus arteriosus.

MANAGEMENT.   Management of the premature infant with symptomatic patent ductus arteriosus must be considered in terms of (1) general supportive care, (2) specific medical therapy directed toward closure of the patent ductus arteriosus and control of congestive cardiac failure, and (3) operative ligation.

Supportive care includes fluid restriction, correction of anemia, and treatment of hypoxemia and acidemia. Total fluid intake should be limited to 70 to 100 ml/kg/day, so long as adequate hydration and urine output are maintained. Packed red blood cell transfusions may be necessary to maintain the hemoglobin concentration at about 12.0 g%. Occasionally, an anemic infant will markedly improve following blood transfusion, presumably due to increased oxygen-carrying capacity. Oxygen therapy, whether administered in a headbox or by a mechanical ventilator, should be adjusted to maintain a Po_2 from 60 to 85 torr. A lower Po_2 may not stimulate ductal constriction, and a higher Po_2 should be avoided because of the risk of retrolental fibroplasia. Ventilatory assistance is necessary if the infant has either severe respiratory distress syndrome or fulminant congestive cardiac failure. Ventilatory assistance improves oxygenation, diminished hypercarbia, and respiratory acidosis and reduces venous return to the heart.

Until recently, pharmacologic treatment consisted solely of digitalis and diuretics. The use of digoxin alone does not often result in dramatic clinical improvement. There are experimental data which suggest that higher doses than those commonly used are needed to effect a positive ionotropic response in prematures due to differences in drug sensitivity.[69]

There is little question that diuretics are effective in controlling congestive cardiac failure in premature infants. Furosemide and chlorothiazide are most commonly used. However, an occasional patient is refractory to these diuretic agents but will respond to the addition of an aldosterone antagonist.[19]

Sharpe and co-workers[70] first suggested the exciting possibility of pharmacologic closure of the ductus arteriosus with indomethacin inhibition of prostaglandin synthesis. Initial reports of the clinical use of indomethacin were encouraging because of the high incidence of successful treatment and the relatively low associated morbidity.[71-73] Our experience with this drug has been less satisfactory, though we used it in more severely ill infants and somewhat later in the course of the disease.[74] Of 18 premature infants with severe respiratory distress syndrome and symptomatic ductus arteriosus treated at West Virginia University, in only 2 did the patent ductus arteriosus close with indomethacin administration.

Indomethacin, when given relatively early and to a symptomatic premature infant, is effective in about half the patients. Therefore, the risk of such treatment must be considered against the risk of operative ligation of the ductus arteriosus. Serious complications of indomethacin therapy have occurred, including massive gastrointestinal hemorrhage and renal failure. Dosage should not exceed 0.1 mg/kg/dose. Two or three doses, given 24 hours apart, may be necessary. Until more data regarding the effectiveness and safety of this therapy are available, no infant should be given indomethacin except as dictated by strict experimental protocol and human subjects review.[75] Perhaps more effective, less toxic prostaglandin synthetase inhibitors will be available in the future.

Operative ligation of a patent ductus arteriosus must still be considered the preferred method of treatment. Selection of the premature infant likely to benefit from closure of the ductus and timing of the operation are difficult for reasons previously discussed. Currently, we recommend ligation of a patent ductus arteriosus only for those premature infants with evident congestive cardiac failure, who are unresponsive to digitalis or who show either no improvement or worsening pulmonary status. Operative ligation performed prior to 1 week of age leads to less morbidity than does protracted medical management.[76] As surgeons and anesthesiologists have gained more experience with ligation of patent ductus arteriosus in the small premature infants, operative complications have decreased. The outcome is related to the gestational age of the infant, the presence of other disease processes, such as hyaline membrane disease, sepsis, necrotizing enterocolitis, or intracranial hemorrhage, and the quality of perioperative care.

Persistence of the Ductus Arteriosus in the Term Infant

The incidence of persistent ductus arteriosus in term infants is considerably less than in premature infants. A study in the nurseries of the Toronto General Hospital revealed characteristic murmurs of patent ductus arteriosus in 14 percent of healthy newborns,[77] but in almost all, the murmur disappeared within 24 hours of birth. Based upon data collected by Campbell,[40] less than 1 per 1,000 term infants would be expected to have persistence of the ductus arteriosus beyond 3 months of age.

CLINICAL FEATURES.   The clinical course of full-term infants is quite different from that of prematures. The term infant with a patent ductus arteriosus is less likely to become symptomatic during childhood, although a few develop congestive cardiac failure during infancy. There are several reasons why a ductus is not as serious in these infants. Respiratory distress syndrome, with its accompanying ventilatory insufficiency and hypoxia, is less common. Pulmonary vascular resistance at 40 weeks gestation is higher than in the premature infant, and, therefore, the magnitude of the left-to-right shunt through the ductus is less. Finally, the ability of the mature myocardium to respond to volume stress is not as impaired.

Cyanosis is not present, and the infant appears healthy. Slight precordial bulging may be present by the end of the first year of life but not before. A suprasternal notch thrill is sometimes palpable by 1 year of age. The cardiac murmur is typically systolic, loudest beneath the left clavicle, and radiates well to the back in early infancy. As the child approaches 1 year of age, the characteristic continuous murmur becomes audible and usually is at least grade 3/6 in loudness. It is described as a "machinery murmur," since continuous left-to-right shunting of blood occurs. In contrast with the continuous murmur of a venous hum, the ductus murmur is constant and varies little with respiration or change in body position. Peripheral pulses are brisk due to the wide pulse pressure, and we have found it helpful to palpate digital and palmar pulses as well as the larger brachial and femoral vessels.

ELECTROCARDIOGRAPHIC AND ROENTGENOGRAPHIC FEATURES.   The roentgenographic and electrocardiographic findings depend upon the magnitude of the left-to-right shunt. Essentially normal data may be acquired from an infant with a small shunt. More commonly, the thoracic roentgenogram reveals mild left ventricular and left atrial enlargement and increased pulmonary vascular markings, and this is substantiated by electrocardiography.

CARDIAC CATHETERIZATION AND ANGIOCARDIOGRAM.   Cardiac catheterization is rarely necessary to substantiate the diagnosis of patent ductus arteriosus in infancy. In addition to the very characteristic clinical findings, the chest roentgenogram, electrocardiogram, and when necessary, echo and technetium[99] radioisotopic flow study provide enough presumptive evidence of the correct diagnosis to proceed with surgery. Cardiac catheterization is indicated when the diagnosis cannot be made with certainty otherwise or when congestive cardiac failure or evidence of pulmonary hypertension occurs.

In those unusual cases where cardiac catheterization is performed, it is often possible to advance the catheter from the pulmonary artery through the ductus into the descending aorta. If the ductus is small, the diagnosis is documented by an increase in oxygen saturation of at least 5 percent in the pulmonary artery and by aortography. Nadas[78] found that 30 percent of patients catheterized for a patent ductus arteriosus at Boston Children's Hospital had elevated pulmonary vascular resistance, but he points out that this figure is skewed by selection of patients who are atypical.

MANAGEMENT.   Since infants with patent ductus arteriosus are usually asymptomatic, no specific treatment is indicated until approximately 1 year of age, when operative ligation should be performed. Spontaneous closure beyond 6 months of age is uncommon and beyond 1 year of age reportable. Thus, there is no particular benefit to be gained by postponing surgery beyond infancy, and the operative risk is extremely low.

The complications of unoperated patent ductus arteriosus include pulmonary vascular disease, subacute bacterial endocarditis, and, rarely, congestive cardiac failure.

The development of irreversible pulmonary vascular disease at an early age secondary to patent ductus arteriosus is unusual but does occur. It is unpredictable and does not seem to be simply related to increased flow through the pulmonary bed. Rather, an occasional infant does not seem to experience the predictable fall in pulmonary vascular resistance after birth which occurs with maturation of the pulmonary vascular bed. Keith et al.[79] reported that 11 percent of patients with isolated patent ductus arteriosus from 1 month to 15 years of age had severe pulmonary hypertension.

Subacute bacterial endocarditis (SBE) is likewise rare, especially during the first decade, but occurred in 38 of 1,433 patients reviewed at the Institute of Cardiology in Mexico City.[80]

Pulmonary vascular disease and subacute bacterial endocarditis account for the majority of deaths in patients with patent ductus arteriosus. The average life expectancy without surgery is 35 to 40 years.[81]

Congestive cardiac failure can develop in some full-term infants. These should be treated with digitalis and diuretics, followed by ligation of the ductus.

Patent Ductus Arteriosus in Association with Other Congenital Cardiac Anomalies

Patency of the ductus arteriosus in association with other congenital heart defects is poorly understood. Though it is known that the incidence of patent ductus arteriosus is substantially increased in the presence of intracardiac anomalies, the reasons remain unclear. Cassels and co-workers[82] have concluded that in some situations, especially cyanotic congenital heart disease, low oxygen tension plays a significant role in maintaining patency, but in others a primary defect in the ductal wall may exist as a part of the congenital heart disease complex.

Patients with pulmonary atresia, tricuspid atresia, and hypoplastic right ventricle may be almost entirely dependent upon ductal patency for the maintenance of pulmonary blood flow. Continued patency of the ductus is also required in interrupted aortic arch to ensure adequate blood flow to the aorta. The patient becomes symptomatic when obliteration of the aortic end of the ductus lumen contributes to the development of critical obstruction.[83]

In 1973, Coceani and Olley[84] demonstrated that the E series prostaglandins were potent relaxants of the ductus arteriosus. Elliott and co-workers[85] infused PGE₁ into two neonates with ductus-dependent cyanotic congenital cardiac anomalies, and arterial oxygen saturation improved. These results have been confirmed by additional clinical trials,[86,87] and the indications for prostaglandin infusion have been extended to include left-sided obstructive lesions, such as coarctation of the aorta, interrupted aortic arch, and critical aortic stenosis. Potentially, very hypoxemic, acidotic infants with transposition of the great vessels may benefit from prostaglandin E₁ infusion by opening the ductus arteriosus and improving shunting from the left to right atrium.

PGE₁ is the preferred drug because it is a weak pulmonary vasodilator as well as a mediator of ductal relaxation. The initial recommended dose of 0.1 μg/kg/min in 5 percent dextrose is infused either intravenously or intraarterially. Heart rate, blood pressure, respiratory rate, and temperature must be closely monitored and the infusion rate reduced to 0.05 μg/kg/min if possible. At least a 50 percent rise in Po_2 should occur within 10 minutes.

Prostaglandin E₁ infusion is of greatest potential benefit to the critically ill, hypoxemic, acidotic infant in need of further diagnostic study and operative correction or palliation. It, therefore, may be indicated while awaiting and effecting transport of the infant to a cardiac center, during cardiac catheterization, and while preparing for cardiac surgery.

CONGENITALLY CORRECTED TRANSPOSITION OF THE GREAT VESSELS

Congenitally corrected transposition of the great vessels is a cardiac malformation that derives its name from the fact that the circulation is correct, i.e., systemic venous blood is delivered to the lungs and pulmonary blood to the body, and transposition of the great vessels is present because the aorta lies anteriorly and arises from an infundibulum. In itself, this malformation should not cause cardiac symptoms, but it is almost always associated with other cardiac anomalies, and it is these that alert the physician to the presence of a congenital cardiac malformation. The most prevalent coexistent anomalies are ventricular septal defect, pulmonary stenosis, left atrioventricular valvular insufficiency, and cardiac malpositions. It is the clinical picture of these associated anomalies that mimics and must be distinguished from ventricular septal defect, tetralogy of Fallot, mitral insufficiency, and dextrocardia, respectively. Although a general introduction to congenitally corrected transposition of the great vessels will be presented in this chapter, the condition will be discussed in each chapter in which it must be considered in the differential diagnosis.

PATHOLOGY.   In congenitally corrected transposition of the great vessels, the great vessels are transposed so that the aorta lies anteriorly and to the left of the pulmonary trunk (Fig. 9-9). In addition, the ventricles are inverted so that the anatomic left ventricle lies to the right and the anatomic right ventricle lies to the left.[88,89]

The vena cavae connect normally to an anatomic right atrium. The right atrium connects with a ventricle with the anatomic features of a left ventricle, i.e., it is smooth walled and lacks an infundibulum, semilunar and atrioventricular valves are continuous, it has a mitral valve, and the outflow tract is posterior. The pulmonary trunk originates from this ventricle and is posteriorly placed.

The pulmonary veins join the left atrium, which communicates with a ventricle having the anatomic features of a right ventricle, i.e., it is trabeculated and has an infundibulum, an anterior outflow tract, and a tricuspid atrioventricular valve. The aorta arises from this ventricle in an anterior position. Because of the relationship of the great vessels, with the aorta being positioned to the left of the pulmonary artery, this condition has also been called "*l*-transposition."

The inversion of the ventricles is believed to result from looping of the primitive cardiac tube toward the left rather than toward the right. Two other

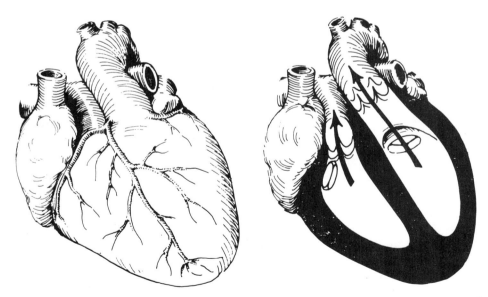

FIG. 9-9.   Diagram showing anatomic relationship in congenitally corrected transposition of great vessels. Aorta lies anteriorly and to left of pulmonary trunk and arises from an infundibulum. Left atrioventricular valve has three cusps. Pulmonary trunk arises posteriorly and rightward. There is continuity between pulmonary and right atrioventricular valve, which is bicuspid. Anterior descending coronary artery arises from right coronary artery.

anatomic features of congenitally corrected transposition have clinical importance: (1) the anterior descending coronary artery arising from the right coronary artery, and (2) abnormalities of the conducting tissues, leading to inversion of the bundles of His.[90,91]

In patients with coexistent ventricular septal defect, the defect is usually large and located in the position of the membranous ventricular septum, immediately below the pulmonary valve and below the crista supraventricularis.[89]

CLINICAL FEATURES.   Most patients with congenitally corrected transposition of the great vessels develop cardiac symptoms in the first year of life.[89] Those with ventricular septal defect present with a murmur of a ventricular septal defect, and if the defect is large, congestive cardiac failure develops.

Aside from the murmur of ventricular septal defect, the important auscultatory finding which indicates the presence of congenitally corrected transposition of the great vessels is a loud, single second sound along the upper left sternal border. This sound represents the closure of the anteriorly placed aortic valve. The loudest second heart sounds we have heard are in patients with congenitally corrected transposition of the great vessels.

ELECTROCARDIOGRAM.   The electrocardiogram also provides a major clue for recognition of congenitally corrected transposition of the great vessels as the underlying cardiac malformation (Fig. 9-10). Typically, lead V_1 shows a q wave, and V_6 shows no q wave.[92,93] Although occasionally V_1 has an R wave, there is not a q wave in lead V_6 of such cases.[89] This abnormality of the initial QRS forces reflects the inversion of the bundles of His. The remainder of the QRS complex reflects this hemodynamic load upon the ventricles, such as elevated pulmonary arterial pressures or excess volume loads.

THORACIC ROENTGENOGRAM.   The thoracic roentgenogram, as expected in a patient with ventricular septal defect, shows increased pulmonary vascularity, cardiomegaly, and left atrial enlargement. The left cardiac border, however, is either straight or shows only two curves (Fig. 9-11), since it is composed of a ventricular border and ascending aorta, instead of an aortic knob, pulmonary trunk, and ventricle, as in normally related great vessels.[94]

ECHOCARDIOGRAM.   Echocardiographic diagnosis of congenitally corrected transposition of the great vessels is difficult to make. One difficulty is that the interventricular septum may not be identified because it lies in a plane parallel to the echo beam. The diagnosis can be suspected if the anterior vessel lies leftward and the posterior vessel rightward, and if the posterior atrioventricular valve (inverted tricuspid) is not in continuity with either semilunar valve.

CARDIAC CATHETERIZATION AND ANGIOCARDIOGRAM.   Definitive diagnosis of congenitally corrected transposition of the great vessels is made by cardiac catheterization and angiocardiography. The catheter course shows the pulmonary trunk to be located medially and posteriorly and the aorta to be located anteriorly and laterally.

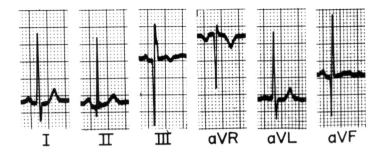

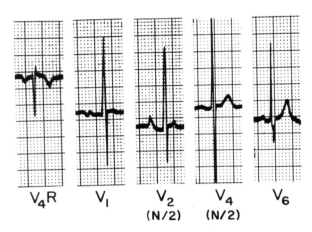

FIG. 9-10.   Electrocardiogram of congenitally corrected transposition of great vessels. Three-month-old infant with left atrioventricular valve insufficiency. Deep q waves in leads III and aVF. Absence of q wave in lead V_6.

Angiography demonstrates the relationship of the great vessels, the anatomy of the inverted ventricles, and the characteristic position of the interventricular septum in the frontal plane (Fig. 9-12). The septum lies perpendicular to the chest wall. The venous ventricle is triangular and lies inferior to the septum, while the arterial ventricle is rounded and forms the superior and left cardiac border.

MANAGEMENT.   Digitalis and diuretics are administered as they are to any infant with congestive cardiac failure. If the infant does not respond to medical management, pulmonary arterial banding should be performed. Previously, corrective operations have been avoided, primarily because of the propensity

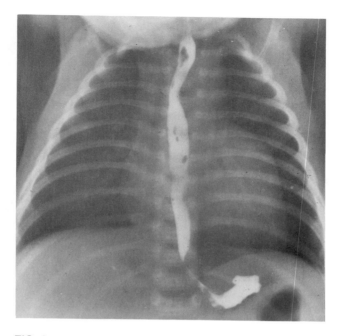

FIG. 9-11.   Thoracic roentgenogram of congenitally corrected transposition of great vessels. Posteroanterior view. Single hump along left cardiac border, which is location of infundibulum. Pulmonary arterial segment is concave.

to develop complete heart block and the difficulties encountered by the abnormal coronary arterial pattern. With the use of His bundle electrocardiography[95] and intracardiac mapping,[91,96,97] identification of the conduction tissue is possible, and, therefore, it can be avoided at operation and correction can be carried out.[98,99] There is little experience to date with corrective procedures in infancy.

AORTICOPULMONARY SEPTAL DEFECT

Aorticopulmonary septal defect is a rare condition in which a communication exists between the ascending aorta and the pulmonary trunk. Usually large, the defect permits free transmission of pressure into the pulmonary arteries. The hemodynamics resemble those of a large patent ductus arteriosus.

Clinical diagnosis is difficult, since the findings resemble those of a large ventricular septal defect or patent ductus, coexisting with pulmonary hypertension and congestive cardiac failure. The peripheral pulses, as expected, are accentuated. A grade 3/6 systolic murmur is present along the left sternal border. Rarely, a continuous murmur is found. The electrocardiogram shows biventricular hypertrophy. Cardiomegaly, left atrial enlargement, and increased

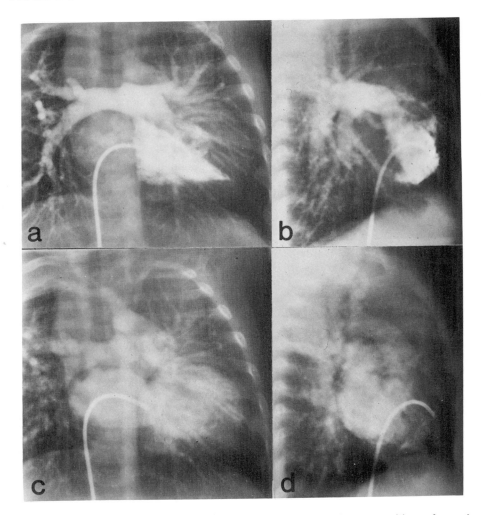

FIG. 9-12. Angiocardiograms of congenitally corrected transposition of great vessels. Early phase. **a.** Anteroposterior view. **b.** Lateral view. Injection into triangular, inverted left ventricle. Pulmonary trunk, medial and posterior. Late view. **c.** Anteroposterior view. **d.** Lateral view. Opacification of left atrium and inverted right ventricle. Aorta, anterior and lateral.

pulmonary blood flow are observed on the thoracic roentgenogram. Occasionally, a right aortic arch is present.

The diagnosis is made by injection of contrast material into the ascending aorta. This shows prompt opacification of the pulmonary arteries. The angiographic picture must be distinguished from persistent truncus arteriosus. In aorticopulmonary septal defect, the aorta is not as wide as in truncus arteriosus. Furthermore, right ventriculography helps to distinguish the two conditions by showing a distinct right ventricular outflow tract and pulmonary artery and by not showing a ventricular septal defect. Since a patent ductus arteriosus may coexist, an aortogram should also be performed in the proximal descending aorta.

Operation should be performed by closing the defect through the ascending aorta.

Patients should be carefully investigated, since aorticopulmonary window can coexist with other conditions, such as tetralogy of Fallot or interruption of the aorta.[100]

AORTIC ORIGIN OF PULMONARY ARTERY

In this rare condition, a pulmonary artery arises from the ascending aorta, usually within a centimeter of the aortic valve. The aortic origin occurs opposite the side of the aortic arch, thus, almost always, the right pulmonary artery arises from the ascending aorta. With right aortic arch, the left pulmonary artery may have ascending aortic origin, except in patients with tetralogy of Fallot,[101] when it arises on the ipsilateral side. This condition usually presents in infancy with a picture of congestive cardiac failure and must be considered in the differential diagnosis of extracardiac left-to-right shunts.

PATHOLOGY. Aortic origin of the pulmonary artery is believed to result from uneven division of the primitive truncus arteriosus, leading to a pulmonary artery arising from the ascending aorta. The pulmonary trunk supplies only the contralateral lung. The involved lung has normal size and structure. This anomaly may coexist with tetralogy of Fallot, ventricular septal defect, or, most frequently, patent ductus arteriosus. The last situation occurred in 38 of 44 patients reviewed by Keane and associates.[102]

Histologic examination of the lungs shows either of two pictures. Usually both lungs show medial hypertrophy,[103,104] but if the pulmonary artery arising from the aorta is narrowed, that lung shows thin-walled arterioles.[105] With age, progressive pulmonary vascular changes occur.

HEMODYNAMICS. The normally connected lung receives the entire systemic venous return, so its flow is at least twice normal. The lung connected to the aorta receives fully oxygenated blood, the volume of pulmonary blood flow being determined by the size of the orifice and the relative vascular resistances. Pulmonary hypertension is found in both lungs, understandably in the lung with aortic origin, since it communicates with the aorta. The reason for the pulmonary hypertension in the contralateral lung is unknown, but the high obligatory pulmonary blood flow from birth probably delays the regression of the neonatal pulmonary vasculature.

Cyanosis may be present, and in one patient, Cumming et al.[106] demonstrated small right-to-left shunts through a patent foramen ovale and a patent ductus arteriosus.

CLINICAL FEATURES.   Within the first month of life, most patients are symptomatic, with tachypnea, dyspnea, and congestive cardiac failure. These symptoms may be associated with a pulmonary infection. Slight or intermittent cyanosis is common.

The auscultatory findings are uncharacteristic and variable. In most infants, a grade 3/6 midsystolic murmur is heard along the left sternal border and a diastolic murmur at the apex.[103,104,107] Because blood flows from the aorta during diastole, accentuated peripheral pulses might be expected, but congestive cardiac failure and reduced cardiac output diminish them. The pulmonary second heart sound is accentuated. Cardiac activity is increased.

ELECTROCARDIOGRAM.   The electrocardiogram shows right ventricular hypertrophy, which may be combined with left ventricular hypertrophy. Right atrial enlargement may be present.

THORACIC ROENTGENOGRAM.   Cardiomegaly and left atrial enlargement are found. Increased pulmonary arterial vasculature is found in the lung field with the aortic origin. Frequently, the contralateral lung also shows increased markings, presumably because it receives twice the normal volume of blood flow.

CARDIAC CATHETERIZATION AND ANGIOCARDIOGRAM.   On right-sided cardiac catheterization, the catheter can be advanced only into one lung from the pulmonary trunk, while a catheter in the ascending aorta may be advanced into the opposite lung.

Oximetry data show no evidence of a left-to-right shunt, although as indicated by Cumming and co-workers,[106] indicator dilution curves show a pattern of left-to-right shunt. Slight systemic arterial desaturation may be present.[102,108] Pulmonary arterial hypertension is found in the pulmonary trunk, and the pulmonary arterial pressures are similar to those of the aorta.

Angiography from the pulmonary trunk shows opacification of a single pulmonary artery, while the opposite pulmonary artery is visualized following aortography from the ascending aorta (Fig. 9-13).

The presence of a coexistent patent ductus arteriosus should be sought.

TREATMENT.   Following the usual management for congestive cardiac failure and appropriate diagnostic studies, attempts should be made to anastomose the pulmonary artery to the pulmonary trunk.[102,106,108] If anastomosis is performed in infancy, the pulmonary arterial pressure and vascular resistance become normal.

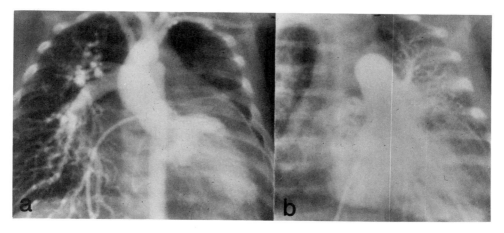

FIG. 9-13.   Aortic origin of right pulmonary artery. Anteroposterior views: **a.** Left ventriculogram. **b.** Right ventriculogram. Right pulmonary artery arises from ascending aorta. Right ventriculogram opacifies pulmonary trunk and only the left pulmonary artery.

SHUNTS AT THE ATRIAL LEVEL

In two conditions, endocardial cushion defect and atrial septal defect, a communication exists at the atrial level which allows a left-to-right shunt. During the first year of life, endocardial cushion defect leads to congestive cardiac failure in a number of patients, while isolated atrial septal defect often escapes detection and rarely leads to symptoms.

As indicated in Chapter 8, flow through atrial communications is dependent upon relative ventricular compliances, and this principle is well illustrated in children with atrial septal defect. In infants with endocardial cushion defect, the hemodynamics are more complex and vary with the form of the defect. They may be governed by relative compliances or vascular resistances or depend upon an obligatory shunt, or a combination of these factors.

ENDOCARDIAL CUSHION DEFECT

Endocardial cushion defect represents a spectrum of cardiac anomalies resulting from maldevelopment of structures formed by endocardial cushion tissue, i.e., lower portion of the atrial septum, posterior-superior portion of the ventricular septum, and septal leaflets of the mitral and the tricuspid valves. Although each of these four structures may be involved individually or in combination, yielding a possibility of 14 different malformations, in most instances, endocardial cushion defects involve the lower part of the atrial septum, a variable extent of the subjacent ventricular septum, and the septal leaflet of the mitral valve. Therefore, most patients with endocardial cushion defect have a combination of left-to-right shunt at the atrial (and ventricular) level and mitral insufficiency.

DEVELOPMENTAL ANATOMY.   A review of the embryology of the endocardial cushion tissue and the structures formed by this tissue will aid in understanding the anatomic details of the anomaly.[109] Early in development, the heart is two chambered, having a common atria and ventricle, which communicate through the primitive atrioventricular canal. The septum primum and the ventricular septum form and partially divide the atria and the ventricles, respectively. The septum primum forms from the posterior superior aspect of the common atrium, and its crescent-shaped free edge grows forward toward the atrioventricular canal.

During this time, masses of endocardial cushion tissue develop from the anterior and posterior aspects of the atrioventricular canal, and these projections grow toward each other in the midline of the atrioventricular canal, meet, and fuse. The fused endocardial cushions arch, so that the convexity is directed toward the atria, and the concavity is directed toward the left ventricle. The superior part of the endocardial cushion tissue fuses with the inferior margin of the septum primum, sealing the septum primum. The right aspect of the arched endocardial cushion tissue fuses with the ventricular septum, closing the secondary interventricular foramen.

The left-sided aspect of the fused endocardial cushion tissue differentiates to form the septal (anterior) leaflet of the mitral valve, while portions of the right side of the fused endocardial cushion tissue contribute to the septal leaflet of the tricuspid valve.

Endocardial cushion defects result from faulty development of this process. Depending upon the extent of malformation of the endocardial cushion tissue, the resultant cardiac malformations range from a partial form, ostium primum defect, to complete atrioventricular canal. The pathologic details have been described.[110-112] In the partial form, there is almost complete fusion of the anterior and posterior endocardial cushions, except for the left-sided aspects. The incomplete fusion causes a cleft in the anterior leaflet of the mitral valve. In addition, the cushion tissue fails to fuse with the septum primum, thus leaving a defect in the lower part of the atrial septum adjacent to the mitral and tricuspid valves. The subjacent portion of the ventricular septum is also deficient, so that an elliptical defect is formed, involving principally the atrial septum.

In the complete form of endocardial cushion defect, complete atrioventricular canal, the process is arrested at an early stage. The endocardial cushion tissue fails to fuse in the midline and causes a large defect involving the lower portion of the atrial septum and adjacent portion of the posterior superior aspect of the ventricular septum (Fig. 9-14).

Because of failure of the cushions to fuse, the mitral and tricuspid valves are significantly malformed. The anterior endocardial cushion begins to differentiate into the atrioventricular valves, the left side into the mitral valve, and

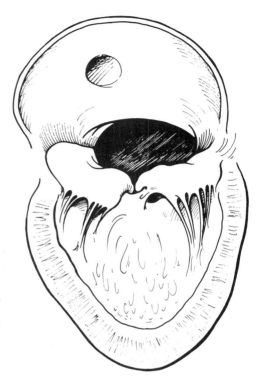

FIG. 9-14.   Diagram of complete atrioventricular canal, left atrial and left ventricular aspect. Defect involving lower atrial septum and adjacent portion of ventricular septum. Portions of anterior leaflet of mitral valve continuous through defect with tricuspid valve.

the right side into the tricuspid valve. The posterior tissue does also. The anterior aspects of each valve fuse with one another through the defect, and a similar process occurs with the posterior aspects, forming a common anterior and common posterior atrioventricular valve leaflet (Fig. 9-15). Each leaflet is comprised of tissue originally designed to be mitral and tricuspid tissue. These common leaflets bridge the defect from the left ventricle to the right ventricle and have chordal attachment to both ventricles and, at times, to the rim of the ventricular septum. The size of the ventricular component of the defect is variable.

Despite the fact that the ventricular septum is involved, the common anterior and posterior atrioventricular valve leaflets may be tethered to the ventricular septum by chordae tendineae, so that no ventricular communication is present.

HEMODYNAMICS.   The hemodynamics of endocardial cushion defects are not well understood. In individual patients, the hemodynamics demonstrated at cardiac catheterization cannot always be correlated with the anatomic details found at autopsy. On the other hand, similar hemodynamic data may be found in patients with endocardial cushion defects which anatomically are quite dissimilar. Furthermore, because shunts may occur at both the atrial and the ven-

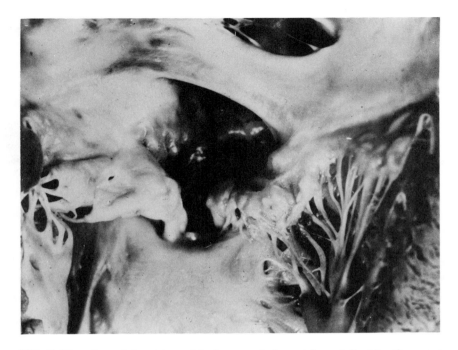

FIG. 9-15. Complete atrioventricular canal viewed from left side. Common atrioventricular valve leaflets pass through the defect.

tricular levels, the flow through each defect cannot be separately quantitated. Atrioventricular valve insufficiency, particularly of the mitral valve, is commonly present, and the degree of regurgitation cannot be quantitated by the usual angiographic techniques. An additional factor complicating understanding of the hemodynamics is the spectrum of abnormalities found among patients with endocardial cushion defect. For these reasons, it is difficult to make definitive statements about the hemodynamics of this anomaly.

Four major hemodynamic abnormalities may be present:

1. Shunt at the atrial level
2. Shunt at the ventricular level
3. Atrioventricular valvular insufficiency, particularly of the mitral valve
4. Pulmonary valvular insufficiency

The direction and magnitude of the shunt at the atrial level occurring through the atrial defect (ostium primum) depend upon the relative ventricular compliances. At birth, the right ventricle is thick walled, but as the pulmonary vascular resistance falls, it thins and becomes more complaint, so that the left-to-right shunt increases. In infants with pulmonary hypertension, the right ventricular hypertrophy may persist and limit the left-to-right shunt. However, the left ventricle may shunt directly into the right atrium in any form of endo-cardial cushion defect because of the proximity of the abnormal anterior leaflet of the mitral valve and the endocardial cushion defect. This obligatory shunt occurs independently of ventricular compliances and depends upon flow from the high-pressure left ventricle into the low-pressure right atrium.

A shunt can also occur at the ventricular level, i.e., through the endocardial cushion defect below the level of the atrioventricular valves, and, when present, indicates complete atrioventricular canal. This shunt depends upon the relative pulmonary and systemic vascular resistances. As the pulmonary vascular resistance falls following birth, the volume of left-to-right shunt through the defect and the volume of pulmonary blood flow increase.

Either atrioventricular valve can be insufficient. Regurgitation through the mitral valve may be a dominant hemodynamic factor in many infants, whereas tricuspid valve regurgitation is not considered an important hemodynamic factor. Perhaps this is because at the time of cardiac catheterization, left ventri-culography is routinely performed, whereas right ventriculography is not. Even with right ventriculography, it may be difficult to separate true from artifactual tricuspid insufficiency. Mitral regurgitation may be directed primarily into either atrium. Even when it occurs into the left atrium, the regurgitant flow may pass principally into the right atrium because of the coexistent left-to-right atrial shunt, and, therefore, the left atrium does not enlarge.

Mitral insufficiency progresses because it causes left ventricular enlarge-ment and dilatation of the mitral annulus. These effects lead to a greater de-gree of mitral insufficiency and further left ventricular dilatation.

Pulmonary hypertension is often present in infants with endocardial cush-ion defect. In infants without a ventricular communication, the elevated pul-monary arterial pressure results primarily from the increased pulmonary blood flow, while in those with a ventricular communication, the ventricular systolic pressures equilibrate because of the defect. With age, pulmonary vascular re-sistance can rise, but this rarely happens during infancy.

The hemodynamics in infants with ostium primum defect resemble those in atrial septal defect and mitral insufficiency. Pulmonary arterial pressures are normal or mildly elevated.

Among infants with complete forms of endocardial cushion defect and a ventricular communication, the left ventricle is submitted to a volume overload because of the mitral regurgitation and the left-to-right shunt through the ven-tricular septal defect. The right ventricle also has increased volume load be-cause of the shunt into the right atrium. The right ventricle in these infants must then eject the blood against the elevated pulmonary arterial pressure. The hemodynamic effect on either ventricle can lead to congestive cardiac fail-ure, which, once present, is usually progressive.

CLINICAL FEATURES.   In most patients with endocardial cushion defect, the pres-ence of congenital cardiac disease is initially recognized during infancy because of the presence of a murmur. Infants with a partial form are asymptomatic or have few symptoms. In contrast, those with complete atrioventricular canal often develop severe symptoms in infancy, even within the first month of life.[113,114] The symptoms of tachypnea, dyspnea, feeding difficulties, repeated respiratory infections, and retarded growth relate to congestive cardiac failure.

The severity and age of onset of congestive cardiac failure relate more closely to the degree of mitral regurgitation than to any other single anatomic factor. Infants with significant mitral regurgitation may develop symptoms in the first month of life, while those with a ventricular septal defect and minimal mitral regurgitation may develop symptoms later in infancy. Infants with a complete atrioventricular canal but without a ventricular communication follow a more benign course, resembling that of ostium primum defect.

Cardiac examination shows a precordial bulge. The cardiac activity is increased, and the apex impulse is displaced downward and laterally. Thrills may be present.

The auscultatory findings vary, depending upon the type of hemodynamic abnormality, but at times they correlate poorly with anatomic or hemodynamic details. We have seen infants with complete atrioventricular canal in whom no murmur was heard.

As in any patient with a shunt at the atrial level, the first heart sound is accentuated in the tricuspid area. The second heart sound should appear fixed and widely split, but if pulmonary hypertension is present, the degree of splitting narrows, and the pulmonary component is accentuated.

Several types of murmurs may be heard. If there is no ventricular component, a grade 2–3/6 pulmonary systolic ejection murmur is present and related to the increased pulmonary blood flow secondary to the atrial left-to-right shunt. An apical pansystolic murmur could also be heard in this patient and indicates mitral regurgitation, the loudness of the murmur reflecting the amount of regurgitation. If a ventricular communication is present, a loud pansystolic murmur is present along the lower left sternal border and radiates well through the precordium. Because of its loudness and radiation, it may be difficult to distinguish a separate murmur of mitral insufficiency.

Low-pitched middiastolic murmurs are usually present and related to increased blood flow across the tricuspid or mitral valve.

ELECTROCARDIOGRAM. The electrocardiographic features in endocardial cushion defect are diagnostic (Fig. 9-16), and it is difficult to make a diagnosis without the characteristic features being present. Left axis deviation is present in 98 percent of patients, and this is caused by an abnormality of the atrioventricular conduction system. In a histologic study of the conduction system in endocardial cushion defect, Feldt and Titus[115] describe five abnormalities: (1) posterior displacement of the atrioventricular node, (2) posterior displacement of the common bundle of His by the endocardial cushion defect, (3) early origin of the left bundle, (4) displacement of the distal left bundle branch fascicle to the posterior aspect of the ventricular septum, and (5) apparent hypoplasia of the anterior portion of the left fasciculus. These abnormalities, defined on careful

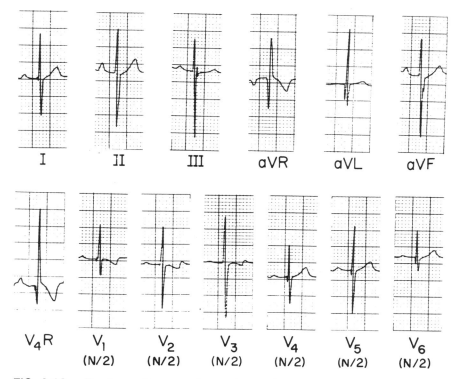

FIG. 9-16. Electrocardiogram of complete atrioventricular canal in 6-month-old infant. QRS axis is $-90°$. PR is 0.18 sec. Biventricular hypertrophy. N/2, half-standardization.

histopathologic studies, probably account for the left axis deviation. Their observations are substantiated by epicardial mapping studies performed at the time of operation which show early depolarization of the posterior portion of the ventricles.[116] The degree of left axis deviation varies from $0°$ to $-150°$, greater degrees being associated with higher levels of right ventricular pressure and, presumably, more complete forms of atrioventricular canal. Ongley and associates[117] indicated that a QRS axis greater than $-90°$ is almost always indicative of a complete atrioventricular canal, and if it is less than $-60°$, it is almost always indicative of partial atrioventricular canal.

Usually the QRS voltage in each of the standard leads is increased. The PR interval is often prolonged. P waves show a pattern of right atrial enlargement by being tall in leads II, III, or the right precordial leads. P waves frequently are broad, but not sufficiently broad for a diagnosis of left atrial enlargement.

The precordial leads may show different patterns of ventricular hypertrophy. In lead V_1, an rSR' or rR' pattern is almost invariably present. Biventricular hypertrophy is common, the left ventricular component reflecting the volume overload on the left ventricle and the right ventricular component reflecting pressure or volume loads. It is difficult to correlate these patterns precisely with the hemodynamics.

THORACIC ROENTGENOGRAM.   Although cardiac size may be normal at birth or within the first month of life, cardiac enlargement is the rule and can involve both ventricles and the right atrium (Fig. 9-17). The left atrium may be normal or minimally enlarged, even in the face of significant mitral regurgitation, since the regurgitant flow is not directed into the body of the left atrium.

In our experience, the cardiac silhouette is enlarged out of proportion to the pulmonary arterial markings. The difference is that cardiac enlargement depends not only on the amount of left-to-right shunt but also upon the degree of atrioventricular valvular insufficiency that contributes to cardiac chamber enlargement. In an occasional patient, the thoracic roentgenogram closely resembles that of cardiomyopathy, since there is diffuse enlargement and the pulmonary vascular markings may appear normal or hazy, as in pulmonary edema.

ECHOCARDIOGRAM.   The echocardiogram in endocardial cushion defect has a high degree of diagnostic specificity, principally because of the echocardiographic abnormalities of the mitral valve. The most common finding is diastolic apposition of the anterior leaflet of the valve to the interventricular septum and, occasionally, apparent movement of the mitral valve across the interventricular septum. Although the movement across the ventricular septum was originally described for complete atrioventricular canal (Fig. 9-18), Hagler[118] indicates that this may be present in partial atrioventricular canal. The mitral valve does not actually move across the interventricular septum, but this appearance is produced by movement of the tricuspid and mitral valve portions of the common valve leaflets into the echocardiographic beam.[119]

Other echocardiographic findings of endocardial cushion defect[120] include (1) multiple systolic echoes of the mitral valve, but this is not specific for this anomaly, for it may be recorded in other conditions such as mitral stenosis, (2) abnormal echoes from the posterior leaflet of the mitral valve, showing deeper posterior movement, especially the a dip, (3) narrowing of the left ventricular outflow tract, which supposedly correlates with the gooseneck deformity observed in left ventriculography, and (4) increased amplitude of mitral valve excursion, but this may be observed in other causes of mitral insufficiency.

Attempts have been made to distinguish partial from complete forms of endocardial cushion defect. The results of studies have varied because of differences in criteria and of difficulties in precisely identifying and distinguishing forms of endocardial cushion defect from clinical, operative, or autopsy data.

Our experience is different from that reported by Hagler.[118] We have found a high correlation of certain echocardiographic findings with partial and complete atrioventricular canal. In partial atrioventricular canal, the following features are observed: (1) lack of continuity between the mitral and tricuspid valves through the septum—by carefully identifying the timing of each valve

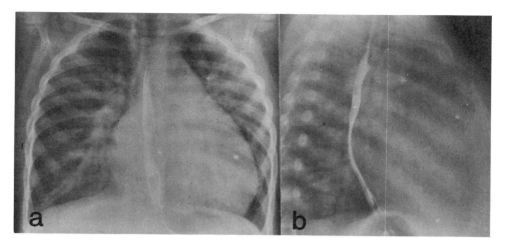

FIG. 9-17. Thoracic roentgenograms of complete atrioventricular canal. **a.** Posteroanterior view. **b.** Lateral view. Moderate cardiomegaly. Increased pulmonary arterial vasculature. Mild left atrial enlargement.

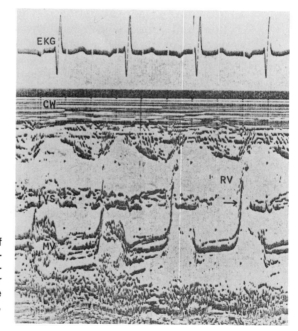

FIG. 9-18. Echocardiogram of complete atrioventricular canal. Mitral valve (MV) leaflet (arrow) appears to cross interventricular septum (IVS) into right ventricle (RV). CW, chest wall; EKG, electrocardiogram.

opening, we found that the mitral and the tricuspid valves open at different times, (2) paradoxical septal motion—present in 80 percent of our patients but in only 42 percent of those reported by Hagler,[118] (3) essentially normal movement of the anterior leaflet of the mitral valve, and (4) late systolic anterior motion of the mitral valve.

In complete atrioventricular canal, we observed (1) continuity of the mitral and tricuspid valves through the ventricular septum, (2) normal movement of the interventricular septum, (3) abnormal motion of the anterior leaflet of the mitral valve, (4) normal systolic motion of the mitral valve, and (5) absence of the interventricular septum separating the mitral and tricuspid valves.

CARDIAC CATHETERIZATION AND ANGIOCARDIOGRAM.   Performance of the catheterization from the inguinal region allows easy manipulation of the catheter tip into the left atrium and left ventricle, although there may be some difficulty entering the right ventricle and pulmonary arteries. This difficulty relates to the fact that the catheter course, either into the right ventricle or through the endocardial cushion defect into the left ventricle, appears identical on the fluoroscopic screen. The catheter course into the left ventricle is characteristic and follows a low straight path rather than the arching course seen in patients in whom the left ventricle is catheterized through a foramen ovale or secundum type atrial septal defect.

Careful oximetry series should be performed through the right atrium and also upon withdrawal from the pulmonary artery. Serial sampling shows a large increase in oxygen saturation at the right atrial level, indicating the left-to-right shunt from either or both the left atrium and left ventricle. The oxygen saturation of the inferior vena cava may be elevated because of reflux of blood from the right atrium, and, therefore, the superior vena caval sample should be used as the mixed venous site for calculation of blood flows. An additional increase in oxygen saturation almost always occurs at the right ventricular level[121] and may be as large as 8 or 9 percent. This increase does not indicate an associated ventricular septal defect but can occur from streaming of the imperfectly mixed blood from the right atrium into the right ventricle.

The atrial pressures are equal and show similar wave forms, with either a or v predominating.[121] In infants with cardiac failure, atrial pressures may be elevated to a level of 15 mm Hg. Although, among the entire group of patients with endocardial cushion defect, right ventricular and pulmonary arterial pressures may range from normal to systemic levels, most symptomatic infants have right ventricular and pulmonary arterial systolic pressures that are at least 75 percent of systemic systolic pressure. Generally, with more extensive forms of endocardial cushion defect, there is a greater degree of pulmonary hypertension. This elevation is usually associated with a ventricular septal defect which allows equalization of ventricular pressures. We have, however, studied young infants and found systemic levels of pulmonary arterial pressure associated with a significant mitral insufficiency and a large left-to-right atrial shunt but no shunt at the ventricular level. If right ventricular systolic pressure is much less than left ventricular systolic pressure and a ventricular communication is present, the defect cannot be large.

The most important diagnostic aspect of the cardiac catheterization is the left ventriculogram, which demonstrates the characteristic gooseneck deformity.[122-124] This term describes the appearance of the left ventricle, subaortic area, and ascending aorta. Although there remains some question regarding the anatomic details causing this appearance, it is likely that the attachment of the septal leaflet tissue of the mitral valve to the lower rim of the canal defect involves and hollows out the ventricular septum beneath the normal location of the mitral annulus.

Normally on an anteroposterior view of the left ventriculogram, the medial border of the left ventricle is straight or slightly convex toward the right ventricle, but in endocardial cushion defect it is concave, and the subaortic area is narrowed. This margin appears scalloped, and in its mid-portion, there may be a nonopaque indentation that presumably represents the cleft of the mitral valve (Fig. 9-19). Following left ventriculography, there is reflux of opaque material, frequently at the site of the cleft, and this passes predominantly and rapidly into the right atrium. It can also pass directly from the left ventricle to the right atrium or from the ventricle to the left atrium and into the right atrium

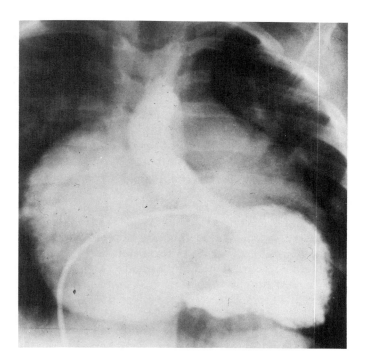

FIG. 9-19.   Left ventriculogram, anteroposterior view, of endocardial cushion defect. Medial border of left ventricle shows concavity, representing lower margin of the cushion defect. This has been called "gooseneck" deformity. Right atrium opacified from mitral insufficiency and left-to-right atrial shunt.

because of the left-to-right shunt. It is difficult to quantitate the degree of mitral regurgitation.

Furthermore, the presence of mitral regurgitation and opacification of the right atria can obscure the identification of a ventricular septal defect. On lateral views of the left ventriculogram, a ventricular septal defect may be suspected if the column of opaque medium is broad and the right ventricle is identified, whereas in mitral regurgitation the jet usually fans out. Often, however, because of the volume of shunt and regurgitation, the opaque material is diluted, making careful delineation not possible. A large volume of opaque material should be delivered as quickly as possible to obtain satisfactory visualization of the anatomic detail. In either projection, ventricular septal defect can be suspected if the pulmonary artery opacifies more densely than or simultaneously with the right atrium. As with any patient with systemic pressure in the right ventricle, an aortogram should be performed to identify a silent patent ductus arteriosus.

MANAGEMENT.   Although many children with endocardial cushion defect are asymptomatic during childhood, those with more extensive defects, such as complete atrioventricular canal, develop congestive cardiac failure during the first year of life and at times within the first month. At least 50 percent of patients with complete atrioventricular canal die in the first year of life.

Prompt and vigorous therapy with a digitalis preparation and diuretics should be given to treat congestive cardiac failure. In our experience, half of infants with endocardial cushion defect developing congestive cardiac failure respond to treatment and can be maintained satisfactorily into childhood, at which time a corrective operation can be performed.

Neonates or infants who do not respond to treatment present a difficult management problem. We have treated such patients extensively and with large doses of medication before undertaking operation. Some die despite extensive medical management.

In patients with a large ventricular septal defect, banding of the pulmonary artery can be performed. All of our patients who have been banded have survived. If there is a small or no ventricular septal defect and congestive cardiac failure results principally from mitral insufficiency, banding is not helpful, and the infants do not survive banding because the mitral reflux is unimproved by banding. Furthermore, if the shunt is obligatory, the right ventricle must eject the large right ventricular volume against the added resistance of the pulmonary arterial band.

We believe that infants who are unresponsive to digitalization and who remain in cardiac failure and have no significant ventricular defect should undergo corrective procedures as described by McGoon et al.[125] and others.[126,127] McGoon and associates[125] have operated on eight infants less than 1 year of age, weighing 2.9 to 6.5 kg, and had one operative and one late death. Frequently, findings of mitral regurgitation are present postoperatively. Correction should be performed (1) in infancy if medical management fails or (2) at 1 to 2 years of age as an elective procedure for all patients with pulmonary hypertension.

ATRIAL SEPTAL DEFECT

Among congenital cardiac anomalies affecting neonates or infants, atrial septal defect is thought to be rare, since few infants with atrial septal defect are symptomatic, and the condition is rarely diagnosed during the first year of life. Yet, a review of atrial septal defect is needed to be able to recognize the facets of this condition as they occur in infancy. In this section, three problems of atrial septal defect in infancy are discussed:

1. The symptomatic infant with atrial septal defect
2. Asymptomatic atrial septal defect
3. Spontaneous closure of atrial septal defect

A brief review of the development of the atrial septum following closure of the ostium primum is helpful. As the ostium primum is being closed by endocardial cushion tissue, perforations develop in the septum primum, coalesce, and form the ostium secundum. Subsequently, the septum secundum develops in the posterior and superior parts of the right atrium and grows anteriorly and inferiorly. The leading edge of the septum secundum is crescent shaped and grows inferiorly until it covers the ostium secundum.

The leading edge of the septum secundum forms the crista dividens of the fetal heart, so named because it divides the returning inferior vena caval blood and directs blood into the left atrium. Following birth, the rise in left atrial pressure forces the septum primum against the septum secundum, hemodynamically closing the foramen ovale, but, anatomically, a probe may be passed from the right to the left atrium for about a month and in one fourth of the population throughout life—this condition is valvular competent foramen ovale.

Atrial septal defects occurring in this area are called "ostium secundum defects" or "fossa ovalis defects." The defect may result from either too large an ostium secundum or too short a septum secundum.

Three other types of atrial septal defect occur:[128] (1) sinus venosus defect, which lies close to the right atrial ostium of the superior vena cava and may be associated with partial anomalous pulmonary venous connection of the right upper pulmonary vein, (2) defect in the area of the coronary sinus, as described by Raghib and associates,[129] in which there is absence of the coronary sinus and persistence of left superior vena cava to the left atrium, and (3) inferior vena caval type, in which the defect is located low in the atrial septum, adjacent to the inferior vena caval ostium in the right atrium.

The left atrium is not enlarged, but the right atrium and right ventricle are dilated. Their walls are usually not hypertrophied. The pulmonary trunk and the central pulmonary vessels are dilated.

There is little anatomic information about atrial septal defect in infancy[130] because, as an isolated lesion, it rarely causes death. It may be found as an incidental finding in infants dying of noncardiac causes, but it is almost always at the fossa ovalis. Tandon and Edwards[131] reviewed the status of the atrial septum in necropsy specimens of infants who died under 1 year of age. Among infants with anatomic evidence of an atrial septal defect, it almost invariably occurred at the fosa ovalis, took the form of a valvular incompetent foramen ovale, and was associated with other cardiac anomalies.

In reviewing 210 specimens of infants dying under 1 year of age, the status of the atrial septum was studied:[131] (1) of 66 specimens with conditions associated with left-to-right shunt, 12 (18 percent) showed a defect of fossa ovalis, presumably the left atrium enlarged from the increased pulmonary blood flow, stretching the valve of the foramen ovale, so that the ostium secundum and the fossa ovalis became enlarged, (2) of 72 specimens with right-sided obstructive anomalies, 22 (30 percent) had a defect at the foramen ovale from enlargement of the foramen ovale, (3) in 49 specimens of left-sided obstructive lesions, 14 (28 percent) also had a defect.

HEMODYNAMICS.   In most patients, the atrial septal defect is large and allows equalization of the atrial pressures, but if the defect is small, left atrial pressure exceeds right atrial pressure, and flow occurs from left to right because of the pressure difference. In infants with equal pressure in the atria, the direction and magnitude of shunt is dependent upon the relative resistances to ventricular inflow. In most patients, ventricular compliance is the determining factor influencing inflow resistance, but it should be remembered that a stenotic lesion in the region of an AV valve may be present and influence the shunt.

Ventricular compliance or distensibility in infants is believed to be determined principally by ventricular wall thickness. At birth, right ventricular weight exceeds left ventricular weight, but the wall thicknesses are equal. Therefore, at birth, no net shunt occurs, although patients with atrial septal defect may have a history of neonatal cyanosis, indicating a right-to-left shunt at this time. Following birth, pulmonary vascular resistance decreases, and, consequently, the right ventricle thins and becomes more compliant. On the other hand, systemic vascular resistance rises, and the left ventricle thickens and becomes less compliant. These changes favor increasing the left-to-right shunt. It has been believed that this process takes some time to take place, which would account for the infrequency of findings of atrial septal defect in infancy.

Because of the catheterization finding of a large left-to-right shunt in infants with atrial septal defect within a few days of life, Rudolph[132] has proposed an explanation based upon relative systemic and pulmonary vascular resistances. The volume of blood a ventricle ejects is dependent upon (1) preload (end-diastolic pressure), (2) afterload (outflow resistances), and (3) myocardial contractility. In atrial septal defect, preload is equal for both ventricles, and myocardial contractility should be equal, since the ventricles would be influenced by the same adrenergic factors. At birth, the afterloads, however, would be nearly equal, since the vascular resistances are similar. As the pulmonary vascular resistance drops, right ventricular stroke volume becomes larger than that of the left ventricle, so that right ventricular end-systolic volume is less than that of the left ventricle. Therefore, a greater volume will flow into the right ventricle during diastole. As pulmonary resistance falls further, the left-to-right shunt increases. These changes could take place without the normal changes in compliances.

The right ventricle tolerates large volumes of blood, since it ejects large volumes of blood against the low pulmonary resistance. Cardiac failure, therefore, rarely occurs, but when it does, such additional abnormalities as mitral stenosis, supravalvular stenosing ring, left ventricular myocardiopathy, or outflow obstruction should be sought. However, no explanation for the cardiac failure is usually found.

Symptomatic Atrial Septal Defect

For over a decade, reports[130,133–139] have appeared describing the clinical and laboratory features of atrial septal defect causing symptoms during the first year of life. Perhaps only 2 percent of patients with atrial septal defects present the picture of congestive cardiac failure in infancy.

CLINICAL FEATURES.   The onset of cardiac symptoms may occur within the first week of life,[129,133,137,138] even being present at birth.[130] The usual symptoms are related to congestive cardiac failure, with difficulty in breathing and feeding. These may occur in the neonatal period or be present over a period of time before the cardiac disease is diagnosed. Respiratory infections, including pneumonia, are frequent and may exacerbate or initiate the congestive cardiac failure. Weight gain is slow.

On physical examination, the features of congestive cardiac failure are present, including tachypnea, tachycardia, hepatomegaly, and cardiomegaly. There may be rales. Frequently, a left precordial bulge, increased cardiac activity, and right ventricular heave are found.

The auscultatory findings have been reported as typical for atrial septal defect by some authors,[130,139] while others[133,138] indicate that the findings were atypical and variable. We have found that the first heart sound is loud in the tricuspid area and believe this is an extremely valuable finding, indicating a shunt at the atrial level. A systolic murmur is present, usually a pulmonary ejection type. It may be louder and longer than typical for atrial septal defect in older patients. Grade 4/6 systolic murmurs have been described. Because of the characteristics, the murmur has been initially considered as being from a ventricular septal defect.[133,137] The second sound may show wide fixed splitting, but this finding is often not present.[132,137,138] The pulmonary second heart sound is often accentuated. A valuable finding is a low-pitched middiastolic murmur in the tricuspid area, reflecting the large volume of blood flow, but this can be overlooked because of tachypnea or noisy breathing. The atypical auscultatory features in infants usually become typical for atrial septal defect by 2 years of age.

ELECTROCARDIOGRAM. The QRS axis ranges from +90° to +150° but, occasionally, may show an indeterminate axis in the frontal plane. Right atrial enlargement is found in half of the patients. As anticipated, a pattern of right ventricular hypertrophy is found in most infants (Fig. 9-20), showing either an rSR' or Rs pattern in lead V_1.[130,137,138]

THORACIC ROENTGENOGRAM. Moderate to marked cardiomegaly is present, and the pulmonary artery is prominent (Fig. 9-21). Left atrial enlargement is not found. Arterial pulmonary vascular markings are accentuated. The cardiac contour, although not classic, appears globular. Pneumonia may be observed.

ECHOCARDIOGRAM. At this time, we are aware of no reports of echocardiographic findings in infants with symptomatic atrial septal defect. Because of the left-to-right shunt at the atrial level, the right ventricle is enlarged. On echocardiogram, the right ventricular dimensions should be increased, and paradoxical septal motion develops once pulmonary vascular resistance falls.

Echocardiographic studies should be performed in each infant with symptomatic atrial septal defect in an attempt to recognize coexistent lesions of the left atrium or left ventricle. Supravalvular stenosing ring of the left atrium or mitral stenosis are two conditions which, in the presence of an atrial septal defect, increase the shunt and which are difficult to diagnose by cardiac catheterization, since the atrial pressures are equal, and left atriograms show prompt opacification of the right atrium, and details of the mitral area cannot be clearly visualized. Similarly, attention should be directed at left ventricular thickness and wall motion to identify a cardiomyopathy.

CARDIAC CATHETERIZATION AND ANGIOCARDIOGRAM. Because of its rarity as a cause of congestive cardiac failure in infancy and the common occurrence of atypical or nonspecific auscultatory or laboratory findings, the diagnosis of atrial septal defect may not have been made or suspected prior to cardiac catheterization. The diagnostic procedure is carried out to diagnose the cardiac anomaly producing the congestive cardiac failure.

At cardiac catheterization, the presence of an atrial septal defect is initially suspected by the oximetry finding of a marked increase in oxygen saturation at the right atrial level, indicating a left-to-right shunt. Usually, the shunt is large and, in our experience, ranges from 52 to 80 percent (average 64 percent). Careful serial sampling should be made through the right side of the heart to exclude other shunts, including anomalous pulmonary venous connection. Systemic arterial blood is fully saturated, helping to exclude total anomalous pul-

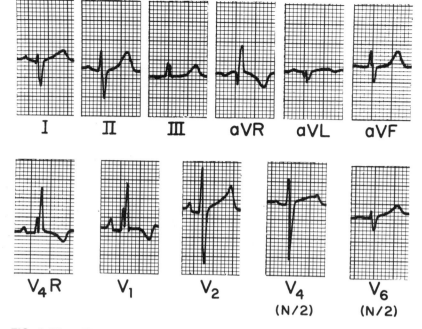

I II III aVR aVL aVF

V₄R V₁ V₂ V₄ (N/2) V₆ (N/2)

FIG. 9-20. Electrocardiogram of atrial septal defect in 4-month-old infant. QRS axis is +180°. Right atrial enlargement and right ventricular hypertrophy. Terminal delay of QRS complex. N/2, half-standardization.

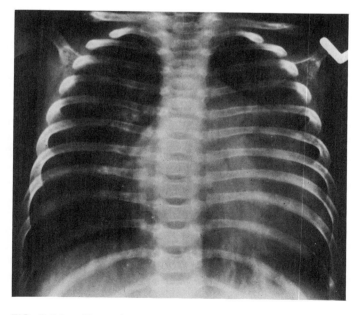

FIG. 9-21. Thoracic roentgenogram of atrial septal defect in 3-month-old infant. Posteroanterior view. Massive cardiomegaly. Increased pulmonary arterial markings.

monary venous connection, the most common lesion leading to increased oxygen saturation at the right atrial level in infants.

The atrial pressures are equal in mean value and wave form. Right atrial pressures have been reported in the normal range,[130,137] but Hunt and Lucas[133] found elevated pressures in most of the infants they reported.

In most infants, moderate elevation of pulmonary arterial pressure is present, the systolic pressure being less than 50 mm Hg, although in one report,[133] infants were described with pulmonary arterial systolic pressure of 70 and 85 mm Hg. Despite the elevation, the pulmonary vascular resistance was normal.[130,133,137] A small gradient can be found across the right ventricular outflow area. Left ventricular pressure should be measured to exclude conditions causing left ventricular outflow obstruction.

In each patient, pulmonary angiography should be performed. The pulmonary venous phase is helpful in identifying the course of the pulmonary veins to make certain it is normal, thereby excluding anomalous pulmonary venous connection. As in any patient with an atrial septal defect, it may be difficult to determine if the right upper pulmonary vein drains normally. Once the opaque material returns to the left atrium, the shunt is delineated. Because of the large pulmonary blood flow, a large amount of opaque material should be injected, and even then, the details of the left atrium are not clearly seen because of dilution and rapid flow. Left ventriculography should be performed to (1) exclude shunts at the ventricular level, (2) exclude left ventricular outflow obstruction, (3) visualize wall thickness and chamber size, (4) visualize details of mitral valve apparatus and annulus, (5) outline the undersurface of a supravalvular stenosis ring if inadvertent mitral reflux occurs, and (6) exclude a gooseneck deformity of the atrioventricular canal.

Because of the rarity of isolated atrial septal defect causing congestive cardiac failure in infancy, a high degree of suspicion must be maintained and every effort made to investigate and exclude conditions that may coexist with an atrial left-to-right shunt.

MANAGEMENT.   For the symptomatic infant, attention must be directed to careful management with digitalis and diuretics. Because of the frequency of respiratory infections and pneumonia and the deleterious effect on cardiac failure, these infections should be promptly and aggressively treated. Most patients respond to treatment and can be followed until an optimum age for operative closure. Usually, the requirement for digitalis diminishes, the number of respiratory infections lessens, and growth improves. We believe digitalis should be continued for at least a year. Deaths have been noted in symptomatic infants with atrial septal defect,[130,133] but this is unusual after 6 months of age. Although closure of atrial septal defect can be successfully performed in infants, the morbidity and mortality are higher than in older children. Closure should be deferred if possible, since most infants improve, and spontaneous closure of the defect may occur. However, operative closure should be performed on any infant with persistent congestive cardiac failure who does not respond to adequate therapy. Phillips and associates[134] have reported successful closure of atrial septal defect in three infants aged 7, 7, and 8 months, respectively.

The reason for the development of congestive cardiac failure in some infants is unknown. The following factors have been considered: (1) size of left-to-right shunt, but it is no different from that found in older asymptomatic children,[130,133] (2) early decrease in pulmonary vascular resistance, but there is no evidence to support this hypothesis, and (3) abnormal ventricular or atrial compliance, but this is difficult to determine.

Asymptomatic Atrial Septal Defect

Although atrial septal defect accounts for about 8 percent of congenital cardiac disease, it is not commonly diagnosed during infancy. Most infants are asymptomatic, and the physical findings are recognized later in childhood, often at the time of preschool physical examination. This occurs despite the fact that the atrial shunt is of the same size as in older children.[135,137] This speaks against the theory that the failure to recognize atrial septal defect could be attributed to the delay in development of the shunt. The failure to recognize it is most likely accounted for by the fact that the auscultatory findings are subtle, and the murmurs are soft or atypical and must be heard in an active, cooing, or crying infant. The typical auscultatory findings are (1) pulmonary systolic ejection murmur may be soft and inseparable from functional pulmonary flow murmur, (2) the typical wide fixed splitting is often not heard in infants, even with a large left-to-right shunt, and (3) the diastolic murmur is low-pitched and may be missed because of tachycardia or noisy breathing.

Spontaneous Closure of Atrial Septal Defect

Clinical reports[140,141] and catheterization studies[137,142] indicate that atrial septal defects may close spontaneously. The defect may be present in patients with left-sided obstructive lesion or left-to-right shunt at the ventricular level. In both situations, the dilated left atrium can stretch open the foramen ovale. Subsequently, perhaps because of operation, the left-to-right shunt at the atrial level disappears.

Isolated atrial septal defect may also undergo closure. Mody[142] described the cardiac catheterization results of 40 patients with atrial septal defect who underwent serial study. Of 20 patients older than 1 year on the initial study, each had persistence of the shunt, whereas among 20 initially catheterized before 1 year, 11 showed spontaneous closure. Likewise, Hoffman and associates[137] found that the shunt had disappeared in 9 of 12 infants who underwent recatheterization and was no longer clinically detectable in the other 3.

The exact mechanism by which this occurs is unknown, but given the frequency with which spontaneous closure occurs and with which atypical features are common, the incidence of atrial septal defect in infancy is probably underestimated.

SYSTEMIC ARTERIOVENOUS FISTULOUS COMMUNICATION

Systemic arteriovenous fistulous communications are a rare cause of congestive cardiac failure in the neonatal period and must be considered in the differential diagnosis of other conditions, such as aortic atresia. The classic picture is mild cyanosis, sharp peripheral arterial pulses, congestive cardiac failure, and increased precordial activity.

PATHOLOGY.   Fistulous communications between arteries and veins are of two general types: (1) fistulae, direct communications between arteries and veins, or (2) angiomas, multiple vascular channels, larger than capillaries, between an artery and vein. The afferent arteries and efferent veins of fistulous communications are dilated and tortuous.

Although systemic arteriovenous communications can be located at various sites, the location of those most commonly occurring in the neonatal period are (1) intracranially, usually between a major cerebral artery and the great vein of Galen,[143-149] (2) between the left subclavian artery and left innominate vein,[150] (3) hepatoportal arteriovenous fistula,[151] (4) internal mammary artery and ductus venosus,[152] (5) extralobar pulmonary sequestration,[153] (6) hemangiomas in skin,[154] (7) pelvic hemangioma,[155] (8) combined cutaneous and visceral hemangioma,[156] and (9) hemangioendothelioma.[157-159]

Smaller systemic arteriovenous fistulous communications may cause a variety of symptoms, depending upon the location of the fistula, but may not have major systemic effects. In this chapter, however, only those fistulae causing neonatal cardiac failure are discussed.

Cardiac enlargement and hypertrophy develop proportionally to the degree of blood flow through the fistula.

HEMODYNAMICS.   The major hemodynamic abnormality results from the shunt of blood from the artery to a vein, with the amount of shunt being proportional to the size of the communicating vessels. Arteriovenous fistulae lower systemic vascular resistance and lead to three effects—increased cardiac output from increased stroke volume, increased heart rate, and increased blood volume (which serves to maintain systemic arterial pressure). The lowered systemic vascular resistance leads to a widened pulse pressure. The physiologic effects are related to high output cardiac failure.

The systemic venous return is increased and causes volume overloading of both the right and left sides of the heart. If the heart is unable to maintain this volume overload, congestive cardiac failure develops.

We are aware of no patient in whom congestive cardiac failure developed in utero, but the symptoms of large systemic arteriovenous fistulae typically appear during the first day of life. During fetal life, the systemic arteriovenous fistula is in parallel circulation with the low resistance placenta. Systemic vascular resistance is low in utero, and the flow through the fistula is small. Following birth and the elimination of the placenta from the circulation, systemic vascular resistance doubles. Therefore, the volume of blood flow through the fistula increases. Holden and Alexander[160] indicate, however, that the fistulae may affect the fetal circulation, since the heart is dilated and hypertrophied in neonates dying with systemic arteriovenous fistulae soon after birth.

Systemic arteriovenous fistulae elevate pulmonary arterial pressure, in neonates usually to the level of the systemic circulation. The elevation is caused by a combination of the normal neonatal increased pulmonary vascular resistance and the increased pulmonary blood flow from the arteriovenous fistula. The right ventricle ejects an increased volume of blood against the elevated pulmonary arterial pressure, and congestive cardiac failure results. If the ductus arteriosus remains patent, a right-to-left shunt can occur because of the elevated pulmonary vascular resistance and lowered systemic vascular resistance. A right-to-left shunt may also occur at the atrial level because the foramen ovale is stretched open by the elevated right atrial pressure.

In a neonate with a cerebral arteriovenous fistula described by Deverall and associates,[149] catheterization findings indicate coarctation of the aorta. The fistula diverted blood from the proximal aorta toward the head, and the distal aorta was supplied by the ductus arteriosus. The aortic isthmus was narrowed, and as the ductus arteriosus closed postnatally, features of coarctation appeared.

CLINICAL FEATURES.   Although congestive cardiac failure may develop by 3 months of age, most instances occur during the first week and often the first day of life. Congestive cardiac failure is profound and manifested by tachypnea, dyspnea, and tachycardia. Cyanosis may be present because of mechanisms discussed previously, although Holden and associates[143] believe that the cyanosis is peripheral rather than central. In the neonates we have seen studied, cyanosis was not present, but the infants developed a mottled appearance.

Cutaneous hemangiomas may indicate visceral hemangiomas. In infants with hepatic hemangioendothelioma, there are multiple small cutaneous raspberry hemangiomas. Dilated veins or nonpulsatile masses may be found at the sites of the fistulae.

Although brisk peripheral arterial pulses are expected, once congestive cardiac failure develops, the pulses become weak, except over the arteries near the site of the fistula. These arteries are sharp and may have a soft thrill.

Cardiomegaly is evident on cardiac examination, and cardiac activity is increased. There are soft ejection systolic murmurs and middiastolic murmurs. P_2 is accentuated. There may be murmurs over the site of the arteriovenous fistula, but we have been disappointed in not hearing them over the head in neonates with intracranial fistulae.

Hepatomegaly accompanies congestive cardiac failure and may be particularly enlarged in infants with hepatic hemangioendotheliomas.

ELECTROCARDIOGRAM.   The electrocardiogram in neonates shows right atrial enlargement and right ventricular hypertrophy occasionally associated with T wave inversion across the precordium (Fig. 9-22). This is in contrast to the findings in older children or adults with systemic arteriovenous fistulae in whom a pattern of left ventricular hypertrophy is present.[161]

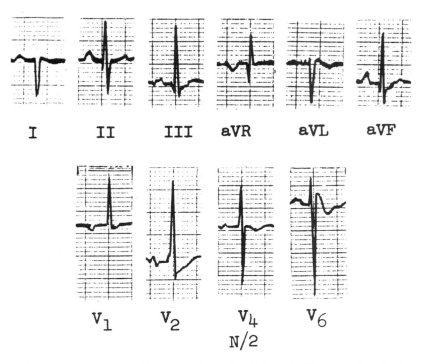

FIG. 9-22. Electrocardiogram in 2-week-old infant with systemic arterio-venous fistula involving subclavian artery and subclavian vein. Right axis deviation. Right ventricular hypertrophy. T waves inverted across precordium. ST segment deviation.

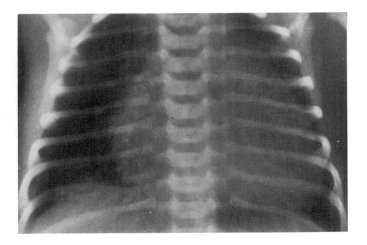

FIG. 9-23. Thoracic roentgenogram of systemic arterio-venous fistula involving great vein of Galen in 1-day-old infant. Severe cardiomegaly.

THORACIC ROENTGENOGRAM.   Moderate to marked cardiomegaly is present and involves each cardiac chamber (Fig. 9-23). The lung fields show increased pulmonary arterial markings or a mixed pattern of arterial and venous markings. There is no characteristic cardiac contour.

ECHOCARDIOGRAM.   We are aware of no description of echocardiograms in systemic arteriovenous fistulae, although normal cardiac structures and relationships should be found, but both ventricles and left atrium should be dilated.

CARDIAC CATHETERIZATION AND ANGIOCARDIOGRAM.   The oximetry data show a high saturation of venous blood draining from the area of the arteriovenous fistula and a large difference of oxygen saturations between the venae cavae. For instance, if there is a cerebral arteriovenous fistula, the superior vena caval saturation may exceed 80 percent, while the inferior vena caval saturation is low. Finding a narrow arteriovenous oxygen difference is paradoxical in the presence of congestive cardiac failure and suggests arteriovenous fistulae. Mild systemic arterial desaturation is present frequently.[143,150]

The pulse pressure is wide. Pulmonary arterial pressure is elevated, often to systemic levels.[145] Right atrial and left atrial pressures are elevated.

Cardiac angiography shows dilatation of the cardiac chambers and great vessels. Aortography or selective arteriography is used to establish the diagnosis (Figs. 9-24 and 9-25). There is rapid circulation through the fistula, and

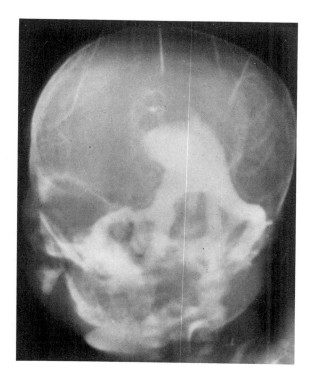

FIG. 9-24. Cerebral angiogram. Cerebral arteriovenous fistula to great vein of Galen.

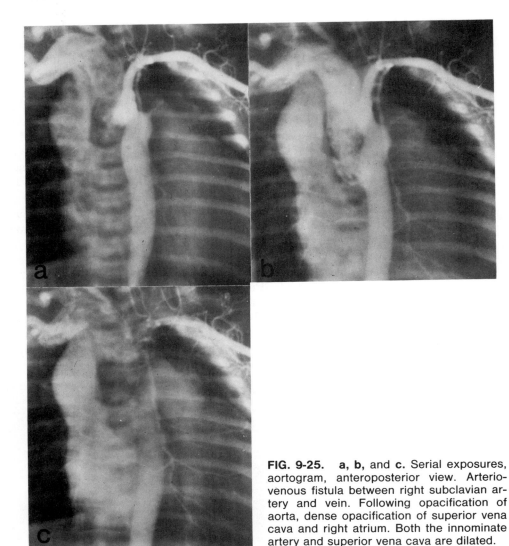

FIG. 9-25.   **a, b,** and **c.** Serial exposures, aortogram, anteroposterior view. Arteriovenous fistula between right subclavian artery and vein. Following opacification of aorta, dense opacification of superior vena cava and right atrium. Both the innominate artery and superior vena cava are dilated.

the contrast material appears in the draining vena cava within a second. The vena cava opacifies much more densely than normal. The afferent arterial and efferent venous vessels are dilated.

Holden and associates[143] suggest that the combination of wide systemic pulse pressure, high oxygen saturation in the superior vena cava, and a narrow arteriovenous oxygen difference is diagnostic of cerebral arteriovenous fistula. They indicate that, rather than perform an angiogram to merely confirm the diagnosis, it is preferable to carry out selective cerebral angiography to outline the details of the vessels in order to plan an operative approach.

TREATMENT. Following treatment with digitalis and diuretics, the arterio-venous fistula should be visualized, noting particularly the afferent arteries, and operation should be undertaken if possible. Intracranial fistulae have been considered inoperable, but Holden and associates[143] report six cases in which arterial vessels were clipped, and congestive cardiac failure resolved in four survivors, although neurologic problems existed in two of these.

Arteriovenous fistulae located at other sites should also be approached operatively. The long-term results of operation in infants are unknown. Because of the difficulty in dividing all of the vessels involved, arteriovenous fistulae tend to recur.

Recently, we have obliterated arteriovenous fistulae in children using a catheter technique.[162] A catheter is passed into the arterial end of the fistula, and metallic coils or brushes and then compressed gel foam are inserted through the catheter into the fistula. Successful closure has been accomplished without embolization through the fistula. This technique may become a method of approaching some arteriovenous fistulae in infants and may avoid an operation.

Hepatic hemangioendothelioma (Fig. 9-26) is a unique form of arteriovenous fistula which is characterized by hepatomegaly out of proportion to the degree of congestive cardiac failure and the presence of cutaneous hemangioma. The survival rate of this condition is 32 percent,[159] despite anticongestive measures. Although operative approaches, such as hepatic arterial ligation, hepatic lobectomy, and radiation, have been suggested, there are risks

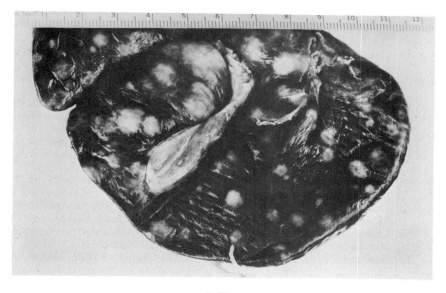

FIG. 9-26.   Liver, visceral surface, showing hepatic hemangioendotheliomas. Multiple nodules throughout liver.

and complications in these treatments. Treatment with prednisone has successfully caused involution of the hemangioendotheliomas.[157,158] Surviving patients show spontaneous involution of the hemangioma.

REFERENCES

Ventricular Septal Defect

1. Hoffman JIE: Natural history of congenital heart disease. Problems in its assessment with special reference to ventricular septal defects. Circulation 37:97, 1968
2. Keith JD, Rose V, Collins G, Kidd BSL: Ventricular septal defect. Incidence, morbidity and mortality in various age groups. Br Heart J 33[Suppl]:81, 1971
3. Fontana RS, Edwards JE: Congenital Cardiac Disease: A Review of 357 Cases Studied Pathologically. Philadelphia, Saunders, 1962, pp 28–29
4. Landtman B: Clinical and morphological studies in congenital heart disease. A review of 777 cases. Acta Paediatr Scand 213[Suppl]:1, 1971
5. Goor DA, Edwards JE, Lillehei CW: The development of the interventricular septum of the human heart: Correlative morphogenetic study. Chest 58:453, 1970
6. Rowe RD, Mehrizi A: The Neonate with Congenital Heart Disease. Philadelphia, Saunders, 1968, p 165
7. Haworth SG, Sauer U, Buhlmeyer K, Reid L: Development of the pulmonary circulation in ventricular septal defect: A quantitative structural study. Circulation 40:781, 1977
8. Heath D, Edwards JE: The pathology of hypertensive pulmonary vascular disease. A description of six grades of structural changes in the pulmonary arteries with special reference to congenital cardiac septal defects. Circulation 18:533, 1958
9. Wood P: The Eisenmenger syndrome. Or pulmonary hypertension with reversed control shunt. Br Med J 2:701, 755, 1958
10. Dammann JF Jr, Ferencz C: The significance of the pulmonary vascular bed in congenital heart disease. III. Defects between the ventricles or great vessels in which both increased pressure and flow may act upon the lungs and in which there is a common ejectile force. Am Heart J 52:210, 1956
11. Adams P Jr, Lucas RV Jr, Ferguson DK, Lillehei CW: Significance of pulmonary vascular pathology in ventricular septal defect as determined by lung biopsy. Am J Dis Child 94:476, 1957 (Abstr)
12. Edwards JE: The Lewis A. Connor Memorial Lecture. Functional pathology of the pulmonary vascular tree in congenital cardiac disease. Circulation 15:164, 1957
13. Wagenvoort CA: Vasoconstriction and medial hypertrophy in pulmonary hypertension. Circulation 22:535, 1960
14. Lucas RV Jr, Adams P Jr, Anderson RC, et al.: The natural history of isolated ventricular septal defect. A serial physiologic study. Circulation 24:1372, 1961
15. Levin AR, Spach MS, Canent RV Jr, et al.: Intracardiac pressure-flow dynamics in isolated ventricular septal defects. Circulation 35:430, 1967
16. Graham TP Jr, Bender HW, Spach MS: Defects of the ventricular septum. In Moss AJ, Adams FA, Emmanouilides GC (eds): Heart Disease in Infants, Children and Adolescents, 2nd ed. Baltimore, Williams & Wilkins, 1977, pp 143–146
17. DuShane JW, Weidman WH, Brandenburg RO, Kirklin JW: The electrocardiogram in children with ventricular septal defect and severe pulmonary hyperten-

sion. Correlation with response of pulmonary arterial pressure to surgical repair. Circulation 22:49, 1960

18. Keith JD, Collins GFN, Rose V, Calder L, Kidd BSL: Improved prognosis in ventricular septal defect. In Kidd BSL, Keith JD (eds): The Natural History and Progress in Treatment of Congenital Heart Defects. Springfield, Ill, Thomas, 1971, pp 5–13
19. Baylen B, Johnson G, Tsang RC, Srivastava L, Kaplan S: Hyperaldosteronism and aldosterone antagonists in congestive heart failure (CHF) and cor pulmonale in infancy. Pediatr Res 10:310, 1976 (Abstr)
20. Hirschfeld S, Meyer R, Schwartz DC, Korfhagen J, Kaplan S: The echocardiographic assessment of pulmonary artery pressure and pulmonary vascular resistance. Circulation 52:642, 1975
21. Corone P, Doyon F, Gaudeau S, et al.: Natural history of ventricular septal defect: A study involving 790 cases. Circulation 55:908, 1977
22. Jain V. Subramanian S, Lambert EC: Concomitant development of infundibular pulmonary stenosis and spontaneous closure of ventricular septal defect. An unusual variant in the natural history of ventricular septal defect. Am J Cardiol 24:247, 1969
23. Nadas AS, Thilenius OG, LaFarge CG, Hauck AJ: Ventricular septal defect with aortic regurgitation: Medical and pathologic aspects. Circulation 29:862, 1964
24. Van Praagh R, McNamara JJ: Anatomic types of ventricular septal defect with aortic insufficiency. Diagnostic and surgical considerations. Am Heart J 75:604, 1968
25. McNicholas KW, Bowman FO Jr, Hayes CJ, Edie RN, Malm JR: Surgical management of ventricular septal defects in infants. J Thorac Cardiovasc Surg 75:346, 1978
26. Lauer RM, Ongley PA, DuShane JW, Kirklin JW: Heart block after repair of ventricular septal defect in children. Circulation 22:526, 1960
27. Cartmill TB, DuShane JW, McGoon DC, Kirklin JW: Results of repair of ventricular septal defect. J Thorac Cardiovasc Surg 52:486, 1966
28. DuShane JW, Krongrad E, Ritter DG, McGoon DC: The fate of raised pulmonary vascular resistance after surgery in ventricular septal defect. In Rowe RD, Kidd BSL (eds): The Child with Congenital Heart Disease after Surgery. Mount Kisco, NY, Futura, 1976, pp 299–312
29. Hallidie-Smith KA, Hollman A, Cleland WP, Bentall HH, Goodwin JF: Effects of surgical closure of ventricular septal defects upon pulmonary vascular disease. Br Heart J 31:246, 1969
30. Allen HD, Anderson RC, Noren GR, Moller JH: Postoperative follow-up of patients with ventricular septal defect. Circulation 50:465, 1974
31. Weidman WH, Blount SG Jr, DuShane JW, et al.: Natural history study: Clinical course in ventricular septal defect. Circulation 56[Suppl 1]:56, 1977
32. Barratt-Boyes BG, Neutze JM, Clarkson PM, Shardey GC, Brandt PWT: Repair of ventricular septal defect in the first two years of life using profound hypothermia-circulatory arrest techniques. Ann Surg 184:376, 1976
33. Rein JG, Freed MD, Norwood WI, Castaneda AR: Early and late results of closure of ventricular septal defect in infancy. Ann Thorac Surg 24:19, 1977
34. Muller WH Jr, Dammann JF Jr: The treatment of certain congenital malformations of the heart by the creation of pulmonic stenosis to reduce pulmonary hypertension and excessive pulmonary blood flow. A preliminary study. Surg Gynecol Obstet 95:213, 1952
35. Hunt CE, Formanek G, Levin MA, Castaneda AR, Moller JH: Banding of the pulmonary artery. Results in 111 children. Circulation 43:395, 1971
36. Griepp E, French JW, Shumway NE, Baum D: Is pulmonary artery banding for ventricular septal defect obsolete? Circulation 50[Suppl 2]:14, 1974

37. Rittenhouse EA, Mohri H, Dillard DH, Merendino KA: Deep hypothermia in cardiovascular surgery. Ann Thorac Surg 17:63, 1974
38. Sade RM, William RG, Castaneda AR: Corrective surgery for congenital cardiovascular defects in infancy. Am Heart J 90:656, 1975
39. Stevenson JG, Stone EF, Dillard DH, Morgan BC: Intellectual development of children subjected to prolonged circulatory arrest during hypothermia open heart surgery in infancy. Circulation 50 [Suppl 2]:54, 1974

Patent Ductus Arteriosus

40. Campbell M: Incidence of cardiac malformation at birth and later, and neonatal mortality. Br Heart J 35:189, 1973
41. Siassi B, Blanco C, Cabal LA, Coran AG: Incidence and clinical features of patent ductus arteriosus in low-birthweight infants: A prospective analysis of 150 consecutively born infants. Pediatrics 57:347, 1976
42. Thibeault DW, Emmanouilides G, Nelson RJ, et al.: Patent ductus arteriosus complicating the respiratory distress syndrome in preterm infants. J Pediatr 86:120, 1975
43. Kitterman JA, Edmunds LH Jr, Gregory GA, et al.: Patent ductus arteriosus in premature infants. Incidence, relation to pulmonary disease and management. N Engl J Med 287:473, 1972
44. Neal WA, Bessinger FB Jr, Hunt CE, Lucas RV Jr: Patent ductus arteriosus complicating respiratory distress syndrome. J Pediatr 86:127, 1975
45. Blanco CE, Siassi B, Cabal LA: Persistent patency of ductus arteriosus in premature newborn infants. Am J Cardiol 31:121, 1973 (Abstr)
46. Thibeault DW, Emmanouilides GC: Prolonged rupture of fetal membranes and decreased frequency of respiratory distress syndrome and patent ductus arteriosus in preterm infants. Am J Obstet Gynecol 129:43, 1977
47. Rudolph AM: Congenital Diseases of the Heart. Chicago, Year Book, 1974, pp 1–16
48. Moss AJ, Emmanouilides G, Duffie ER Jr: Closure of the ductus arteriosus in the newborn infant. Pediatrics 32:25, 1963
49. Mitchell S: The ductus arteriosus in the neonatal period. J Pediatr 51:12, 1957
50. Buchanan JW, Patterson DF, Pyle RL: Morphologic studies in dogs with hereditary patent ductus arteriosus. Circulation 44 [Suppl 2]:147, 1971
51. Gittenberger-deGroot AC: Persistent ductus arteriosus: Most probably a primary congenital malformation. Br Heart J 39:610, 1977
52. Born GVR, Dawes GS, Mott JC, Rennick B: The constriction of the ductus arteriosus caused by oxygen and by asphyxia in newborn lambs. J Physiol 132:304, 1956
53. Moss AJ, Emmanouilides GC, Adams FH, Chuang K: Response of ductus arteriosus and pulmonary and systemic arterial pressure to changes in oxygen environment in newborn infants. Pediatrics 33:937, 1964
54. McMurphy DM, Heymann MA, Rudolph AM, Melmon KL: Developmental changes in constriction of the ductus arteriosus: Responses to oxygen and vasoactive agents in the isolated ductus arteriosus of the fetal lamb. Pediatr Res 6:231, 1972
55. Boreus LO, Malmfors T, McMurphy DM, Olson L: Demonstration of adrenergic receptor function and innervation in the ductus arteriosus of the human fetus. Acta Physiol Scand 77:316, 1969
56. Melmon KL, Cline MJ, Hughes T, Nies AS: Kinins: Possible mediators of neonatal circulatory changes in man. J Clin Invest 47:1295, 1968
57. Heymann MA, Rudolph AM: Effects of acetylsalicylic acid on the ductus arteriosus and circulation in fetal lambs in utero. Circ Res 38:418, 1976
58. Wagenvoort CA, Neufeld HN, Edwards JE: The structure of the pulmonary ar-

terial tree in fetal and early postnatal life. Lab Invest 10:751, 1961
59. Levin DL, Rudolph AM, Heymann MA, Phibbs RH: Morphological development of the pulmonary vascular bed in fetal lambs. Circulation 53:144, 1976
60. Hoffman JIE, Buckberg GD: The myocardial supply:demand ratio—a critical review. Am J Cardiol 41:327, 1978
61. Sreenivasan VV, Fisher BJ, Liebman J, Downs TD: Longitudinal study of the standard electrocardiogram in the healthy premature infant during the first year of life. Am J Cardiol 31:57, 1973
62. Silverman NH, Lewis AB, Heymann MA, Rudolph AM: Echocardiographic assessment of ductus arteriosus shunt in premature infants. Circulation 50:821, 1974
63. Baylen BG, Meyer RA, Kaplan S, Ringenburg WE, Korfhagen J: The critically ill premature infant with patent ductus arteriosus and pulmonary disease—an echocardiographic assessment. J Pediatr 86:423, 1975
64. Baylen BG, Meyer RA, Korfhagen J, et al.: Evaluation of left ventricular function in critically ill premature infants with patent ductus arteriosus and pulmonary disease. Circulation 55:182, 1977
65. Hirschklau MJ, Kirkpatrick SE, Higgins CB, Friedman WF: Echocardiographic pitfalls in the premature with large patent ductus arteriosus. Pediatr Res 11:392, 1977 (Abstr)
66. Neal WA, Reynolds JW, Jarvis CW, Williams HJ: Umbilical artery catheterization: Demonstration of arterial thrombosis by aortography. Pediatrics 50:6, 1972
67. Williams HJ, Jarvis CW, Neal WA, Reynolds JW: Vascular thromboembolism complicating umbilical artery catheterization. Am J Roentgenol Radium Ther Nucl Med 116:475, 1972
68. Bessinger FB Jr, Neal WA, Hunt CE, Lucas RV Jr: Catheterization and pulmonary function studies in 10 infants with respiratory distress syndrome (RDS) and patent ductus arteriosus (PDA). Pediatr Res 3:347, 1974 (Abstr)
69. Berman W, Ravenscroft PJ, Sheiner LB, et al.: The relationship of age to the distribution and physiologic effects of digoxin in sheep. Pediatr Res 11:414, 1977 (Abstr)
70. Sharpe GL, Thalme B, Larsson K: Studies on closure of the ductus arteriosus. XI. Ductal closure in utero by a prostaglandin synthetase inhibition. Prostaglandins 8:363, 1974
71. Friedman WF, Hirschklau MJ, Printz MP, Pitlick PT, Kirkpatrick SE: Pharmacologic closure of patent ductus arteriosus in the premature infant. N Engl J Med 295:526, 1976
72. Heymann MA, Rudolph AM, Silverman NH: Closure of the ductus arteriosus in infants by inhibition of prostaglandin synthesis. N Engl J Med 295:530, 1976
73. Friedman WF, Heymann MA, Rudolph AM: Commentary: New thought on an old problem—patent ductus arteriosus in the premature infant. J Pediatr 90:338, 1977
74. Neal WA, Kyle JM, Mullett MD: Failure of indomethacin therapy to induce closure of patent ductus arteriosus in premature infants with respiratory distress syndrome. J Pediatr 91:621, 1977
75. Nadas AS: Patent ductus revisited (Commentary). N Engl J Med 295:563, 1976
76. Cotton RB, Stahlman MT, Bender HW, et al.: Randomized trial of early closure of patent ductus arteriosus in small preterm infants. J Pediatr 93:647, 1978
77. Braudo M, Rowe RD: Auscultation of the heart—early newborn period. Am J Dis Child 101:575, 1961
78. Nadas AS, Fyler DC: Pediatric Cardiology, 3rd ed. Philadelphia, Saunders, 1972, pp 405–431
79. Keith JD, Rowe RD, Vlad P: Heart Disease in Infancy and Childhood, 2nd ed. New York, Macmillan, 1967, pp 164–212

80. Espino-Vela J, Zamora C: Patent ductus arteriosus—The natural history after the first year of life. In Kidd BSL, Keith JD (eds): The Natural History and Progress in Treatment of Congenital Heart Defects. Springfield, Ill, Thomas, 1971, p 42

81. Keys A, Shapiro MJ: Patency of the ductus arteriosus in adults. Am Heart J 25:158, 1943

82. Cassels DE, Bharati S, Lev M: The natural history of the ductus arteriosus in association with other congenital heart defects. Perspect Biol Med 18:541, 1975

83. Rudolph AM, Heymann MA, Spitznas U: Hemodynamic considerations in the development of narrowing of the aorta. Am J Cardiol 30:514, 1972

84. Coceani F, Olley PM: The response of the ductus arteriosus to prostaglandin. Can J Physiol Pharmacol 51:220, 1973

85. Elliott RB, Starling MB, Neutze JM: Medical manipulation of the ductus arteriosus. Lancet 1:140, 1975

86. Coceani F, Olley PM, Bodach E: Prostaglandins: A possible regulator of muscle tone in the ductus arteriosus. Adv Prostaglandin Thromboxane Res 1:417, 1976

87. Olley PM, Coceani F, Bodach E: E-type prostaglandins—a new emergency therapy for certain cyanotic congenital heart malformations. Circulation 53:728, 1976

Congenitally Corrected Transposition of the Great Vessels

88. Allwork SP, Bentall HH, Becker AE, et al.: Congenitally corrected transposition of the great arteries: Morphologic study of 32 cases. Am J Cardiol 38:910, 1976

89. Schiebler GL, Edwards JE, Burchell HB, et al.: Congenital corrected transposition of the great vessels: A study of 33 cases. Pediatrics 27[Suppl 5, Part 2]:851, 1961

90. Anderson RH, Becker AE, Arnold R, Wilkinson JL: The conducting tissues in congenitally corrected transposition. Circulation 50:911, 1974

91. Waldo AL, Pacifico AD, Bargeron LM Jr, James TN, Kirklin JW: Electrophysiological delineation of the specialized A-V conduction system in patients with corrected transposition of the great vessels and ventricular septal defect. Circulation 52:435, 1975

92. Anderson RC, Lillehei CW, Lester RG: Corrected transposition of the great vessels of the heart. A review of 17 cases. Pediatrics 20:626, 1957

93. Ruttenberg HD, Elliott LP, Anderson RC, Adams P Jr, Tuna N: Congenital corrected transposition of the great vessels. Correlation of electrocardiograms and vectorcardiograms with associated cardiac malformations and hemodynamic states. Am J Cardiol 17:339, 1966

94. Lester RG, Anderson RC, Amplatz K, Adams P: Roentgenologic diagnosis of congenitally corrected transposition of the great vessels. Am J Roentgenol Radium Ther Nucl Med 83:985, 1960

95. Foster JR, Damato AN, Kline LE, Akhtar M, Ruskin JN: Congenitally corrected transposition of the great vessels: Localization of the site of complete atrioventricular block using His bundle electrograms. Am J Cardiol 38:383, 1976

96. Maloney JD, Ritter DG, McGoon DC, Danielson GK: Identification of the conduction system in corrected transposition and common ventricle at operation. Mayo Clin Proc 50:387, 1975

97. Kupersmith J, Krongrad E, Gersony WM, Bowman FO Jr: Electrophysiologic identification of the specialized conduction system in corrected transposition of the great arteries. Circulation 50:795, 1974

98. Fox LS, Kirklin JW, Pacifico AD, Waldo AL, Bargeron LM Jr: Intracardiac repair of cardiac malformations with atrioventricular discordance. Circulation 54:123, 1976

99. Olinger GN, Maloney JV Jr: Transpulmonary artery repair of ventricular septal defect associated with congenitally corrected transposition of the great arteries. J Thorac Cardiovasc Surg 73:353, 1977

Aorticopulmonary Septal Defect

100. Blieden LC, Moller JH: Aorticopulmonary septal defect. An experience with 17 patients. Br Heart J 36:630, 1974

Aortic Origin of Pulmonary Artery

101. Robin E, Silberg B, Ganguly SN, Magnisalis K: Aortic origin of the left pulmonary artery. Variant of tetralogy of Fallot. Am J Cardiol 35:324, 1975
102. Keane JF, Maltz D, Bernhard WF, Corwin RD, Nadas AS: Anomalous origin of one pulmonary artery from the ascending aorta. Diagnostic, physiological and surgical considerations. Circulation 50:588, 1974
103. Rosenberg HS, Hallman GL, Wolfe RR, Latson JR: Origin of the right pulmonary artery from the aorta. Am Heart J 72:106, 1966
104. Griffiths SP, Levine OR, Andersen DH: Aortic origin of the right pulmonary artery. Circulation 25:73, 1962
105. Wagenvoort CA, Neufeld HN, Birge RF, Caffrey JA, Edwards JE: Origin of right pulmonary artery from ascending aorta. Circulation 23:84, 1961
106. Cumming GR, Ferguson CC, Sanchez J: Aortic origin of the right pulmonary artery. Am J Cardiol 30:674, 1972
107. Porter DD, Canent RV Jr, Spach MS, Baylin GJ: Origin of the right pulmonary artery from the ascending aorta. Unusual cineangiocardiographic and pathologic findings. Circulation 27:589, 1963
108. Kirkpatrick SE, Girod DA, King H: Aortic origin of the right pulmonary artery. Surgical repair without a graft. Circulation 36:777, 1967

Endocardial Cushion Defect

109. Van Mierop LHS: Embryology of the atrioventricular canal region and pathogenesis of endocardial cushion defects. In Feldt RH (ed): Atrioventricular Canal Defects. Philadelphia, Saunders, 1976, pp 1–12
110. Wakai CS, Edwards JE: Developmental and pathologic considerations in persistent common atrioventricular canal. Mayo Clin Proc 31:487, 1956
111. Wakai CS, Edwards JE: Pathological study of persistent common atrioventricular canal. Am Heart J 56:779, 1958
112. Titus JL, Rastelli GC: Anatomic features of persistent common atrioventricular canal. In Feldt RH (ed): Atrioventricular Canal Defects. Philadelphia, Saunders, 1976, pp 13–35
113. Ongley PA, Pongpanich B, Feldt RH: The clinical profile of the atrioventricular canal defects. In Feldt RH (ed): Atrioventricular Canal Defects. Philadelphia, Saunders, 1976, pp 44–50
114. Weyn AS, Bartle SH, Nolan TB, Dammann JF Jr: Atrial septal defect—primum type. Circulation 32[Suppl 3]:13, 1965
115. Feldt RH, Titus JL: The conduction system in persistent common atrioventricular canal. In Feldt RH (ed): Atrioventricular Canal Defects. Philadelphia, Saunders, 1976, pp 36–43
116. Durrer D, Roos JP, vanDam RT: The genesis of the electrocardiogram of patients with ostium primum defects (ventral atrial septal defects). Am Heart J 71:642, 1966
117. Ongley PA, Pongpanich B, Spangler JG, Feldt RH: The electrocardiogram in

atrioventricular canal. In Feldt RH (ed): Atrioventricular Canal Defects. Philadelphia, Saunders, 1976, pp 51–75

118. Hagler DJ: Echocardiographic findings in atrioventricular canal defect. In Feldt RH (ed): Atrioventricular Canal Defects. Philadelphia, Saunders, 1976, pp 87–109
119. Williams RG, Rudd M: Echocardiographic features of endocardial cushion defects. Circulation 49:418, 1974
120. Bass JL, Bessinger FB Jr, Lawrence C: Echocardiographic differentiation of partial and complete atrioventricular canal. Circulation 57:1144, 1978
121. Park JM, Ritter DG, Mair DD: Cardiac catheterization findings in persistent common atrioventricular canal. In Feldt RH (ed): Atrioventricular Canal Defects. Philadelphia, Saunders, 1976, pp 76–86
122. Girod D, Raghib G, Wang Y, Adams P Jr, Amplatz K: Angiocardiographic characteristics of persistent common atrioventricular canal. Radiology 85:442, 1965
123. Rastelli GC, Kincaid OW, Ritter DG: Angiocardiography of persistent common atrioventricular canal. In Feldt RH (ed): Atrioventricular Canal Defects. Philadelphia, Saunders, 1976, pp 110–118
124. Baron MG: Abnormalities of the mitral valve in endocardial cushion defects. Circulation 45:672, 1972
125. McGoon DC, McMullan MH, Mair DD, Danielson GK: Correction of complete atrioventricular canal in infants. Mayo Clin Proc 48:769, 1973
126. Mair DD, McGoon DC: Surgical correction of atrioventricular canal during the first year of life. Am J Cardiol 40:66, 1977
127. Berger TJ, Kirklin JW, Blackstone EH, Pacifico AD, Kouchoukos NT: Primary repair of complete atrioventricular canal in patients less than 2 years old. Am J Cardiol 41:906, 1978

Atrial Septal Defect

128. Edwards JE: The pathology of atrial septal defect. Semin Roentgenol 1:24, 1966
129. Raghib G, Ruttenberg HD, Anderson RC, et al.: Termination of left superior vena cava in left atrium, atrial septal defect, and absence of coronary sinus. A developmental complex. Circulation 31:906, 1965
130. Hastreiter AR, Wennemark JR, Miller RA, Paul MH: Secundum atrial septal defects with congestive heart failure during infancy and early childhood. Am Heart J 64:467, 1962
131. Tandon R, Edwards JE: Atrial septal defect in infancy. Common association with other anomalies. Circulation 49:1005, 1974
132. Rudolph AM: Congenital Diseases of the Heart. Chicago, Year Book, 1974, pp 246–248
133. Hunt CE, Lucas RV Jr: Symptomatic atrial septal defect in infancy. Circulation 47:1042, 1973
134. Phillips SJ, Okies JE, Henken D, Sunderlund CO, Starr A: Complex of secundum atrial septal defect and congestive heart failure in infants. J Thorac Cardiovasc Surg 70:696, 1975
135. Nakamura FF, Hauck AJ, Nadas AS: Atrial septal defect in infants. Pediatrics 34:101, 1964
136. Kavanagh-Gray D: Atrial septal defect in infancy. Mod Med 31:132, 1963 (Abstr)
137. Hoffman JIE, Rudolph AM, Danilowicz D: Left to right atrial shunts in infants. Am J Cardiol 30:868, 1972
138. Dimich I, Steinfeld L, Park SC: Symptomatic atrial septal defect in infants. Am Heart J 85:601, 1973
139. Ainger LE, Pate JW: Ostium secundum atrial septal defects and congestive heart failure in infancy. Am J Cardiol 15:380, 1965

140. Cayler GG: Spontaneous functional closure of symptomatic atrial septal defects. N Engl J Med 276:65, 1967
141. Cumming GR: Functional closure of atrial septal defects. Am J Cardiol 22:888, 1968
142. Mody MR: Serial hemodynamic observations in secundum atrial septal defect with special reference to spontaneous closure. Am J Cardiol 32:978, 1973

Systemic Arteriovenous Fistulous Communication

143. Holden AM, Fyler DC, Shillito J Jr, Nadas AS: Congestive heart failure from intracranial arteriovenous fistula in infancy. Pediatrics 49:30, 1972
144. Gomez MR, Whitten CF, Nolke A, Bernstein J, Meyer JS: Aneurysmal malformation of the great vein of Galen causing heart failure in early infancy. Report of five cases. Pediatrics 31:400, 1963
145. Hamby RI, Desposito F: Congenital intradural arteriovenous fistula and congestive heart failure in infancy. J Pediatr 61:590, 1962
146. Hernandez A Jr, Schwartz HG, Goldring D: Cerebral arteriovenous fistulas and congenital heart disease. J Pediatr 66:722, 1965
147. Levin OR, Jameson AG, Nellhaus G, Gold AP: Cardiac complications of cerebral arteriovenous fistula in infancy. Pediatrics 30:563, 1962
148. Glatt BS, Rowe RD: Cerebral arteriovenous fistula associated with congestive heart failure in the newborn. Report of two cases. Pediatrics 26:596, 1960
149. Deverall PB, Taylor JFN, Sturrock GS, Aberdeen E: Coarctation-like physiology with cerebral arteriovenous fistula. Pediatrics 44:1024, 1969
150. Walker WJ, Mullins CE, Knovick GC: Cyanosis, cardiomegaly, and weak pulses. A manifestation of massive congenital systemic arteriovenous fistula. Circulation 29:777, 1964
151. Helikson MA, Shapiro DL, Seashore JH: Hepatoportal arteriovenous fistula and portal hypertension in an infant. Pediatrics 60:921, 1977
152. Glass IH, Rowe RD, Duckworth JWA: Congenital arteriovenous fistula between the left internal mammary artery and the ductus venosus: Unusual case of congestive heart failure in the newborn infant. Pediatrics 26:604, 1960
153. Goldblatt E, Vimpani G, Brown JH: Extralobar pulmonary sequestration. Presentation as an arteriovenous aneurysm with cardiac failure in infancy. Am J Cardiol 29:100, 1972
154. Cohen MI, Sinclair JC: Neonatal death from congestive heart failure associated with large cutaneous cavernous hemangioma. Pediatrics 32:924, 1963
155. Price AC, Coran AG, Mattern AL, Cochran RL: Hemangioendothelioma of the pelvis. A cause of cardiac failure in the newborn. N Engl J Med 286:647, 1972
156. Cooper AM, Bolande RP: Multiple hemangiomas in an infant with cardiac hypertrophy. Postmortem angiographic demonstration of the arteriovenous fistulae. Pediatrics 35:27, 1965
157. Rocchini AP, Rosenthal A, Issenberg HJ, Nadas AS: Hepatic hemangioendothelioma: Hemodynamic observations and treatment. Pediatrics 57:131, 1976
158. Touloukian RJ: Hepatic hemangioendothelioma during infancy: Pathology, diagnosis and treatment with prednisone. Pediatrics 45:71, 1970
159. McLean RH, Moller JH, Warwick WJ, Satran L, Lucas RV Jr: Multinodular hemangiomatosis of the liver in infancy. Pediatrics 49:563, 1972
160. Holden KR, Alexander F: Diffuse neonatal hemangiomatosis. Pediatrics 46:411, 1970
161. Amorim D de S, Burchell HB: The electrocardiogram in systemic arteriovenous fistulas. Cardiologia 38:319, 1961
162. Tadavarthy SM, Moller JH, Amplatz K: Polyvinyl alcohol (Ivalon)—a new embolic material. Radiology 125:609, 1975

10 Acyanosis and Normal Pulmonary Blood Flow

Three types of conditions occur in infants who are acyanotic and have normal pulmonary vascular markings: obstruction to ventricular outflow, diseases affecting the myocardium, and pericardial disease.

Infants with right ventricular outflow obstruction may be either acyanotic or appear cyanotic if a shunt occurs at the atrial level. This latter situation is discussed in Chapter 12.

Infants with left ventricular outflow obstruction and those with diseases affecting the myocardium can present a similar clinical picture of congestive cardiac failure, which may be profound, a soft murmur, left ventricular hypertrophy with ST and T wave changes of strain, and cardiomegaly with a left ventricular contour. The pulmonary vascular markings may show a venous pattern and in this case must be distinguished from other diseases that may present with pulmonary venous obstruction (Chap. 13).

CONGENITAL CARDIAC ANOMALIES CAUSING OUTFLOW OBSTRUCTION

Obstruction to outflow can occur on either the left or the right side of the heart. The principal response to the increased preload is ventricular hypertrophy. In infants, however, symptoms of congestive cardiac failure can develop in these cardiac anomalies, whereas it is uncommon later in life. There are three factors that can influence the ventricular response to the increased afterload: (1) the severity of the degree of obstruction, (2) the limitations of the neonatal myocardium in its contractile ability, and (3) a disequilibrium between myocardial oxygen consumption and supply, leading to myocardial ischemia.

Therefore, in the infant or neonate, ventricular dilatation is common, whereas in older children, it is uncommon.

PULMONARY STENOSIS

Obstruction to right ventricular outflow in neonates and infants with intact ventricular septum occurs almost always at the level of the pulmonary valve. Isolated infundibular stenosis is rare in this age group. Although clinical findings of peripheral pulmonary arterial stenosis may be found in infants, particularly in prematures, this condition infrequently causes symptoms.

Obstruction at the level of the pulmonary valve can occur as either atresia or stenosis and with either a hypoplastic or normal-sized right ventricle. In this section, patients with pulmonary valvular stenosis and normal-sized right ventricle will be discussed. The severity of pulmonary stenosis is variable, but the severe forms can cause congestive cardiac failure and lead to cyanosis.

ANATOMY.   Pulmonary valvular stenosis occurs in two anatomic forms. In the classic form, the pulmonary valve is dome shaped (Fig. 10-1a) and has a central orifice,[1] presumably from fusion of the valve cusps. Usually three raphes, representing the margins of the cusps, are present. The size of the orifice varies considerably among patients, and this variation directly affects the severity of the condition. In severe cases, the orifice may be pinpoint. Although in the classic form, the valvular leaflets are thin, in severe cases, the leaflets may be thickened and immobile and form a platelike obstruction.

In the other form of pulmonary valvular stenosis described by Koretzky and others,[2] the pulmonary valve is dysplastic. The valvular leaflets are greatly thickened and redundant, but the commissures are not fused (Fig. 10-1b). The bulk of pulmonary valvular tissue obstructs right ventricular outflow and causes stenosis. The diameter of the annulus may be reduced in both anatomic forms of pulmonary stenosis, particularly the latter.

Poststenotic dilatation of the pulmonary trunk and the left pulmonary artery, present in infants with a dome-shaped stenotic pulmonary valve, is only minimal in infants with dysplastic pulmonary valve. In neonates, since the pulmonary artery is normally large, poststenotic dilatation in pulmonary stenosis is absent and tends to develop with age.

In patients with mild pulmonary stenosis, the right ventricle is normal, but with increasing degrees of stenosis, the right ventricular wall and interventricular septum thicken. With significant degrees of hypertrophy, the right ventricular cavity may be reduced in size, particularly in severe forms in which the apical region of the right ventricle may be obliterated by hypertrophied trabeculae and papillary muscles. Hypertrophy of the crista supraventricularis also occurs in severe forms.

The tricuspid valve is normal, but in patients with severe stenosis, the valve may be abnormal, resembling Ebstein's malformation or showing dysplastic changes of the leaflets and chordae tendineae. These abnormalities can lead to tricuspid regurgitation.

In severe forms, the right atrium is dilated, and its walls show striking hypertrophy and trabeculation because of altered right ventricular compliance or

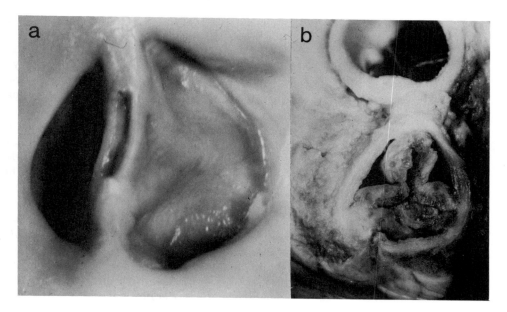

FIG. 10-1.   Pulmonary valvular stenosis, anatomic forms. **a.** Dome-shaped pulmonary valve, superior aspect. Commissural fusion. Small central orifice. **b.** Dysplastic pulmonary valve, superior aspect. No commissural fusion. Three distinct leaflets seen, which are thickened and redundant.

tricuspid insufficiency. The atrial septum may be intact, but in severe cases, a valvular competent foramen ovale may be stretched open because of right atrial dilatation. An atrial septal defect may be present in an occasional case. The ductus arteriosus usually closes at the anticipated time, regardless of the severity of the stenosis. The ductus may remain patent in an occasional infant and, if the stenosis is severe, provide a major source of pulmonary blood flow.

The media of the pulmonary vasculature may be normal or thinned.[3]

HEMODYNAMICS.   The principal hemodynamic effect of the pulmonary stenosis is elevation of right ventricular systolic pressure. The amount of pressure elevation is determined by the size of the stenotic pulmonary valvular orifice and the cardiac output according to:

$$PVA = \frac{\dfrac{CO}{SEP \times HR}}{K \sqrt{RVSP\text{-}PA}}$$

PVA = pulmonary valvular area; CO = cardiac output; SEP = systolic ejection period; HR = heart rate; K = constant (44.5); RVSP = mean right ventricular systolic pressure; PA = mean pulmonary arterial pressure.

This relationship indicates that the more severe the stenosis (i.e., smaller pulmonary valvular area), the larger the gradient across the pulmonary valve must be to maintain a normal cardiac output. Since pulmonary arterial pressure is low, the gradient is developed by increase in right ventricular systolic pressure. Furthermore, the equation also illustrates that in a given patient, if the cardiac output increases for any reason, such as fever or exertion, the right ventricular systolic pressure also increases.

In infants with mild or moderate pulmonary stenosis, the cardiac output is maintained by hypertrophy of the right ventricular myocardium and elevated right ventricular systolic pressure. In neonates with severe stenosis, however, the immature myocardium may be unable to develop right ventricular systolic pressure to maintain normal cardiac output even though the right ventricle is hypertrophied.

In patients with more severe forms of pulmonary stenosis, right atrial pressure may increase for several reasons: (1) significant right ventricular hypertrophy, raising the right ventricular end-diastolic pressure, (2) right ventricular failure, or (3) tricuspid insufficiency. The elevated right atrial pressure and dilatation stretch the foramen ovale open. Because right atrial pressure exceeds left atrial pressure and right ventricular compliance is less than left ventricular compliance, a right-to-left shunt occurs at the atrial level. Once a right-to-left shunt develops, the volume of pulmonary blood flow is decreased. Therefore, according to the formula for pulmonary valvular area, the right ventricular systolic pressure should also decrease.

The degree of cyanosis varies according to the volume of right-to-left shunt.

An abnormal relationship between right ventricular myocardial blood flow and myocardial oxygen demands[4] may contribute to right ventricular failure and a decrease in right ventricular compliance. The myocardial oxygen requirements of the right ventricle are increased in patients with pulmonary stenosis, and the blood flow to the subendocardial region is compromised by elevated intraventricular systolic pressures. This combination of increased oxygen requirements and decreased myocardial perfusion can lead to ischemia and, ultimately, myocardial fibrosis, decreasing myocardial contractility and increasing ventricular compliance. We have observed histologic changes of ischemia and fibrosis in the right ventricular myocardium of several infants with severe pulmonary stenosis.[5]

In the first year of life, right ventricular systolic pressure rarely exceeds 200 mm Hg. Although we have not recorded a right ventricular systolic pressure greater than 200 mm Hg in the first year of life, we have recorded 165 mm Hg at 2 weeks of age.

Symptoms progress in some infants. Deterioration may result from decreased right ventricular performance or failure of the stenotic pulmonary valvular orifice to grow in relation to the child. In older children, the orifice increases with body growth,[6] but comparable data in infants are limited. Danilowicz and associates[7] address this question by the study of 35 children with pulmonary stenosis with serial cardiac catheterization. Most children were initially catheterized in the first year of life and then restudied, 10 after 1 year of age. During the interval, right ventricular systolic pressure often increased in 1 patient from 72 mm Hg at 4 days of age to 200 mm Hg at 13 months, and the calculated pulmonary valvular area decreased. Often, this was associated with infundibular hypertrophy, which could have led to the increased right ventricular systolic pressure. Although right ventricular systolic pressure increased with age in some infants, whether this was related to infundibular obstruction or to failure of the valve orifice to grow remains uncertain. In infants with thickened immobile valves, it is unlikely that the orifice grows as compared to infants with dome-shaped, more pliable pulmonary valves.

Severe Stenosis

CLINICAL FEATURES.   Patients with pulmonary stenosis appear normal at birth. A murmur may be detected in the neonatal period but may not be discovered until the first postnatal visit to the physician. Patients with pulmonary stenosis usually show normal growth and development, even those who subsequently develop congestive cardiac failure. If severe cyanosis is present, however, growth may be retarded.

Patients with severe stenosis may present a history of progressive cyanosis because of a right-to-left shunt through a patent foramen ovale. The cyanosis may be associated with congestive cardiac failure. Severe pulmonary stenosis may occasionally present with congestive cardiac failure but without cyanosis because the foramen ovale is sealed. Acrocyanosis, however, may be present because of diminished cardiac output and increased tissue extraction of oxygen. The development of either cyanosis or congestive cardiac failure demands immediate investigation of the patient, for these symptoms precede hypoxic spells or sudden death. The symptoms of cyanosis and/or congestive cardiac failure may be present shortly following birth or may develop subsequently in the first year of life.

Hepatomegaly is present in patients with congestive cardiac failure. Luke[8] describes that patients deteriorate in a characteristic pattern. Initially, the infant gains weight and progresses normally but later develops restlessness, irritability, poor feeding, and slow weight gain. Subsequently, motor development slows, and cyanosis deepens. Cyanotic spells associated with rapid respirations, limpness, and transient unconsciousness occur and may lead to death.

On conducting physical examination, we have been struck by the severe dyspnea and breathlessness which infants with severe symptomatic pulmonary stenosis manifest. The facies appear anxious, the cheeks are suffused, and there may be diffuse cyanosis. They otherwise appear healthy and have a round, chubby face.

The chest is symmetrical, and the cardiac activity is normal. A right ventricular heave is present. A systolic ejection-type murmur is heard along the left sternal border but not invariably in the pulmonary area, and, if it is loud, it transmits to the left upper back. In perhaps a third of the patients, a systolic thrill coexists. Although commonly loud (grade 4/6), it becomes softer in patients with congestive cardiac failure. Occasionally, patients have a high-pitched pansystolic murmur along the lower left sternal border. This murmur, reflecting tricuspid insufficiency, may be the only murmur present. In the neonatal period, a continuous murmur of patent ductus arteriosus may indicate severe pulmonary stenosis. The second heart sound appears single in most infants with pulmonary stenosis. In older infants, the murmur may be associated with a pulmonary systolic ejection click.

Prominent a waves have been described in the jugular venous pulse,[9] but we have found this difficult to identify because the necks of neonates and infants are short and fat.

ELECTROCARDIOGRAM. The P waves show right atrial enlargement with tall, peaked P waves in leads II, III, and VI. Right axis deviation up to +210° is present. A pattern of right ventricular hypertrophy is found (Fig. 10-2) and manifested by either a pure R wave or qR pattern in leads V_1 and V_4R and a deep S wave in lead V_6. There is a rough correlation between the height of the

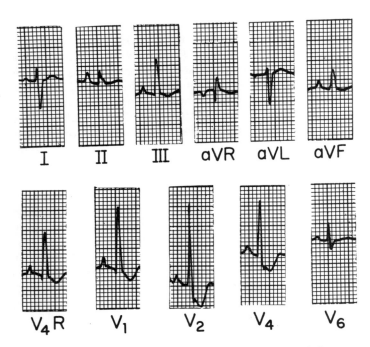

FIG. 10-2. Electrocardiogram of pulmonary stenosis in neonate with dome-shaped valve. QRS axis is +120°. Right atrial enlargement, and right ventricular hypertrophy.

R wave in the right precordial leads and the level of right ventricular systolic pressure.

With time, the amplitude of the R wave in the right precordial leads may increase, indicating increasing severity of the stenosis, but, more commonly, change is reflected by abnormalities of ventricular repolarization. A pattern of right ventricular strain may develop, as reflected by ST segment depression and deeply inverted T waves in the right precordial leads. Although the T waves are normally inverted in leads V_1 to V_4 in infants and upright in leads V_5 and V_6, as right ventricular strain develops, the T waves in lead V_5 and then lead V_6 become inverted.

THORACIC ROENTGENOGRAM.   The cardiac size is larger than normal (Fig. 10-3) and may be greatly enlarged in patients with coexistent tricuspid insufficiency. The cardiac contour is globular, and the right cardiac border (right atrium) is prominent if tricuspid regurgitation is present. The pulmonary arterial segment is normal or concave but does not show poststenotic dilatation. The pulmonary vasculature is usually diminished, sparse, and stringy. An increase in cardiac size reflects the increasing severity.

CARDIAC CATHETERIZATION AND ANGIOCARDIOGRAM.   Cardiac catheterization is performed through the saphenous vein, and the initial efforts should be made to direct the catheter tip into the right ventricle, for at this site, the critical information is obtained. Right ventricular pressure is recorded to determine the severity of the stenosis. The contour of the right ventricular systolic pressure characteristically shows a peaked, symmetrical wave form as contrasted to the

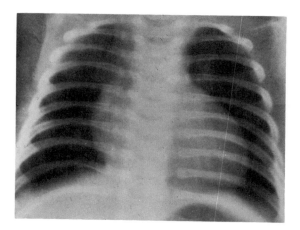

FIG. 10-3.   Thoracic roentgenogram of pulmonary valvular stenosis. Moderate cardiac enlargement. Concave pulmonary arterial segment. Pulmonary arterial markings diminished.

square-topped wave form in patients with pulmonary stenosis and coexistent ventricular septal communication. Attempts should not be made to advance the catheter tip into the pulmonary artery, for it may occlude the narrowed pulmonary orifice, as described by Paul and Rudolph,[10] and cause severe hypoxic symptoms. Furthermore, in most instances, information about pulmonary arterial pressure is not needed to make management decisions, and in a critically ill infant, valuable time may be wasted trying to obtain these data.

Once pressure is recorded, preparations should be made to perform an angiocardiogram. Care must be taken to properly position the catheter in the right ventricle because it is highly trabeculated. Furthermore, the right ventricular cavity may be small. In performing a test injection, ventricular size and catheter position should be observed. If the cavity is small, the amount of contrast should be reduced and the catheter repositioned if located in a trabeculated portion of the ventricle.

Right ventriculography is needed to define right ventricular size and visualize the details of the pulmonary valve and pulmonary trunk. The crista supraventricularis narrows in systole but usually widens during diastole. We have not considered such systolic narrowing as indicative of significant subvalvular obstruction.

The pulmonary valve often appears thickened and domed during systole (Fig. 10-4). A central jet of contrast material passes through the pulmonary valve. The pulmonary annulus is usually normal, and the pulmonary trunk and left pulmonary artery may be enlarged.

After angiography, other data can be gathered, such as right atrial pressure and left atrial or systemic arterial saturation.

Tricuspid insufficiency may be recognized on the right ventriculogram. At times, it is difficult to determine if tricuspid insufficiency is significant because the catheter passes across the tricuspid valve to enter the right ventricle. If, however, a large amount of contrast material appears in the right atrium and remains for several frames, and the right atrium and right ventricle are ex-

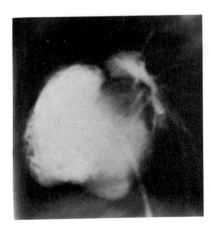

FIG. 10-4. Right ventriculogram, lateral view, of pulmonary valvular stenosis. Domed pulmonary valve, with minute jet through valve.

tremely pulsatile, the tricuspid insufficiency is not artifactual but of major degree.

The pulmonary valvular area can be calculated by assuming or measuring the oxygen consumption and by using the arteriovenous oxygen difference across the pulmonary circulation.

The catheterization procedure should be expedited in infants with pulmonary stenosis, since they are often critically ill. Care should be taken to avoid arrhythmias, particularly tachyarrhythmias, since they decrease cardiac output, especially pulmonary perfusion, significantly.

MANAGEMENT. Following the catheterization, neonates or infants with cyanosis and/or congestive cardiac failure should undergo a transpulmonary arterial pulmonary valvotomy. We utilize inflow venous stasis for pulmonary valvotomy and have had very satisfactory results.[11,12] The infundibular area does not need to be operated upon. Many centers use cardiopulmonary bypass with equally satisfactory results.

The results of operation are very gratifying, cyanosis disappears, cardiac size decreases, and congestive cardiac failure is relieved. Postoperative cardiac catheterization data[8,11,12] show reduction of right ventricular systolic pressure, usually to a value less than 50 mm Hg. In some patients, arterial desaturation may persist, although it is minimal and the patient appears acyanotic.

Pulmonary Valvular Dysplasia

Previously in this section, the anatomic details of pulmonary valvular dysplasia were described. There are several distinctive clinical features which should lead the physician to suspect this form of pulmonary stenosis. The family history is often positive; there may be one or more siblings or parents with pulmonary stenosis.[2] Children with dysplastic pulmonary valve are small and have an abnormal facies, showing ptosis and a triangular shape. Since poststenotic dilatation does not develop, a systolic ejection click is not heard, and the pulmonary arterial segment is of normal size on thoracic roentgenogram. The electrocardiogram is abnormal (Fig. 10-5) and characteristically shows the QRS axis directed markedly leftward (-60 to $-120°$). This finding is unexpected for pulmonary stenosis and is valuable for recognizing this form of pulmonary stenosis.

Dysplastic pulmonary valve has distinctive angiographic features (Fig. 10-6): the pulmonary annulus is smaller than normal, the valve leaflets are thickened and do not dome, and the sinuses of Valsalva are slitlike.

Recognition of this anatomic type of pulmonary stenosis is important because the operative approach is different from that used with dome-shaped pulmonary stenosis. Rather than a pulmonary valvotomy, one or two pulmonary valvular leaflets must be excised and, at times, a patch placed across the pulmonary annulus. The indications for operation for this form are similar to those for operative dome-shaped pulmonary valve.

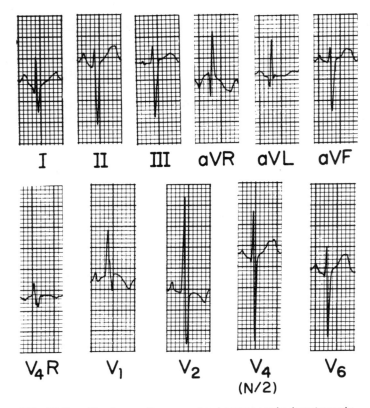

FIG. 10-5. Electrocardiogram of pulmonary valvular stenosis from dysplastic pulmonary valve. QRS axis is −90°. Right ventricular hypertrophy. N/2, half-standardization.

Mild to Moderate Pulmonary Stenosis

Infants with mild to moderate pulmonary stenosis are asymptomatic and come to the physician's attention because of a murmur. Although the murmur may be present at birth, it more often is initially heard later in infancy.

Rowe and Mehrizi[9] state that neonates with pulmonary stenosis may have a pulmonary systolic ejection murmur but no ejection click. With time, the murmur becomes louder and is associated with a click and a delayed pulmonary second sound.

In infants with mild or moderate pulmonary stenosis, physical examination reveals no cyanosis. The chest is symmetrical, and there is no clinical evidence of cardiomegaly. A grade 3–4/6 pulmonary systolic ejection murmur is present and may be associated with a thrill along the upper left sternal border and in the suprasternal notch. A pulmonary systolic ejection click is present except in patients with a dysplastic valve. The pulmonary component of the second sound may be delayed. The liver is normal sized.

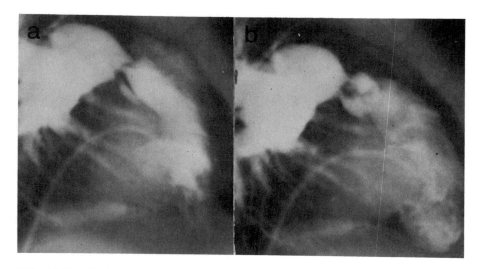

FIG. 10-6.   Right ventriculogram of dysplastic pulmonary valve, lateral views. **a.** Systole. **b.** Diastole. Thickened pulmonary valve cusps. No doming. Narrowed sinuses of Valsalva.

ELECTROCARDIOGRAM.   The electrocardiogram may be normal or show varying degrees of right ventricular hypertrophy, but the ST and T waves are normal. Usually, right atrial enlargement is not found.

THORACIC ROENTGENOGRAM.   Cardiac size and pulmonary vasculature are normal. The pulmonary arterial segment is dilated, and the left pulmonary artery is enlarged.

MANAGEMENT.   Patients considered to have mild to moderate pulmonary stenosis do not require investigation by cardiac catheterization in infancy, and it is best to delay study until they are older. The patients should be observed periodically during the first year of life, for the pulmonary stenosis may progress, the signs of progression being the development of cyanosis or other symptoms, and increasing severity of right ventricular hypertrophy or cardiomegaly. If these findings develop, cardiac catheterization should be undertaken.

Should they be studied, the criteria for pulmonary valvotomy are more stringent than in older children. Operation should be delayed until at least 1 year of age, unless the right ventricular systolic pressure exceeds 125 mm Hg.

Peripheral Pulmonary Arterial Stenosis

Peripheral pulmonary arterial stenosis is a congenital cardiac anomaly that is frequently recognized in infancy but rarely causes symptoms. Although it may occur as an isolated lesion or may coexist with other conditions, in this section, isolated peripheral pulmonary stenosis will be emphasized. In patients with coexistent peripheral pulmonary arterial stenosis, the clinical and laboratory findings are usually those of the primary cardiac anomaly.

ETIOLOGY.   Peripheral pulmonary arterial stenosis is associated with several syndromes or other factors, and these relationships may indicate an etiology in many patients. Although the association of congenital cardiac anomalies with maternal rubella infection was well known, it was not until the early 1960s that peripheral pulmonary arterial stenosis was fully recognized and described[13,14] in infants with rubella syndrome. In fact, the incidence of peripheral pulmonary arterial stenosis in infants with rubella syndrome equals that of patent ductus arteriosus.

Beuren and co-workers[15] described the presence of peripheral pulmonary arterial stenosis in patients with Williams syndrome, i.e., the combination of supravalvular aortic stenosis, mental retardation, and abnormal facies. Subsequent reports [16,17] have reemphasized this association.

Murmurs suggesting peripheral pulmonary stenosis may be heard in otherwise normal neonates and young infants, and these murmurs subsequently disappear. Danilowicz and associates[18] described the cardiac catheterization findings in these infants and called the condition "physiologic" bilateral peripheral pulmonic stenosis. In these infants, a small pressure gradient was found between the pulmonary trunk and the peripheral pulmonary arteries. However, no anatomic lesion was found on pulmonary angiography to account for the gradient other than the fact that the caliber of the peripheral pulmonary arteries was significantly smaller than that of the pulmonary trunk, and the pulmonary arteries arose at an acute angle. With growth, the angle between the pulmonary trunk and the branch pulmonary arteries becomes less, and the branch pulmonary arteries increase in size.

Finally, families with peripheral pulmonary arterial stenosis have been described.[19]

PATHOLOGY.   Peripheral pulmonary arterial stenosis has been classified by Gay and others[20] into four types:

Type I   Single, central stenosis involving the pulmonary trunk or one of the main pulmonary arteries

Type II   Bifurcation stenosis involving the origin of the pulmonary arteries

Type III   Multiple, peripheral stenosis involving segmental arteries, with normal pulmonary trunk and major pulmonary arteries

Type IV   Central and peripheral stenosis

Of these types, stenosis rarely involves the pulmonary trunk. Type II is most common, and type III is least frequent. The obstruction rarely occurs as a membrane, as in coarctation of the aorta, but rather takes the form of either short segmental tubular narrowing or elongated narrowing or hypoplasia of the pulmonary artery. In our experience, the nature and extent of peripheral pulmonary arterial stenosis are better demonstrated by angiography than by autopsy. Although the stenosis may involve only one lung, in most patients it is bilateral.

Usually, the external appearance of the pulmonary arteries is normal, but when the artery is opened, the intima appears greatly thickened. Histologic examination shows intimal thickening by fibrous tissue proliferation and diminished amounts of elastic tissue in the media. In our experience, the media does not show a normal laminar arrangement, but the bundles of media course in different directions, forming a mosaic pattern.

Rowe and Mehrizi[21] believe that the severity of stenosis increases with age in some patients because the increasing blood flowing across the stenotic area increases intimal proliferation and causes poststenotic dilatation.

As in valvular pulmonary stenosis, right ventricular hypertrophy develops proportionally to the degree of obstruction.

HEMODYNAMICS.   In most respects, the hemodynamics of peripheral pulmonary arterial stenosis resemble those of valvular pulmonary stenosis, with the level of right ventricular systolic pressure being related to the degree of obstruction. The right ventricle ejects blood into the pulmonary arterial tree proximal to the stenosis. During systole, this segment serves as a continuation of the right ventricle because systolic pressure is elevated and blood is forced through the stenotic areas to the lower pressure distal pulmonary arteries. Right ventricular ejection may be delayed, as in patients with valvular pulmonary stenosis, since the pulmonary valve remains open as long as a pressure difference exists in the pulmonary arteries proximal and distal to the stenosis. Diastolic pressures are identical proximally and distally to the obstruction. Thus, the pulse pressure proximal to the obstruction is characteristically widened.

If unilateral peripheral pulmonary arterial stenosis is present, right ventricular systolic pressure remains normal. The peripheral pulmonary arterial stenosis causes blood to be shunted away from the involved lung, but the capacity of the normal contralateral lung is such that the increased flow is unassociated with a pressure rise. In such patients, a discrepancy of blood flow exists between the lungs, which could be shown by radioactive scintillation scanning.

CLINICAL FEATURES.   Neonates and infants with peripheral pulmonary arterial stenosis are most always asymptomatic, since the stenosis is rarely of such severity as to lead to right ventricular failure. The condition is almost always recognized by the presence of a systolic murmur. The murmur may be from grade 1–3/6 in loudness and is heard well throughout the chest, particularly in the back, and in the axilla. It is rarely continuous in timing. The only continuous murmur we have heard in a patient with peripheral pulmonary arterial stenosis occurred when a ventricular septal defect coexisted. Presumably, the increased pulmonary blood flow caused a gradient across the stenosis throughout the cardiac cycle. The presence of a continuous murmur in patients with peripheral pulmonary arterial stenosis and coexistent lesions with increased pulmonary blood flow has been described by others.[21,22] A systolic ejection click is not heard because the pulmonary trunk is normal sized. The second heart sound shows either normal or wide splitting. The intensity of the pulmonary component of the second heart sound is normal because the pulmonary arterial pressure and the resistance beyond the obstruction are normal. Therefore, the pulmonary valvular closure occurs at a normal level of diastolic pressure.

In patients with peripheral pulmonary arterial stenosis secondary to the rubella syndrome, a patent ductus arteriosus may mask the murmur of peripheral pulmonary arterial stenosis.

The findings on general examination may indicate either the rubella or Williams' syndrome (Fig. 10-7).

ELECTROCARDIOGRAM.   The electrocardiogram reflects the degree of right ventricular hypertension. Accordingly, it is often normal but may show right atrial enlargement, right axis deviation, and right ventricular hypertrophy, as in valvular pulmonary stenosis (Fig. 10-8).

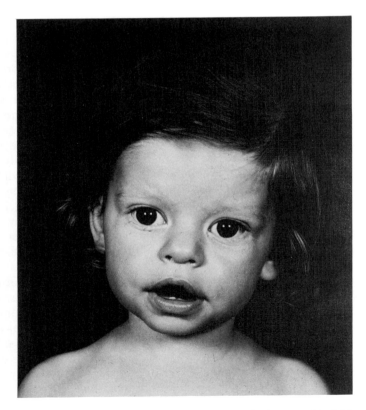

FIG. 10-7.   Facies of Williams' syndrome in 1-year-old child.

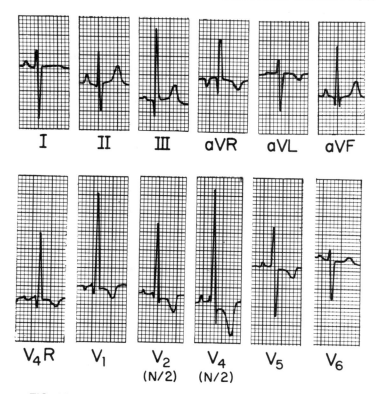

I   II   III   aVR   aVL   aVF

V₄R   V₁   V₂   V₄   V₅   V₆
                   (N/2) (N/2)

FIG. 10-8. Electrocardiogram of peripheral pulmonary arterial stenosis in 5-month-old infant. Right ventricular pressure is 160/0mm Hg. QRS axis is +150°. Right ventricular hypertrophy and strain. N/2 = half-standardization.

THORACIC ROENTGENOGRAM.   In patients with isolated peripheral pulmonary arterial stenosis, the thoracic roentgenogram is normal. Cardiac size and contour are normal, and unlike valvular pulmonary stenosis, the pulmonary trunk is not dilated. The peripheral pulmonary vasculature is also normal. In case of severe peripheral pulmonary arterial stenosis, cardiac enlargement is present, but severe stenosis is rare in infants.

CARDIAC CATHETERIZATION AND ANGIOCARDIOGRAM.   The diagnosis may be confirmed by cardiac catheterization and angiography. The crucial catheterization data are supplied by a continuous pressure tracing recorded from the distal pulmonary artery into the right ventricle. Analysis of the tracing in patients with peripheral pulmonary arterial stenosis shows several characteristic findings[23]: (1) proximal pulmonary arterial tracings show a wide pulse pressure, rapid systolic upstroke, and low diastolic pressure; and (2) distal tracings show narrow pulse pressure, slower upstroke, and diastolic pressure similar to that proximally.

The right ventricular systolic and right atrial pressures may be elevated according to the level of obstruction. Data from infants[13,14] usually show the right ventricular systolic pressure to be less than 100 mm Hg, although we have studied one child with peripheral pulmonary arterial stenosis at 14 months whose pressure was 200 mm Hg.

Pulmonary angiography can demonstrate the anatomy of the lesion (Fig. 10-9). Usually an anteroposterior projection best defines the lesions, although stenosis of the proximal left pulmonary artery may only be visualized on oblique or lateral projections.

During infancy, cardiac catheterization and angiocardiography are not indicated, unless the infants become symptomatic, and/or the diagnosis is uncertain.

MANAGEMENT. No treatment is required during infancy, and even in older patients, it is rarely indicated. Although the suggestion has been made that the condition may become more severe, we know of no long-term data that indicate that this occurs after infancy, but more data are needed before the natural history is clarified.

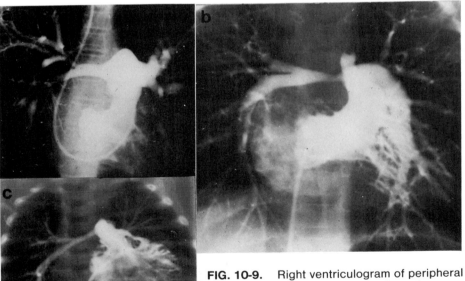

FIG. 10-9. Right ventriculogram of peripheral pulmonary arterial stenosis. **a.** Stenotic areas and poststenotic dilatation present in major branches of right pulmonary artery. **b.** Stenotic area in proximal right pulmonary artery. **c.** Diffuse hypoplasia of pulmonary arterial branches.

OBSTRUCTION TO LEFT VENTRICULAR OUTFLOW

Four conditions can cause left ventricular outflow obstruction in infants:

1. Coarctation of the aorta
2. Interruption of the aortic arch
3. Valvular aortic stenosis
4. Systemic hypertension

Although aortic atresia also is associated with left ventricular obstruction, it is discussed elsewhere because its clinical picture differs from the conditions discussed in this section.

The clinical picture of these four conditions resembles cardiomyopathy, since there are symptoms of congestive cardiac failure, a soft murmur, electrocardiographic changes of left ventricular hypertrophy associated with ST segment and T wave changes, and roentgenographic findings of generalized cardiomegaly. Often after digitalization, the murmur becomes louder.

In this chapter, emphasis will be placed upon infants who become symptomatic from the obstruction. Milder forms of these conditions may be discovered in infancy but are asymptomatic. The clinical features in asymptomatic infants resemble those occurring in older children.

COARCTATION OF THE AORTA

Coarctation of the aorta is a congenital cardiac anomaly in which obstruction or narrowing occurs in the distal aortic arch or proximal descending aorta (Fig. 10-10). It occurs as either an isolated lesion or coexisting with a variety of other congenital cardiac anomalies. Patent ductus arteriosus is one of the most important of these coexistent conditions. Coarctation has been classified according to the position relative to the ductus, and in many infants, the ductus contributes a major hemodynamic role.

Coarctation of the aorta has been classified in several ways. One classification divides coarctation of the aorta into the adult and infantile types.[24] Clinical and hemodynamic differences exist between the two forms. The adult type is localized and occurs opposite the ductus arteriosus (patent or ligamentous), while the infantile type is associated with tubular hypoplasia usually of the distal arch and proximal descending aorta, and the ductus enters the aorta below the narrowing. There is a high incidence of coexistent cardiac malformations in patients with the infantile type. The terms "infantile" and "adult" are misnomers because the infantile type, although usually leading to symptoms in infancy, can cause problems later, and the adult type may cause major symptoms in infancy. We prefer the terminology of Rudolph,[25] who classified coarctation of the aorta as localized (juxtaductal) aortic obstruction or aortic isthmus narrowing.

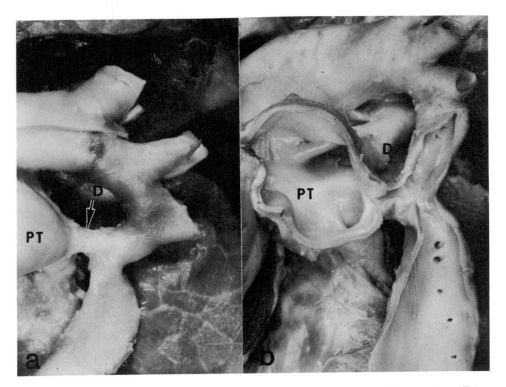

FIG. 10-10.   Coarctation of aorta. Aortic arch and proximal descending aorta. **a.** External appearance. Localized indentation opposite ductus arteriosus (D). **b.** Internal appearance. Coarctation opposite ductus arteriosus (D). PT, pulmonary trunk.

Localized (Juxtaductal) Aortic Obstruction

In this form of coarctation of the aorta, the aorta is narrowed opposite the ductus arteriosus. The exterior of the aorta shows posterolateral indentation. Interiorly, an eccentric shelf projects into the lumen, although occasionally the narrowing may be concentric. The orifice of the coarctation is immediately opposite the ductus.[26]

The caliber of the ductus arteriosus, if patent, is usually small, and as its aortic orifice narrows, the extent of aortic obstruction is accentuated.

Although associated cardiac anomalies are uncommon in this form of coarctation of the aorta, small infracristal ventricular septal defect is the most prevalent.

The aortic arch is of normal caliber, although between the left subclavian artery and the coarctation, it may have slight tubular hypoplasia. Poststenotic dilatation occurs in the aorta below the coarctation. The left subclavian artery arises at or proximal to the coarctation.

In patients who develop congestive cardiac failure, the left atrium and left ventricle are dilated and hypertrophied. The endocardial surface of the left ventricle frequently shows changes of endocardial fibroelastosis.[27] The papillary muscles may be abnormal, and anatomic findings suggest coexistent mitral insufficiency.

HEMODYNAMICS.   Prior to birth, the coarctation interferes little with the normal fetal circulation. Following birth, as long as the ductus arteriosus remains patent, ductal blood flow resembles the normal pattern during the transition from fetal to adult type circulation. During this phase, the coarctation does not obstruct aortic flow because the patency of the ductus widens the effective orifice at the site of the coarctation, and blood can pass freely from the ascending to the descending aorta. Closure of the ductus arteriosus progresses from the pulmonary arterial end toward the aortic end. When the aortic orifice of the ductus eventually occludes, the coarctation becomes obstructive. The normal sequence of ductal closure in infants with coarctation of the aorta may be delayed for several days or weeks,[25] and severe symptoms do not appear in the immediate neonatal period. Because of the responsiveness of the ductus arteriosus to oxygen,[28] the administration of oxygen to an infant can constrict the ductus and accentuate the findings of coarctation of the aorta. As long as the ductus remains patent, a small left-to-right shunt may occur.

The rate at which aortic obstruction develops depends upon the rate of ductal closure and the severity upon the extent of the aortic shelf. Because of the obstruction, the systolic pressure in the proximal aorta and left ventricle increases, while that in the descending aorta remains normal or falls. In the neonatal period, because myocardial response to increased afterload is limited, left ventricular failure occurs. The left ventricle and left atrium dilate, and the end-diastolic and left atrial pressures are elevated. Modest elevation of pulmonary arterial and right ventricular pressures occurs.

In infancy, coarctation of the aorta is tolerated better by the left ventricle, and the presence of collateral vessels permit escape of some blood from the proximal aorta. Cardiac failure, however, can develop within the first year of life, usually between 1 to 3 months, because of severe coarctation.

COLLATERAL ARTERIAL VESSEL DEVELOPMENT.   In any arterial system when the pressure differs between two components, the naturally occurring vessels which communicate around the obstruction enlarge and serve as collateral vessels. In coarctation of the aorta, collateral arterial vessels, such as between the internal mammary and hypogastric arteries and within the intercostal system, enlarge between the high pressure proximal aorta and the lower pressure descending aorta. These communications assist in the transfer of blood from the ascending to the descending aorta. The collateral arterial vessels enlarge and become tortuous. The changes are particularly striking in the intercostal arteries.

While others have noted the relative lack of collateral vessels in neonates, we found extensive collateral arteries in infants 1 week of age,[29] but we could not correlate the extent of collaterals with either blood pressure levels or age.

CLINICAL FEATURES.   Coarctation of the aorta is not clinically evident at birth, but signs and symptoms develop subsequently. The first sign of cardiac disease may be the development of congestive cardiac failure, perhaps precipitated by an acute respiratory infection. The infant may, however, have had a history of heavy breathing, perspiration, poor feeding, and irritability before developing overt signs of congestive cardiac failure. Neonates or infants with the sudden onset of symptoms show features of cardiogenic shock, such as poor perfusion and mottled skin.

The neonate or infant appears in respiratory distress and may have mottled skin, or mild to moderate cyanosis may be present from a combination of poor peripheral perfusion and pulmonary edema. Rales are heard.

If the infant has congestive cardiac failure, the blood pressure may be low (30 mm Hg), with no pressure difference found between the arms and legs. Following digitalization, as cardiac output improves, a blood pressure difference develops, although even in treated infants with congestive cardiac failure, the blood pressure proximal to the obstruction is rarely elevated.

Cardiomegaly is clinically evident, the cardiac apex being displaced laterally to the anterior axillary line. A precordial bulge may be found in older infants. The first heart sound may be normal or accentuated, while the second heart sound is usually accentuated. A third heart sound giving the appearance of a gallop rhythm is found. When the infant is in cardiac failure, no murmur may be found, but following digitalization, a grade 2–3/6 systolic ejection murmur may be heard in the interscapular area or at the apex or lower left sternal border.

ELECTROCARDIOGRAM.   The electrocardiographic findings vary considerably, depending in part on the age of the infant. In symptomatic neonates and some young infants, a pattern of right axis deviation and right ventricular hypertrophy is present and associated with depressed ST segment and inverted T waves in leads V_5 and V_6[30] (Fig. 10-11). As such infants grow, a pattern of left ventricular hypertrophy develops. In older infants with coarctation of the aorta or in those infants with a coexistent large patent ductus arteriosus, a pattern of left or combined ventricular hypertrophy is found.

THORACIC ROENTGENOGRAM.   Diffuse cardiac enlargement is present in symptomatic neonates, and while symptomatic infants also show cardiac enlargement, the cardiac silhouette has a left ventricular contour (Fig. 10-12a). Left atrial enlargement may be found (Fig. 10-12b). The lung fields show either venous obstruction or a pattern of both venous and arterial markings.[30]

Rib notching does not occur in infancy.

CARDIAC CATHETERIZATION AND ANGIOCARDIOGRAM.   After treatment of the infant for congestive cardiac failure, diagnostic studies should be performed. In the infant who clearly has findings of isolated coarctation of the aorta and no coex-

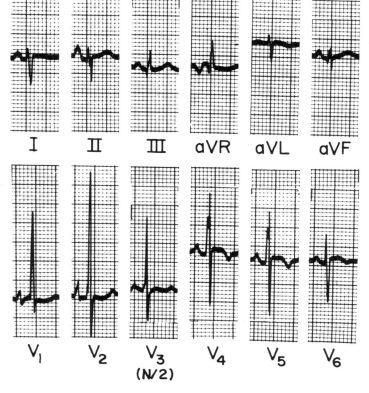

FIG. 10-11. Electrocardiogram of coarctation of aorta in 1-month-old infant. QRS axis is +180°, right atrial enlargement, and right ventricular hypertrophy. Inverted T waves in left precordial leads. N/2, half-standardization.

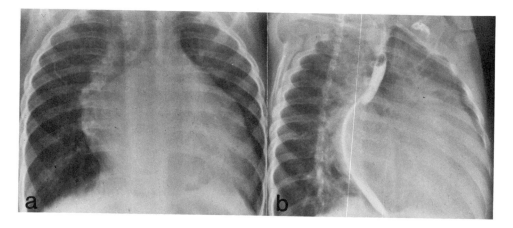

FIG. 10-12. Thoracic roentgenogram of coarctation of aorta. a. Posteroanterior view. b. Right anterior oblique view. Marked cardiomegaly and left atrial enlargement. Slight pulmonary venous obstruction.

istent cardiac lesion, we often perform only a retrograde aortogram through a brachial artery (Fig. 10-13). If blood pressures are equal in the arms, we prefer using the left arm.

In most neonates or infants, cardiac catheterization should be performed because of the difficulty in distinguishing narrowing of the aortic isthmus from isolated coarctation of the aorta and because of the necessity of excluding associated malformations.[31] We prefer to perform a cutdown in the saphenous vein and use this approach to the heart. Others use the percutaneous method. On occasion, we have used an umbilical artery to catheterize the aorta and injected contrast material and visualized the aortic arch and proximal aspect of the coarctation. We have sometimes experienced difficulty passing the catheter beyond the coarctation, and if an aortogram is performed, in this instance, only the descending aorta and arch are visualized. The information provided by such a study is inadequate to decide operative approaches, and further angiographic studies are indicated.

If cardiac catheterization is performed in infants with coarctation of the aorta, right ventricular systolic and pulmonary arterial pressures are elevated

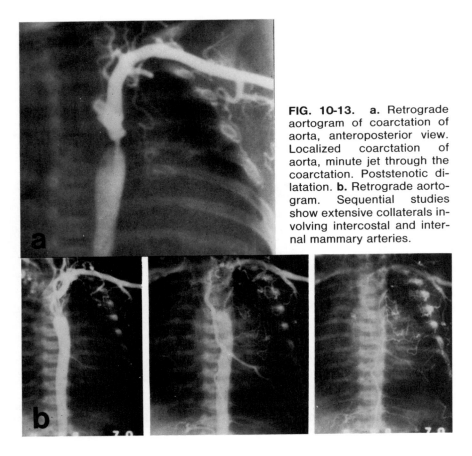

FIG. 10-13. **a.** Retrograde aortogram of coarctation of aorta, anteroposterior view. Localized coarctation of aorta, minute jet through the coarctation. Poststenotic dilatation. **b.** Retrograde aortogram. Sequential studies show extensive collaterals involving intercostal and internal mammary arteries.

to 40 to 60 mm Hg.[30,31] Left atrial and pulmonary capillary pressures may be elevated to a mean of 20 to 25 mm Hg, and left ventricular end-diastolic pressure is also elevated. Pressures in the two components of the aorta vary considerably. In the presence of severe cardiac failure, the mean pressures may be 30 to 40 mm Hg, with little difference between the ascending and decending aorta. In the infant without cardiac failure, the pressure in the ascending aorta may be 180/100 mm Hg.

Oximetry data may show no shunt or a small left-to-right shunt through the foramen ovale. Peripheral arterial blood may be desaturated because of pulmonary edema. The arteriovenous oxygen difference is wide in patients with cardiac failure.

During cardiac catheterization, angiocardiography should be performed. If a ventricular septal defect coexists, the catheter may be passed through it into the ascending aorta, and an aortogram can be performed in the ascending aorta. Otherwise, a left ventriculogram can outline the aorta. If the ductus is patent, a balloon angiocatheter can be passed through the right side of the heart into the descending aorta immediately beyond the insertion of the ductus. The balloon is momentarily inflated occluding the descending aorta and contrast material injected to visualize the coarctation and aortic arch. The balloon is then deflated. Usually, angiography is not indicated on the right side of the heart unless the right ventricular systolic pressure is elevated to systemic levels. Right ventriculography is then indicated to determine if there is a ventricular septal defect, reversing ductus arteriosus or such conditions as double outlet right ventricle.

MANAGEMENT. The initial steps in the management of congestive cardiac failure should be directed toward stabilization of the infant by placing him in a neutral environment and starting an intravenous line for administration of drugs.

Metabolic acidosis, which is frequently present and coexists with disseminated intravascular coagulation, should be treated. Rudolph[32] is concerned about administering oxygen in concentrations greater than 30 to 35 percent, since the oxygen may increase the obstruction by constricting the ductus arteriosus further. The infant should be digitalized, and in the severely ill infant, rapid digitalization is necessary, with total digitalization accomplished in 6 to 8 hours. Diuretics should be given also. In severely ill infants with cardiac failure and inadequate systemic perfusion, prostaglandin E_1 often dilates the ductus arteriosus, improving perfusion and reducing left ventricular failure.[33] This allows stabilization of the infant before proceeding with diagnostic or operative procedures.

If the infant's condition deteriorates, angiography should be undertaken within 6 to 8 hours, but if improvement occurs, studies can be delayed until 24 hours following initiation of therapy.

Following angiography, if the infant shows no signs of persistent congestive cardiac failure, such as tachypnea, tachycardia, or hepatomegaly, and feeds well without tiring, we believe operation is not indicated at that time. The infant can be discharged, maintained on a digitalis preparation, and followed periodically. At an older age, elective resection of the coarctation can be performed.

If the infant's condition deteriorates further or does not improve, however, operation to resect the coarctation should be undertaken immediately. If localized, the coarctation can be resected and the aorta reanastomosed. Another approach is to incise the aorta longitudinally through the site of the coarctation and place a patch over the area.

The operative mortality in infants with a localized coarctation of the aorta, with or without an associated patent ductus arteriosus and with other major cardiac anomalies, is about 10 percent.

We have not observed the complication of mesenteric arteritis in neonates or infants.

Some patients operated in infancy will probably require reoperation in later childhood because the anastomotic site may not grow at the same rate as the aorta, or there may be restenosis. In our experience,[34] 8.5 percent required reoperation, but no study has followed a large number of infants into adolescence to determine the true incidence of this complication. Several studies[35-37] have addressed the issue of recoarctation.

Aortic Isthmus Narrowing

This form of coarctation of the aorta has also been called "infantile coarctation" because it usually appears in infancy and rarely does it initially cause symptoms in older children. Nadas[38] has called it "coarctation of the aorta with systemic right ventricle," since the right ventricle communicates through a patent ductus arteriosus with the descending aorta.

PATHOLOGY.   In this form of coarctation of the aorta, the aorta shows tubular hypoplasia from the left subclavian artery to the area of the ductus arteriosus. Frequently, there is also a localized constriction immediately proximal to the ductus arteriosus. Occasionally, the aortic arch is also narrowed between the left subclavian and left carotid arteries. The ductus is almost always patent, and its diameter is the same as that of the descending aorta.

A ventricular septal defect is often present as well, and although Rudolph[32] indicates that there is a high incidence of the supracristal type, this has not been our experience. Occasionally, subaortic stenosis coexists.

HEMODYNAMICS.   Following birth, the systemic vascular resistance rises, and the pulmonary vascular resistance falls. Because of the coexistent ventricular septal defect, the decrease in pulmonary resistance causes an increase in pulmonary blood flow. In the postnatal period, pulmonary resistance falls less than in normal infants, in part because of the increased arterial mass in the pulmonary arterioles as described by Naeye.[39] Because of the ventricular septal defect, right ventricular, pulmonary arterial, and ascending aortic systolic pressures are identical. Since the ductus arteriosus is widely patent, the pressure in the descending aorta and perfusion of the lower portion of the body are maintained. For the right-to-left shunt to occur through the ductus arteriosus, the pulmonary vascular resistance must exceed the resistance in the vascular system of the descending aorta.

At this time, the circulation resembles that in the fetus.

Two events cause the patient's condition to deteriorate: constriction of the ductus arteriosus and decrease in pulmonary vascular resistance. Both factors have a profound effect upon perfusion of the descending aorta, and a pressure difference develops between the pulmonary artery and the descending aorta. The blood in the pulmonary trunk flows predominantly through the lungs, and little flows through the narrowed ductus. The fall of pulmonary vascular resistance further enhances pulmonary blood flow.

As a result of the large volume of pulmonary blood flow, the left atrium and left ventricle dilate, and the left ventricular end-diastolic pressure rises. Congestive cardiac failure develops not only because of left ventricular enlargement but also because the left ventricle is ejecting blood against the increased resistance imposed by the coarctation. Rudolph[32] indicates that administration of 100 percent oxygen to these patients may be harmful by further constricting the ductus, thereby interfering with perfusion to the descending aorta and its effect on further narrowing the coarctation. The oxygen also has an effect on lowering pulmonary vascular resistance and increasing pulmonary blood flow.

Perfusion of the lower extremities is limited, and metabolic acidosis and its consequences can develop.

CLINICAL FEATURES.   Most patients develop congestive cardiac failure and die in the neonatal period or in early infancy unless treated. Patients are usually asymptomatic at birth but develop symptoms according to the rate of ductal closure, degree of aortic obstruction, and type of coexistent cardiac condition.

The presenting features are those of congestive cardiac failure and they develop in the first few days or within 2 weeks of birth. Initially, tachypnea and poor feeding occur. Cardiac failure may progress slowly or occur abruptly, perhaps being precipitated by a respiratory illness. There may be a history of cyanosis or irritability.

On physical examination, the infant appears dyspneic, tachypneic, and often mildly or moderately cyanotic. The infant may be mottled because of markedly reduced cardiac output.

When congestive cardiac failure is present, the peripheral pulses are weak or impalpable. Blood pressure readings are low, and in our experience, usually no significant difference is found between the upper and lower extremities. Following digitalization, the pulses and blood pressure readings improve, and a difference is noted between the upper and lower extremities. Blood pressure readings must be obtained in both upper arms and compared to readings obtained in the legs, for there may be a blood pressure difference between the right and left arms if the origin of the left subclavian artery is narrowed in conjunction with the coarctation of the aorta.

The chest is symmetrical, and rales may be heard. Cardiomegaly is clinically evident. The first heart sound is normal, and the second heart sound is accentuated. A third heart sound, giving the appearance of a gallop, is regularly heard. No murmur may be present in the patient with severe congestive cardiac failure, or a short, soft, ejection-type murmur may be heard over the precordium or in the interscapular area. Following digitalization, the murmur may become louder, probably caused by both the coarctation of the aorta and the ventricular septal defect.

Hepatomegaly is a prominent finding, with the enlargment often being below the level of the umbilicus. Peripheral edema may also be evident.

Differential cyanosis is rare, probably because of several factors. If a left-to-right shunt is present through a ventricular septal defect, pulmonary arterial and, therefore, descending aortic oxygen saturations are increased. If pulmonary edema is present, cyanosis is present throughout. Poor peripheral perfusion also causes cyanosis and obscures differential cyanosis.

ELECTROCARDIOGRAM.   The electrocardiogram is rather characteristic in showing a pattern of right ventricular hypertrophy and flat or inverted T waves in the left precordial leads. Right atrial enlargement is usually present, but the QRS axis is normal.

The reason for the seemingly paradoxical right ventricular hypertrophy in a patient with left ventricular outflow obstruction is not fully understood. It might be attributed to a relatively hypoplastic left ventricle present in some patients or to the elevated pulmonary arterial pressure and the pulmonary vascular resistance.

The right ventricular hypertrophy is usually manifested by an rR', pure R, or Rs complex in lead V_1. In older infants, left ventricular hypertrophy may coexist.

THORACIC ROENTGENOGRAM.   Diffuse cardiomegaly is present, and the pulmonary arterial markings are increased. Prominent pulmonary venous markings are found if cardiac failure is present. Left atrial enlargement is present. Classic findings of an E or 3 sign on the barium-filled esophagus, common in older patients with coarctation, are rarely seen in infants.

CARDIAC CATHETERIZATION AND ANGIOCARDIOGRAM.   Cardiac catheterization is performed via the saphenous vein, and the information to be obtained is identical to that in patients with isolated coarctation of the aorta.

Since patent ductus arteriosus shows a right-to-left shunt, particular studies must be performed. The wedge pressure, pulmonary veins, and left atrium should be carefully evaluated to make certain there is no obstruction to pulmonary venous return. Furthermore, the site of obstruction in the aorta must be carefully evaluated.

Cardiac catheterization data may also show evidence of a left-to-right shunt at the ventricular level.[30, 31]

MANAGEMENT.   The steps and principles of management of these patients are identical to those taken for patients with localized coarctation of the aorta. The operative approach may be different, however. Formerly, we believed that the initial step should be the relief of aortic obstruction by resection of the coarctation, thereby reducing left ventricular outflow obstruction and reducing the volume of the left-to-right shunt. Unfortunately, this rarely had the desired effect. As an alternative, we combined resection with banding of the pulmonary artery, but there was still frequently a prolonged and often unsatisfactory convalescence.

Some surgeons now approach these lesions by resecting the coarctation of the aorta, dividing the ductus arteriosus, and repairing the ventricular septal defect. Usually, the aorta has sufficient elasticity so that even when a section of the aorta must be resected, the proximal and distal components can be drawn together. Occasionally, graft material, the left subclavian artery or the left carotid artery has been used to form a conduit to bypass the obstruction.

The operative mortality for these infants is greater than for infants with localized coarctation of the aorta.[40-42] The mortality rate is also higher in infants with multiple cardiac anomalies and in those operated within the first 6 weeks of life. Many of the deaths are related to cardiac and respiratory failure which continue postoperatively and result in hyperkalemia, hypoxemia, and acidosis.

Our follow-up data of 45 survivors indicate that 3 survivors died unexpectedly within 9 months of the operation. Three others died 2, 4, and 8 years following resection, during procedures to correct an intracardiac lesion.

The long-term prognosis is unknown, since many patients will require at least one other operation, such as correction of an intracardiac lesion or reoperation of a recurrent coarctation of the aorta.

Coarctation of the aorta may coexist with transposition of the great vessels,[43] but in these patients, tricuspid atresia or hypoplastic right ventricle coexists. Origin of both great vessels from the right ventricle with a supracristal ventricular septal defect (Taussig-Bing heart) has a frequent association with coarctation of the aorta.

Coarctation of the aorta has also been associated with the development complex described by Shone et al.[44] In this complex, two or more of the following lesions on the left side of the heart may coexist: coarctation of the aorta, subaortic stenosis, parachute mitral valve, and supravalvular stenosis ring of the left atrium. These may lead to pulmonary venous obstruction, usually later in life.

Bicuspid aortic valve coexists in patients with coarctation of the aorta but does not cause additional findings. Aortic valvular stenosis occasionally coexists.

INTERRUPTION OF THE AORTIC ARCH

Interruption of the aortic arch is an uncommon congenital cardiac anomaly, which is usually symptomatic in the neonatal period. Clinically and functionally, it resembles aortic isthmus narrowing.

PATHOLOGY.   In this anomaly, there is a lack of continuity in the aortic arch or isthmus between the proximal and distal portions of the aorta. The descending aorta is continuous with a patent ductus arteriosus and, through it, receives blood from the right ventricle. Two forms of interruption of the aortic arch may be recognized. Usually, there is a lack of tissue between the proximal and distal segments of the aorta, while in the other uncommon form, also called "atresia of the aortic arch," a fibrous strand connects the two segments.

The pattern of origin of brachiocephalic vessels and the site of interruption vary considerably. From our review of 105 cases,[45] in 46 percent the interruption occurred immediately beyond the left subclavian artery, and in one 1 of these patients, the right subclavian artery arose from the descending aorta. In 50 percent, the interruption was located between the left common carotid and left subclavian arteries, with the left subclavian artery arising from the descending aorta. The site of origin of the right subclavian artery was variable. In most patients, it arose from the innominate artery, in about 20 percent of these patients, it arose from the descending aorta, and rarely, it arose from the right pulmonary artery through a right-sided ductus arteriosus.

Rarely, the interruption occurs distal to the innominate artery, and both the left subclavian and carotid arteries arise from the descending aorta.

In almost every patient, a ventricular septal defect is present, and its regular association with interruption and patent ductus arteriosus was considered the third component of a triad. The ventricular septal defect is often located superior and anterior to the membranous septum and may involve the crista supraventricularis. This defect is associated with a subaortic muscle bundle, which leads to subaortic stenosis.[46] Interruption of the aortic arch may occur in patients with complete transposition of the great vessels, persistent truncus arteriosus, origin of both great vessels from the right ventricle, and other less common cardiac malformations.

Rarely, the ventricular septum is intact. In 2 older patients, interruption occurred without a patent ductus arteriosus.[47,48]

Bicuspid aortic valve occurs in about 50 percent of the patients.

HEMODYNAMICS.   The hemodynamics resemble the hemodynamics of preductal coarctation of the aorta with aortic isthmus narrowing and ventricular septal defect.

Left ventricular output is directed into the ascending aorta and into the brachiocephalic vessels arising from the proximal component of the aorta. In addition, flow occurs in a left-to-right direction through the ventricular septal defect into the right ventricle. Right ventricular output is directed into the pulmonary trunk, and a portion flows through the ductus arteriosus into the descending aorta. The remainder flows through the pulmonary arterial system.

The hemodynamics and volume of blood flow through the shunts and the volume of left ventricular flow depend upon three factors: (1) the status of the pulmonary vasculature—as it decreases, the volume of pulmonary blood flow and the left ventricular volume increase and cardiac failure can ensue; (2) the presence of subaortic stenosis, which increases the resistance to left ventricular output and augments the left-to-right shunt; and (3) the caliber of the ductus arteriosus—if it narrows, a pressure difference develops between the pulmonary artery and the descending aorta. In infants with a narrowed ductus, the pressure in the ascending aorta and the pulmonary artery remains equal because of the ventricular septal defect, but the pulmonary blood flow further increases because of the constriction of the ductus. Collateral arterial vessels develop between segments of the aorta proximal and distal to the interruption.

Because the descending aorta is isolated from the ascending aorta and is supplied through the ductus arteriosus, with desaturated blood, various patterns of differential cyanosis might be expected,[49] depending upon the location of the interruption and origin of the various brachiocephalic vessels. Differential cyanosis is rarely recognized, however, because the oxygen saturations of blood in the two aortic compartments are nearly equal, since the ventricular septal defect and associated left-to-right shunt raise the saturation of pulmonary arterial blood.

CLINICAL FEATURES.   Regardless of the type of associated cardiac anomaly or the site of aortic interruption,[50] the clinical and laboratory features are similar. In two thirds of the patients, symptoms develop within the first week of life, and in almost all, congestive cardiac failure develops by 1 month of age. The clinical picture is one of respiratory distress, tachypnea, mild cyanosis, cardiac failure, and early death. The presentation is not distinctive and resembles coarctation of the aorta but differs from other conditions, such as aortic atresia or complete transposition of the great vessels, which can cause cardiac symptoms within the first week of life.

Differential cyanosis is rarely described, but in infants who show this finding, complete transposition of the great vessels frequently coexists, leading to cyanosis of the head, trunk, and arms, and pink lower extremities.

In one third of our patients,[50] a blood pressure difference was found between the arms and legs, indicating a narrowed ductus. We have considered constriction of the ductus a major factor leading to death.

A soft to moderately loud nonspecific murmur is present in about two thirds of the patients and is usually located along the left sternal border. An apical diastolic murmur, due to increased pulmonary blood flow, is infrequently heard. The pulmonary component of the second heart sound is accentuated. Hepatomegaly related to cardiac failure is found.

ELECTROCARDIOGRAM.   The QRS axis is either normal or shows right axis deviation. Right atrial enlargement and right ventricular hypertrophy are present, as expected, since the right ventricle is developing systemic levels of pressure. Left ventricular hypertrophy coexists in older patients and is related to increased pulmonary blood flow and consequent left ventricular dilatation. It might also develop secondary to subaortic stenosis.

THORACIC ROENTGENOGRAM.   There is no distinctive cardiac silhouette. Generalized cardiomegaly is present and related to dilatation of each cardiac chamber. The pulmonary trunk is enlarged, and the pulmonary vasculature is increased.

ECHOCARDIOGRAM.   The echocardiogram does not, of course, indicate the interruption but shows nondiagnostic features of left ventricular dilatation and right ventricular hypertrophy.

CARDIAC CATHETERIZATION AND ANGIOCARDIOGRAM.   Cardiac catheterization data obtained from the right side of the heart show pulmonary hypertension and elevation of right ventricular systolic pressure to the same level as the left ventricular systolic pressure. Oximetry data reveal a left-to-right shunt at the ventricular level. The catheter passes easily and often repeatedly through the patent ductus arteriosus into the descending aorta. Blood is desaturated at this site.

Angiography reveals the diagnosis (Fig. 10-14). As in any patient with systemic levels of pressure in the right ventricle, a right ventriculogram should be performed. This study shows a reversing ductus arteriosus and opacification of the descending aorta. Remembering the anatomic variations of the brachiocephalic vessels, the right subclavian artery may arise from the descending aorta. The left subclavian artery may also arise from the descending aorta, and when it does, this finding is highly suggestive of interruption, since, in coarctation of the aorta, the left subclavian artery lies proximal to the obstruction.

As in any patient with a reversing ductus arteriosus, further studies must determine if (1) pulmonary venous pressure is elevated or (2) severe obstruction in the aortic arch exists. The former can be excluded by measurement of the pulmonary wedge pressure and careful review of the late films of the right ventriculogram to visualize the pulmonary veins, left atrium, and left ventricle. The second factor needs to be studied by aortography to visualize the brachiocephalic vessels and demonstrate the site of interruption of the aortic arch. Left ventriculography can be performed, but often it is not diagnostic, since following injection, the right ventricle, pulmonary artery, and descending aorta opacify through the ventricular septal defect, while the ascending aorta and arch fill from the left ventricle. Thus, it may be difficult to identify the discontinuity of the aorta.

Two additional findings we have observed only in patients with interruption of the aortic arch: (1) On the lateral views of the ascending aorta, the aorta passes superiorly and does not arch posteriorly. (2) On the anteroposterior views of the aorta, the right subclavian artery often appears to arise not from an innominate artery in the normal fashion but often from the carotid artery.

MANAGEMENT.   In our review, among 66 patients,[50] 41 deaths occurred in the first month of life, and 11 more occurred between 1 month and 1 year. Death usually results from congestive cardiac failure, but we have also had several infants with cardiogenic shock.

Because of the high mortality rate in infancy, medical management has little to offer for these infants. Following digitalization and other decongestive measures, diagnostic procedures should be performed and operation undertaken. The infusion of prostaglandin E. helps maintain patency of the ductus arteriosus and adequate perfusion of the descending aorta. It should be admin-

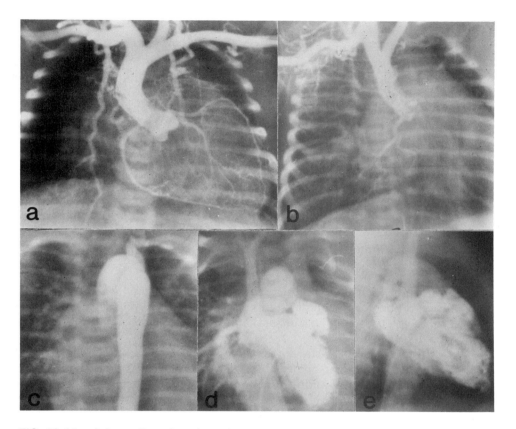

FIG. 10-14.   Interruption of aortic arch, angiographic studies. **a.** Aortogram, anteroposterior view, in 2-week-old infant. Interruption beyond left subclavian artery. **b.** Ascending aortogram and, **c,** descending aortogram in a 1-month-old infant with interruption occurring between left common carotid and left subclavian arteries. Only left subclavian artery opacifies from descending aorta. **d.** Anteroposterior and, **e,** lateral views of left atriogram. Ascending aorta gives rise only to common carotid arteries. On lateral view **(e)**, ascending aorta passes directly cephalad without an arch directed posteriorly as in normal aortic arch.

istered, if needed, during cardiac cathetherization and in preparation for operation.

Several operative procedures have been suggested for infants with interruption of the aortic arch, but in principle, they are designed to establish continuity of the aorta and relieve the excessive pulmonary blood flow. Currently, in neonates with interruption beyond the left carotid artery, we connect the ascending and descending portions of the aorta with a graft, divide the patent ductus arteriosus, and band the pulmonary artery. If the interruption is beyond the left subclavian, we would perform direct anastomosis of the ascending and descending portions of the aorta, divide the ductus, and band the pulmonary artery. Others have used the subclavian artery[51] or have combined the left subclavian and left carotid arteries[52] to connect the ascending and descending portions of the aorta.

Recently, attempts have been made to correct the three components of this condition simultaneously, using cardiopulmonary bypass. The operation includes establishing aortic continuity, dividing the ductus arteriosus, and repairing the intracardiac defect. Barratt-Boyes and co-workers[53] described one instance, and Gomes and McGoon[54] described another.

The operative mortality for this condition remains high, in part because the patients are critically ill at the time of operation.

VALVULAR AORTIC STENOSIS

Aortic stenosis causing symptoms in infancy almost always results from a valvular lesion. Supravalvular or subvalvular forms of aortic stenosis rarely lead to symptoms at this age. The infant with valvular aortic stenosis presents a picture of congestive cardiac failure, systolic murmur, left ventricular hypertrophy and strain, and cardiomegaly.

PATHOLOGY. Although in infancy, aortic stenosis may be associated with coarctation of the aorta, patent ductus arteriosus, and hypoplastic left ventricle, the form being presented in this section is associated with a normal or enlarged left ventricle.

In most patients, the aortic valve is unicuspid and unicommissural[55] (Fig. 10-15). Among 11 personally observed patients, it was unicommissural in 9, bicuspid in the tenth, and a membrane with stellate central orifice in the eleventh. The valvular leaflets are thickened and often severely deformed.

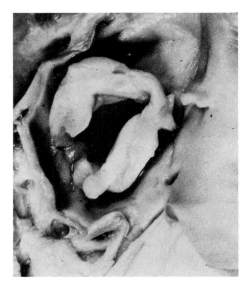

FIG. 10-15. Valvular aortic stenosis, with unicommissural valve, superior aspect.

Histologically, the valvular tissue may show large clear cells similar to myxomatous tissue rather than a regular arrangement of fibrous tissue.

The left ventricle is dilated and hypertrophied, and the heart weighs two to three times the norm. In almost all patients, the left ventricular endocardium is apparent as a distinct, grayish white layer of endocardial fibroelastosis.[27] Histologically, the endocardium is thickened many times the norm by a proliferation of fibrous and elastic tissue, and the subjacent myocardium may show evidence of recent or healed myocardial fibrosis. The fibrosis can also involve the papillary muscles, so that they appear thin and atrophic.[56] These changes are considered secondary to myocardial hypoxia from inadequate perfusion of the subendocardial regions secondary to the severe myocardial hypertrophy.[57] The free edge of the anterior leaflet of the mitral valve is thickened and nodular.

CLINICAL FEATURES.   Although in our experience, aortic stenosis in infants occurred more commonly in females, the reports of Keane[58] and Lakier[59] show a male predominance of approximately 2:1. The infant usually appears normal at birth but may have a murmur on the initial neonatal examination. If infants develop symptoms, they occur by 2 months of age and at times in the neonatal period.[59] The major presenting symptoms of respiratory distress, dyspnea, and tachycardia are related to congestive cardiac failure. Signs of decreased cardiac output, such as pallor, may be observed.

Cardiac examination usually shows a grade 2–4/6 murmur, but in infants with severe cardiac failure, the murmur may be absent but appear following digitalization. In half of the infants, the murmur is heard best in the third and fourth left intercostal spaces, and in the other infants, it is heard best in the aortic area. Because of the location of the murmur, a diagnosis of ventricular septal defect may be made mistakenly. The murmur is rarely associated with a precordial thrill, but in about half of our patients, a suprasternal notch thrill was present. Likewise, only half of such infants have an aortic systolic ejection click.

Palpation of the thorax rarely reveals a left ventricular heave, but a right ventricular heave has been described, particularly in neonates with poor perfusion. A gallop thythm may be present.

ELECTROCARDIOGRAM.   The QRS axis is usually normal but, occasionally, may show mild left or right axis deviation.

Four precordial lead patterns have been described. The most frequent is a pattern of left ventricular hypertrophy and inverted T waves in the left precordial leads[55,58] (Fig. 10-16). Patterns of right ventricular hypertrophy have also been reported [58,59] but usually in infants with a hypoplastic left ventricle or in neonates. Biventricular hypertrophy has rarely been reported.[55]

We were able to find two reports of infants who showed a pattern of anterolateral myocardial infarction resembling anomalous left coronary artery.[55,60] Right or left atrial enlargement may be present.

Arrhythmias and conduction abnormalities are rare.

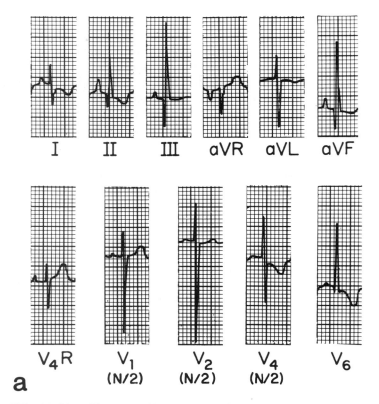

FIG. 10-16. Electrocardiograms of valvular aortic stenosis. **a.** One-day-old infant. QRS axis is +90°, right atrial enlargement, and left ventricular hypertrophy. Inverted T waves in left precordial leads (*Cont.*).

THORACIC ROENTGENOGRAM. In symptomatic infants, cardiomegaly is regularly present and usually massive. The cardiac silhouette has a left ventricular contour (Fig. 10-17). Variable degrees of left atrial enlargement are present. The ascending aorta does not appear dilated, perhaps because it is hidden by the thymus.

The pulmonary vasculature may be normal or show a fine reticular pattern of pulmonary venous obstruction.

ECHOCARDIOGRAM. In aortic stenosis, several echocardiographic features (Fig. 10-18) suggest the diagnosis: (1) the aortic valve closure is eccentric within the aortic root, (2) the aortic valve shows multiple diastolic echos, and (3) the interventricular septum and left ventricular posterior wall are thickened. Although in children with aortic stenosis a number of studies have investigated the relationship between various echocardiographic measurements and data obtained from cardiac catheterization, such correlations have not been made in infants.

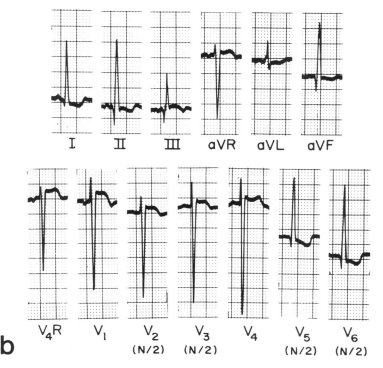

I   II   III   aVR   aVL   aVF

V₄R   V₁   V₂   V₃   V₄   V₅   V₆
(N/2)   (N/2)   (N/2)   (N/2)

b

FIG. 10-6 (*Cont.*)   **b.** Six-month-old infant. QRS axis is +45°, left ventricular hypertrophy. ST segment and T wave changes of strain. N/2, half-standardization.

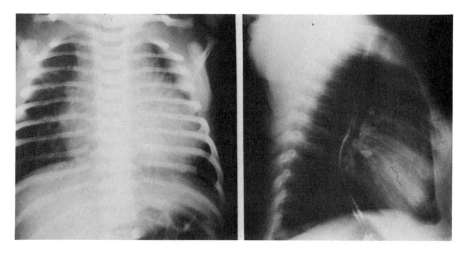

FIG. 10-17.   Thoracic roentgenogram of valvular aortic stenosis. **a.** Posteroanterior projection. **b.** Lateral projection. Marked cardiomegaly. Left atrial enlargement.

CARDIAC CATHETERIZATION AND ANGIOCARDIOGRAM.   Diagnosis rests upon measurement of left ventricular systolic pressure and performance of a left ventriculogram. The left ventricle is usually catheterized through the foramen ovale or, on occasion, in retrograde direction across the aortic valve.

The major finding is a systolic gradient across the aortic valve. This may reach 130 mm Hg, with left ventricular peak systolic pressure being as high as 220 mm Hg. Left ventricular end-diastolic pressure is elevated, and in the experience in neonates reported by Lakier,[59] it ranged from 15 mm Hg to 37 mm Hg, and from 12 mm Hg to 28 mm Hg in the experience of Keane et al.[58] Variable degrees of pulmonary hypertension are present and result, in part, from the elevated left ventricular end-diastolic pressure.

The cardiac output is either normal or slightly reduced.

In the neonatal period, a left-to-right shunt may be found at the atrial level, presumably through a stretched patent foramen ovale, and may be as large as a QP:QS>3:1.

Left ventricular angiography can outline the details of the stenotic valve and show the left ventricular size (Fig. 10-19). Following injection of contrast medium into the left ventricle, variable degrees of mitral insufficiency [55] can be observed and are believed to be related to the previously described changes in the left ventricular papillary muscles.

The ascending aorta shows poststenotic dilatation, and the aortic valve domes.

MANAGEMENT.   The initial efforts should be made to promptly treat the congestive cardiac failure. Cardiogenic shock and metabolic acidosis may coexist and require immediate therapy. Following stabilization, cardiac catheterization should be performed. In our experience, infants with aortic stenosis do not tolerate procedures well, so catheterization should be performed expeditiously.

Aortic valvular stenosis in infancy, associated with congestive cardiac failure, should be treated by aortic valvotomy. Any infant who develops failure should have surgery, regardless of response to digitalization. In our experience, no infant managed medically alone has survived.

The operative risk is high.[55,58,59,61,62] The operative approach in most centers uses cardiopulmonary bypass and incision of the valve or, occasionally, excision of a valve cusp. Among survivors of the operation, recovery is slow, perhaps because of the alterations of the myocardium reflecting hypoxia.

The largest group of survivors has been described by Keane and co-workers.[58] They followed 18 patients from 6 months to 11 years, and only 4 were asymptomatic postoperatively. Residual abnormalities were present in most patients (aortic regurgitation in 8, left ventricular hypertrophy in 14). Six of their patients have been reoperated because of peak systolic gradients across the aortic valve, ranging from 60 mm Hg to 140 mm Hg. In 5, the valve could be incised, but in the sixth, the valve was replaced because of severe aortic regurgitation. Therefore, the valvotomy can be considered a palliative procedure, since most patients will require another operation subsequently.

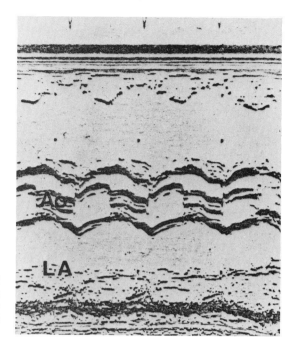

FIG. 10-18. Echocardiogram of valvular aortic stenosis. Aortic valve shows multiple diastolic echoes. Eccentric diastolic closure. Ao, aorta; LA, left atrium.

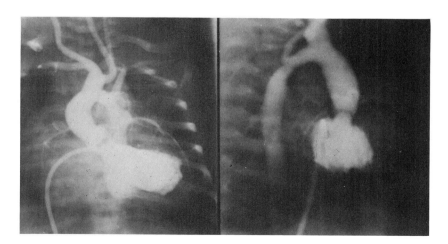

FIG. 10-19. Left ventriculogram, AP (left) and lateral (right) views of valvular aortic stenosis. Left ventricular hypertrophy. Aortic valve domes. Poststenotic dilatation ascending aorta.

SYSTEMIC HYPERTENSION

Renal Arterial Stenosis

Renal arterial stenosis appears in the first year of life as systemic hypertension. The hypertension may be of such severity as to lead to cardiomegaly and congestive cardiac failure.

Renal arterial stenosis with systemic hypertension must be considered in the differential diagnosis of cardiomyopathy. This condition indicates the importance of obtaining blood pressures in infants with cardiorespiratory or genitourinary symptoms.

PATHOLOGY AND ETIOLOGY. Renal arterial stenosis can occur as an isolated condition or as part of a generalized disease process involving systemic arteries. Several syndromes have been associated with renal arterial stenosis.

In the congenital rubella syndrome, renal arterial stenosis has been described,[63-65] and one of these patients had systemic hypertension. In the rubella syndrome, intimal fibromuscular proliferation narrows the renal arterial lumen, generally external to the kidney.

Renal arterial stenosis has been reported in infants with the syndrome associated with idiopathic hypercalcemia and supravalvular aortic stenosis.[66] Marked hyperplasia of the renal arterial media occurs.

Renal arterial stenosis also occurs in instances of abdominal coarctation of the aorta. This condition, more frequent in females than in males, involves the abdominal aorta, usually about the origin of the renal arteries. The aorta, over some distance, is narrowed by a proliferation of the intima. This narrowing encroaches upon the renal arteries. Usually the aorta is not narrowed sufficiently to cause a blood pressure difference between the arms and legs. We have seen one infant with cardiac failure and hypertension secondary to Turner's syndrome and renal arterial stenosis.

The renal arteries may be narrowed in patients with no evidence of abnormalities of other arteries or organs. The renal arteries may show diffuse hypoplasia of congenital origin,[67] or there may be various combinations of thickening of the adventia, destruction of elastic fibers in the media, or gross thickening of the intima.[68]

Unilateral or bilateral involvement occurs equally. Unilateral involvement can lead to severe hypertension in the neonatal period,[69] presumably through a Goldblatt mechanism.

The heart in autopsied cases shows left ventricular hypertrophy and increased cardiac weight, often twice normal.[70]

CLINICAL FEATURES. There is no typical clinical picture of renal arterial stenosis and hypertension, but symptoms may include failure to thrive, vomiting, polydipsia, polyuria, and dyspnea.[71,72] The presenting signs and symptoms are often those of cardiac disease and congestive cardiac failure. Because of such clinical presentation, our initial diagnostic impression was endocardial fibroelastosis in three personally observed cases, and this has also been described by Makker.[72]

There may be features of rubella or hypercalcemia syndromes. Renal arterial stenosis occurs more commonly in males, although coarctation of the abdominal aorta occurs more frequently in females.

Blood pressure values to 250/130 mm Hg may be present. Rahill and co-workers[73] reported a mean value of 200/115 mm Hg in 13 infants, indicating the severe degree of blood pressure elevation present in the condition. The blood pressure may be normal when the infant is in cardiac failure, but following digitalization, blood pressure may rise to hypertensive levels as the cardiac output increases.

Systolic murmurs as loud as grade 3/6 have been described[67] and were found in our patients. A third heart sound may be present, and hepatomegaly is found.

ELECTROCARDIOGRAM.   The electrocardiogram characteristically shows left ventricular hypertrophy. This may be associated with ST segment and T wave changes in the left precordial leads (Fig. 10-20) and is indistinguishable from that of aortic stenosis or endocardial fibroelastosis. Occasionally, the precordial leads are normal.

THORACIC ROENTGENOGRAM.   Thoracic roentgenograms show either mild or marked cardiomegaly, predominantly of the left ventricle, yielding a prominent left heart contour. The lungs may show a pattern of pulmonary venous obstruction.

DIAGNOSIS.   The diagnosis rests upon the recognition of elevated blood pressure in a child who has cardiorespiratory or urinary tract symptoms. As indicated, the hypertension may be first recognized only after digitalization.

Urinalysis and urine culture are usually normal in infants with renal arterial stenosis. BUN, electrolyte determination, and intravenous pyelography should be performed. If the pyelogram shows no major structural abnormality of the kidney, the renal arteries should be visualized.[71] Aortography (Fig. 10-21) adequately visualizes the details of the renal arteries, especially in instances of abdominal coarctation.[74] In some infants, selective renal arteriograms, perhaps involving oblique views, may be necessary to visualize the renal arteries better, but they are difficult to perform in patients of this age and have a higher complication rate.

MANAGEMENT.   Digoxin should be administered as the initial step in treatment of infants with renal arterial stenosis and cardiac failure. Diuretics benefit the cardiac failure and the hypertension, the latter through increasing sodium excretion. Efforts also should be made to lower blood pressure. The following agents have been useful to us in managing these patients, both during infancy and over a period of follow-up: alpha-methyldopa, spironolactone, and hydrochlorothiazide.

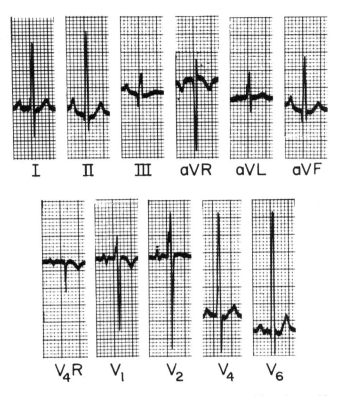

FIG. 10-20. Electrocardiogram of 1-year-old patient with systemic hypertension secondary to renal arterial stenosis. Left ventricular hypertrophy.

If renal arterial stenosis is present, the optimum treatment is repair of the renal arterial stenosis, but the anatomic details or the complications of thrombosis of the repaired artery frequently limit the usefulness of this technique, commonly used in adults.[71] Renal autotransplantation offers a solution for these patients.[75]

DIFFERENTIAL DIAGNOSIS. As indicated, renal arterial stenosis and hypertension may mimic cardiomyopathy, but the condition is easily distinguished by obtaining a blood pressure recording. Once hypertension is recognized, the origin must be sought, since, frequently, a treatable cause may be present. Ordinary parenchymal abnormalities or structural abnormalities[76] are other causes of hypertension in infancy. The reports by Cook et al.[77] and Snyder et al.[78] describe instances of hypertension related to renal arterial thrombosis that may complicate another serious condition in neonates.

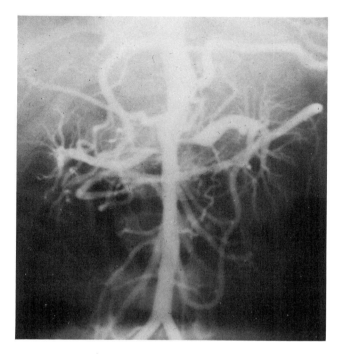

FIG. 10-21.   Abdominal aortogram shows marked stenosis at origin of both renal arteries.

DISEASES AFFECTING THE MYOCARDIUM

Several cardiac conditions affect primarily the myocardium in such a way that myocardial function is depressed. Such conditions are unassociated with (1) left-to-right shunt, (2) primary valvular abnormalities, (3) hypertension, or (4) bacterial infections.

Although some of the diseases affecting the myocardium have been clearly identified and described so that a clinical diagnosis can be made, in many cases a precise description of the disease is lacking, and the pathogenesis is unknown. Slowly, information is being obtained about diseases that involve the myocardium, but much is yet to be learned. As a result, the term "cardiomyopathy" has been applied to a variety of cardiac conditions involving the myocardium because they cannot be described more exactly.

This uncertainty applies to infants also, as in the example of the conditions, endocardial fibroelastosis and myocarditis. In most patients, the etiology of each condition is unknown, the clinical features may be similar, and the pathologic features overlap.

Although many cardiomyopathies have been described, we will consider only the most prevalent and those with discrete clinical pictures. The conditions to be discussed include:

1. Endocardial fibroelastosis
2. Myocarditis
3. Anomalous origin of the left coronary artery
4. Other causes of myocardial infarction
5. Glycogen storage disease of the heart
6. Other storage diseases
7. Rhabdomyoma

ENDOCARDIAL FIBROELASTOSIS

Endocardial fibroelastosis describes a pathologic state in which the endocardium is thickened by a proliferation of fibrous and elastic tissue. It has been considered to exist in two forms: primary—in which there is no other recognized cardiac anomaly, and secondary—in which the endocardium is believed to be thickened in response to some other abnormality of the heart. The following conditions in infants have been associated with endocardial fibroelastosis: severe aortic stenosis,[79,80] severe coarctation of the aorta,[81,82] hypoplastic left ventricle,[83,84] anomalous origin of the left coronary artery,[85,86] and certain myocardial storage diseases.[87,88] In patients with these cardiac anomalies, the coexistent endocardial fibroelastosis is believed to result from the anomaly and not cause it. The endocardial fibroelastosis does not alter the clinical picture of the underlying anomaly; it may lead to inverted T waves in the left precordial leads.

PATHOLOGY. Although any cardiac chamber may show diffuse endocardial thickening by fibrous and elastic tissue, the changes most frequently involve the left ventricle and left atrium (Fig. 10-22). The endocardium has a creamy white color and often appears as a distinct layer, being many times thicker than the normal one-two cell layers. Composed of collagenous fibrous and elastic tissue (Fig. 10-23), the thickened endocardium may extend into the myocardial sinusoids. The underlying myocardium appears normal, although it may show chronic inflammatory reaction.[89] There is no gross or histologic difference between the primary and secondary forms.[27]

In patients showing endocardial fibroelastosis, the size of the left ventricle varies and has been grouped as dilated, contracted, or hypoplastic.[90] Most of the primary and secondary cases are associated with a dilated left ventricle. The overall heart size and weight is increased two- to fourfold, and this is accounted for primarily by the enlarged left atrium and ventricle. The left ventricle is dilated but has a normal wall thickness. The contracted type of endocardial fibroelastosis, in which the left ventricle is smaller than normal, accounts for less than 5 percent of all the cases.[91] The hypoplastic left ventricle

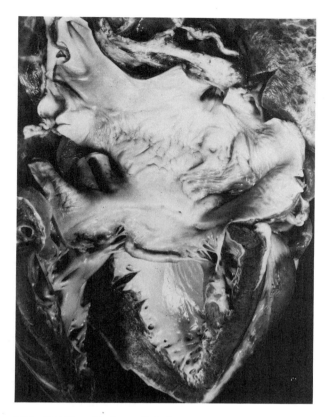

FIG. 10-22. Endocardial fibroelastosis of left side of heart. Left atrium above, left ventricle below. Endocardium white, thickened, appears as distinct layer. Anterior mitral valve leaflet thickened.

with endocardial fibroelastosis is associated with a unicuspid stenotic aortic valve, and tubular hypoplasia will be discussed in Chapter 13.

The mitral valve is abnormal in patients with the dilated form of endocardial fibroelastosis, whether primary or secondary.[27] The papillary muscles, instead of originating from the junction of the lower and middle thirds of the left ventricular wall, originate higher on the left ventricular wall. This change may be caused by dilatation of the left ventricle. From the apex of the papillary muscles, shortened chordae tendineae pass to the leaflets of the mitral valve. The orientation of the papillary muscle chordal mechanism, with respect to the long axis of the ventricle, is horizontal. This orientation tethers the mitral valve and leads to mitral regurgitation.

Anatomic evidence, such as thickened anterior leaflet of the mitral valve, left atrial enlargement, and on occasion, jet lesions in the left atrium,[27] sup-

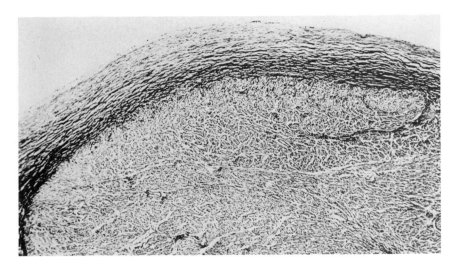

FIG. 10-23.   Endocardial fibroelastosis. Histologic appearance showing thickened endocardium.

ports the presence of mitral insufficiency in patients with endocardial fibroelastosis. There may be anatomic changes of pulmonary venous obstruction as well.

In this section, the clinical features of primary endocardial fibroelastosis will be presented. The secondary forms will be discussed in relation to associated cardiac malformation. Those patients with secondary endocardial fibroelastosis usually have severe cardiac symptoms, including congestive cardiac failure in infancy. The role of endocardial fibroelastosis in altering the clinical picture is unknown.

ETIOLOGY.   The etiology of endocardial fibroelastosis remains unknown. Although many theories of pathogenesis have been presented, none satisfactorily explains all instances of its presence.[92] Some consider the endocardial proliferation a response to left ventricular dilatation.[27,93] The dilatation may result from severe obstructive lesions, such as aortic stenosis, from myocardial damage, as in anomalous origin of the left coronary artery, or from other conditions that affect the left ventricle. The presence of endocardial fibroelastosis in Hurler's and Sandhoff's syndromes, both involving the left ventricle and its presence in patients who have recovered from myocarditis, supports the view that the endocardial change may be secondary to alteration of the left ventricle. The left ventricle, perhaps, has a limited way of responding to stress. There remain, however, cases with no known cause for left ventricular disease.

In many cases of endocardial fibroelastosis, the cause of the proliferation is unclear. The role of intrauterine mumps viral infection in the pathogenesis of endocardial fibroelastosis is controversial.[94-96] Although a high incidence of positive mumps skin tests has been reported by some authors, the lack of serologic evidence of mumps infections cast doubt on the mumps virus being an etiologic agent. Kline,[97] by ligating cardiac lymphatics in experimental animals, produced a condition similar to endocardial fibroelastosis, but this pathogenesis remains unclear.

CLINICAL FEATURES. The clinical features of endocardial fibroelastosis, consisting of congestive cardiac failure, cardiomegaly, and absence of a loud murmur, resemble those of myocarditis. The onset of endocardial fibroelastosis is during the first year of life, usually by 6 months of age.[27,89,98] One of our patients showed congestive cardiac failure at birth. Often, infants appear normal for a period of time, and then the symptoms of congestive cardiac failure develop. Although symptoms may occur acutely, in our experience, they more commonly develop gradually and are accompanied by a history of frequent respiratory infections, including pneumonia. Prominent symptoms include a history of difficulty in feeding, respiratory difficulties, easy fatigability, and failure to gain weight.

PHYSICAL EXAMINATION. The children are small and may appear malnourished. Evidence of low cardiac output, such as pallor and weak pulses, is present and is marked in acutely ill infants. Prominent features are those of congestive cardiac failure, particularly hepatomegaly, dyspnea, and tachypnea. Although peripheral edema is uncommon in infants with cardiac failure, we have treated two children with endocardial fibroelastosis who showed massive peripheral edema, one of whom was admitted with a provisional diagnosis of nephrosis.

Rales from cardiac failure or pneumonia may be auscultated. Cardiomegaly is evident on physical examination as a left precordial bulge and can be present even at 3 months of age. The cardiac apex is displaced into the fifth or sixth left intercostal space in the anterior or even midaxillary line. The first and second heart sounds are usually normal, although in three of our older patients with significant pulmonary hypertension, the pulmonary component of the second heart sound was accentuated. An apical third heart sound is nearly always present and becomes louder in patients with congestive cardiac failure. Most of our patients have shown an apical systolic murmur. Although these have usually been soft, we believe they originate from mitral insufficiency.[27] Diastolic murmurs are rare.

ELECTROCARDIOGRAM. The typical electrocardiogram shows a pattern of left ventricular hypertrophy and strain. The QRS axis is normal, and the QRS voltage is almost never reduced in magnitude, as in cases of myocarditis. The precordial leads usually show a deep S wave in lead V_1 and a tall R wave in lead V_6 (Figure 10-24). The latter may be accompanied by a deep Q wave. We have observed single instances of Wolff-Parkinson-White syndrome and of a QRS pattern of anterolateral myocardial infarction. Other authors have described these

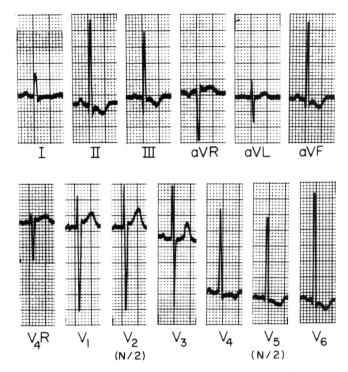

FIG. 10-24. Electrocardiogram of endocardial fibroelastosis in 8-month-old infant. QRS axis is +75°, left ventricular hypertrophy. Inverted T waves in left precordial leads. N/2, half-standardization.

patterns in this condition.[98,99] Almost all patients show flattening or inversion of T wave in leads V_5 and V_6. P waves may show left, right, or biatrial enlargement. After treatment with digitalis preparation, prolongation of the PR interval and depression of the ST segments are common.

Nearly 20 percent of our patients have shown rhythm or conduction disturbances.[27] Atrial fibrillation or flutter has developed in long-standing cases. Complete heart block was observed in three patients. In one, the heart block was a presenting sign, while in two others, it developed over the period of observation. In the latter, histologic examinations of the conduction system revealed interruption of the His bundle by the endocardial fibroelastosis.[100]

THORACIC ROENTGENOGRAM. The cardiac silhouette is massively enlarged, and the cardiac apex extends to the left thoracic border (Fig. 10-25). The enlargement, due principally to left ventricular dilatation, is best seen on a left anterior oblique view. Left atrial enlargement is uniformly present and recognized by posterior displacement of the barium-filled esophagus. Left atrial enlarge-

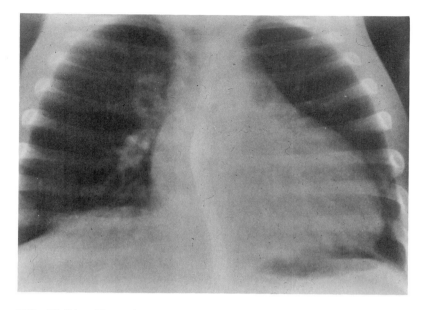

FIG. 10-25. Thoracic roentgenogram, posteroanterior view, of endocardial fibroelastosis. Cardiomegaly. Left ventricular contour. Pulmonary venous obstruction.

ment is frequently great enough to elevate the left main stem bronchus. Elevation and compression of the bronchus can lead to left lower lobe atelectasis,[101] a finding that may be associated with any cardiomyopathy in infancy.

The pulmonary vasculature may be normal or show a fine reticular pattern if congestive cardiac failure is present.

ECHOCARDIOGRAM. The echocardiogram shows normal septal and left ventricular posterior wall thickness, but the left ventricle and left atrium are dilated (Fig. 10-26). Left ventricular diameter changes little between systole and diastole. The mitral valve leaflets are displaced posteriorly in the left ventricle but separate from the left ventricular posterior wall. The preejection period is prolonged, and ejection time is shortened.

CARDIAC CATHETERIZATION AND ANGIOCARDIOGRAM. Cardiac catheterization and angiography reflect the hemodynamics of endocardial fibroelastosis. The cardiac output and stroke volume are usually normal.[27,102] Left ventricular end-diastolic pressure may be as high as 25 mm Hg. As a consequence, left atrial and pulmonary wedge pressures are elevated. In infants, pulmonary arterial pressures are rarely elevated above levels of 40/20 mm Hg,[27,102] although we have seen levels of 140/75 mm Hg in older children with this condition. Angiography demonstrates a dilated left ventricular cavity.[103] In the report by

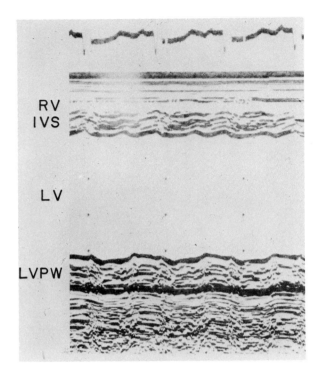

FIG. 10-26. Echocardiogram of endocardial fibroelastosis. Greatly dilated left ventricle (LV), markedly decreased contractility. LVPW, left ventricular posterior wall; IVS, interventricular septum; RV, right ventricle.

McLoughlin and co-workers,[102] 16 of their 22 patients showed the left ventricular cavity size more than 2 standard deviations above normal. Little change in the left ventricular volume occurs between systole and diastole. The left ventricular wall may be thicker than normal, but this is not striking, particularly in comparison to the left ventricular volume.

In our experience, the left ventricular cavity has a round contour (Fig. 10-27). Many patients show mitral regurgitation, which may be of significant degree. Although the left atrium and pulmonary veins are enlarged, the right-sided cardiac chambers are usually normal.

MANAGEMENT. Digitalis is the cornerstone of treatment of patients with endocardial fibroelastosis.[104] Patients often respond promptly to digitalization and, when maintained on this medication, remain clinically well for considerable periods of time. Controversy exists concerning duration of digitalis therapy. We believe it should be continued as long as there is cardiomegaly or electrocardiographic abnormalities.

During the acute episode, diuretics and the limitation of sodium intake are useful adjuncts to management.

COURSE AND PROGNOSIS. It is difficult to state the prognosis of endocardial fibroelastosis exactly, since the clinical picture may be mimicked by myocarditis or, perhaps, other myocardial diseases that improve spontaneously. Previously,

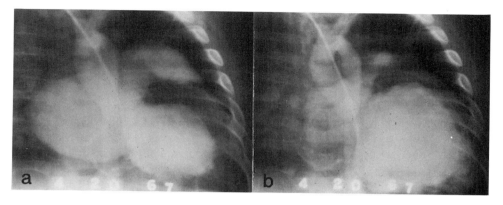

FIG. 10-27. Left ventriculogram. **a.** Systolic view. **b.** Diastolic view. Endocardial fibroelastosis of 3-month-old female. Left ventricle dilated. During systole, dense opacification of enlarged left atrium and left atrial appendage, indicating mitral insufficiency.

the diagnosis of endocardial fibroelastosis carried a poor prognosis, and the condition was nearly always fatal in the first year of life. Partially, this was related to the inclusion of all patients with thickened endocardium, many of whom had primary cardiac conditions, such as aortic stenosis, coarctation of the aorta, or anomalous left coronary artery. By excluding such cases from consideration and studying only cases of primary endocardial fibroelastosis, the prognosis is considerably better, and many patients survive beyond 1 year of age. Manning and associates[104] report the improved outlook for these patients when treated vigorously early in their course, particularly before massive cardiomegaly is present and when using adequate amounts of digitalis.

Despite vigorous treatment, some patients fail to respond and die in infancy with congestive cardiac failure. With improved survival beyond infancy, the ultimate outcome remains unknown. We have observed three children with endocardial fibroelastosis treated since infancy. They showed clinical improvement, but during adolescence, developed progressive congestive cardiac failure and died.

In some older patients, mitral insufficiency may play a major role in the signs and symptoms. In two of our patients, at ages 10 and 12, respectively, a valve replacement and annuloplasty were performed, and, in each, considerable improvement resulted.

MYOCARDITIS

Myocarditis presents a clinical picture of cardiac enlargement, congestive failure—often acute and severe, no clinical evidence of cardiac valvular abnormalities, and absence of electrocardiographic evidence of ventricular hypertrophy.

Myocarditis often occurs as part of a generalized systemic disease, although the heart may appear to be the major organ involved. Many etiologic agents can cause myocarditis, but most cases in the first year of life are believed to be of infectious origin. Of infectious agents, viruses have been most frequently identified as etiologic agents, but rickettsia, bacteria, and protozoa (toxoplasmosis) may also infect the myocardium. In the last 2 decades, much information has been obtained about the relationship between viruses and myocarditis, and specific viruses have been identified. Still, in many infants with myocarditis, an etiologic agent is never identified.

In infants, Coxsackie B[105-108] and rubella virus[109] are the viruses most frequently identified as involving the heart. Coxsackie B myocarditis specifically occurs in the neonatal period, may be either sporadic or epidemic, and has a high mortality. Rubella, recognized as causing structural anomalies of the heart, can also cause myocarditis.

Aside from the neonatal period, the incidence of myocarditis is low during the remainder of the first year of life, although slightly higher after 6 months of age. Myocarditis bears a low mortality beyond the neonatal period. Inflammation of the heart occurs during the course of many viral infections, but the number of patients who present the clinical picture of myocarditis is probably small.

PATHOLOGY.   The cardiac chambers are enlarged but usually show no other abnormalities. Histologically, there is varying interstitial infiltration of inflammatory cells, lymphocytes, and mononuclear cells. A spectrum of myocardial changes occurs, ranging from swelling of myocardial cells to necrosis. With long-standing disease, fibrosis may be present. At autopsy, the heart may be the only organ involved, but there may be inflammation of other tissues, especially in those neonates with Coxsackie B infection. In these neonates, encephalitis and hepatitis may coexist.

CLINICAL FEATURES.   There are two clinical presentations of myocarditis in children under 1 year of age. In the neonatal period, infants become acutely and severely ill within the first 2 weeks of age. Frequently, there is a maternal history of respiratory infection. The infants have fever, lethargy, hepatomegaly, cardiac failure, cyanosis, shock, and respiratory distress. Central nervous system symptoms may be prominent. In older infants, particularly over 6 months of age, the clinical picture is more variable.[110] The onset consists of a prodromal illness of several days duration, in which upper respiratory symptoms, cough, fever, and anorexia are prominent. Then, there may be the sudden onset of respiratory distress, tachycardia, and congestive cardiac failure or a more insidious illness of lethargy, ectopic rhythm, and low-grade fever.

PHYSICAL EXAMINATION.   In the neonate, lethargy, cardiovascular collapse, pallor, and subnormal temperatures are the major features. Cyanosis and, occasionally, jaundice are also present. Respirations are difficult and rapid.

Cardiac enlargement is present, although this may be difficult to recognize clinically in neonates. The heart sounds are diminished. A prominent gallop is frequent. A gallop without other auscultatory findings is very suggestive of myocarditis or myocardiopathy. Tachycardia is out of proportion to fever. Although in most patients, no murmur is heard, a soft systolic murmur may be present at the apex. The cardiac rhythm may be irregular. Hepatomegaly is invariably present.

The clinical picture in infants is usually not as severe as in neonates, although patients in this age group may also show profound cardiovascular collapse.

ELECTROCARDIOGRAM. Electrocardiographic changes are important in the diagnosis of myocarditis and in distinguishing this condition from other cardiomyopathies, particularly endocardial fibroelastosis.[111] The magnitudes of QRS voltages in both the standard and precordial leads are reduced (Fig. 10-28), although, occasionally, they may be normal. Patterns of left ventricular hypertrophy or anterior myocardial infarction have been described infrequently. The Q wave in lead V_6 is small. In the left precordial leads, T waves are flat or slightly inverted. The ST segment depression may coexist. The PR interval may be prolonged. Occasionally, AV nodal conduction is delayed, so that more advanced degrees of heart block develop. Premature ventricular contractions are common.

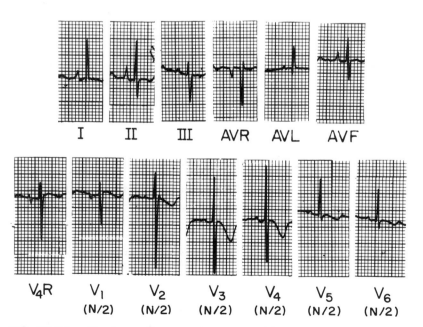

FIG. 10-28.   Electrocardiogram of neonate with myocarditis. Pattern of left ventricular hypertrophy and inverted T waves in left precordium. N/2, half-standardization. (Courtesy of Dr. Richard Schienken)

THORACIC ROENTGENOGRAM. Typically, the cardiac silhouette is enlarged and indistinguishable from other forms of myocardial disease. All cardiac chambers may be enlarged, principally the left ventricle. Occasionally, the heart size may be near normal in patients who die suddenly early in the course of the illness.

Pulmonary congestion, manifested by a diffuse reticular pattern and haziness of the hila, is observed. Kerley's B lines are uncommon except in patients with a chronic course.

ECHOCARDIOGRAM. Echocardiograms show features similar to those of endocardial fibroelastosis.

MANAGEMENT. Myocarditis should be treated vigorously with digoxin, diuretics, and oxygen. Acutely ill infants should be digitalized by the intravenous route and, depending upon the response to the initial dose, may require the total digitalizing dose in less than 24 hours.[112] The response of the congestive cardiac failure is variable, but some infants show remarkable improvement. Careful monitoring of the electrocardiogram should be carried out.

COURSE AND PROGNOSIS. In neonates, the prognosis is poor, with 50 to 75 percent of the patients dying, frequently within 48 to 72 hours. The prognosis is better in the older infant. Many show remarkable improvement within hours after initiation of treatment, while others require prolonged treatment with digitalis and diuretics.[89] In patients showing clinical improvement, pulmonary congestion disappears promptly, although cardiomegaly and electrocardiographic changes take perhaps a year to return to normal. We believe digitalis should be continued until heart size is normal on thoracic roentgenogram. In some patients, cardiomegaly persists, and the prognosis of these patients is guarded. These patients may redevelop signs of cardiac failure and ultimately die, the heart showing diffuse fibrosis.

ANOMALOUS ORIGIN OF LEFT CORONARY ARTERY FROM PULMONARY TRUNK

Anomalous left coronary artery presents a picture of cardiac enlargement, sudden episodes of crying, and an electrocardiographic pattern of myocardial infarction.

PATHOLOGY. In this condition, the left coronary artery arises from the pulmonary trunk, while the right coronary artery arises, as usual, from the aortic root. The wall of the left coronary artery is thin and veinlike. The left ventricle is greatly dilated, and although the heart weight may be twice normal,[113] the wall is usually not hypertrophied. In fact, the apex or lateral wall of the left ventricle may be thin because of myocardial infarction. In all personally observed patients, the left ventricle and often the left atrium were thickened by endocardial fibroelastosis.[114]

The left ventricular papillary muscles also show myocardial infarction. They are thinned and scarred. Frequently, the chordae tendineae of the mitral valve are short, and the free edge of the mitral valve is thickened.[114] The left atrium may be enlarged. Histologically, necrosis and fibrosis are present in the left ventricle. Other cardiac or visceral anomalies are extremely rare.

Three developmental stages in the coronary blood flow have been described.[113,115] The first stage is the state during fetal life and in the immediate neonatal period. Because of the high pulmonary arterial pressure and pulmonary vasculature, blood flows into the left coronary artery from the pulmonary trunk. With the postnatal fall in pulmonary resistance, perfusion of the left coronary arterial system from the pulmonary trunk diminishes and depends, to a progressively greater extent, on collateral blood flow from the right coronary arterial system. In the second stage, ischemia of the left ventricular myocardium occurs because of inadequate perfusion through the small collaterals. In the third stage, larger collaterals have developed between the right and left coronary arteries, and the magnitude of shunt increases from the right to the left coronary artery through the collaterals. Blood flow increases in a retrograde direction to the pulmonary trunk. Myocardial ischemia can also occur at this stage because the collaterals and left coronary artery act as an arteriovenous fistula and carry blood away from the left ventricular myocardium.

In 1888, Hilary St. John Brooks,[116] in studying a specimen of an anomalously arising coronary artery, speculated that blood flow was in a retrograde direction through that coronary artery. Subsequently, this pathway of blood flow was confirmed both by the observation at the time of operation of fully saturated blood in the left coronary artery and by angiography.

CLINICAL FEATURES.   Most patients with anomalous left coronary artery are symptomatic in infancy. They are normal at birth and, typically, develop symptoms after 1 month of age, although Rowe and Mehrizi[117] stress that careful questioning often reveals symptoms prior to that age.

Many infants have symptoms interpreted as angina.[118,119] They have episodes of distress crying, as in pain, pallor, and sweating. These often occur in relation to feeding. The episode lasts several minutes, following which the infant appears happy. The nurses' observations of hospitalized patients often record such episodes.

PHYSICAL EXAMINATION.   Generally, the infants show normal growth, in contrast to infants with endocardial fibroelastosis where growth is retarded. Infants may appear healthy, except when they have an episode in which they may appear pale, sweaty, and have anxious facies.

The clinical evidence of cardiomegaly is manifested by displacement of the cardiac apex inferiorly and laterally as far as the midaxillary line.

Although anomalous left coronary artery has been considered a condition without a significant cardiac murmur, several of our patients have had grade 1–3/6 apical systolic murmurs.[114,119,120] These murmurs present on initial examination, persist in childhood, and we believe are from mitral regurgitation secondary to infarction of left ventricular papillary muscles. The second heart sound may be prominent, and a third heart sound may be present.

Additional findings on physical examination, which are related to congestive cardiac failure, include rales, weak arterial pulses, and hepatomegaly.

ELECTROCARDIOGRAM.   The electrocardiogram in anomalous origin of the left coronary artery is usually diagnostic of this condition, since it almost always shows a pattern of anterolateral myocardial infarction and features of left ventricular hypertrophy[114,121] (Fig. 10-29). In lead aVL and often in lead I, a qR pattern is present, with the Q wave being large in comparison to the height of the R wave. A qR pattern is usually present in leads V_5 and V_6 also. T waves are almost always inverted in each of these four leads.

Left ventricular hypertrophy usually coexists and is manifested by deep S waves in lead V_1 and tall R waves in lead V_6. One of our patients showed a pattern of complete left bundle-branch block. There may also be failure of QRS progression across the precordial leads.

The electrocardiogram usually serves to distinguish anomalous left coronary artery from endocardial fibroelastosis. In cases where the diagnosis is un-

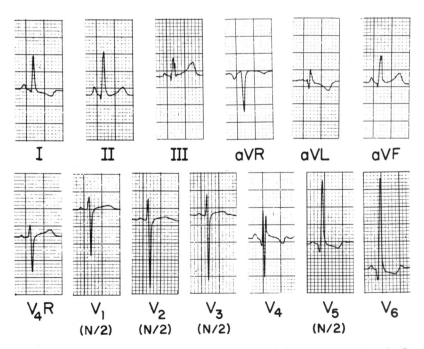

FIG. 10-29.   Electrocardiogram of anomalous left coronary artery in 3-month-old infant. QRS axis is +60°. Deep, broad q waves in leads V_5 and V_6. Abnormal T waves. Bizarre q Rsr′ in lead V_4. Pattern of anterolated myocardial infarction. N/2 = half standardization.

certain, a vectorcardiographic tracing will be helpful. In our experience, the vectorcardiogram has always shown a pattern of anterolateral myocardial infarction.[114]

In the horizontal plane, the initial QRS forces are normal, but the 0.02 to 0.05 sec vectors are abnormal, so that most of the QRS loop is inscribed in a clockwise rotation rather than in a counterclockwise direction. We have not observed this in patients with endocardial fibroelastosis or other cardiomyopathies.

THORACIC ROENTGENOGRAM.   The thoracic roentgenogram shows gross cardiomegaly, principally of the left ventricle (Fig. 10-30). The cardiac apex is directed downward and leftward, and left atrial enlargement may be present. The pulmonary vasculature is usually normal but may show pulmonary congestion if the patient is in congestive cardiac failure.

ECHOCARDIOGRAM.   The echocardiogram resembles endocardial fibroelastosis.

CARDIAC CATHETERIZATION AND ANGIOCARDIOGRAM.   Cardiac catheterization data may be normal in patients with anomalous left coronary artery. The pulmonary arterial wedge, pulmonary arterial, and left ventricular end-diastolic pressures may be moderately elevated but are usually normal.[122] Cardiac output is normal. Using sensitive indicators, such as hydrogen, the shunt into the pulmonary artery can be detected, although it is usually not detected by oximetry.

The diagnosis is established by selective injection of contrast material into the ascending aorta.[114] (Fig. 10-31). Only the right coronary artery opacifies

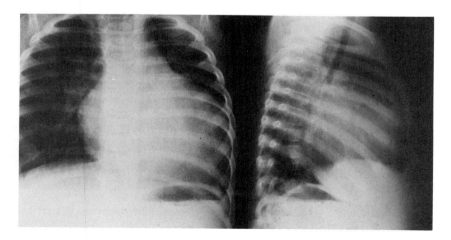

FIG. 10-30.   Thoracic roentgenograms of anomalous left coronary artery (same patient as in Fig. 10-29). Anterior view (right) and lateral view (left). Marked cardiomegaly. Left ventricular contour.

from the aorta, and it is enlarged. Collateral vessels, particularly about the apex, opacify. The left coronary artery then fills, and the opaque material then passes into the pulmonary trunk. The transit time from the aorta to the pulmonary trunk is rapid (about 0.5 sec). We misinterpreted the angiograms in one of our patients, for there was a slight delay in our filming sequence, so that the first film showed opacification of both coronary arteries, and we had missed the rapid transit through the right coronary and collaterals to the left coronary artery. Others report no false negative or false positive studies.[122]

Left ventricular angiocardiogram shows dilatation and diminished contractility of the left ventricle. Mitral regurgitation may be present.

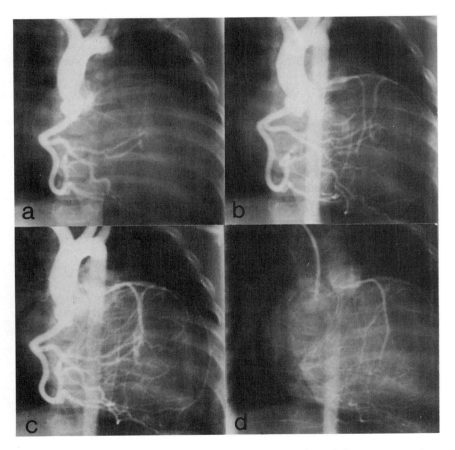

FIG. 10-31. Aortogram, serial AP views, of anomalous left coronary artery. Same patient as in Figures 10-29 and 10-30. **a.** Injection of contrast material into aortic root. Opacification only of right coronary artery, which is enlarged. **b.** Visualization of left coronary arterial system. **c.** Numerous collateral arteries seen between two coronary arterial systems. **d.** Late film. Predominant opacification of left coronary artery. Opacification of pulmonary trunk.

MANAGEMENT.   Infants with congestive cardiac failure should be treated with digitalis and diuretics. The infants should be managed according to the principles of the coronary care unit, including careful monitoring and prompt treatment of complications.

COURSE AND PROGNOSIS.   The prognosis for infants with anomalous left coronary artery is guarded, for many patients die in infancy,[113] often during an episode of irritability. Some, however, may live well into childhood after early onset of chest pain and cardiac failure. In fact, our experience and that of others[119,122,123] suggest a more favorable outcome. In two of our patients, the chest pain disappeared with age. Sudden death from ischemia and persistent cardiomegaly are two important complications.

Debate exists concerning the role of surgery in patients with anomalous left coronary artery. Formerly, ligation of the left coronary artery was recommended for all patients with a left-to-right shunt through the coronary arterial system. This procedure eliminates the arteriovenous fistula of the anomalous left coronary artery and improves perfusion of the left ventricular myocardium. This procedure does not create a physiologic single coronary artery, since the left coronary arterial system must still be perfused through collateral vessels. In a review by Wesselhoeft and associates,[113] of 20 infants treated by ligation of the anomalous left coronary artery, 10 survived, and in the survivors, the symptoms improved. Congestive cardiac failure disappeared, and heart size became smaller. Usually, the electrocardiogram or vectorcardiogram persists in showing myocardial infarction. Four of our survivors of this operation improved symptomatically and radiographically. Exercise treadmill in two showed significant ST segment depression on mild to moderate exercise; it was normal in the other two.

Because of observations[119,122,123] that patients with moderate left-to-right shunts have a relatively good prognosis, recommendations have been made that the patients be followed, and when older, cardiac bypass surgery be done. These authors suggest that if the infant's condition deteriorates, surgery should be undertaken sooner.

OTHER CAUSES OF MYOCARDIAL INFARCTION

There are several causes of myocardial infarction in neonates and infants.

CORONARY THROMBOSIS OR EMBOLISM.   Several reports[124-127] have described anatomic findings of myocardial infarction and thrombosis or embolism in neonates with normal coronary arteries. Electrocardiograms may show evidence of myocardial infarction.

The etiology of these acquired coronary arterial lesions is unknown, but frequently they occurred in infants with deliveries complicated by prolapsed or nuchal cord, evidence of fetal distress, or breech delivery. In some, paradoxical embolism to the coronary artery was considered. Death may be sudden or follow a brief illness.

CALCIFICATION OF THE CORONARY ARTERIES.   Calcification of the coronary arteries has been described by Baggenstoss and Keith,[128] Stryker,[129] Beuren et al.,[130] and Cochrane and Bowden.[131] The arterial lesions show calcification of the media and fibrous thickening of the intima. The etiology of this is unknown. No abnormality of calcium metabolism has been found. Calcification can occur in other arteries and in the glomeruli.

Death may occur in the neonatal period or late in the first year of life. The onset of symptoms was often sudden, and the duration of illness was short, with cardiovascular collapse and congestive cardiac failure.

THROMBOCYTOSIS.   Sanyal and co-workers[132] described two infants—one 6 days old and one 6 weeks old—with thrombocytosis, central nervous system signs, and electrocardiographic evidence of apical myocardial infarction. One patient showed isoenzymatic evidence of myocardial necrosis, while in the other patient, isoenzyme levels were normal, suggesting that the electrocardiographic abnormalities might be related to central nervous system disease. The origin of the thrombocytosis is unknown, but similar findings have been described in an older patient.[133] Neither of the infants died, so anatomic information is not available.

MUCOCUTANEOUS LYMPH NODE SYNDROME (KAWASAKI DISEASE).   In the 1960s, Kawasaki identified a number of children who had striking features that appeared to represent a new disease that was appearing in epidemic proportions in Japan.[134] He named it "mucocutaneous lymph node syndrome" after the predominant clinical features. It is of interest to cardiologists because in 2 percent of patients, severe cardiac complications occur that can be fatal months after the acute illness. Subsequently, the disease has been reported widely in the United States and other portions of the world. This condition is probably the same as that described by Munro-Faure,[135] discussing necrotizing arteritis of the coronary arteries in infants.

Pathology.   The pathologic findings cannot be distinguished from infantile periarteritis nodosa.[136] Arteritis is present primarily in nonparenchymal vessels of many organs, particularly the heart, kidneys, spleen, and lungs. Inflammatory and necrotic lesions are seen initially, and, subsequently, there may be obliterative changes or the development of aneurysms, which can thrombose.

The coronary arteries at any level may be involved and associated with myocardial inflammation or infarction.

Typically, the vessels show periarterial inflammation, medial necrosis, and destruction and intimal proliferation.

Clinical Features.   Kawasaki disease occurs in childhood. In the United States, it occurs from 3 months to 13 years of age, with a mean age of 3.8 years,[137] while in Japan, the median age was 1 year. The male to female ratio is 1.5:1.

Kawasaki disease is an acute febrile illness with characteristic conjunctival erythema, erythema of oral mucosa, anterior cervical adenopathy, and erythema, induration, rash, and desquamation of the extremities. Thrombocytosis (to 2,000,000/mm^3), elevated leukocyte count, and elevated erythrocyte sedimentation rate are present.

Diagnostic criteria, based upon the studies of Kawasaki,[134] have been established to diagnose this condition. Following the exclusion of other diseases, such as juvenile rheumatoid arthritis, Stevens-Johnson syndrome, or childhood diseases, such as scarlatina, rubella, or measles, five of the following six criteria should be met:

1. Fever—at least 5 days, may last to 3 weeks, is high and spiking (present in 95 percent of patients)
2. Bilateral conjunctival injection—individual bulbar conjunctival vessels engorged and prominent (90 percent)
3. Changes in oral-pharyngeal mucous membranes (90 percent)
    Redness and fissuring of lips
    Strawberry tongue
    Redness of oropharynx
4. Change in peripheral extremities (90 to 95 percent)
    Induration and swelling of hands and feet
    Erythematous or magenta-colored palms and soles
    Subsequent desquamation, particularly fingertips
5. Truncal polymorphic erythematous rash (90 percent)
6. Cervical lymphadenopathy (75 percent)

Other findings may include diarrhea, vomiting, arthritis or arthralgia, urethritis, and aseptic meningitis.

Laboratory abnormalities include leukocytosis with shift to the left, slight anemia, thrombocytosis in second or third week, mild pyuria and proteinuria, and elevated acute phase reactants (ESR, CRP, and alpha$_2$-globulin).

Cardiac manifestations may be apparent throughout the course of the illness. During the acute phase, tachycardia is observed, but this would be expected because of the fever. More importantly, the heart sounds appear distant, and cardiac enlargement is found on thoracic roentgenograms (one third of cases). During the acute phase, there may be a gallop. Cardiac dysrhythmia, reduction in QRS voltage, and ST and T wave changes may occur. Cardiac murmurs of mitral insufficiency may develop during the course of the disease. The findings of myocarditis and pericarditis are present.

Deaths can occur from the coronary arterial anomalies, approximately three fourths of these within the first 2 months of the acute illness.

Coronary arteriography should be performed and may show aneurysms (Fig. 10-32), which may be present even with normal electrocardiographic and cardiac findings.[138] Coronary aneurysms may regress following the acute illness.[138] Recently, a real-time cross-sectional echocardiographic study[139] demonstrated the aneurysms.

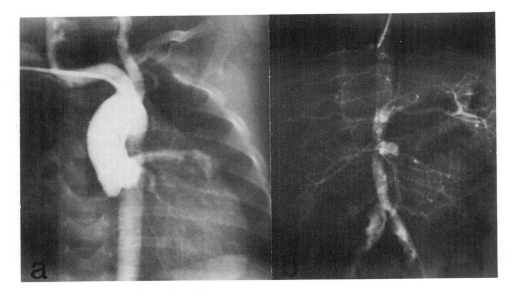

FIG. 10-32. Mucocutaneous lymph node syndrome in 10-month-old infant. **a.** Ascending aortogram, dilatation of left coronary artery. **b.** Abdominal aortogram, aneurysm of renal artery and thrombosis in right iliac artery.

Proper therapy remains to be defined. While corticosteroids have been used and result in prompt disappearance of the acute aspects of sepsis, symptoms, and acute phase reactants, the study by Kato and associates[138] indicates that 65 percent of patients treated with corticosteroids had angiographic evidence of coronary aneurysms, compared to 11 percent of patients treated with aspirin alone.

Their recommendation is to perform an angiogram following the acute illness.[138] If the coronary arteries are normal, aspirin is discontinued; if abnormal, aspirin is continued, and coronary angiography is repeated in 1 to 2 years to confirm regression, identify obstruction, and assess left ventricular function. If the arteries are still abnormal, aspirin probably should be continued.

GLYCOGEN STORAGE DISEASE OF THE HEART

Of the several types of glycogen storage disease, type II (Pompe's disease) has the most striking cardiac findings. Minor cardiac abnormalities have been described in other types.[140] Glycogen storage disease type II is characterized by congestive cardiac failure, muscular hypotonia, and greatly increased QRS voltages on the electrocardiogram.

In type II glycogen storage disease, a lysosomal enzyme, acid maltase (alpha 1,4-glucosidase), is deficient.[141] As a result of this enzymatic deficiency, glycogen accumulates in the lysomes of various organs, particularly the heart, liver, skeletal muscle, and central nervous system.[142] The glycogen content of these organs is many times normal—for example, the glycogen content of skeletal muscles and heart may reach 10 percent, whereas normal values are 0.01 and 0.10 percent, respectively.[142-144] This deposition of glycogen alters organ function and increases organ size.

Inherited as an autosomal recessive trait, Pompe's disease can be diagnosed biochemically by demonstrating the enzymatic deficiency in leukocytes.[145]

Studies of carbohydrate metabolism are normal.

PATHOLOGY.   The heart is greatly enlarged and weighs at least twice as much as normal. The ventricular walls and interventricular septum are thickened, and the left ventricular wall may approach 20 mm in thickness (Fig. 10-33). The atria are usually normal.

The interventricular septum bulges into the right ventricular cavity. The endocardial surface is usually lined by endocardial fibroelastosis. Other structural anomalies are usually absent.

The microscopic findings are striking. The myocardium shows extensive vacuolization of myocardial fibers which, in formalin-fixed tissues, gives a lacework pattern.[146] The vacuoles contain glycogen, which appear on Best carmine stain of nonformalin-fixed tissue. The glycogen in myocardial cells displaces myofibrils to the periphery. Electron microscopic studies show the glycogen in membrane-lined sacs.[147,148] Skeletal muscle, including that of the tongue, also shows histologic evidence of glycogen deposition.

Subaortic and subpulmonary pressure differences have been described in this condition, presumably from the thickened interventricular septum. Myocardial function is altered from the glycogen deposition and leads to congestive cardiac failure.

CLINICAL FEATURES.   Because the disease is rare, the experience of any center with glycogen storage disease type II is limited. The reported cases have been reviewed by Ehlers[144] and the clinical features summarized. In five personally observed patients, symptoms developed in the first month of life. The predominant symptoms of difficulty in feeding and respiratory difficulties are related to skeletal muscle weakness. The symptoms progress as the infant develops congestive cardiac failure.

PHYSICAL EXAMINATION.   Physical examination shows striking muscular hypotonia but usually a normal muscle mass. The infant's cry is weak. The growth is delayed. The facies have been described as doll-like, and macroglossia is present. Cardiac enlargement is found, and although cardiac murmurs have been described, they are not specific. Hepatomegaly accompanies congestive cardiac failure and is accentuated by glycogen deposition.

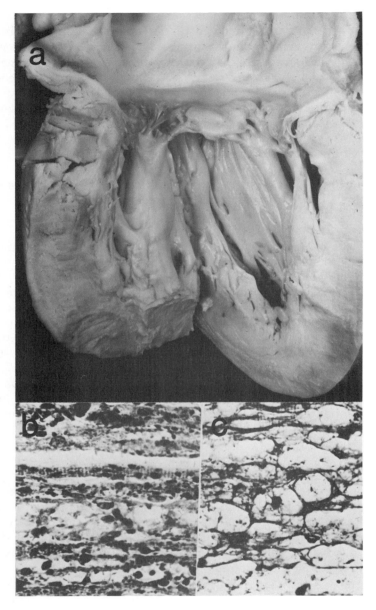

FIG. 10-33.   Glycogen storage disease type II. **a.** Left side of heart. Left ventricle below and left atrium above. Left ventricular myocardium greatly thickened. Anterior leaflet of mitral valve thickened. **b** and **c.** Histologic appearance. Extensive vacuolization displacing myocardial fibers.

ELECTROCARDIOGRAM.   The electrocardiogram is characteristic—shortened PR interval and greatly enlarged QRS voltages.[143] Ehlers[144] found a short PR interval (0.05 to 0.09 sec) in 80 percent of cases reviewed. There is no explanation for this finding, although it has been found in other storage diseases. The striking feature is greatly accentuated QRS voltages (Fig. 10-34). In one of our patients, the QRS voltage reached 25 mv, presumably because of increased ventricular wall thickness. The electrocardiogram, even the standard leads, may have to be recorded at 0.5 or even 0.2 standardization. The QRS axis is usually normal. The voltages are usually larger in the left precordial leads and may be accompanied by inverted T waves.

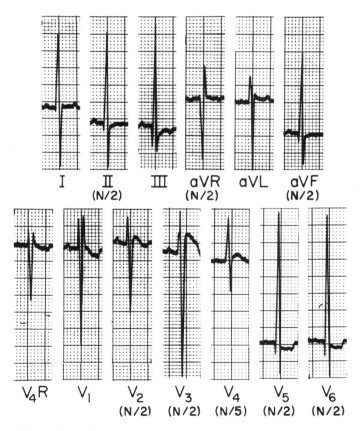

FIG. 10-34.   Electrocardiogram of glycogen storage disease type II in a 7-month-old infant. Large QRS voltages. Several leads recorded at half-standardization (N/2) and lead V₄ at one-fifth standardization (N/5). Left ventricular hypertrophy. T wave inverted in left precordial leads.

THORACIC ROENTGENOGRAM.   The thoracic roentgenogram shows massive cardiomegaly related to left ventricular and left atrial enlargement and is indistinguishable from endocardial fibroelastosis (Fig. 10-35).

ECHOCARDIOGRAM.   One instance of an echocardiogram in Pompe's disease has been described.[149] This showed greatly thickened interventricular septum and posterior left ventricular wall (Fig. 10-36). There was abnormal anterior movement of the mitral valve leaflets during systole, causing narrowing of the subaortic area.

CARDIAC CATHETERIZATION AND ANGIOCARDIOGRAM.   There are few hemodynamic data.[146] Cardiac output is at lower limits of normal. Left ventricular end-diastolic pressure is elevated and leads to elevation of pulmonary capillary pressure. Pulmonary arterial pressures are also mildly elevated (40/25 mm Hg in our patients).

Rees[149] described a 7-month-old infant with 69 mm Hg across the left ventricular outflow area and 20 mm Hg across the right ventricular area. Ehlers,[144] in studying a 10-month-old infant, found a left ventricular pressure of 255 mm Hg and a femoral arterial pressure of 97/41. Hohn[140] reported a 4-month-old infant with gradients of 43 mm Hg on the right and 73 mm Hg on the left, following Isuprel infusion. The angiograms show a dilated left ventricle which has a thickened wall (Fig. 10-37).

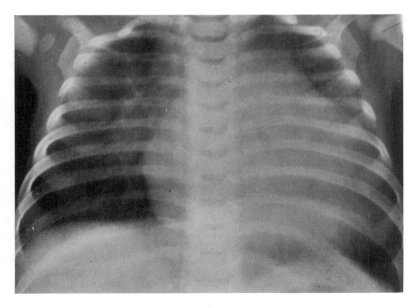

FIG. 10-35.   Thoracic roentgenogram of glycogen storage disease type II. Massive cardiomegaly.

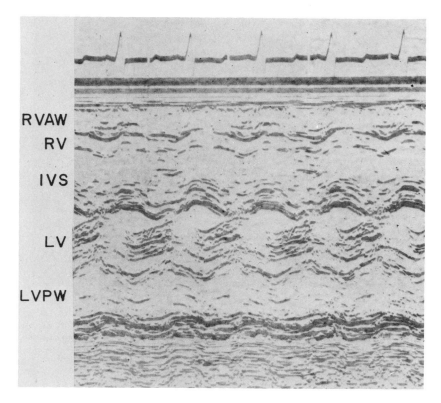

FIG. 10-36.   Echocardiogram of glycogen storage disease type II in a 4-month-old infant. Greatly thickened left ventricular posterior wall (LVPW), interventricular septum (IVS), and right ventricular anterior wall (RVAW). LV, left ventricle; RV, right ventricle.

MANAGEMENT. There is no specific treatment for the enzymatic deficiency. Management is based upon treatment of congestive cardiac failure with digitalis and diuretics. Care must be taken that aspiration not occur during feeding, and the child should be observed for respiratory infection.

COURSE AND PROGNOSIS. The onset of the disease is insidious, and the course progressive. Most patients die by 6 months of age, although a few survive until 1 year of age.

OTHER STORAGE DISEASES

Other than those with glycogen storage disease of the heart, few other patients with myocardial storage diseases have been reported in infancy.[88] There are, however, several inherited metabolic diseases in which the heart may be involved.

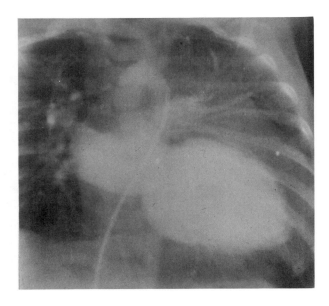

FIG. 10-37. Pulmonary arteriogram, levogram phase, of glycogen storage disease type II (same patient as in Fig. 10-34). Left atrium, left ventricle, and aorta opacified. Left ventricle dilated. Left ventricular wall greatly thickened.

In disorders of sphingolipid or mucolipid metabolism, lipids accumulate in the myocardium. Sandhoff's disease is a sphingolipidosis caused by deficiency of hexosaminidases A and B that causes cardiac symptoms in infancy.[150] In two personally observed infants, the clinical and laboratory features were those of endocardial fibroelastosis, except that both patients showed developmental retardation and cherry-red macula. At postmortem examination, the gross cardiac findings resembled endocardial fibroelastosis, but increased concentrations of sphingolipid were found in the myocardium.

Among the mucolipidoses, we have seen an infant with a mucolipidosis type III variant and another with gangliosidosis type II, each with cardiomegaly and murmur of mitral insufficiency. In these patients, facial characteristics resemble those in Hurler-Hunter syndromes.

With further identification and characterization of metabolic diseases, perhaps the etiology of more instances of cardiomyopathy will be understood.

RHABDOMYOMA

Rhabdomyoma, although the second most frequently occurring cardiac tumor, is the most common primary tumor of the heart occurring in infancy. Although it can present several clinical features, most frequently it mimics cardiomyopathy[151,152] and, therefore, is discussed in this chapter. It should also, however, be considered in the differential diagnosis of tricuspid or pulmonary valvular stenosis or atresia.[151,152]

PATHOLOGY. Rhabdomyomas usually occur as multiple discrete intramural tumors but may be a single localized mass (Fig. 10-38). The tumor nodules are firm and grayish white. Any layer of the heart may be involved, and although considered an intramural tumor, rhabdomyoma may project into cardiac cavities, causing obstruction to blood flow. This occurred in two of our cases and in cases reported by others.[152,153] Either ventricle and the interventricular septum may be involved.

The tumor has distinctive histologic features. The tumors show spider cells, i.e., enlarged cardiac myocardial cells with abundant cytoplasm and enlarged vacuoles. The material in the vacuoles is PAS positive and is glycogen. Because the tumor cells have a large glycogen content, rhabdomyomas have also been called "glycogen tumors of the heart."[154]

It is probable that most patients with rhabdomyomas have the tuberous sclerosis complex.[151] In most patients, characteristic lesions are found in the central nervous system. Splenic histiocytosis, renal cysts, and renal tumors may also be present.

CLINICAL FEATURES. The clinical presentation is variable[151,152,155] but includes the development of congestive cardiac failure in the first 2 days of life. Four of our five personally observed cases presented cardiac failure, one in utero, two on the first day of life, and the fourth at age 4 months. The latter patient was diagnosed as having cardiomyopathy. In neonates, a right-to-left shunt at the

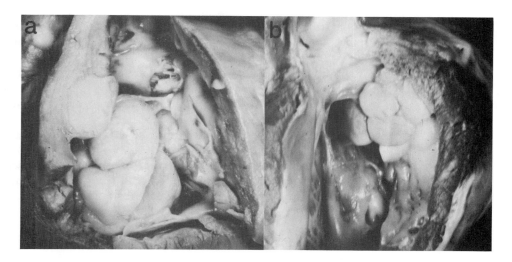

FIG. 10-38. Rhabdomyoma. **a.** Right ventricular cavity. Nodular tumor in tricuspid orifice. **b.** Left ventricular cavity. Nodular tumor encroaches on mitral valve.

atrial level, leading to cyanosis, may occur if the tumor obstructs the tricuspid valve or the right ventricle.[152]

Cardiac findings include tachypnea, tachycardia, cardiomegaly, and hepatomegaly. Usually no murmurs are present, although they may be heard in infants with intracavity tumors, leading to subaortic and subpulmonary stenosis.

Since most patients die early in life, developmental and mental retardation have been infrequently described. One of our patients has shown developmental retardation, believed to be a manifestation of tuberous sclerosis. Adenoma sebaceum are uncommon in neonates. Since as many as 85 percent of cases of tuberous sclerosis may represent new mutants, the family history is frequently negative.[157] A family history of tuberous sclerosis or findings suggesting this familial occurrence should be sought. Questions should relate to seizures, adenoma sebaceum, shagreen skin lesions, or renal cysts.

ELECTROCARDIOGRAM.   There were no characteristic findings among the electrocardiograms of our patients. One showed left ventricular hypertrophy and ST and T wave changes; a second, right atrial enlargement, prolonged PR interval, and intraventricular conduction defect; a third, Wolff-Parkinson-White syndrome; and a fourth, right ventricular hypertrophy or intraventricular conduction abnormality. This diversity of electrocardiographic findings is similar to the experience of others.[152] Cardiac arrhythmias, such as supraventricular or ventricular tachycardia or atrioventricular block, can occur.

THORACIC ROENTGENOGRAM.   Cardiomegaly is almost always present and may be massive. Irregularity of the cardiac contour has been described but must be an infrequent finding.

ECHOCARDIOGRAM.   The echocardiogram can identify intraluminal tumor masses[156] by demonstrating a mass of echoes originating within a cardiac chamber or valve orifice.

CARDIAC CATHETERIZATION AND ANGIOCARDIOGRAM.   Few catheterization data are available in infants with rhabdomyomas, and they show no consistent pattern. Of the four neonates we have studied, pulmonary arterial pressure was elevated in two and normal in the other two.

Angiography reliably demonstrates the tumor as either a distinct intracardiac filling defect or a thickened septum or ventricular wall (Fig. 10-39). The ventricular cavities may be narrowed as the tumor encroaches, and this may lead to subaortic or subpulmonary narrowing.[152] Small tumors may escape detection. One of our patients showed tricuspid valve obstruction and a right-to-left atrial shunt.

MANAGEMENT.   Management includes digitalis and diuretics, but the response to such treatment in our experience has been poor. Three of our patients showed no response. In the fourth, digoxin was discontinued at age 9 months without change occurring in the patient's condition. In the fifth patient, con-

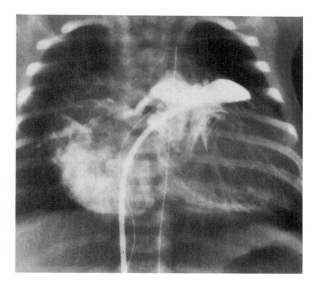

FIG. 10-39. Right ventriculogram, anteroposterior view of rhabdomyoma in a 2-day-old infant. Injection in outflow area of right ventricle with reflux into right atrium. Body of right ventricle not opacified because of large tumor involving septum.

gestive cardiac failure was present at birth, and the neonate died shortly later. Tumors obstructing blood flow should be resected, but if they are multiple, complete excision is impossible.

COURSE AND PROGNOSIS.   Most patients with rhabdomyomas die by 1 year of age, and few live beyond 5 years of age. The latter show developmental retardation.

DIAGNOSIS.   The diagnosis of rhabdomyoma depends upon angiocardiography. The diagnosis should be considered in infants with (1) unusual congestive cardiac failure, (2) unusual cardiac arrhythmias or conduction abnormalities, and (3) unusual cardiac findings with outflow tract murmurs.

PERICARDIAL DISEASE

The combination of normal pulmonary vasculature, enlarged cardiac silhouette, and absence of cyanosis can be caused by pericardial effusion. Although the typical cardiac contour of pericardial effusion on thoracic roentgenogram is a globular-shaped heart which lacks distinct anatomic outlines, the x-ray may be indistinguishable from cardiomyopathy. With the development of echocardiography, the ability to correctly diagnose and distinguish pericardial effusion from cardiomyopathy has increased considerably.

Pericarditis and pericardial effusion in the neonate are rare,[158,159] and, even in infancy, are uncommon conditions. Pericardial disease in this age group is almost always related to either purulent pericarditis or intrapericardial teratoma. Pericarditis may rarely occur in viral infections in infants, especially

Coxsackie B, but this virus usually causes severe or fatal myocarditis.[160,161]

One infant with endarteritis, myocardial infarction, and pericardial effusion has been described.[162]

Regardless of the etiology of pericardial effusion, cardiac tamponade can be a major hemodynamic consequence. The development of cardiac tamponade depends upon the volume of pericardial fluid, the rate of accumulation, the distensibility of the pericardium, and the presence of associated cardiac anomalies.

If fluid is accumulated slowly over a long period of time, there may be no cardiac embarrassment, despite the presence of a large effusion. On the other hand, the rapid accumulation of a small amount of fluid in a relatively nondistensible pericardial sac can cause tamponade.

Therefore, some infants with pericardial effusion may be asymptomatic. The incidence of pericardial disease in the first year of life is difficult to determine because almost all reported cases have had cardiac tamponade or major symptoms of the underlying condition.

Depending upon the factors described above, pericardial effusion can impair ventricular filling because of the limited volume of the pericardial sac and compression on the heart. As a result, ventricular filling pressure elevates and is clinically manifested by distended neck veins and hepatomegaly. Impaired ventricular filling reduces stroke volume, which is compensated for by increased heart rate. Systemic blood pressure is maintained by peripheral vasoconstriction, but the pulse pressure narrows.

One of the classic clinical features of pericardial tamponade is pulsus paradoxus, a term given by Kussmaul to the phenomenon of varying intensity of peripheral pulses in the presence of unchanged heart sounds and rhythm. Subsequently, the term has been applied to an accentuation of a normal phenomenon of diminution of arterial pulses during inspiration. The cause of the accentuated respiratory variation has been disputed, but new insight has been gained with the aid of echocardiographic studies.[163,164] During inspiration, two factors decreased left ventricular filling—one is the augmented systemic venous return, which increases right ventricular filling and causes a shift of the ventricular septum toward the left ventricle, and the other is the increased capacity of pulmonary veins. Consequently, left ventricular filling is decreased and so is systemic blood flow and pressure. As a result, a more marked reduction in blood pressure occurs on inspiration, than in a normal individual.

PURULENT PERICARDITIS

Purulent pericarditis, particularly in an infant, is a medical and surgical emergency because this disease is fatal in nearly 50 percent of infants and children.

Generally, a site of infection, such as pneumonia or osteomyelitis or altered immunologic status, is found. It is unclear whether the pericarditis develops by hematogenous origin or by direct spread in the presence of pneumonia.

Staphylococcus aureus is the principal organism involved in infants, but

Haemophilus influenzae B[165] and the meningococcus[166–168] have been described. Staphylococcal pericarditis has a high mortality rate.

Because of its rarity, pericarditis may be overlooked clinically and only found at postmortem examination. Usually, the finding of an enlarged cardiac silhouette during the diagnostic evaluation of an acutely ill infant should focus attention on the possibility of purulent pericarditis.

CLINICAL FEATURES. The presenting symptoms are usually fever and those of a respiratory infection.[166,167,169] There is tachypnea, difficulty in breathing, and cough. The infant appears acutely ill and febrile. We have been impressed by the anxious facies, fretful appearance, and grunting of these infants. Tachypnea and tachycardia are regularly present. Nadas and Levy[162] found that the pulse rate was between 150 and 165 beats per min in each of their patients. The presence of hepatomegaly helps round out the findings normally associated with congestive cardiac failure, but in this instance, they represent pericardial tamponade.

The diagnosis of pericarditis can be firmly made on the finding of a pericardial rub, but in infants, a rub is inconsistently found and may be present only after pericardiocentesis.[166,167,169] The physical findings of cardiac tamponade have been reported in one half of the infants. In addition to hepatomegaly, these include distended neck veins, which may be difficult to observe in the short plump neck of an infant, muffled heart tones, and pulsus paradoxus. The latter may also be difficult to detect in an infant who has a rapid respiratory rate. We have felt that a narrowed pulse pressure and weak peripheral arterial pulses are more reliable indices of pericardial effusion in the infant than is pulsus paradoxus.

There may be other physical findings related to infection at another site.

ELECTROCARDIOGRAM. In almost every infant, the electrocardiogram shows changes of acute pericarditis. Initially, ST segment elevation occurs and is typically found in the II, III, aVF, and left precordial leads[166,167,169] (Fig. 10-40). These may return to normal within days after[165] initiation of therapy. T waves may become inverted later and gradually return to an upright deflection. A few infants show significantly low QRS voltages, but in most infants, the voltages are reduced from their normal pattern but are still in normal range. Following treatment, the QRS voltages become larger.

THORACIC ROENTGENOGRAM. The cardiac silhouette is enlarged (Fig. 10-41a) and enlargement occurs rapidly. The shape is characteristically described as water bottle or globular but may not be dissimilar to that found in myocarditis.

ECHOCARDIOGRAM. The echocardiogram makes a major contribution to the diagnosis of pericarditis and pericardial effusion and often obviates the need for more invasive studies. The effusion is demonstrated by an echofree space behind the left ventricle and at times between the echoes of the chest wall and the right ventricle.[170]

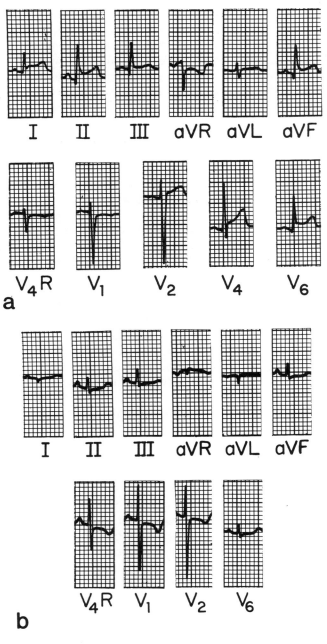

FIG. 10-40. Electrocardiograms of patients with pericardial disease. **a.** Purulent pericarditis due to *Haemophilus influenzae* in a 7-month-old infant. ST segment elevation leads I, II, III, V_4, and V_5. QRS voltages within normal limits. **b.** Pericardial effusion of unknown etiology. Reduced QRS voltages in standard leads and lead V_6.

CARDIAC CATHETERIZATION AND ANGIOCARDIOGRAM.   Cardiac catheterization is not necessary to diagnose pericardial effusion or cardiac tamponade. There are important clues at cardiac catheterization that should indicate to the physician the presence of pericardial effusion, namely, the fact that in manipulating the catheter in the right atrium, the catheter tip does not touch the lateral wall of the cardiac silhouette. If cardiac tamponade is present, atrial pressure is elevated, and the ventricular pressure shows an abrupt elevation in early diastole, followed by a plateau during the remaining portion of diastole and square root sign.[171]

Angiography has been used to diagnose pericardial effusion. Contrast material, such as Renografin, can be injected into a peripheral vein or vena caval catheter, and the distance between the opacified right atrium and the cardiac contour on the right heart border can be noted (Fig. 10-41b). This distance should not exceed 2 mm. CO_2 can also be injected into the vena cava with the patient in the left lateral projection. The CO_2 gravitates to the most superior aspect of the right atrium and delineates its wall. Another method employing the same principle is the injection of technetium and performance of scintillation scans of the heart. These methods have largely been supplemented by echocardiography.

MANAGEMENT.   The diagnosis is established by obtaining and analyzing the pericardial fluid. The removal of pericardial fluid has therapeutic effects as well. Subxiphoid pericardiocentesis or pericardial drainage through a small anterior thoracotomy are the two approaches. The technique used depends upon the preference of the individual physician and the experience of the institution.

Optimum treatment combines medical and surgical therapy. Once the or-

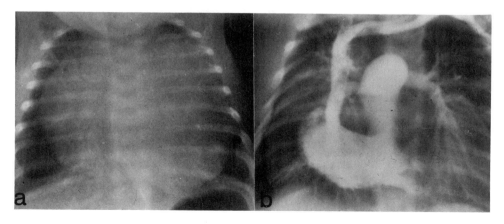

FIG. 10-41.   Pericardial effusion in 3-week-old infant. **a.** Thoracic roentgenogram, massive cardiomegaly. **b.** Venous angiogram, opacification of right side of heart. Large distance between wall of right atrium and right side of cardiac silhouette from a large pericardial effusion.

ganism has been identified and sensitivities have been determined, large doses of appropriate antibiotics should be given intravenously and continued for 2 to 4 weeks, depending upon the infant's response. It is difficult to clear any infection in a closed space, such as the pericardium. Drainage must also be obtained. Repeated pericardiocenteses are an inadequate means, since the thick, tenacious, purulent material plugs the small cannulae and tends to loculate and become inaccessible. Open and continuous surgical drainage must be established.

The mortality rate is higher in infants and children with purulent pericarditis treated with antibiotics alone, as compared to those patients in whom surgical drainage is also used.[166,167]

Constrictive pericarditis has been reported as a complication of purulent pericarditis by several authors.[166,172-174] Constriction can occur within weeks of the acute illness and develops more commonly in patients not treated by pericardial drainage.

SUMMARY.   The diagnosis of purulent pericarditis rests on a high index of suspicion in an acutely ill febrile infant with respiratory symptoms. Signs of congestive cardiac failure, i.e., tachypnea, tachycardia, and hepatomegaly, are found, but combined with muffled heart sounds, narrow pulse pressure, ST segment elevation, and enlarging heart size. Echocardiography can noninvasively establish the diagnosis of pericardial effusion, but diagnosis of its origin and decisions regarding its management must await analysis of the pericardial fluid.

INTRAPERICARDIAL TERATOMA

Intrapericardial teratoma is one of the two frequently occurring cardiac tumors of infancy, and of all reported cases of this tumor, nearly half have occurred in infants less than 3 months of age. It can even be present in the neonate. Two reviews of the literature have summarized the information about these uncommon tumors.[159,174]

The tumors may be large, up to three times the size of the heart. The shape varies, but usually it is pedunculated and attached to the adventitia of the aorta and/or pulmonary artery near their origin.[175,176] The tumor may lie over the right or the left side of the heart. Usually, the tumors are cystic, and the cysts contain mucoid material. The histologic appearance, as in any teratoma, can show a variety of tissue derivatives, which may appear immature. Almost all intrapericardial teratomas are benign.

A large volume of pericardial fluid is present in infants with this tumor, and the fluid is usually clear and pale yellow, but occasionally it has been described as serosanguineous following pericardiocentesis.

CLINICAL FEATURES.   The major clinical features are those of pericardial tamponade and are present in almost every patient with this tumor. The effusion can apparently develop rapidly and the infant can present with respiratory distress, cyanosis, and occasionally apnea. The electrocardiogram shows low voltage QRS complex but no ST segment deviation.[159]

Thoracic roentgenograms show an enlarged globular cardiac contour and normal pulmonary vasculature.

DIAGNOSIS. Diagnosis of pericardial effusion can be made by echocardiographic findings. Pericardiocentesis should be performed to determine the nature of the fluid. Perhaps after pericardiocentesis, an irregular outline of the tumor will be evident on thoracic roentgenogram. Pneumopericardium or angiography may be helpful in diagnosing the tumor, by either outlining the tumor or showing displacement of the heart.[159]

TREATMENT. Since Beck[177] performed the first operation to remove an intrapericardial tumor, successful operations have been reported. Care must be taken in removing the tumor from the great vessel. Approach should be made by shaving it off the vessel rather than by taking a cuff of tissue.

REFERENCES

Pulmonary Stenosis

1. Edwards JE: Congenital malformations in the heart and great vessels. In Gould SE (ed): Pathology of the Heart, 2nd ed. Springfield, Ill, Thomas, 1960, pp 391–397
2. Koretzky E, Moller JH, Korns ME, Schwartz CJ, Edwards JE: Congenital pulmonary stenosis resulting from dysplasia of valve. Circulation 40:43, 1969
3. Naeye RL: Perinatal changes in the pulmonary vascular bed with stenosis and atresia of the pulmonic valve. Am Heart J 61:586, 1961
4. Archie JP, Fixler DE, Ullyot DJ, Buckberg GD, Hoffman JIE: Regional myocardial blood flow in lambs with concentric right ventricular hypertrophy. Circ Res 34:143, 1974
5. Moller JH, Arosemena E, Edwards JE: Right ventricular myocardial fibrosis in pulmonary stenosis. Unpublished observations
6. Moller JH, Adams P Jr: The natural history of pulmonary valvular stenosis. Serial cardiac catheterizations in 21 children. Am J Cardiol 16:654, 1965
7. Danilowicz D, Hoffman JIE, Rudolph AM: Serial studies of pulmonary stenosis in infancy and childhood. Br Heart J 37:808, 1975
8. Luke MJ: Valvular pulmonic stenosis in infancy. J Pediatr 68:90, 1966
9. Rowe RD, Mehrizi A: The Neonate with Congenital Heart Disease. Philadelphia, Saunders, 1968, p 277
10. Paul MH, Rudolph AM: Pulmonary valve obstruction during cardiac catheterization. Circulation 18:53, 1958
11. Mustard WT, Jain SC, Trusler GA: Pulmonary stenosis in the first year of life. Br Heart J 30:255, 1968
12. Mistrot J, Neal W, Lyons G, et al.: Pulmonary valvulotomy under inflow stasis for isolated pulmonary stenosis. Ann Thorac Surg 21:30, 1976

Peripheral Pulmonary Arterial Stenosis

13. Rowe RD: Maternal rubella and pulmonary artery stenoses. Report of eleven cases. Pediatrics 32:180, 1963
14. Emmanouilides GC, Linde LM, Crittenden IH: Pulmonary artery stenosis associated with ductus arteriosus following maternal rubella. Circulation 29:514, 1964
15. Beuren AJ, Schulze C, Eberle P, Harmjanz D, Apitz J: The syndrome of supravalvular aortic stenosis, peripheral pulmonary stenosis, mental retardation and similar facial appearance. Am J Cardiol 13:471, 1964
16. Ottesen OE, Antia AU, Rowe RD: Peripheral vascular anomalies associated with the supravalvular aortic stenosis syndrome. Cardiology 86:430, 1966
17. Jones KL, Smith DW: The Williams elfin facies syndrome. A new perspective. J Pediatr 86:718, 1975
18. Danilowicz D, Rudolph AM, Hoffman JIE: Vascular resistance in the large pulmonary arteries in infancy. Circulation 31, 32[Suppl 2]:74, 1965
19. McCue CM, Robertson LW, Lester RG, Mauck HP Jr: Pulmonary artery coarctations. A report of 20 cases with review of 319 cases from the literature. J Pediatr 67:222, 1965
20. Gay BB Jr, Franch RH, Shuford WH, Rogers JV: The roentgenologic features of single and multiple coarctations of the pulmonary artery and branches. Am J Roentgenol Radium Ther Nucl Med 90:599, 1963
21. Rowe RD, Mehrizi A: The Neonate with Congenital Heart Disease. Philadelphia, Saunders, 1968, pp 318–324
22. D'Cruz IA, Agustsson MH, Bicoff JP, Weinberg M Jr, Arcilla RA: Stenotic lesions of the pulmonary arteries. Clinical and hemodynamic findings in 84 cases. Am J Cardiol 13:441, 1964
23. Agustsson MH, Arcilla RA, Gasul BM, et al.: The diagnosis of bilateral stenosis of the primary pulmonary artery branches based on characteristic pulmonary trunk pressure curves. A hemodynamic and angiocardiographic study. Circulation 26:421, 1962

Coarctation of the Aorta

24. Lev M: Autopsy Diagnosis of Congenitally Malformed Hearts. Springfield, Ill, Thomas, 1953, p 58
25. Rudolph AM, Heymann MA, Spitznas U: Hemodynamic considerations in the development of narrowing of the aorta. Am J Cardiol 30:514, 1972
26. Edwards JE: Congenital malformations of the heart and great vessels. In Gould SE (ed): Pathology of the Heart, 2nd ed. Springfield, Ill, Thomas, 1960, pp 450–451
27. Moller JH, Lucas RV Jr, Adams P Jr, et al.: Endocardial fibroelastosis. A clinical and anatomic study of 47 patients with emphasis on its relationship to mitral insufficiency. Circulation 30:759, 1964
28. Moss AJ, Emmanouilides GC, Adams FH, Chaung K: Response of ductus arteriosus and pulmonary and systemic arterial pressure to changes in oxygen environment in newborn infants. Pediatrics 33:937, 1964
29. Knight LC, Tadavarthy M, Moller JH: Angiographic study of collateral arterial circulation in 33 infants with coarctation of the aorta. Unpublished
30. Sinha SN, Kardatzke ML, Cole RB, et al.: Coarctation of the aorta in infancy. Circulation 40:385, 1969
31. Hartmann AF Jr, Goldring D, Staple TW: Coarctation of the aorta in infancy. Hemodynamic studies. J Pediatr 70:95, 1967

32. Rudolph AM: Congenital Diseases of the Heart. Chicago, Year Book, 1974, p 357
33. Heymann MA, Berman W Jr, Rudolph AM, Whitman V: Dilatation of the ductus arteriosus by prostaglandin E_1 in aortic arch abnormalities. Circulation 59:169, 1979
34. Ibarra-Perez C, Castaneda AR, Varco RL, Lillehei CW: Recoarctation of the aorta. Nineteen year clinical experience. Am J Cardiol 23:778, 1969
35. Khoury GH, Hawes CR: Recurrent coarctation of the aorta in infancy and childhood. J Pediatr 72:801, 1968
36. Hartmann AF Jr, Goldring D, Hernandez A, et al.: Recurrent coarctation of the aorta after successful repair in infancy. Am J Cardiol 25:405, 1970
37. Pelletier C, Davignon A, Ethier MF, Stanley P: Coarctation of the aorta in infancy. Postoperative follow-up. J Thorac Cardiovasc Surg 57:171, 1969
38. Nadas AS: Pediatric Cardiology. Philadelphia, Saunders, 1964, p 524
39. Naeye RL: Perinatal vascular changes in coarctation of the aorta with distal patent ductus arteriosus. Circulation 24:754, 1961
40. Shinebourne EA, Tam ASY, Elseed AM, et al.: Coarctation of the aorta in infancy and childhood. Br Heart J 38:375, 1976
41. Tawes RL Jr, Aberdeen E, Waterston DJ, Bonham-Carter RE: Coarctation of the aorta in infants and children. A review of 333 operative cases, including 179 infants. Circulation 39[Suppl 1]:173, 1969
42. Howard R, Moller J, Bessinger B, et al.: Coarctation of the aorta in infancy. Circulation 48[Suppl 4]:4, 1973 (Abstr)
43. Becker AE, Becker MJ, Edwards JE: Anomalies associated with coarctation of aorta. Particular reference to infancy. Circulation 41:1067,1970
44. Shone JD, Sellers RD, Anderson RC, et al.: The developmental complex of "parachute mitral valve," supravalvular ring of left atrium, subaortic stenosis, and coarctation of aorta. Am J Cardiol 11:714, 1963

Interruption of the Aortic Arch

45. Moller JH, Edwards JE: Interruption of the aortic arch. Anatomic patterns and associated cardiac malformations. Am J Roentgenol Radium Ther Nucl Med 95:557, 1965
46. Becu LM, Tauxe WN, DuShane JW, Edwards JE: A complex of congenital cardiac anomalies: Ventricular septal defect, biventricular origin of the pulmonary trunk, and subaortic stenosis. Am Heart J 50:901, 1955
47. Evans W: Congenital stenosis (coarctation), atresia, and interruption of the aortic arch. (Study of twenty-eight cases.) Q J Med 26:1, 1933
48. Pillsbury RC, Lower RR, Shumway NE: Atresia of the aortic arch. Circulation 30:749, 1964
49. Chesler E, Moller JH, Edwards JE: Anatomic basis for delivery of right ventricular blood into localized segments of the systemic arterial system. Am J Cardiol 21:72, 1968
50. Immagoulou A, Anderson RC, Moller JH: Interruption of the aortic arch: Clinical features in 20 patients. Chest 61:276, 1972
51. Tyson KRT, Harris LC, Nghiem QX: Repair of aortic arch interruption in the neonate. Surgery 67:1006, 1970
52. Sirak HD, Ressallat M, Hosier DM, de Lorimier AA: A new operation for repairing aortic arch atresia in infancy. Report of 3 cases. Circulation 37[Suppl 2]:43, 1968
53. Barratt-Boyes BG, Nicholls TT, Brandt PW, Neutze, JM: Aortic arch interruption associated with patent ductus arteriosus, ventricular septal defect, and total anomalous pulmonary venous connection. Total correction in an 8-day-old in-

fant by means of profound hypothermia and limited cardiopulmonary bypass. J Thorac Cardiovasc Surg 63:367, 1972

54. Gomes MMR, McGoon DC: Truncus arteriosus with interruption of the aortic arch: Report of a case successfully repaired. Mayo Clin Proc 46:40, 1971

Valvular Aortic Stenosis

55. Moller JH, Nakib A, Eliot RS, Edwards JE: Symptomatic congenital aortic stenosis in the first year of life. J Pediatr 69:728, 1966
56. Moller JH, Nakib A, Edwards JE: Infarction of papillary muscles and mitral insufficiency associated with congenital aortic stenosis. Circulation 34:87, 1966
57. Vincent WR, Buckberg GD, Hoffman JIE: Left ventricular subendocardial ischemia in severe valvar and supravalvar aortic stenosis. A common mechanism. Circulation 49:326, 1974
58. Keane JF, Bernhard WF, Nadas AS: Aortic stenosis surgery in infancy. Circulation 52:1138, 1975
59. Lakier JB, Lewis AB, Heymann MA, et al.: Isolated aortic stenosis in the neonate. Natural history and hemodynamic considerations. Circulation 50:801, 1974
60. Price AC, Lee DA, Kagan KE, Baker WP: Aortic dysplasia in infancy simulating anomalous origin of the left coronary artery. Circulation 48:434, 1973
61. Mody MR, Nadas AS, Bernhard WF: Aortic stenosis in infants. N Engl J Med 276:832, 1967
62. Coran AG, Bernhard WF: The surgical management of valvular aortic stenosis during infancy. J Thorac Cardiovasc Surg 58:401, 1969

Systemic Hypertension

63. Esterly JR, Oppenheimer EH: Vascular lesions in infants with congenital rubella. Circulation 36:544, 1967
64. Menser MA, Dorman DC, Reye RDK, Reid RR: Renal-artery stenosis in the rubella syndrome. Lancet 1:790, 1966
65. Menser MA, Dorman DC, Reye RDK, Reid RR: Renal-artery stenosis in rubella. Lancet 1:571, 1967
66. Antia AU, Wiltse HE, Rowe RD, et al.: Pathogenesis of the supravalvular aortic stenosis syndrome. J Pediatr 71:431, 1967
67. Angella JJ, Sommer LS, Poole C, Fogel BJ: Neonatal hypertension associated with renal artery hypoplasia. Pediatrics 41:524, 1968
68. Dawson IMP, Nabarro S: A case of intimal hyperplasia of arteries with hypertension in a male infant. J Pathol 66:493, 1953
69. Ljungqvist A, Wallgren G: Unilateral renal artery stenosis and fatal arterial hypertension in a newborn infant. Acta Paediatr Scand 51:575, 1962
70. Oppenheimer EH, Esterly JR: Cardiac lesions in hypertensive infants and children. Arch Pathol 84:318, 1967
71. Korobkin M, Perloff DL, Palubinskas AJ: Renal arteriography in the evaluation of unexplained hypertension in children and adolescents. J Pediatr 88:388, 1976
72. Makker SP, Lubahn JD: Clinical features of renovascular hypertension in infancy: Report of a 9-month-old infant. Pediatrics 56:108, 1975
73. Rahill WJ, Molteni A, Hawking KM, Koo JH, Menon VA: Hypertension and narrowing of the renal arteries in infancy. J Pediatr 84:39, 1974
74. Robicsek F, Sanger PW, Daugherty HR: Coarctation of the abdominal aorta diagnosed by aortography. Report of three cases. Ann Surg 162:227, 1965
75. Sinaiko A, Najarian J, Michael AF, Mirkin BL: Renal autotransplantation in the treatment of bilateral renal artery stenosis: Relief of hypertension in an 8-year-old boy. J Pediatr 83:409, 1973

76. Mininberg DT, Roze S, Yoon HJ, Pearl M: Hypertension associated with crossed renal ectopia in an infant. Pediatrics 48:454, 1971
77. Cook GT, Marshall VF, Todd JE: Malignant renovascular hypertension in a newborn. J Urol 96:863, 1966
78. Snyder CH, Bost RB, Platou RV: Hypertension in infancy, with anomalous renal artery. Diagnosis by renal arteriogram, apparent cure after nephrectomy. Pediatrics 15:88, 1955

Endocardial Fibroelastosis

79. DuShane JW, Edwards JE: Congenital aortic stenosis in association with endocardial sclerosis of the left ventricle. Proc Staff Meet Mayo Clin 29:102, 1954
80. Farber S, Hubbard J: Fetal endomyocarditis: Intrauterine infection as the cause of congenital cardiac anomalies. Am J Med Sci 186:705, 1933
81. Levine HD: Cardiac hypertrophy in infancy associated with thickened endocardium and coarctation of the aorta. Am J Dis Child 48:1072, 1934
82. Oppenheimer EH: The association of adult-type coarctation of the aorta with endocardial fibroelastosis of infancy. Bull Johns Hopkins Hosp 93:309, 1953
83. MacGregor RR, McKendry R: Fetal endocarditis. (Report of a case.) Can Med Assoc J 50:433, 1944
84. Andersen DH, Kelly J: Endocardial fibroelastosis. I. Endocardial fibroelastosis associated with congenital malformations of the heart. Pediatrics 18:513, 1956
85. Johnson FR: Anoxia as a cause of endocardial fibroelastosis in infancy. Arch Pathol 54:237, 1952
86. Paul RN, Robbins SG: A surgical treatment proposed for either endocardial fibroelastosis or anomalous left coronary artery. Pediatrics 16:147, 1955
87. Wilson RA, Clark N: Endocardial fibroelastosis associated with generalized glycogenosis. Occurrence in siblings. Pediatrics 26:86, 1960
88. Blieden LC, Moller JH: Cardiac involvement in inherited disorders of metabolism. Prog Cardiovasc Dis 16:615, 1974
89. Hastreiter AR, Miller RA: Management of primary endomyocardial disease. The myocarditis-endocardial fibroelastosis syndrome. Pediatr Clin North Am 11:401, 1964
90. Edwards JE: Congenital malformations of heart and great vessels. In Gould SC (ed): Pathology of the Heart. Springfield, Ill, Thomas, 1953, p 420
91. Edwards JE: An Atlas of Congenital Anomalies of the Heart and Great Vessels. Springfield, Ill, Thomas, 1954
92. Mitchell SC, Froehlich LA, Banas JS Jr, Gilkeson MR: An epidemiologic assessment of primary endocardial fibroelastosis. Am J Cardiol 18:859, 1966
93. Black-Schaffer B, Turner ME: Hyperplastic infantile cardiomegaly. A form of "idiopathic hypertrophy" with or without endocardial fibroelastosis; and a comment on cardiac "atrophy." Am J Pathol 34:745, 1958
94. Shone JD, Muñoz-Armas S, Manning JA, Keith JD: The mumps antigen skin test in endocardial fibroelastosis. Pediatrics 37:423, 1966
95. Gersony WM, Katz SL, Nadas AS: Endocardial fibroelastosis and mumps virus. Pediatrics 37:430, 1966
96. St. Geme JW Jr, Noren GR, Adams P Jr: Proposed embryopathic relation between mumps virus and primary endocardial fibroelastosis. N Engl J Med 275:339, 1966
97. Kline IK, Miller AJ, Pick R, Katz LN: Relationship between human endocardial fibroelastosis and obstruction of cardiac lymphatics. Circulation 30:728, 1964
98. Vlad P, Rowe RD, Keith JD: The electrocardiogram in primary endocardial fibroelastosis. Br Heart J 17:189, 1955

99. Lintermans JP, Kaplan EL, Morgan BC, Baum D, Guntheroth WG: Infarction patterns in endocardial fibroelastosis. Circulation 33:202, 1966

100. Carter JB, Blieden LC, Edwards JE: Congenital heart block. Anatomic correlations and review of the literature. Arch Pathol 97:51, 1974

101. Stanger P, Lucas RV Jr, Edwards JE: Anatomic factors causing respiratory distress in acyanotic congenital cardiac disease. Special reference to bronchial obstruction. Pediatrics 43:760, 1969

102. McLoughlin TG, Schiebler GL, Krovetz LJ: Hemodynamic findings in children with endocardial fibroelastosis. Analysis of 22 cases. Am Heart J 75:162, 1968

103. Miller GAH, Rahimtoola SH, Ongley PA, Swan HJC: Left ventricular volume and volume change in endocardial fibroelastosis. Am J Cardiol 15:631, 1965

104. Manning JA, Sellers FJ, Bynum RS, Keith JD: The medical management of clinical endocardial fibroelastosis. Circulation 29:60, 1964

Myocarditis

105. Brightman VJ, Scott TFM, Westphal M, Boggs TR: An outbreak of Coxsackie B-5 virus infection in a newborn nursery. J Pediatr 69:179, 1966

106. Javett SN, Heymann S, Mundel B, et al.: Myocarditis in the newborn infant. A study of an outbreak associated with Coxsackie Group B virus infection in a maternity house in Johannesburg. J Pediatr 48:1, 1956

107. Kibrick S, Benirschke K: Acute aseptic myocarditis and meningoencephalitis in the newborn child infected with Coxsackie virus Group B, type 3. N Engl J Med 255:883, 1956

108. Van Creveld S, DeJager H: Myocarditis in newborns, caused by Coxsackie virus. Clinical and pathological data. Ann Paediatr 187:100, 1956

109. Ainger LE, Lawyer NG, Fitch CW: Neonatal rubella myocarditis. Br Heart J 28:691, 1966

110. Rosenberg HS, McNamara DG: Acute myocarditis in infancy and childhood. Prog Cardiovasc Dis 7:179, 1964

111. Keith JD, Rowe RD, Vlad P: Heart Disease in Infancy and Childhood, 2nd ed. New York, Macmillan, 1967, pp 866–867

112. Silber EN: Respiratory viruses and heart disease. Ann Intern Med 48:228, 1958

Anomalous Origin of Left Coronary Artery from Pulmonary Trunk

113. Wesselhoeft H, Fawcett JS, Johnson AL: Anomalous origin of the left coronary artery from the pulmonary trunk. Its clinical spectrum, pathology, and pathophysiology, based on a review of 140 cases with seven further cases. Circulation 38:403, 1968

114. Noren GR, Raghib G, Moller JH, et al.: Anomalous origin of the left coronary artery from the pulmonary trunk with special reference to the occurrence of mitral insufficiency. Circulation 30:171, 1964

115. Edwards JE: The direction of blood flow in coronary arteries arising from the pulmonary trunk. Circulation 29:163, 1964

116. St. John Brooks H: Two cases of an abnormal coronary artery of the heart arising from the pulmonary artery. With some remarks upon the effect of this in producing cirsoid dilatation of the vessels. J Anat Physiol 20:26, 1886

117. Rowe RD, Mehrizi A: The Neonate with Congenital Heart Disease. Philadelphia, Saunders, 1968, p 256

118. Bland EF, White PD, Garland J: Congenital anomalies of the coronary arteries: Report of an unusual case associated with cardiac hypertrophy. Am Heart J 8:787, 1933

119. Nora JJ, McNamara DG, Hallman GL, Sommerville RJ, Cooley DA: Medical and surgical management of anomalous origin of the left coronary artery from the pulmonary artery. Pediatrics 42:405, 1968
120. Foster HR Jr, Hagstrom JWC, Ehlers KH, Engle MA: Mitral insufficiency due to anomalous origin of the left coronary artery from the pulmonary artery. Pediatrics 34:649, 1964
121. Keith JD: The anomalous origin of the left coronary artery from the pulmonary artery. Br Heart J 21:149, 1959
122. Askenazi J, Nadas AS: Anomalous left coronary artery originating from the pulmonary artery. Report on 15 cases. Circulation 51:976, 1975
123. Perry LW, Scott LP: Anomalous left coronary artery from pulmonary artery. Report of 11 cases. Review of indications for and results of surgery. Circulation 41:1043, 1970

Other Causes of Myocardial Infarction

124. Arthur A, Cottom D, Evans R, Spencer H: Myocardial infarction in a newborn infant. J Pediatr 73:110, 1968
125. Gault MH, Usher R: Coronary thrombosis with myocardial infarction in a newborn infant. Clinical, electrocardiographic, and post-mortem findings. N Engl J Med 263:379, 1960
126. Martelle RR: Coronary thrombosis in a five month old infant. J Pediatr 46:322, 1955
127. Ramsay RE, Crumrine RM: Coronary thrombosis in an infant aged four months. Am J Dis Child 42:107, 1931
128. Baggenstoss AH, Keith HM: Calcification of the arteries of an infant. Report of a case. J Pediatr 18:95, 1941
129. Stryker WA: Arterial calcification in infancy with special reference to the coronary arteries. Am J Pathol 22:1007, 1946
130. Beuren AJ, Schultz R, Sinapius D, Stoermer J: Calcinosis of the arteries with coronary calcification in infancy. Am Heart J 78:87, 1969
131. Cochrane WA, Bowden DH: Calcification of the arteries in infancy and childhood. Pediatrics 14:222, 1954
132. Sanyal SK, Yules RB, Eidelman AI, Talner NS: Thrombocytosis, central nervous system disease, and myocardial infarction pattern in infancy. Pediatrics 38:629, 1966
133. Spach MS, Howell DA, Harris JS: Myocardial infarction and multiple thromboses in a child with primary thrombocytosis. Pediatrics 31:268, 1963
134. Kawasaki T, Kosaki F, Okawa S, Shigematsu I, Yanagawa H: A new infantile acute febrile mucocutaneous lymph node syndrome (MLNS) prevailing in Japan. Pediatrics 54:271, 1974
135. Munro-Faure H: Necrotizing arteritis of the coronary vessels in infancy. Case report and review of the literature. Pediatrics 23:914, 1959
136. Landing BH, Larson EJ: Are infantile periarteritis nodosa with coronary artery involvement and fatal mucocutaneous lymph node syndrome the same? Comparison of 20 patients from North America with patients from Hawaii and Japan. Pediatrics 59:651, 1977
137. Morens DM, O'Brien RJ: Kawasaki disease in the United States. J Infect Dis 137:91, 1978
138. Kato H, Koike S, Yokoyama T: Kawasaki disease: Effect of treatment on coronary artery involvement. Pediatrics 63:175, 1979
139. Yoshikawa J, Yanagihara K, Owaki T, et al.: Cross-sectional echocardiographic diagnosis of coronary artery aneurysms in patients with mucocutaneous lymph node syndrome. Circulation 59:133, 1979

Storage Diseases

140. Hohn AR, Lowe CU, Sokal JE, Lambert EC: Cardiac problems in the glycogenoses with specific reference to Pompe's disease. Pediatrics 35:313, 1965
141. Hers HG: α-glucosidase deficiency in generalized glycogen storage disease (Pompe's disease). Biochem J 86:11, 1963
142. Kahana D, Telem C, Steinitz K, Solomon M: Generalized glycogenosis. Report of a case with deficiency of alpha glucosidase. J Pediatr 65:243, 1964
143. Caddell JL, Wittemore R: Observations on generalized glycogenosis with emphasis on electrocardiographic changes. Pediatrics 29:743, 1962
144. Ehlers KH, Hagstrom JWC, Lukas DS, Redo SF, Engle MA: Glycogen-storage disease of the myocardium with obstruction to left ventricular outflow. Circulation 25:96, 1962
145. Huijing F, van Creveld S, Losekoot G: Diagnosis of generalized glycogen storage disease (Pompe's disease). J Pediatr 63:984, 1963
146. Ruttenberg HD, Steidl RM, Carey LS, Edwards, JE: Glycogen storage disease of the heart. Hemodynamic and angiocardiographic features in 2 cases. Am Heart J 67:469, 1964
147. Cardiff RD: A histochemical and electron microscopic study of skeletal muscle in a case of Pompe's disease (glycogenosis II). Pediatrics 37:249, 1966
148. Hernandez A Jr, Marchesi V, Goldring D, Kissane J, Hartman AF Jr: Cardiac glycogenosis. Hemodynamic, angiocardiographic, and electron microscopic findings—report of a case. J Pediatr 68:400, 1966
149. Rees A, Elbl R, Minhas K, Solinger R: Echocardiographic evidence of outflow tract obstruction in Pompe's disease (glycogen storage disease of the heart). Am J Cardiol 37:1103, 1976
150. Blieden LC, Desnick RJ, Carter JB, et al.: Cardiac involvement in Sandhoff's disease. Inborn error of glycosphingolipid metabolism. Am J Cardiol 34:83, 1974

Rhabdomyoma

151. Tsakraklides V, Burke B, Mastri A, et al.: Rhabdomyomas of heart. A report of four cases. Am J Dis Child 128:639, 1974
152. Shaher RM, Mintzer J, Farina M, Alley R, Bishop M: Clinical presentation of rhabdomyoma of the heart in infancy and childhood. Am J Cardiol 30:95, 1972
153. Van der Hauwaert LG: Cardiac tumors in infancy and childhood. Br Heart J 33:125, 1971
154. Batchelor TM, Maun ME: Congenital glycogenic tumors of the heart. Arch Pathol 39:67, 1945
155. Nadas AS, Ellison RC: Cardiac tumors in infancy. Am J Cardiol 21:363, 1968
156. Allen HD, Blieden L, Stone FM, Bessinger FB Jr, Lucas RV Jr: Echocardiographic demonstration of a right ventricular tumor in a neonate. J Pediatr 84:854, 1974
157. Haslam RHA: Tuberous sclerosis. In Bergsma D (ed): Birth Defects Atlas and Compendium. Baltimore, Williams & Wilkins, 1973, p 868

Pericardial Disease

158. Valdes-Dapena M, Miller WH: Pericarditis in the newborn. Pediatrics 16:673, 1955
159. Pernot PC, Frisch R, Mathieu P, Olive MD, Vidailhet M: Les tératomes intrapéricardiques du nourrisson. A propos de deux observations avec succès chirurgical. Arch Mal Coeur 61:546, 1968
160. Dery P, Marks ML, Shapera R: Clinical manifestations of coxsackievirus infections in children. Am J Dis Child 128:464, 1974

161. Bain HW, McLean DM, Walker SJ: Epidemic pleurodynia (Bornholm disease) due to coxsackie B-5 virus. The interrelationship of pleurodynia, benign pericarditis and aspectic meningitis. Pediatrics 27:889, 1961
162. Nadas AS, Levy JM: Pericarditis in children. Am J Cardiol 7:109, 1961
163. Fowler NO: Physiology of cardiac tamponade and pulsus paradoxus. I. Mechanisms of pulsus paradoxus in cardiac tamponade. Mod Concepts Cardiovasc Dis 47:109, 1978
164. Fowler NO: Physiology of cardiac tamponade and pulsus paradoxus. II. Physiological, circulatory, and pharmacological responses in cardiac tamponade. Mod Concepts Cardiovasc Dis 47:115, 1978
165. Echeverria P, Smith EWP, Ingram D, Sade RM, Gardner P: *Haemophilus influenzae* b pericarditis in children. Pediatrics 56:808, 1975
166. Gersony WM, McCracken GH Jr: Purulent pericarditis in infancy. Pediatrics 40:224, 1967
167. Okoroma EO, Perry LW, Scott LP: Acute bacterial pericarditis in children: Report of 25 cases. Am Heart J 90:709, 1975
168. Van Reken D, Strauss A, Hernandez A, Feigin RD: Infectious pericarditis in children. J Pediatr 85:165, 1974
169. Benzing G III, Kaplan S: Purulent pericarditis. Am J Dis Child 106:289, 1963
170. Feigenbaum H: Echocardiographic diagnosis of pericardial effusion. Am J Cardiol 26:475, 1970
171. Shabeti R, Fowler NO, Guntheroth WG: The hemodynamics of cardiac tamponade and constrictive pericarditis. Am J Cardiol 26:480, 1970
172. Strauss AW, Stana-Maria M, Goldring D: Constrictive pericarditis in children. Am J Dis Child 129:822, 1975
173. Rubenstein JJ, Goldblatt A, Daggett WM: Acute constriction complicating purulent pericarditis in infancy. Am J Dis Child 124:591, 1972
174. Caird R, Conway N, McMillan IKR: Purulent pericarditis followed by early constriction in young children. Br Heart J 35:201, 1973
175. Reynolds JL, Donahue JK, Pearce CW: Intrapericardial teratoma: A cause of acute pericardial effusion in infancy. Pediatrics 43:71, 1969
176. Bigelow NH, Klinger S, Wright AW: Primary tumors of the heart in infancy and early childhood. Cancer 7:549, 1954
177. Beck CS: An intrapericardial teratoma and a tumor of the heart: Both removed operatively. Ann Surg 116:161, 1942

11 Cyanosis and Increased Pulmonary Blood Flow

Malformations with cyanosis and increased pulmonary blood flow are termed "admixture lesions" because there is both a left-to-right and a right-to-left shunt. In most of the conditions, there is a chamber in which both the pulmonary venous return and the systemic venous return mix and then are ejected into the great vessels.

In almost all admixture lesions, there is an inverse relationship between the degree of cyanosis and pulmonary blood flow, the exception being complete transposition of the great vessels. As the volume of pulmonary blood flow increases, the total volume of pulmonary venous return, which is fully saturated, increases, so that the volume of fully saturated blood mixing with systemic venous blood increases, and this raises systemic arterial saturation. This fact is useful in following the course of patients with admixture lesions, for as the infant becomes more cyanotic, the volume of pulmonary blood flow is decreasing for whatever reasons influence the blood flows in an individual patient.

The admixture lesions discussed are:

1. Truncus arteriosus
2. Transposition of the great vessels
3. Single ventricle
4. Tricuspid atresia
5. Total anomalous pulmonary venous connection

In the first three conditions, the magnitude of pulmonary blood flow depends upon the relative resistances to pulmonary and systemic blood flows, whereas total anomalous pulmonary venous connection flow is determined by relative ventricular compliance.

In transposition of the great vessels, there is no direct relation between pulmonary blood flow and degree of cyanosis, and the mechanisms influencing the shunts are unknown.

Congestive cardiac failure is common in infants with admixture lesions because the increased pulmonary blood leads to ventricular volume overloads. There may be additional factors that influence the development of congestive cardiac failure in certain infants.

PERSISTENT TRUNCUS ARTERIOSUS

In persistent truncus arteriosus, a single arterial vessel leaves the heart through a single semilunar valve and supplies the systemic, pulmonary, and coronary arterial systems.[1] This vessel overlies a ventricular septal defect and receives the entire output from both ventricles.

PATHOLOGY.   Persistent truncus arteriosus results from failure of the spiral septum to divide the embryonic truncus arteriosus into a separate aorta and pulmonary trunk. This septum is also responsible for closing the superior portion of the ventricular septum. Thus, in this anomaly, the single arterial trunk overrides an interventricular septal defect.

The ventricular septal defect is located superiorly and anteriorly and immediately below the truncal valve. The truncal and mitral valves are in continuity, and sometimes the tricuspid valve is also in continuity with the truncal valve and the mitral valve through the defect.[1,2] Although the truncus generally overrides the ventricular septal defect, occasionally, it may arise predominantly from either the right or left ventricle. In this situation, the outflow area from the opposite ventricle may be restrictive.[1]

The truncal valve, in about two thirds of the cases, is tricuspid and is tetracuspid in about one fourth of the cases, with bicuspid or pentacuspid forms making up the remaining cases. Study of the pathologic changes in the semilunar valve reveals a number of abnormalities, including variation in size of individual cusps, prolapse of cusps, and imperfectly formed commissures. Nodularity and thickening of the cusps by mucoid connective tissue are the most common changes. The nodularity increases with age,[2,3] but such changes can be found in the first week of life.[2] The truncal valve may be either stenotic[4,5] or insufficient,[6] and nodular thickened cusps are associated with truncal insufficiency.[6]

Because of recent operative success in correcting this lesion, it is important to understand the coronary arterial pattern. Anderson and associates[7] have emphasized that in about two thirds of the patients, large branches of the right coronary artery cross the upper anterior surface of the right ventricle, supplying both ventricles and the interventricular septum. These coronary vessels are vulnerable in procedures requiring a conduit from the right ventricle. The left coronary artery tends to arise more posteriorly than from a normal aorta. In some patients, the posterior descending coronary artery may arise from the left circumflex coronary artery.[8]

The truncus gives rise to a right aortic arch in about 30 percent of the instances.[2,9] Interruption of the aortic arch may coexist with truncus arteriosus and left aortic arch.

The origin of the pulmonary arteries from the truncus arteriosus is variable, and although Collett and Edwards[10] developed a classification based upon the anatomic details of the pulmonary arteries, this has not been useful clinically, and it may be difficult even with the specimen in hand to clearly classify a specimen into a particular type.

The pulmonary arteries usually arise from the left posterior aspect of the truncus a short distance above the truncal valve. The pulmonary arteries may originate from a short pulmonary trunk or from separate but adjacent orifices in the truncus. In about 10 percent of the patients, there is unilateral absence of a pulmonary artery, being more frequent on the same side as the aortic arch.[2,9] There may occasionally be stenosis of the origin of the pulmonary arteries.

Collett and Edwards[10] describe a type of truncus arteriosus (type IV) in which the pulmonary blood supply originated from the descending aorta. Subsequently, it has been felt that these patients are better classified as tetralogy of Fallot with coexistent pulmonary atresia, since the anatomy of the right ventricle differs from that of truncus arteriosus.[1]

HEMODYNAMICS. The hemodynamics of truncus arteriosus resemble those of ventricular septal defect in that relative resistances to blood flow govern the volume of pulmonary blood flow. Both ventricles eject blood into the truncus arteriosus, and blood is distributed into the aorta and into the pulmonary arteries according to the relative resistances. Resistance to pulmonary blood flow is affected by the status of the pulmonary arterioles and the caliber of the pulmonary arteries. If the pulmonary arteries arising from the truncus are stenotic, blood flow into the lungs is limited, a pressure difference occurs across the narrowed area, and the pulmonary arterial pressure is less than the aortic pressure.

In most patients, however, the pulmonary arteries are large, so that pulmonary arterial and aortic pressures are equal. Therefore, the volume of pulmonary blood flow is inversely related to the pulmonary vascular resistance. At birth, pulmonary vascular resistance is elevated, but it decreases in early infancy, so that pulmonary blood flow progressively increases. Left ventricular dilatation and, eventually, congestive cardiac failure occur.

Pulmonary vascular disease develops with age in these patients.

As in any admixture lesion, the degree of cyanosis is inversely related to the volume of pulmonary blood flow. In the neonatal period, cyanosis is more intense, but with fall in pulmonary vascular resistances, the degree of cyanosis lessens.

In patients with truncal insufficiency, additional volume load is placed upon the left ventricle that accentuates the congestive cardiac failure.

CLINICAL FEATURES. Although the anatomy and hemodynamics would indicate that cyanosis would be expected, particularly in the neonatal period, this is variable, being present in 79 percent of one series[11] and 50 percent of another.[12] Cyanosis, if present, is mild and may be intermittent and present from birth or appear later in the first year of life. The initial recognition of congenital cardiac disease may be the discovery of a murmur, which is usually recognized by 1 month of age. The symptoms of congestive cardiac failure are also prominent in infants by 3 months of age. Tachypnea, pneumonia, poor feeding, and failure to thrive are symptoms related to the congestive cardiac failure.

The infants are often small for their age, being below the third percentile.[11,12] A wide pulse pressure is found in many patients, and this valuable finding indicates aortic runoff during diastole. A precordial bulge may be present, and a thrill may be palpated along the left sternal border and perhaps in the suprasternal notch as well. The first heart sound is loud and typically is followed by an aortic systolic ejection click. The second heart sound should be loud and single, but phonocardiographic studies[12] have shown variable patterns, including wide second heart sound with multiple components, two discrete components, or a single second heart sound.

A systolic murmur, either ejection type or pansystolic type, is present along the midleft sternal border and is usually grade 3/6 or louder. An early diastolic murmur of truncal insufficiency may be heard in some infants.[2,11] An apical middiastolic murmur is heard in most infants with large pulmonary blood flow.

ELECTROCARDIOGRAM. The QRS axis in the frontal plane is normal or slightly rightward, usually being between +60 and +120°. Right atrial enlargement is found in about half the patients.[11,13] The precordial leads usually show a pattern of biventricular hypertrophy (Fig. 11-1) similar to that in patients with ventricular septal defect, although a few infants show isolated right ventricular hypertrophy.[11,12]

THORACIC ROENTGENOGRAM. The pulmonary arterial markings are increased and often very prominent (Fig. 11-2). Cardiomegaly and left atrial enlargement are present. The cardiac contour resembles that of complete transposition of the great vessels, being described as "egg-shaped."[2,12] Unlike complete transposition of the great vessels, however, the upper mediastinum is wide, due to the enlarged truncus, and the upper left cardiac border may be straighter or show a distinct pulmonary arterial segment. A right aortic arch is found in about one third of the patients.[11-13]

ECHOCARDIOGRAM. The echocardiographic features resemble those of tetralogy of Fallot and typically show an enlarged arterial vessel overriding the interventricular septum, continuity of the posterior aortic wall with the anterior leaflet of the mitral valve, and right ventricular hypertrophy. The identification of a pulmonary valve should serve to distinguish these conditions, but as pointed out by Chung and associates,[14] inability to identify the pulmonary valve does not exclude tetralogy of Fallot. Our studies[15] and those of Assad-Morell and associates[16] indicate that the overriding great artery is not identified in each patient with truncus arteriosus, since this vessel may arise exclusively from the right or left ventricle, and the transducer position can affect the echocardiographic demonstration of overriding.

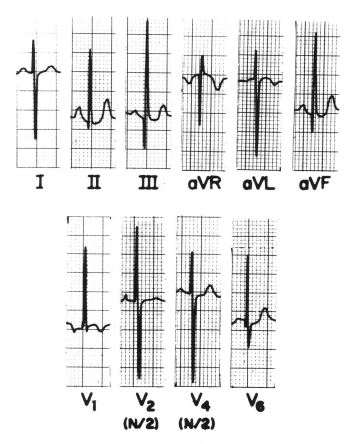

FIG. 11-1. Electrocardiogram of persistent truncus arteriosus in 3-month-old infant. Right atrial enlargement. QRS axis is +120°. Biventricular hypertrophy. N/2, half-standardization.

Left atrial size reflects the volume of pulmonary blood flow and is more likely to be increased in patients with truncus arteriosus, than in patients in tetrology of Fallot.

CARDIAC CATHETERIZATION AND ANGIOCARDIOGRAM. Cardiac catheterization and angiography in persistent truncus arteriosus are performed to (1) establish the diagnosis, (2) identify the origins of the pulmonary arteries, (3) assess the competence of the truncal valve, and (4) determine the volume of pulmonary blood flow and the level of pulmonary vascular resistance. Pressure data indicate elevation of right ventricular systolic pressure to the level of the left ventricle, and this usually equals that of the aorta, although in one third of the cases in one series[2] a gradient was found across the truncal valve, indicating truncal stenosis. A wide pulse pressure (>40 mm Hg) is found in the truncus, systolic

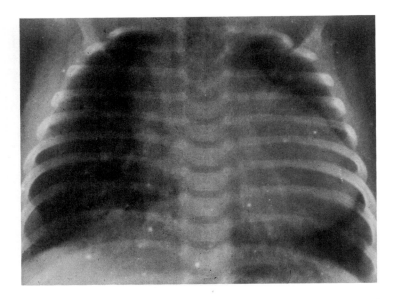

FIG. 11-2. Thoracic roentgenogram, posteroanterior view, of persistent truncus arteriosus. Moderate cardiomegaly. Increased pulmonary arterial blood flow. Right aortic arch.

pressure being elevated by the large stroke volume into the truncus, and diastolic pressure lowered by the free communication with the pulmonary arteries and, in some infants, the presence of truncal regurgitation. Usually, pulmonary arterial pressure equals aortic pressure, but care must be taken to record withdrawal pressure tracings from each pulmonary artery, since a pressure gradient may be present.[2,11] Left atrial and left ventricular end-diastolic pressures are elevated in patients with large pulmonary blood flow.

Oximetry data may show a slight increase of oxygen saturation at the right atrial or right ventricular level. The blood in the truncus arteriosus is desaturated but may be as high as 94 percent, reflecting the large volume of pulmonary blood flow. The pulmonary arterial saturation is usually lower than systemic arterial oxygen saturation,[2,11,12] presumably from streaming within the truncus arteriosus. The oxygen saturation difference between the two vessels may be 10 percent but usually is less. It may be difficult to accurately calculate pulmonary blood flow and vascular resistance because of the narrowed pulmonary arteriovenous oxygen difference.

The diagnosis of truncus arteriosus rests upon angiographic demonstration (Fig. 11-3a). Although right ventriculography can show the diagnosis, the best detail is obtained following aortography. Because of the large volume of blood flowing through the root of the truncus arteriosus, large volumes of contrast material must be injected. Clear detail may not be obtained, but the result is usually sufficient to make the diagnosis. Attention should be directed to the site of origin and size of the pulmonary arteries (Fig. 11-3b). Truncal regurgitation can be recognized on such studies, and if the truncal valve is stenotic, it may be domed or appear thickened.

MANAGEMENT.   Congestive cardiac failure is invariably present and progressive, despite intensive treatment with digitalis and diuretics. Death frequently results in unoperated patients. The median age of death in one series was 5 weeks.[2]

Marcelletti and associates[9] discussed the natural history of 23 patients with truncus arteriosus. Ten infants with congestive cardiac failure died; eight were between the ages of 1 and 7 years. Two had congestive cardiac failure, and the rest had a pulmonary vascular resistance of 10.6 units/m^2. Five patients were older and had more severe pulmonary vascular disease. Their study highlights the problem of management of this condition. Infants die frequently in congestive cardiac failure because of normal pulmonary vascular resistance, but older patients may be inoperable because of pulmonary vascular disease.

Pulmonary arterial banding was the initial operative procedure used to palliate the congestive cardiac failure of infants with truncus arteriosus. It, however, was associated with a high operative mortality, 66 percent in the experience of Singh and associates[17] and 59 percent in a review of 22 published reports.[18] Technical problems may be encountered in banding because of the variations in position of the pulmonary arteries. If the infant survives, banding complications occur,[19] but the band can be highly effective in preventing the development of pulmonary vascular disease and in allowing the infant to sur-

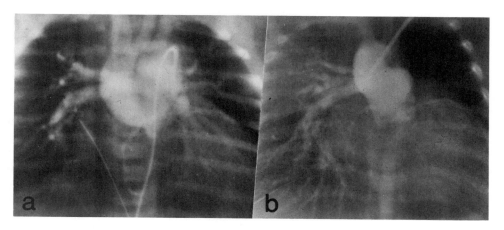

FIG. 11-3.   Angiograms of two infants with persistent truncus arteriosus. **a.** Age, 2 days. Arterial catheter passed through patent ductus arteriosus into pulmonary artery. Injection visualizes truncus arteriosus. **b.** Age, 2 months. Injection into truncus arteriosis. Absence of left pulmonary artery. Opacification of only right pulmonary artery.

vive to an age when correction can be carried out.[20] The presence of a band, however, makes correction with a conduit more difficult.

Because of the problems associated with banding and with the development of conduit-type correction for truncus arteriosus,[21] recent interest has been directed toward correction of this anomaly in infancy.[22] Although successful operations have been performed,[17,23,24] the risk is high in the experience of Marcelletti,[24] being 83 percent (five deaths in six patients under 2 years of age). More experience has been gained with corrective operation, and successful conduit operations are being performed in infants under 6 months of age.[25,26] The survival rate is probably better than with banding, but the long-term results need evaluation.

COMPLETE TRANSPOSITION OF THE GREAT VESSELS

Complete transposition of the great vessels is the most common cardiac anomaly producing cyanosis in the newborn period and represents 8 percent of all congenital cardiac malformations studied by Campbell.[27] It was the second most common catheterization diagnosis among infants studied at Boston Children's Hospital between 1968 and 1971.[28] Despite recorded anatomic observations as early as 1672[29] and clinical recognition of this defect by Fanconi in 1932[30] and Taussig in 1938,[31] treatment was either nonexistent or consisted of only short-term palliation until successful physiologic repair was accomplished in 1964.[32] This signalled a new era in the treatment of complex congenital cardiac disease. Interest in early recognition and aggressive management of these infants was awakened, so that palliation could be quickly effected, followed by definitive operative correction. In less than a generation, the situation has changed from hopelessness to the expectation that the majority of children with transposition of the great vessels will survive for a prolonged period, free of symptoms.

Transposition is a general term referring to a change in anteroposterior relationships and, when applied to the great vessels, indicates that the aorta lies anterior to the pulmonary artery. The prefix *d* or *l* has been applied to transposition of the great vessels to denote the right-to-left relationship of the aortic and pulmonary valves. The presence or absence of associated ventricular inversion is designated by *l* or *d* looping, respectively.

This section will deal principally with *complete* transposition (*d*-transposition), a specific lesion within the broad spectrum of transposition complexes in which the venous connections with the heart are normal and the ventricles occupy normal positions, but the aorta arises anteriorly from the right ventricle and the pulmonary artery posteriorly from the left ventricle. Complete transposition of the great vessels should not be confused with corrected transposition (*l*-transposition), discussed in Chapter 9, which is distinguished by origin of the aorta anterior and to the *left* of the pulmonary artery and is associated with ventricular inversion.

PATHOLOGY.   For many years, investigators attributed transposition of the great vessels to failure of spiraling of the truncal septum. The works of Keith,[33] Lev and Saphir,[34] and Van Praagh and Van Praagh[35] have focused attention on abnormalities of growth and resorption of conal tissue as fundamental to understanding the transposition complexes. The term "conus" refers to the muscular cardiac segment separating the semilunar and atrioventricular valves. Normally, there is preferential growth of the left-sided subpulmonic conus, causing displacement of the pulmonary valve anterior, superior, and to the left of the aortic valve. The right-sided subaortic conus remains undeveloped.

In complete transposition of the great vessels, d-ventricular looping results in normally located ventricles, but the subaortic conus preferentially develops, bringing the aortic valve anterior and higher than the pulmonary valve. The underdeveloped subpulmonic conus allows continuity between the mitral and pulmonary valves. The tricuspid valve is separated from the aorta by a well-developed conus (infundibulum) located anteriorly, just beneath the aortic valve. The result is a heart that is completely normal except for transposed great vessels. In addition to faulty growth and absorption of the conus, Goor and Edwards[36] proposed that defects in counterclockwise conotruncal inversion invariably play a role in the development of transposition complexes.

Among 521 patients with d-transposition of the great vessels treated at the Hospital for Sick Children in Toronto, slightly more than half had an intact ventricular septum.[37] A few of these patients (6 percent) had subpulmonic stenosis. Forty-eight percent had at least a small ventricular septal defect when studied during the neonatal period, and nearly one third of them had associated pulmonary stenosis.

HEMODYNAMICS.   The physiology and life expectancy of infants with transposition of the great vessels are variable and depend upon the presence of associated cardiac defects.

The circulation through the heart and lungs is in parallel rather than in series. Complete transposition of the great vessels would be incompatible with life for more than a few minutes after birth if some degree of mixing of pulmonary and systemic venous return within the heart or great vessels did not exist. In complete transposition of the great vessels with intact ventricular septum, mixing occurs through the foramen ovale primarily and to a lesser extent through the patent ductus arteriosus. The latter means of mixing is unlikely to be effective for more than a few hours because, as pulmonary vascular resistance falls, the shunt is no longer bidirectional and the ductus arteriosus closes shortly following birth. The presence of a ventricular septal defect allows greater mixing to occur, and this may be enhanced on the presence of obstruction to pulmonary blood flow. Patients with transposition of the great vessels, ventricular septal defect, and pulmonary stenosis have substantially higher systemic arterial oxygen saturation than do patients without associated anomalies.

CLINICAL FEATURES.   Complete transposition of the great vessels occurs more commonly in males (2:1), and the condition almost always causes symptoms in the neonatal period.[38,39] The age of onset depends upon the status of the ventricular septum. In neonates with intact ventricular septum, mixing of pulmonary and systemic venous returns is inadequate, and cyanosis appears within the first day of life. In a newborn nursery, the presence of mild cyanosis often does not cause concern for a few hours after birth because acrocyanosis is a normal finding in an otherwise robust, healthy appearing infant.[40] The degree of cyanosis gradually worsens, however, over the first 12 to 24 hours, perhaps due to functional closure of the ductus arteriosus. Symptoms of hypoxemia develop, and the nursing staff is usually the first to recognize that the neonate is becoming more intensely cyanotic and has developed tachypnea. The cry becomes less vigorous, and disinterest in feeding occurs. Oxygen is administered but the baby remains cyanotic.

Infants with a ventricular septal defect usually show symptoms at 1 to 2 weeks of age, presumably because better mixing is accomplished through the defect. Cyanosis is less profound, but signs and symptoms of congestive cardiac failure develop. If subpulmonary stenosis coexists with the ventricular septal defect, cardiac failure does not occur because pulmonary blood flow is limited by the pulmonary stenosis. The pulmonary stenosis favors passage of fully oxygenated blood from the left ventricle into the aorta, and the hemodynamics resemble tetralogy of Fallot.

Physical examination is not diagnostic of transposition of the great vessels but does exclude cyanosis caused by airway obstruction or parenchymal pulmonary disease. The respiratory rate is rapid because of hypoxemia and acidosis, but air entry is normal and vesicular lung sounds are audible. Generalized cyanosis is present.

The precordium and peripheral pulses are normal. In half of the infants, no murmur is present. In the other half, a systolic murmur ranging from grade 1–3/6 is present. The murmur is nonspecific, and it is difficult to determine the origin. Although murmurs occur more commonly in infants with either ventricular septal defect or pulmonary stenosis, their presence is not specific for any lesion. The second heart sound is loud and single, but this in a newborn baby can be a normal finding. Hepatomegaly is present in infants with congestive cardiac failure.

ELECTROCARDIOGRAM.   In the neonate, the electrocardiogram is normal for age, but as the infant grows, the neonatal pattern persists, so that right axis deviation and right ventricular hypertrophy are found[41] (Fig. 11-4). In infants with intact ventricular septum, lead V_1 shows an R wave and lead V_6 shows an rS— presumably because of the right ventricular hypertrophy and the low left ventricular systolic pressure. The R wave in lead V_6 is taller in infants with coexistent ventricular septal defect and/or pulmonary stenosis, but combined ventricular hypertrophy is uncommon in infancy.

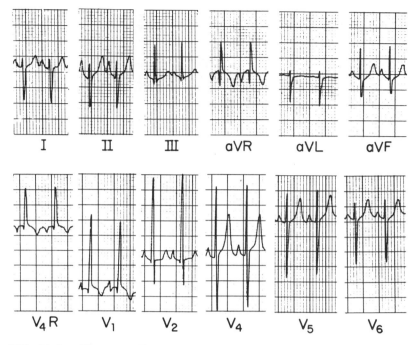

FIG. 11-4. Electrocardiogram of complete transposition of great vessels in 4-month-old infant with intact ventricular septum. Right atrial enlargement. QRS axis is +180°. Right ventricular hypertrophy.

THORACIC ROENTGENOGRAM. The thoracic roentgenogram excludes pulmonary disease or a ductus-dependent cardiac anomaly as a cause of cyanosis. Pulmonary vascular markings are increased to a moderate degree. Cardiomegaly is minimal unless there is large ventricular septal defect and the patient is several weeks old. The contour of the heart is characteristic (Fig. 11-5). The mediastinum appears narrow due to the loss of a thymus shadow and the anterior-posterior relationship of the great vessels. This egg-on-side appearance is present in approximately 75 percent of patients.

ECHOCARDIOGRAM. The echocardiogram of complete transposition of the great vessels resembles in most respects that of a normal heart, in that the relationships among chambers, valves, and great vessels and the aorta and pulmonary artery cannot be distinguished anatomically. In complete transposition of the great vessels, however, the anterior blood vessel (aorta) originates to the right of the other great vessel (pulmonary artery) 75 percent of the time, and this position of the great vessels is opposite of normal. The identification of this position of the great vessels depends upon the echocardiographer's noting the

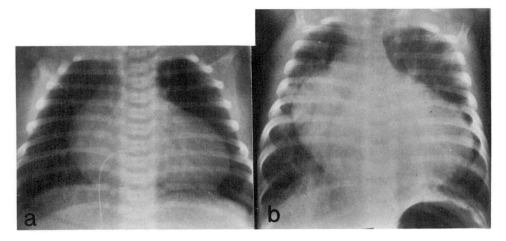

FIG. 11-5. Thoracic roentgenogram, posteroanterior views, of complete transposition of great vessels. **a.** Neonate. **b.** Three-month-old infant. Cardiomegaly. Narrow upper mediastinum. Increased pulmonary arterial markings.

transducer position when he records the great vessels.[42] The aorta and pulmonary artery can be distinguished in most patients with complete transposition of the great vessels by measuring systolic time intervals.

Much time can be spent obtaining an echocardiogram. Since clinical diagnosis is relatively accurate and palliation is an urgent matter, in most instances the echocardiogram can be eliminated.

OXYGEN INHALATION STUDIES. In neonates with complete transposition of the great vessels, arterial Po_2 is nearly identical in room air and following inhalation of 100 percent oxygen for 15 minutes.

The arterial Po_2 rises considerably in infants with parenchymal pulmonary disease. If there is inadequate mixing of systemic and pulmonary venous return, as in infants with an intact ventricular septum, the Po_2 ranges between 15 and 30 torr. A Po_2 less than 20 torr is ominous, particularly when the Pco_2 is greater than 40 torr. This combination indicates profound hypoxemia and metabolic acidosis. Hypercarbia indicates that the infant is tiring and is no longer capable of hyperventilating as a means of respiratory compensation. The infant should be placed on a ventilator.

If a ventricular septal defect is present, arterial Po_2 ranges between 35 and 60 torr.

CARDIAC CATHETERIZATION AND ANGIOCARDIOGRAM. Emergency cardiac catheterization is indicated in all infants with suspected transposition of the great vessels who present with very low arterial oxygen saturation (Po_2 <30). When severe hypoxemia is present, catheterization should not be delayed because the patient is too sick. The purposes of cardiac catheterization are to (1) substantiate the clinical diagnosis, (2) determine the presence of major associated cardiac anomalies, and (3) effect palliation.

The risk of the procedure is minimized by taking the infant to the catheterization laboratory before he or she is moribund, by attention to good supportive care, and by using ventilatory assistance if necessary.

An angiocatheter should be inserted and advanced into the right ventricle. Following measurement of pressure, a blood sample should be drawn for determination of pH, Po_2, and Pco_2. A right ventriculogram should be performed. In transposition of the great vessels, the aorta arises anteriorly and superiorly from a trabeculated right ventricle (Fig. 11-6). If a ventricular septal defect is present, both ventricles opacify, and the pulmonary artery is visualized posteriorly arising from a smooth-walled left ventricle.

Following review of the films, the catheter should be exchanged for a Rashkind catheter. This catheter is advanced into the left atrium through the foramen ovale, the balloon is inflated with 2 to 3 ml of contrast medium, and the catheter is withdrawn vigorously across the atrial septum, producing a tear in the fossa ovalis tissue (Fig. 11-7). The procedure is repeated several times until no resistance is met on pullback. The complications of the Rashkind procedure were discussed in Chapter 7.

Infants with complete transposition require repeat catheterization, at least prior to corrective operation, and perhaps earlier if such symptoms as increasing cyanosis develop. At these times, more detailed studies can be performed, since the catheterization is not being performed as an emergency.

At subsequent catheterization, each cardiac chamber and both great vessels should be catheterized. Oximetry series should be performed from the pulmonary artery through the left side of the heart, including the pulmonary vein, and also through the right side of the heart from the aorta to the venae cavae. The oximetry data permit determination of the site of mixing and allow calculation of blood flows, especially effective pulmonary blood flow. The effective pulmonary blood flow (QEP) represents the portion of the total pulmonary flow derived from the systemic venous return and, therefore, is an important quantitative measure of the adequacy of mixing. Effective pulmonary blood flow is calculated by dividing the pulmonary vein-mixed venous oxygen difference into measured or assumed oxygen consumption. Kidd[43] has reported a threefold increase in effective pulmonary blood flow following successful palliation.

Accurate measurements of systemic and pulmonary blood flows are difficult to achieve for several reasons. The volume of pulmonary blood flow derived from the bronchial circulation is variable and not readily measurable. Other difficulties include (1) erroneously high assumed oxygen consumption, (2) relatively inaccurate measurement of oxygen saturation in the low ranges encountered in transposition of the great vessels, (3) narrow pulmonary vein-pulmonary artery atrioventricular O_2 difference, compounding small errors in measurement, (4) inability to obtain a true mixed venous sample because of shunting at the atrial level, and (5) frequent presence of a patent ductus

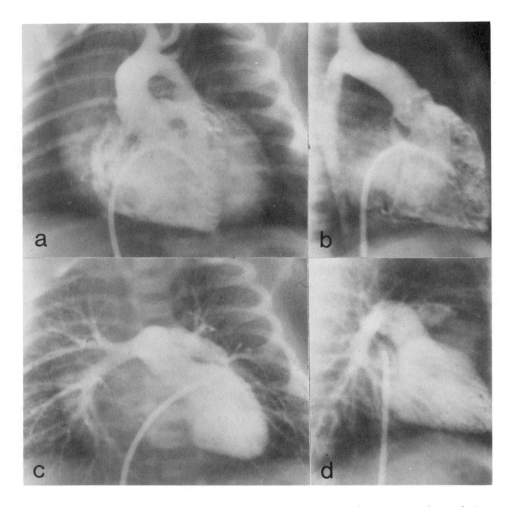

FIG. 11-6.   Right ventriculogram of complete transposition of great vessels. **a.** Antero-posterior. **b.** Lateral. Following injection of right ventricle, aorta, which is anterior, opaci-fies. Left ventriculogram. **c.** Anteroposterior. **d.** Lateral. Following injection, left ventricle opacifies the posteriorly placed pulmonary trunk.

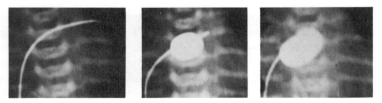

FIG. 11-7.   Complete transposition of great vessels. Rashkind pro-cedure. Sequential films showing passage of catheter through fora-men ovale into left atrium, inflation of balloon, and withdrawal of balloon.

arteriosus, making collection of an accurate pulmonary arterial sample difficult.

During cardiac catheterization, prior to corrective operation, pressures should be remeasured across the left ventricular outflow area, for subpulmonary stenosis develops, particularly if the ventricular septum is intact. If a pressure gradient is measured, left ventriculography should be performed. Right ventriculogram should be repeated if the first one failed to visualize the right ventricle in its entirety or findings suggest a ventricular septal defect.

MANAGEMENT.   Proper management includes early recognition of cyanosis, prompt cardiac catheterization, and performance of the Rashkind procedure.[44]

Success of the Rashkind procedure is evident by rapid clinical improvement of the patient, a 15 to 25 percent increase in oxygen saturation, and a decrease in left atrial pressure.[45] This correlates with approximately a 12 mm tear in the fossa ovalis.[46] It is not uncommon for the arterial Po_2 to drift down within several days of the procedure. We do not feel that this is an indication for repeat septostomy or surgical septectomy as long as the pH remains normal and the patient is asymptomatic.

In one series, the Rashkind procedure improved the 3-month survival rate from 25 percent before the technique was utilized to 84 percent.[47] Complications include arrhythmias, avulsion of an atrioventricular valve or inferior vena cava, perforation of the heart with pericardial tamponade, and embolization of a piece of the rubber balloon.[48] We have experienced one instance of complete left hemothorax, presumably from partial evulsion of a pulmonary vein, successfully treated by thoracentesis and rapid replacement of 80 ml of blood.

The incidence of late Rashkind failure is difficult to determine. At one time, nearly all babies with transposition of the great vessels had physiologic correction deferred until at least 1 year of age, and any infant who required surgical atrial septectomy during infancy was considered a "Rashkind failure." Presently, a number of institutions prefer to perform a corrective operation during infancy, so operative septectomies have become less common. Nevertheless, 20 percent of our patients require a Blalock-Hanlon procedure[49] prior to 3 months of age to insure adequate mixing compatible with normal growth and development. Our present policy is to closely monitor the arterial Po_2 and pH for a week following the Rashkind procedure and, thereafter, follow hemoglobin and hematocrit concentrations and growth monthly. If the patient remains acidotic or the Po_2 consistently falls below 20 torr, operative septectomy is performed prior to discharge from the hospital. After discharge, we consider failure to grow adequately or development of extreme polycythemia (hemoglobin 20.0 g%) as indications for an operative palliation or corrective procedure.

Early attempts to anatomically correct transposition of the great vessels by restitution of the aorta to the left ventricle and the pulmonary artery to the right ventricle were unsuccessful.[50] Blalock was the first to propose transposing the venous return to the heart as a solution,[51] and this idea met with partial success in two of eight patients reported by Lillehei and Varco in 1953.[52] Further modifications were developed by Baffes, Senning, Albert, and Merendino, reaching fruition in 1964 when Mustard reported successful physiologic correction of transposition of the great vessels using an intraatrial baffle.

The Mustard procedure consists of placement of a pantaloon-shaped baffle, made from pericardium or Dacron, around the pulmonary veins in such a manner as to direct the pulmonary venous return through the tricuspid valve and the systemic return behind the baffle to the left side of the heart. The right ventricle continues to deliver blood to the aorta, and the left ventricle delivers blood to the pulmonary artery.

We studied 19 hearts of patients who died following the Mustard procedure performed at the University of Minnesota and found many problems that were encountered during the early application of the intraatrial baffle technique. Four patients had complex-associated anomalies, including endocardial cushion defect, hypoplastic right ventricle, Ebstein's anomaly, and cor triatriatum, which precluded successful outcome. An additional three patients had hypertensive pulmonary vascular disease (two of these had ventricular septal defect). Thus, seven patients' deaths were contributed to incomplete preoperative evaluation, poor patient selection, and delay in referral for operation.

Operative complications contributing to death include redundancy of the intraatrial baffle obstructing venous return (five cases), severe residual obstruction at the site of previous pulmonary arterial banding (four cases), and obstruction of the right ventricular outflow tract with a ventricular septal defect patch (one case).

Early postoperative death was usually related to low cardiac output syndrome associated with redundancy of the baffle, partially obstructing an atrioventricular valve. Late deaths resulted from pulmonary complications or fatal arrhythmias. Mortality was lowest in the group of patients operated upon between 6 and 18 months of age.

Most of these problems have been solved. Presently, the combined early and late mortality related to the Mustard procedure in most centers is less than 10 percent. Postoperative arrhythmias are much less common since the incorporation of minor variations of surgical technique. Tricuspid incompetence has been an infrequent complication.[53] Pulmonary vascular obstructive disease is usually avoided when correction is performed prior to 12 to 18 months of age. Late pulmonary or systemic venous obstruction is occasionally encountered,[54, 55] prompting some institutions to employ a modification of the Senning technique, thereby avoiding the use of an intraatrial baffle.[56] Finally, there is continued concern that the right ventricle is not suited for prolonged function as a systemic pump. Postoperative studies have documented reduced right ventricular ejection fraction and increased end-diastolic volume.[57]

Because of these complications, there has been recent renewed interest in surgically transposing the great vessels to their proper ventricles, resulting in anatomic correction of transposition of the great vessels rather than physiologic correction.[58] A few reports of such operations have been discouraging because of technical difficulties with the coronary arteries. This may become the preferred operation if it can be performed within several days following birth, while the left ventricle is still adapted to elevated resistance.

Patients with transposition of the great vessels, ventricular septal defect, and subpulmonic stenosis generally are deferred for surgical correction until an older age, when a Rastelli procedure is performed. This technique consists of patching the ventricular septal defect so that the left ventricular outflow tract is in continuity with the aorta, and right ventricular flow is diverted through a valved conduit to the pulmonary arteries.

TAUSSIG-BING MALFORMATION

In 1949, Taussig and Bing[59] described a complex congenital cardiac defect in which the aorta arose anteriorly from the right ventricle, the pulmonary artery arose normally, and a ventricular septal defect was present. This variety of double outlet right ventricle is further characterized by fibrous discontinuity between the aortic and mitral valves, bilateral conus, and side-by-side relationship of the great vessels.[60]

Though relatively uncommon, the Taussig-Bing malformation is important because of operative considerations and its frequent association with left-sided obstructive lesions. It must be differentiated from an isolated ventricular septal defect with pulmonary hypertension and transposition of the great vessels with a large ventricular septal defect.

Pulmonary stenosis is rarely present. The ventricular septal defect is located in close proximity to the pulmonary valve, and, therefore, pulmonary arterial saturation is higher than aortic saturation. Six of the nine patients studied by Zamora et al[61] had coarctation of the aorta, and four patients had subaortic stenosis. Mitral valve anomalies may be present,[62,63] but they are more common in patients with subaortic type, double outlet right ventricle.

When coexistent left-sided obstructive lesions are severe, symptoms appear in early infancy and consist of severe congestive cardiac failure and mild cyanosis.[64] Femoral pulses are absent or decreased if coarctation of the aorta is present, and the diagnosis is confirmed by aortography. Unless pulmonary edema is severe, cyanosis is not expected in uncomplicated coarctation of the aorta, and its presence may lead one to expect an intracardiac anomaly, such as the Taussig-Bing malformation. Thoracic roentgenograms show cardiomegaly and increased pulmonary arterial and venous markings. In seven of the eight cases of double outlet right ventricle without pulmonary stenosis, described by Neufeld and co-workers,[65] left axis deviation in the frontal plane of the electrocardiogram was observed. This may be related to abnormalities of the conduction system described by Bharati and Lev.[66] Echocardiographically, double outlet right ventricle is suspect because of extreme overriding of the aorta and aortic-mitral discontinuity.

The diagnosis of Taussig-Bing malformation is substantiated by careful biplane cineangiography (Fig. 11-8). Both semilunar valves appear at the same coronal body plane. The ventricular septal defect is usually supracristal and is

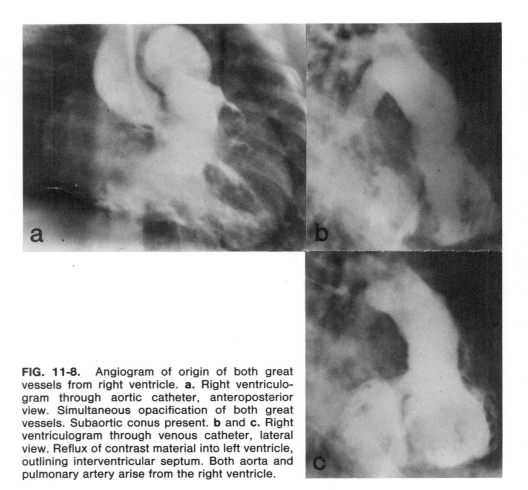

FIG. 11-8. Angiogram of origin of both great vessels from right ventricle. **a.** Right ventriculogram through aortic catheter, anteroposterior view. Simultaneous opacification of both great vessels. Subaortic conus present. **b** and **c.** Right ventriculogram through venous catheter, lateral view. Reflux of contrast material into left ventricle, outlining interventricular septum. Both aorta and pulmonary artery arise from the right ventricle.

located just beneath the pulmonary valve. Left ventriculography demonstrates a smooth-walled left ventricle with a filling defect between the anterior mitral leaflet and the aorta (subaortic conus). Subaortic obstruction as well as coarctation of the aorta may be present, as previously noted. A left atriogram should be performed to exclude an obstructive lesion of the mitral valve or double inlet right ventricle (straddling mitral valve).

Operative correction consists of patching the ventricular septal defect so that the left ventricular outflow tract is in continuity with the pulmonary artery, thereby converting the patient to transposition of the great vessels with an intact ventricular septum. A Mustard procedure is then performed. Unfortunately, the complexity of associated cardiovascular anomalies often precludes successful outcome in infancy.

TRICUSPID ATRESIA WITH INCREASED PULMONARY BLOOD FLOW

Certain anatomic forms of tricuspid atresia are associated with increased blood flow and, therefore, must be considered in the differential diagnosis of cardiac lesions discussed in this section. Occasionally, this form of tricuspid atresia is confused with ventricular septal defect or other conditions associated with left-to-right shunt, since the degree of systemic arterial desaturation may be so mild that the infant does not appear cyanotic. The electrocardiographic findings of left axis deviation should alert the physician to this possibility.

PATHOLOGY. Many of the details of tricuspid atresia will be described in Chapter 12, and a classification of this malformation is given there. Two types of tricuspid atresia associated with increased pulmonary blood flow are discussed in this chapter:

> Type Ic: Normally related great vessels, normal pulmonary valve, and large ventricular septal defect
> Type IIc: Transposition of the great vessels and normal pulmonary valve

In type Ic of tricuspid atresia, the ventricular septal defect is large, subpulmonary stenosis is absent, and the pulmonary valve is normal. The pulmonary artery is larger than the aorta. In type IIc, the aorta arises from the rudimentary chamber, and the pulmonary artery arises from the left ventricle. Therefore, subaortic stenosis may exist because of the size of the ventricular septal defect and the amount of muscular obstruction in the rudimentary chamber. Tandon and Edwards [67] have indicated that the aorta may be positioned anteriorly and either to the right or to the left in relation to the pulmonary artery. Regardless of the relative positions of the great vessels, the anatomic and circulatory relationships are those of complete transposition of the great vessels.

Coarctation of the aorta frequently coexists with type IIc (tricuspid atresia with transposition of the great vessels).[68,69] In our 11 neonates with this condition, 4 had coarctation, and in the Marcano series,[69] each patient had an aortic arch anomaly, such as coarctation, tubular hypoplasia, or interruption of the aortic arch.

HEMODYNAMICS. An obligatory right-to-left shunt occurs at the atrial level, and the two venous returns mix in the left atrium. The left ventricle ejects blood into both the aorta and the pulmonary artery. The relative volume of blood flow into the systemic and pulmonary circuits is dependent upon the relative resistances to flow. At birth, pulmonary blood flow is limited by the normal neonatal elevation of pulmonary vascular resistance. As the resistance falls, pulmonary blood flow increases. The pulmonary blood flow is greater in infants with either subaortic stenosis or coarctation of the aorta than in those without these obstructive lesions.

Since the degree of systemic arterial desaturation is inversely related to the volume of pulmonary blood flow, cyanosis exists in the neonatal period but lessens with age, as pulmonary blood flow increases.

Congestive cardiac failure develops because of the volume load on the left ventricle.

CLINICAL FEATURES.   The infants have mild or, occasionally, no recognizable cyanosis. There is a history of tachypnea, poor feeding, and poor weight gain, with congestive cardiac failure manifested usually after 1 month. It may develop earlier if coarctation of the aorta coexists. There is a tendency for congestive cardiac failure to be more prominent in type IIc,[69,70] while those with normally related great vessels more likely initially present with cyanosis.

On physical examination, a difference in blood pressure may be found between the upper and lower extremities in patients with coexistent coarctation of the aorta, but this may be missed if cardiac failure is present. The cardiac findings are not diagnostic. Cardiomegaly is evident as displacement of the cardiac apex laterally and inferiorly. A grade 2–3/6 systolic murmur is present along the left sternal border and may be either short or pansystolic. A middiastolic rumble is present at the apex, indicating the large pulmonary blood flow. The second heart sound is accentuated and may be single. Hepatomegaly is present.

ELECTROCARDIOGRAM.   Left axis deviation of the QRS complex is the expected finding in tricuspid atresia (Fig. 11-9). In patients with type Ic, the axis is usually leftward, while in those with coexistent transposition of the great vessels, the axis is normal or slightly rightward in about half of the patients.[69,71] We have seen patients with a QRS axis of $+110°$. In both types Ic and IIc, the R wave is often taller in lead V_6 than in infants with tricuspid atresia and diminished pulmonary blood flow. T wave inversion occurs in the left precordial leads.

Left atrial enlargement is evident on the electrocardiogram of many infants with increased flow and is combined with right atrial enlargement.

THORACIC ROENTGENOGRAM.   Cardiomegaly and increased pulmonary blood flow are found, and left atrial enlargement is seen on lateral films. The cardiac contour is not as distinctive as in patients with tricuspid atresia and decreased pulmonary blood flow (Fig. 11-10). In those with normally related great vessels, the pulmonary arterial segment may be prominent, while in those with transposition of the great vessels, the upper mediastinum is narrow.

ECHOCARDIOGRAM.   The echocardiogram shows (1) small anterior chamber without an atrioventricular valve, (2) posterior ventricle and great vessel enlargement, and (3) left atrial enlargement.

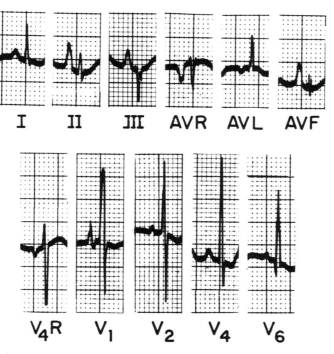

FIG. 11-9. Electrocardiogram of 2-month-old infant with tricuspid atresia and transposition of great vessels. Right atrial enlargement. QRS axis is 0°. Precordial leads show left ventricular hypertrophy and inverted T v aves in left precordial leads.

CARDIAC CATHETERIZATION AND ANGIOCARDIOGRAM. Cardiac catheterization is indicated to diagnose the presence of tricuspid atresia and to identify the associated cardiac conditions. Left ventriculography is necessary to demonstrate the position of the great vessels and to identify coarctation of the aorta. The pulmonary arterial pressure is elevated to systemic levels. The pulmonary blood flow is usually greatly elevated, and systemic artery saturation may be 90 percent.

At cardiac catheterization, a Rashkind procedure should be performed.

MANAGEMENT. Intensive anticongestive measures are indicated. Most patients require banding of the pulmonary artery,[70,72,73] and in some, it must be combined with resection of coarctation of the aorta.

Marcano and colleagues[69] have emphasized that patients with type IIc have a poor prognosis, while those with type Ic show improvement with age, presumably from decrease in pulmonary blood flow by narrowing of the ventricular septal defect and subpulmonary area.

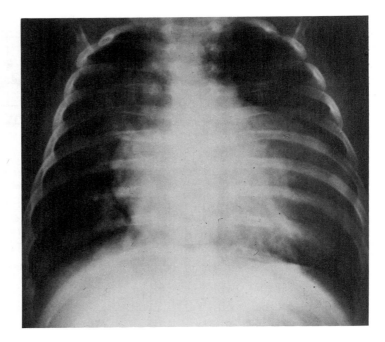

FIG. 11-10. Thoracic roentgenogram of tricuspid atresia and transposition of great vessels. Marked cardiomegaly and increased pulmonary vascularity.

Williams and associates[70] report an experience with 23 patients with tricuspid atresia and increased pulmonary blood flow. Pulmonary arterial banding was performed in 6 infants, and 5 survived. In subsequent palliative procedures of 4 survivors, 2 died. The outlook for infants following banding is not good, for corrective procedures, such as the Fontan procedure, will probably be unavailable because of the development of pulmonary vascular changes.

Palliative shunt surgery was necessary ultimately in 5 other patients[70] (ages 1½ to 16 years) with normally related great vessels. Four survived. Ten of their patients[70] were not operated, and 6 died, 4 of congestive cardiac failure before age 3 months and 2 from hypoxemia at ages 9 and 10 months, respectively. Four survivors have reached childhood.

SINGLE VENTRICLE WITHOUT PULMONARY STENOSIS

This uncommon form of congenital cardiac disease is classified as an admixture lesion, since both the systemic and pulmonary venous returns mix in the ventricle. Although there are conditions with similar hemodynamics, such as mitral atresia, tricuspid atresia, large endocardial cushion defect, and double inlet left ventricle, they should not be classed as single ventricle because of differences in anatomy, clinical features, and management.

ANATOMY.   In single ventricle, the ventricular chamber receives both the mitral and tricuspid valves. In about 80 percent of the patients, the great vessels are transposed, with *l*-transposition and *d*-transposition occurring in equal frequency. In the remaining patients, the great vessels are normally related.

Van Praagh and co-workers[74,75] have classified single ventricle into four types, depending upon anatomic features. Type A—single ventricle—is the most common form,[74-78] and the single ventricle resembles a left ventricle. On one side of the ventricle, the papillary muscles of both atrioventricular valves insert, while the other side of the ventricular wall is smooth. The smooth portion lies below an opening, leading through a bulboventricular foramen into the outlet chamber. The anterior great vessel (either pulmonary artery or aorta) arises from the outlet chamber, while the other great vessel is in continuity with the atrioventricular valves.

In the other types of single ventricle, there is no outflow chamber, and both great vessels are separate from the atrioventricular valves. We have called this form single primitive ventricle.[77,78] Van Praagh and associates[74,75] have classified this form into type B—single right ventricle, having an absence of left ventricular sinus—and type C—undivided ventricle, in which there are approximately equal amounts of left and right ventricular sinus, but they are not divided by a ventricular septum. Type D has absence of right and left ventricular sinuses and the interventricular septum.

Lesions obstructing blood flow from the heart are frequent. Pulmonary stenosis or atresia can coexist with single ventricle, and the details of these conditions are discussed in Chapter 12. Coarctation or interruption of the aorta can occur and augment pulmonary blood flow. A unique form of aortic stenosis can develop in patients with an outflow chamber in which the bulboventricular foramen narrows, creating obstruction of blood flow from the single ventricle into the outflow chamber and, thus, to the transposed aorta.[79]

HEMODYNAMICS.   All of the systemic and pulmonary venous blood returns to the single ventricle. The ventricular blood is ejected into the great vessels, the volume of blood flowing into the aorta and into the pulmonary artery being inversely related to the resistance to flow into that vessel. Since in this section, we are not considering those patients with coexistent pulmonary stenosis, blood flow is determined by the relative pulmonary and systemic vascular resistances. In the few infants with conditions causing obstruction to aortic flow, such as coarctation of the aorta or outflow chamber stenosis, this factor further increases resistance to systemic blood flow. A birth, the pulmonary vascular resistance is elevated, and pulmonary blood flow is limited. As the pulmonary vascular resistance declines, pulmonary blood flow increases. When the pulmonary blood flow increases significantly, congestive cardiac failure develops from volume overload of the single ventricle.

Patients with single ventricle show systemic arterial desaturation. As in other admixture lesions, the aortic saturation is inversely related to the volume of pulmonary blood flow. This fact can be valuable in evaluating patients serially, even though mixing may not be complete in the single ventricle, and streaming may occur. Pulmonary venous return often flows preferentially into the aorta, and the systemic venous return flows preferentially into the pulmonary trunk. This streaming effect occurs more commonly in patients with associated *l*-transposition of the great vessels.[80]

CLINICAL FEATURES.   The clinical features of infants with single ventricle but without obstruction to pulmonary blood flow resemble those of infants with a large left-to-right ventricular shunt. The symptoms of congestive cardiac failure—dyspnea, frequent respiratory infections, difficulty feeding, and slow growth—are prominent. Cyanosis is present and often initially noted at birth. It is mild, and some infants may appear acyanotic.

On physical examination, the infant is small for his age. The features of cardiac failure—tachypnea, tachycardia, excessive perspiration, and hepatomegaly—are present.

Cardiomegaly is clinically evident, and cardiac activity is increased. The first heart sound is normal, and the second heart sound is usually loud and single because of the high incidence of coexistent transposition of the great vessels. A grade 2–4/6 murmur is present along the left sternal border and in a few infants may be associated with a thrill.[77,78] The murmur is ejection type and probably related to blood flow into the pulmonary artery. A third heart sound, which is sometimes followed by a low-pitched middiastolic murmur, may be heard, reflecting the large flow across the mitral valve.[77,78]

ELECTROCARDIOGRAM.   One of four electrocardiographic patterns may be found in an individual infant with single ventricle: (1) right ventricular hypertrophy, (2) left ventricular hypertrophy, (3) an RS pattern across the precordial leads, or (4) pattern of corrected transposition. Because of this wide variation of precordial lead patterns and the QRS axis, the electrocardiogram is not diagnostic of single ventricle but, when combined with other clinical and laboratory features, may lead to a suspicion of the diagnosis. Correlations have been made between the electrocardiographic patterns and the anatomic details of the single ventricle and the relationship of the great vessels, but the patterns observed are not absolute and show variability.

Among patients with single ventricle and with the great vessels in the position of *l*-transposition (Fig. 11-11), there is a strong tendency for the electrocardiogram and vectorcardiogram to resemble those of corrected transposition with ventricular inversion.[78,81–83] In these patients, the initial QRS forces are usually directed posteriorly, superiorly, and leftward, yielding a q wave in the right precordial leads and absence of a q wave in the left precordial leads. The major QRS forces are usually directed anteriorly and rightward, and the QRS axis is usually directed toward the right.

In patients with single ventricle and *d*-transposition of the great vessels, we found that the initial QRS forces were usually directed anteriorly and to the left, yielding a pattern of absence of q waves in both leads V_1 and V_6. Left axis deviation or a QRS axis beyond $-90°$ was common. The precordial leads may

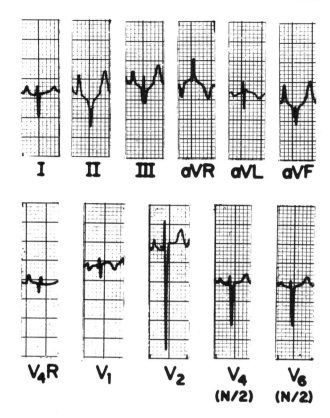

FIG. 11-11. Electrocardiogram of patient with single ventricle and *l*-transposition of great vessels. Right atrial enlargement. Major QRS forces directed posteriorly and superiorly. N/2, half-standardization.

show either left ventricular hypertrophy or right ventricular hypertrophy and, uncommonly, a stereotypic rS. This is at variance with the experience of Gessner,[82] who found the major QRS forces directed leftward, posteriorly, and inferiorly, yielding a pattern of left ventricular hypertrophy.

In our experience,[77,83] patients with single ventricle and normally related great vessels tended to have a QRS axis that ranged from −75° to +120° or a pattern of R, S, Rs, or rS in each of the precordial leads.

Despite these tendencies, there is considerable overlap[78,84] of these ventricular complexes, for the pattern resembling corrected transposition can be found in patients with *d*-transposition. Either right atrial or left atrial enlargement may be found, left atrial enlargement reflecting a large volume of pulmonary blood flow. Complete heart block may occur in infants with either *d*- or *l*-transposition of the great vessels.

THORACIC ROENTGENOGRAM. In infants with single ventricle but without obstruction to pulmonary blood flow, the pulmonary arterial vasculature is increased. Cardiomegaly is present, even in the neonatal period, and may reach a cardiothoracic ratio of 0.75.[85] Left atrial enlargement is present.

The cardiac contour varies. In patients with coexistent *l*-transposition, a bulge is present along the upper left heart border, resembling corrected transposition of the great vessels.[86] A similar contour is present in some patients with *d*-transposition of the great vessels.[78] In the infants with transposition of the great vessels, the pulmonary arterial segment is not identified, since it is located medially.

ECHOCARDIOGRAM. Echocardiography has proven to be a useful diagnostic method for identifying single ventricle. Seward and associates,[87,88] based on an experience with 55 patients, present a set of echocardiographic features to diagnose single ventricle: (1) two atrioventricular valves recorded simultaneously without an intervening ventricular septum, (2) no ventricular septal echo recorded in the usual position, although an echo may be recorded anteriorly to both atrioventricular valves in patients with an outflow chamber, (3) usually mitral continuity with the posterior semilunar valve (Fig. 11-12).

Bini and associates[89] stress that the echocardiographic information, when combined with clinical features, helps distinguish single ventricle from hemodynamically similar conditions and yields information useful in planning cardiac catheterization and angiography.

Seward and associates[87,88] have studied 35 patients with contrast echocardiography and feel that this technique has a greater specificity than standard M mode echocardiography. Following the injection of echo-producing material centrally, with the next diastole, echoes are found anterior to the mitral valve, providing strong evidence of single ventricle. If an outflow chamber is present, it will be filled with echoes during the next systole. This pattern differentiates single ventricle from other conditions with similar clinical features.

CARDIAC CATHETERIZATION AND ANGIOCARDIOGRAM. Cardiac catheterization and angiocardiography in patients with single ventricle must (1) clearly diagnose the single ventricle and separate it from other conditions, (2) determine if outflow obstruction exists, and (3) determine pulmonary vascular resistance.

Cardiac catheterization is performed from the inguinal area, and attempts should be made to pass the catheter into both the aorta and the pulmonary artery. Careful attention should be directed toward the catheter course in both the anteroposterior and lateral views. In the anteroposterior view of patients with coexistent *l*-transposition of the great vessels, the aorta is located along the upper left sternal border, and the pulmonary artery is medially placed. When observed on the lateral view, the catheter in the aorta appears anterior and in the pulmonary artery posterior in infants with transposition of the great vessels.

To identify the presence, site, and severity of outflow obstruction, careful withdrawal pressure tracings should be recorded from both the aorta and the pulmonary artery into the body of the right ventricle. Balloon-tipped flow-guided catheters have made it easier to catheterize the great vessels. Macartney and associates[90] successfully catheterized the pulmonary artery in 71 per-

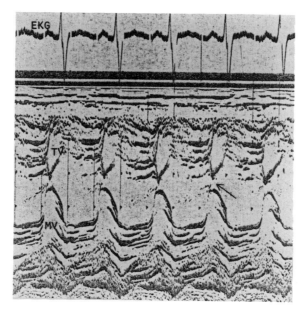

FIG. 11-12. Echocardiogram of infant with single ventricle. Tricuspid valve (TV) and mitral valve (MV) visualized, but there is no intervening ventricular septum (arrow). EKG, electrocardiogram.

cent of patients they studied and were unsuccessful in only two patients without pulmonary stenosis or atresia. In most instances of single ventricle, the systolic pressure is identical in the pulmonary artery, aorta, and single ventricle. In pulmonary stenosis, the pulmonary arterial pressure will be lower than normal, but ventricular pressure will not be altered.

Atrial pressures are normal. In a few patients with narrowing between the single ventricle and the outflow chamber, a gradient is found at that site. Aortic pressure is normal, but ventricular pressure is increased.

Oximetry data show evidence of bidirectional shunt at the ventricular level but rarely a shunt at the atrial level. In infants with single ventricle without pulmonary stenosis, there is usually a large increase in oxygen saturation between the right atrium and the ventricle. The aortic saturation is less than that of the left atrium, reflecting the right-to-left shunt, but may be as high as 97 percent.[90] Theoretically, the pulmonary arterial and aortic oxygen saturations should be equal, but, in general, incomplete mixing occurs so that a difference exists between these two arterial vessels.[78,80,90] Rahimtoola and associates[80] studied 19 patients with single ventricle without pulmonary stenosis and found complete mixing in 3, the systemic arterial saturation greater than the pulmonary arterial saturation in 11 (9 of whom had *l*-transposition), and pulmonary arterial saturation greater than systemic in the other 5. This experience is similar to ours. Macartney and associates[90] found, however, that neither pulmonary stenosis nor the type of transposition influence streaming, but the position of the outflow chamber is important. When it was positioned laterally, aortic saturation was greater than pulmonary arterial saturation as compared to when the chamber was located medially.

From the pressure and oximetry data, pulmonary and systemic blood flows and resistances can be calculated, and the information about pulmonary vascular resistance is needed to make decisions regarding operation.

Selective ventriculography provides the definitive diagnosis. Injection shows the ventricle to occupy the entire area of the ventricular mass in both the anteroposterior and lateral projections. In most patients, this chamber is finely trabeculated and has the appearance of a left ventricle. The outflow chamber immediately opacifies and may be located either along the upper left cardiac border or in the midline. When in the latter position, it may be difficult to visualize. In the former, the outflow chamber is variable in size, trabeculated, and fills through the bulboventricular foramen. The aorta usually arises from the outflow chamber, and, therefore, as in patients with transposition of the great vessels, the aortic valve lies cephalad to the pulmonary valve. In a few cases, the ventricle does not have the appearance of the left ventricle but is much more heavily trabeculated, has a rounder apex, and a conus lies below both semilunar valves.[78]

Both atrioventricular valves must be identified, not only to exclude such conditions as tricuspid or mitral atresia, but to obtain information to reach decisions about operation. On ventriculography, the valves are apparent as round, unopacified filling defects. The right atrioventricular valve is usually identified by passage of the catheter into the ventricle. The left atrioventricular valve can also be identified on the levophase of the study. Following opacification of the left atrium, the ventricle is opacified and shows the same contour and opacification of both great vessels as are shown following the ventriculogram. In patients with atresia of either valve, a large shunt is present at the atrial level in contrast to its absence in patients with single ventricle.

MANAGEMENT. The initial management is directed toward the treatment of the congestive cardiac failure with digitalis and diuretics. Although a few infants will respond, especially those with some degree of pulmonary stenosis, in most, congestive cardiac failure persists. Palliation by pulmonary arterial banding is needed in many infants to reduce pulmonary blood flow and congestive cardiac failure.

Subaortic stenosis has been reported to develop, following pulmonary arterial banding, in patients with single ventricle and transposition of the great vessels.[79,91] The site of obstruction is located at the bulboventricular foramen. In both patients described by Somerville and associates,[79] chest pain was present. The patient's failure to improve clinically, despite reduction of pulmonary blood flow on thoracic roentgenogram, should also alert the physician to this possibility. Although neither paper[79,91] reported electrocardiographic changes, we have observed ST segment and T wave changes of strain. If present, the obstruction can be relieved by opening the outflow chamber and resecting the area of the bulboventricular foramen.

When the patient is older, corrective operations are available to separate the systemic and pulmonary venous returns and redirect them to the appropriate great vessel[92,93] and, in patients with pulmonary stenosis, to use of a valved conduit.[93,94] Because of this operative capability, an aggressive approach to management of infants with single ventricle is indicated.

TOTAL ANOMALOUS PULMONARY VENOUS CONNECTION WITHOUT OBSTRUCTION

Total anomalous pulmonary venous connection presents two clinical pictures. One resembles atrial septal defect, which is discussed here, and the other, in which pulmonary venous obstruction occurs, is discussed in Chapter 13.

In total anomalous pulmonary venous connection, the pulmonary veins connect to the systemic venous side of the circulation and not directly to the left atrium. Although several anatomic variations of total anomalous pulmonary venous connection coexist, the clinical picture is the same as in all admixture lesions—bidirectional shunting occurs, which in this anomaly takes place at the atrial level. The pulmonary vasculature is increased, and the patient shows cyanosis, the intensity being inversely related to the volume of pulmonary blood flow.

Since the left atrium carries a normal volume of blood and is not involved in handling the excess pulmonary blood flow, total anomalous pulmonary venous connection is the major admixture lesion in which left atrial enlargement is not found. In considering the differential diagnosis of admixture lesions, the absence of left atrial enlargement strongly suggests total anomalous pulmonary venous connection.

ANATOMY.   Review of the normal development of the pulmonary veins aids in understanding the anatomic variations of total anomalous pulmonary venous connection (Fig. 11-13). Embryologically, the lung beds develop as outpouchings of the foregut, and their early venous system is derived from the splanchnic plexus and does not connect independently with the heart. The venous blood from the lung buds drains into the anterior cardinal veins, right and left, and the umbilical-vitelline system. Ultimately, a projection, the common pulmonary vein, grows from the dorsal aspect of the left atrial wall toward the lungs and makes contact with the primitive pulmonary venous system. The common pulmonary vein and, then, the individual pulmonary veins are incorporated into the posterior wall of the left atrium, and the earlier communications of the pulmonary venous system to the systemic venous system disappear.

Total anomalous pulmonary venous connection results from a failure of the common pulmonary vein to develop fully from the left atrium or from failure of

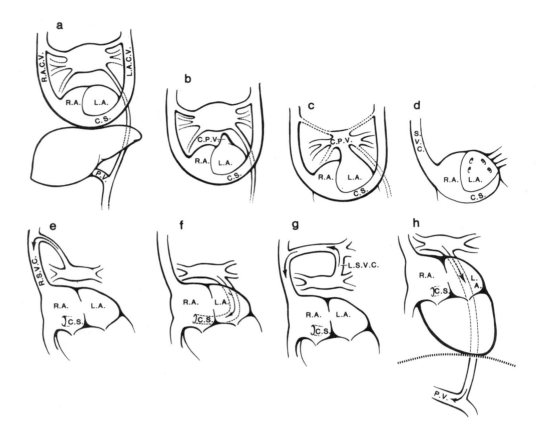

FIG. 11-13.   Development of total anomalous pulmonary venous connection. **a.** Early stage. Pulmonary venous confluence connects with right anterior cardinal vein (R.A.C.V.), left anterior cardinal vein (L.A.C.V.) through coronary sinus (C.S.) to right atrium (R.A.) and portal vein (P.V.). **b.** Common pulmonary vein (C.P.V.) extends from left atrium (L.A.) toward confluence of pulmonary veins. **c.** Communication exists between pulmonary veins and left atrium. Earlier pathways to systemic venous circulation fade. **d.** Pulmonary veins incorporated into left atrium. Several anatomic forms of total anomalous pulmonary venous connection may result. **e.** To right superior vena cava (R.S.V.C.), if communication to right anterior cardinal vein persists. **f.** To coronary sinus, if communication to proximal left anterior cardinal vein persists. **g.** To left superior vena cava (L.S.V.C.), if communication to distal left anterior cardinal vein persists. **h.** To portal vein, if communication persists to umbilical-vitelline system.

appearance, involution, or atresia of the common pulmonary vein.[95] Because of the faulty development of the common pulmonary vein, primitive connections of the pulmonary veins to the systemic venous system persist, but usually only to a single site. The common forms of total anomalous pulmonary venous connection result from persistence to (1) a remnant of right anterior cardinal vein (superior vena cava) (2) a remnant of left anterior cardinal vein (either to coronary sinus or to a left superior vena cava), or (3) the umbilical-vitelline system (to portal venous system[96,97]). Less commonly, each pulmonary vein may connect directly to the right atrium, or the pulmonary veins may connect to more than one site (mixed type).

The pulmonary veins converge behind the left atrium and form a confluence that connects by way of a venous trunk to the systemic venous system.

In the patients with total anomalous pulmonary venous connection discussed in this section, since obstruction to pulmonary venous return does not coexist, the involved venous channels are dilated from the large volume of blood flow. The right atrium, right ventricle, and pulmonary trunk are greatly dilated. In comparison, the left side of the heart appears small but, in most instances, is normal for age. An atrial septal defect is an integral part of this anomaly, and, although usually large, infrequently it may be small.[95]

Total anomalous pulmonary venous connection can coexist with other major cardiac anomalies, particularly those associated with splenic anomalies. In patients with asplenia, total anomalous pulmonary venous connection is common but rarely of major clinical significance, since ventricular septal defect and pulmonary stenosis commonly occur, so that pulmonary blood flow is reduced, and there is little flow through the pulmonary venous system. In polysplenia, total anomalous pulmonary venous connection occurs infrequently and usually directly to the right atrium.

HEMODYNAMICS.   The right atrium receives both the systemic and pulmonary venous returns, and these mix almost completely in this chamber. Blood exits from the right atrium across the tricuspid valve and through the atrial communication into the left atrium. The atrial pressures are equal, and the volume of blood entering each ventricle depends upon their relative ventricular compliances. These, in turn, are influenced principally by ventricular weight and thickness.

Since, prior to birth, the pulmonary arterial and aortic pressures are equal, the thickness of the ventricles and, therefore, relative ventricular compliances are relatively equal. At birth, the systemic and pulmonary blood flow should be similar. As the pulmonary vascular resistance decreases following birth, the pulmonary arterial pressure falls, the right ventricle thins, and the right ventricular compliance increases. These changes favor increased flow into the right ventricle, and the pulmonary blood flow becomes larger than the systemic blood flow. Thus, the hemodynamics resemble those of atrial septal defect, and the volume of pulmonary blood flow may exceed three times the systemic blood flow.

The left atrium has no direct venous return and depends upon an obligatory shunt from the right atrium. In fact, the entire systemic blood flow must pass through the atrial communication, so that the right-to-left shunt equals the systemic blood flow. The degree of cyanosis does not depend upon the volume of the right-to-left shunt but, as in any admixture lesion, is inversely related to the volume of pulmonary blood flow. Therefore, as the pulmonary blood flow increases after birth, a greater volume of pulmonary venous blood returns to mix with a relatively fixed volume of systemic return. The systemic arterial saturation usually exceeds 85 percent and may reach 92 percent.

Since the hemodynamics resemble those of atrial septal defect, the pulmonary arterial pressure should be normal, and congestive cardiac failure should not occur. Indeed, many infants with total anomalous pulmonary venous connection have normal pulmonary arterial pressures and do not develop congestive cardiac failure. Yet, infants may present with congestive cardiac failure and have elevated pulmonary arterial pressures. Although pulmonary arterial pressure is elevated in infants with obstructed total anomalous pulmonary venous connection, why it occurs in infants without obstruction is unknown. Some infants with unobstructed total anomalous pulmonary venous connection develop pulmonary arteriolar changes,[98,99] in which increased arterial musculature extends into small arteries. The incidence and severity of these changes increase with age, but they can occur in early infancy. Eight of 53 infants with total anomalous pulmonary venous connection, less than 8 months of age, had grade III or IV Heath-Edwards changes in the lungs.[99]

Pulmonary arterial pressure could be elevated in two ways. If the anomalously connecting vein is small in comparison to the volume of pulmonary blood flow, pulmonary venous pressure will become elevated to some degree, perhaps only slightly, but may cause pulmonary hypertension. If the atrial communication were small, left ventricular filling would be impaired and cardiac output reduced. The small orifice would also have profound effects upon the right side of the heart, elevating right atrial pressure. Elevated right atrial pressure would raise pulmonary venous and pulmonary arterial pressures. Because of Starling's law, the increased atrial pressure would increase right ventricular contractility, raising right ventricular output and increasing pulmonary blood flow. Therefore, with a small communication, the right ventricle ejects an increased volume of blood at a higher systolic pressure, and right ventricular failure results. The occurrence of a small atrial communication in total anomalous pulmonary venous connection is, however, uncommon.[100]

CLINICAL FEATURES.   The major clinical features are failure to thrive, cyanosis, and congestive cardiac failure.[101-103] The infants grow slowly because of the combination of cyanosis and congestive cardiac failure. They exhibit breathlessness on feeding, a manifestation of congestive cardiac failure.

Although cyanosis is expected, the age of appearance of this symptom is variable. Gathman and Nadas[103] reported 61 percent of their patients had cyanosis by 1 month of age, and in most of these, it was noted at birth. In almost all, cyanosis is discovered by 1 year of age. Because the degree of systemic desaturation is mild, cyanosis may escape casual observation. Often, the infant appears dusky and becomes cyanotic only during exertion, such as crying.

Congestive cardiac failure occurred by 1 month of age in 41 percent of patients described by Gathman and Nadas,[103] predominantly in those with pulmonary hypertension. It developed in most patients by 1 year of age.

On physical examination, the infants appear thin and undernourished. Cyanosis is usually minimal, unless there is pulmonary infection or congestive cardiac failure. Cardiac enlargement is evident as displacement of the cardiac apex inferiorly and leftward. Precordial activity is increased, and there is a right ventricular heave. A precordial bulge may develop in infants.

As in any patient with increased blood flow across the tricuspid valve, the first heart sound (tricuspid component) is accentuated along the lower left sternal border. Although fixed splitting of the second heart sound would be expected, normal respiratory variation is frequently found.[102,103] The pulmonary component of the second heart sound is accentuated in infants with pulmonary hypertension. A grade 2–3/6 pulmonary systolic ejection murmur is usually found, as is a middiastolic low-pitched murmur along the lower left sternal border. In infants with total anomalous pulmonary venous connection to the left superior vena cava, there may be a continuous murmur over the upper anterior right or left chest below the clavicles.

ELECTROCARDIOGRAM.   The electrocardiogram (Fig. 11-14) shows a QRS axis between $+90$ and $+210°$, the average being $+140°$.[103] Right atrial enlargement, manifested by tall peaked P waves, is found in lead II or leads V_1 and V_2. The precordial leads show a pattern of right ventricular hypertrophy. In half of the patients, a qR pattern is present in leads V_4R and V_1 and occurs independently of the site of pulmonary venous connection or the level of pulmonary arterial pressure. In the other half, lead V_1 shows an rR' or rSR' pattern instead. In the first months of life, the T waves may be upright in the right precordial leads and subsequently inverted. Patients with elevated pulmonary vascular resistance tend to have greater degrees of right ventricular hypertrophy,[104] manifested by taller R wave voltages in the right precordial leads.

THORACIC ROENTGENOGRAM.   Moderate to marked cardiomegaly is present and is caused by right atrial and right ventricular enlargement. The pulmonary trunk is prominent. The pulmonary arterial vasculature is increased.

Unlike most other conditions grouped as admixture lesions, left atrial enlargement is not found, since the volume flow through this chamber is normal.

In certain anatomic forms of total anomalous pulmonary venous connection, the cardiac contour may be distinctive enough to permit definition of the site of anomalous connection of the pulmonary veins. In total anomalous pulmonary venous connection to the left superior vena cava, the cardiac silhouette characteristically appears as a figure-of-eight or a snowman (Fig. 11-15a). The lower portion of the snowman represents the bulk of the heart, and the upper portion is formed by the enlarged left superior vena cava, innominate vein, and right superior vena cava. These venous structures are dilated, since they are carrying the large volume of pulmonary blood flow. This cardiac contour may be obscured until 6 months of age by the thymus. The superior mediastinum is normally prominent in neonates and young infants. The enlarged venous structures may be mistakenly diagnosed as the thymus, but the border of the

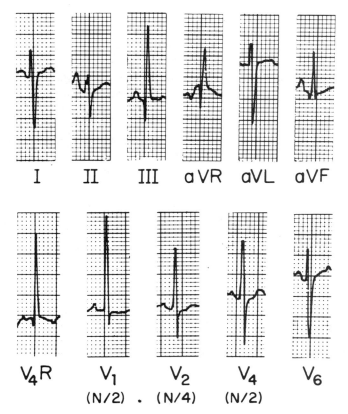

I   II   III   aVR   aVL   aVF

V₄R   V₁   V₂   V₄   V₆
      (N/2) . (N/4) (N/2)

FIG. 11-14. Electrocardiogram of 3-month-old infant with total anomalous pulmonary venous connection. Right atrial enlargement. QRS axis is +150°. Right ventricular hypertrophy. N/2, half-standardization; N/4, quarter-standardization.

enlarged venous structures is smoother and not as distinct as the thymus.

In patients with total anomalous pulmonary venous connection to the right superior vena cava, the supracardiac shadow on the right side is prominent because the superior vena cava is dilated (Fig. 11-15b). In patients with total anomalous pulmonary venous connection to the coronary sinus, the coronary sinus dilates and indents the anterior wall of the barium-filled esophagus. It might be confused with the effects of an enlarged left atrium but occurs at a site lower than expected for the left atrium.

ECHOCARDIOGRAM. The echocardiogram provides valuable diagnostic clues of total anomalous pulmonary venous connection and helps differentiate it from other cyanotic cardiac conditions.

Because total anomalous pulmonary venous connection places excessive

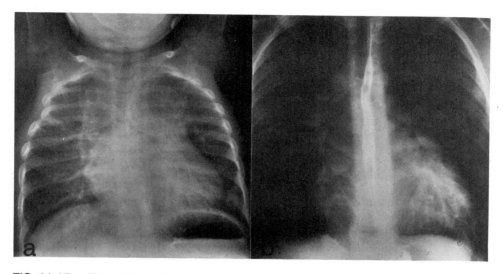

FIG. 11-15.   Thoracic roentgenograms, posteroanterior view, of total anomalous pulmonary venous connection. **a.** Connection to left superior vena cava, giving figure-of-eight appearance. **b.** Connection to right superior vena cava. Prominence of right superior vena cava.

volume in the right ventricle, paradoxical movement of the interventricular septum is expected,[105] but may not be found, in the neonatal period[106] because the volume of pulmonary blood flow has not increased sufficiently at this age.

The left atrium has a normal diameter. The most diagnostic feature of total anomalous pulmonary venous connection is the presence of an echo-free space posterior to the left atrium (Fig. 11-16). This presumably represents the confluence of the pulmonary veins, and since the veins do not always coalesce behind the left atrium, it is not uniformly present. Bozio and Davignon[106] have found an echo-free space behind the left atrium in normal neonates and indicate caution in interpreting this finding.

Total anomalous pulmonary venous connection to the coronary sinus can be recognized as a distinct entity, since in this condition the enlarged coronary sinus can be identified as a linear echo recorded behind the anterior mitral valve leaflet and posterior aortic wall.[107]

CARDIAC CATHETERIZATION AND ANGIOCARDIOGRAM.   At the time of cardiac catheterization, information must be sought that assists in making decisions regarding management and provides details for the surgeon.

The important information obtained at cardiac catheterization is:

1. Site of connection of each pulmonary vein
2. Size of atrial communication
3. Level of pulmonary arterial pressure

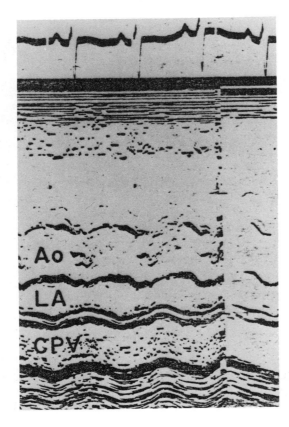

FIG. 11-16. Echocardiogram of total anomalous pulmonary venous connection to coronary sinus. Echo-free space representing common pulmonary vein (CPV) outlined behind left atrium (LA). Ao, aorta.

4. Presence of pulmonary venous obstruction
5. Presence of coexistent conditions

In infants, the inguinal approach facilitates passage of the catheter through the foramen ovale and often permits passage of the catheter into the anomalously connecting pulmonary veins, as in patients with connection to the left superior vena cava or directly to the right atrium. If anomalously connecting veins are catheterized, angiography should be performed from the site, and careful withdrawal pressure tracings should be made to the right atrium to identify sites of obstruction.

Oximetry series through the right side of the heart show a marked increase of oxygen saturation at the site at which the pulmonary venous blood enters the right side of the circulation. This increase may occur in the innominate vein (anomalous connection to the left superior vena cava), right superior vena cava, or within the right atrium (anomalous connection of the coronary sinus or directly to the right atrium). There is also evidence of a right-to-left shunt at the atrial level, with a lower than normal oxygen saturation being found in the left atrium and left ventricle. Because total anomalous pulmonary venous connection is an admixture lesion, the oxygen saturation would be expected to be identical in each cardiac chamber, but this occurs in only half of the infants. In the other half, the pulmonary arterial saturation is higher than the systemic arterial saturation. When the anomalous pulmonary venous connection is directly to the right atrium or to the coronary sinus, the oxygen saturations are more likely to be identical, but when the connection occurs to either superior vena cava, a difference is usually found. In such patients, the blood from the superior vena cava, having a higher oxygen saturation, flows preferentially into the right ventricle, while the inferior vena caval blood flows preferentially into the atrium. The oxygen saturation difference between the aorta and pulmonary artery is usually less than 5 percent but may occasionally reach 10 percent.

It is difficult to accurately calculate systemic blood flow because of the difficulties in obtaining a reliable mixed venous oxygen sample. This is more of a problem with connection to the superior vena cava than with connection to the right atrium or coronary sinus. Yet, even in the two latter instances, there may be a reflux of the fully saturated blood into the inferior vena cava.

The systemic arterial oxygen saturation is inversely related to the volume of pulmonary blood flow and may be as high as 92 percent in infants with greatly increased pulmonary blood flow.

Three specific pressure measurements are necessary in evaluation of an infant with total anomalous pulmonary venous connection. The pulmonary arterial wedge pressure must be measured to determine if pulmonary venous return is obstructed. An alternative is the measurement of pulmonary venous pressure by passing the catheter into the veins, as can be done most easily in patients with connection to the left superior vena cava or to the right atrium. In patients in whom the catheter has been passed into the connecting vein, a careful pressure tracing should be recorded as the catheter is withdrawn to the systemic venous system. A pressure difference may be recorded, as in instances when the left superior vena cava passes between the left main stem bronchus and the left pulmonary artery.

The pulmonary arterial pressure may be elevated from various factors, such as pulmonary arteriolar changes, increased pulmonary blood flow, and elevated pulmonary venous pressure. The pulmonary arterial pressure may be elevated to systemic levels or greater but only in infants with pulmonary venous obstruction. In patients without pulmonary venous obstruction but with congestive cardiac failure, the pulmonary arterial systolic pressure ranges between 40 and 80 mm Hg. In many infants, it is normal. As in patients with atrial septal defect, a pressure difference may be found across the pulmonary outflow area.

Atrial pressure should also be carefully measured. The right atrial pressure may be normal or elevated to a level of twice normal. The atrial pressures may be equal, or right atrial pressure may be greater than left atrial pressure,[100,103,108] but rarely by more than 3 mm Hg. This pressure difference probably reflects a small atrial communication, but its significance is difficult to assess fully because the right atrium is very compliant. Since atrial pressures also depend upon ventricular compliances, if the compliances are equal, atrial pressures are the same even in the presence of a small defect.

El-Said and associates[100] studied the relationship between atrial pressure gradients and anatomic details of the atrial septum and found that only a small gradient may be associated with a small atrial communication. They believed that infants with a small atrial communication have symptoms early and need balloon atrial septostomy at the time of cardiac catheterization. Others[109-111] have also indicated the beneficial effects of balloon atrial septostomy in infants with total anomalous pulmonary venous connection. At the time of initial cardiac catheterization, we insert a balloon-tipped catheter and pass it into the left atrium. Following inflation, the balloon is withdrawn across the atrial septum to determine if resistance is met at the atrial septum. If there is resistance, a balloon atrial septostomy is performed, but if done after 3 months of age, it is unlikely to be successful.

Selective pulmonary angiography should be performed to identify the site of the connection of each of the pulmonary veins. The volume of pulmonary blood flow is greatly increased. Therefore, a large volume of opaque medium should be injected at a rapid rate. Following opacification of the pulmonary veins, the connecting venous channel and the right side of the heart are subsequently visualized. The atrial shunt is demonstrated by opacification of the left atrium. The forms of total anomalous pulmonary venous connection connecting to the left superior vena cava or right superior vena cava are usually clearly visualized (Fig. 11-17). In total anomalous pulmonary venous connection to the coronary sinus, the dilated coronary sinus will be visualized as a large round mass appearing posteriorly on the lateral view and as an ovoid mass immediately to the left of the spine, slightly above the diaphragm. It may be difficult to distinguish total anomalous pulmonary venous connection directly to the right atrium from the atrial septal defect. The presence of a right-to-left atrial shunt and the course of the left pulmonary veins toward the midline distinguish these two conditions.

MANAGEMENT.   Clarke and associates[112] indicate that improved mortality for infants with total anomalous pulmonary venous connection can be accomplished by (1) early recognition and referral, (2) prompt cardiac catheterization, (3) vigorous preoperative care, (4) early complete correction, and (5) intensive postoperative care. Total anomalous pulmonary venous connection is usually recognized in infancy, and many infants manifest congestive cardiac failure, requiring treatment with digitalis and diuretics. Some infants respond well to such treatment, but many show persistent congestive cardiac failure.

Regardless of response to digitalization, cardiac catheterization should be performed to obtain important data. At the time of cardiac catheterization, we believe balloon atrial septostomy should be performed.

Following initiation of medical management and cardiac catheterization, decisions must be reached regarding corrective operation. The indication and

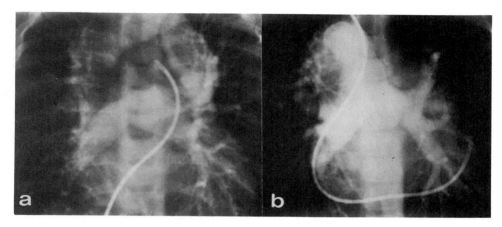

FIG. 11-17. Angiocardiogram, anteroposterior view, of total anomalous pulmonary venous connection. **a.** Connection to left superior vena cava. Late film. Opacification of pulmonary veins, left superior vena cava, and innominate vein. **b.** Connection to right superior vena cava. Late film. Opacification of pulmonary veins and, then, right superior vena cava.

timing for operation vary with the experience of an institution, but, in general, operations are performed during infancy because of the high mortality rate in unoperated patients. Gersony and associates[108] indicate that these infants should not be managed medically for a long period if they are symptomatic.

El-Said and co-workers[100] recommend prolonged medical treatment and delaying corrective operation until at least 6 months of age, unless pulmonary edema persists despite adequate medical management and an adequate atrial septal defect. Wukasch and associates[113] also recommend medical treatment until 6 months of age but realize that congestive cardiac failure may dictate earlier correction.

The operative mortality for total anomalous pulmonary venous connection in infancy has been reported from 35 to 50 percent.[100,101,112–114] Various techniques have been used. Dillard and associates[115] described the successful use of hypothermia and total circulatory arrest for correction of total anomalous pulmonary venous connection for infants, while Castaneda and co-workers[116] use deep hypothermia and limited cardiopulmonary bypass. In contrast, Gersony and associates[108] use normothermia.

Various factors have been investigated to explain this high operative mortality. The role of age, at the time of operation, upon mortality is unclear. The site of anomalous connection influences the operative mortality. A higher mortality rate occurs in infants with connection to the superior vena cava,[112,114] particularly to the right superior vena cava,[100,113] than in infants with connection to the coronary sinus or directly to the right atrium.[112]

El-Said and associates[100] found that the level of systemic arterial oxygen saturation, pulmonary vascular resistance, pulmonary blood flow, or pulmonary arterial pressure did not correlate with operative mortality. Breckenridge and associates[114] and Clarke and co-workers[112] report that severity of pulmonary hypertension does not influence operative mortality, but Behrendt et al.[101] and Wukasch et al.[113] believe that pulmonary hypertension is associated with a higher operative mortality.

Whether left atrial size influences operative mortality has long been a matter of conjecture. Clarke et al.[112] and Breckenridge et al.[114] indicate that it may be a factor, but it is difficult to quantitate left atrial size at autopsy. Recent hemodynamic studies[117] in the postoperative period of infants with total anomalous pulmonary venous connection indicate that reduced left atrial size and compliance may be major factors in the high mortality rate. Parr and associates[117] have carefully monitored nine infants aged 4 months or less in the postoperative period and have determined atrial pressure and cardiac index. Cardiac index and stroke index were low and gradually increased postoperatively. Left atrial volume fluctuated abnormally, suggesting that the left atrial volume was small in relation to the ventricular stroke volume.

Mathew and co-workers[118] studied cardiac volumes angiographically in 12 infants before and following corrective operation for total anomalous pulmonary venous connection. The left ventricular volume was normal, but the ejection fraction of 57 percent was low. Although left atrial volume was 53 percent of predicted normal, they felt that the small left atrial size was not a factor in the operative success. The volume of left atrial appendix was normal, suggesting that reduced left atrial size was related to failure of incorporation of the common pulmonary vein. The small left atrial size may also be the result of hemodynamic factors. During ventricular systole, with the atrioventricular valves closed, filling of the atria depends upon the compliances of the atria, and, therefore, filling of the right atrium is favored over the left atrium. In addition, a restrictive atrial septal communication would limit left atrial filling and, therefore, left atrial size. The finding that left atrial v waves are lower than a waves supports the concept of reduced left atrial filling during systole. In spite of small left atrial volume, left ventricular volumes are normal. Therefore, the left atrium probably functions as a conduit to left ventricular filling, the flow running from the right atrium. This argues for the need of an adequate atrial communication.

From our data and that of others,[108,113,115,116] the left atrium seems of adequate size and not a limiting factor to operative success. At operation, a Dacron or pericardial patch to close the atrial septum can be placed to the right of the atrial septum in an effort to enlarge the left atrium.

Postoperatively, the infants require respiratory support and intensive monitoring of the acid-base and fluid balance.[108]

Silove and co-workers[119] described spontaneous functional closure of an interatrial communication in total anomalous pulmonary venous connection following operative correction, suggesting that the atrial septal defect may not need to be corrected at the time of correction of the confluence to the left atrium.

Whight and others[120] have studied the long-term results following correction of total anomalous pulmonary venous connection and found a significant late mortality and a high incidence of pulmonary venous obstruction in infants with connection to the coronary sinus.

REFERENCES

Persistent Truncus Arteriosus

1. Crupi G, Macartney FJ, Anderson RH: Persistent truncus arteriosus. A study of 66 autopsy cases with special reference to definition and morphogenesis. Am J Cardiol 40:569, 1977
2. Calder L, Van Praagh R, Van Praagh S, et al.: Truncus arteriosus communis. Clinical, angiocardiographic, and pathologic findings in 100 patients. Am Heart J 92:23, 1976
3. Becker AE, Becker MJ, Edwards JE: Pathology of the semilunar valve in persistent truncus arteriosus. J Thorac Cardiovasc Surg 62:16, 1971
4. Farooki ZQ, Brough JA, Green EW: Truncal valve stenosis—a case report. J Pediatr 84:305, 1974
5. Ledbetter MK, Tandon R, Titus JL, Edwards JE: Stenotic semilunar valve in persistent truncus arteriosus. Chest 69:182, 1976
6. Gelband H, Van Meter S, Gersony WM: Truncal valve abnormalities in infants with persistent truncus arteriosus. A clinicopathologic study. Circulation 45:397, 1972
7. Anderson KR, McGoon DC, Lie JT: Surgical significance of the coronary arterial anatomy in truncus arteriosus communis. Am J Cardiol 41:76, 1978
8. Shrivastava S, Edwards JE: Coronary arterial origin in persistent truncus arteriosus. Circulation 55:551, 1977
9. Marcelletti C, McGoon DC, Mair DD: The natural history of truncus arteriosus. Circulation 54:108, 1976
10. Collett RW, Edwards JE: Persistent truncus arteriosus: A classification according to anatomic types. Surg Clin North Am 29:1245, 1949
11. Tandon R, Hauck AJ, Nadas AS: Persistent truncus arteriosus. A clinical, hemodynamic, and autopsy study of nineteen cases. Circulation 28:1050, 1963
12. Victoria BE, Krovetz LJ, Elliott LP et al.: Persistent truncus arteriosus in infancy. A study of 14 cases. Am Heart J 77:13, 1969
13. Anderson RC, Obata W, Lillehei CW: Truncus arteriosus. Clinical study of fourteen cases. Circulation 16:586, 1957
14. Chung KJ, Alexson CG, Manning JA, Gramiak R: Echocardiography in truncus arteriosus. The value of pulmonic valve detection. Circulation 48:281, 1973
15. Orsmond GS, Moller JH, Bessinger FB Jr, Lawrence C, Edwards JE: Echocardiographic-pathologic correlations in young infants with congenital heart disease. Unpublished observations
16. Assad-Morell JL, Seward JB, Tajik AJ, et al.: Echo-phonocardiographic and contrast studies in conditions associated with systemic arterial trunk overriding the ventricular septum. Truncus arteriosus, tetralogy of Fallot, and pulmonary atresia with ventricular septal defect. Circulation 53:663, 1976
17. Singh AK, deLeval MR, Pincott JR, Stark J: Pulmonary artery banding for truncus arteriosus in the first year of life. Circulation 54 [Suppl 3]:17, 1976
18. Poirier RA, Berman MA, Stansel HC Jr: Current status of the surgical treatment of truncus arteriosus. J Thorac Cardiovasc Surg 69:169, 1975

19. Mahle S, Nicoloff DM, Knight L, Moller JH: Pulmonary artery banding: Long-term results in 63 patients. Ann Thorac Surg 27:216, 1978

20. McFaul RC, Mair DD, Feldt RH, Ritter DG, McGoon DC: Truncus arteriosus and previous pulmonary arterial banding: Clinical and hemodynamic assessment. Am J Cardiol 38:626, 1976

21. Wallace RB, Rastelli GC, Ongley PA, Titus JL, McGoon DC: Complete repair of truncus arteriosus defects. J Thorac Cardiovasc Surg 57:95, 1969

22. Appelbaum A, Bargeron LM Jr, Pacifico AD, Kirklin JW: Surgical treatment of truncus arteriosus, with emphasis on infants and small children. J Thorac Cardiovasc Surg 71:436, 1976

23. Sullivan H, Sulayman R, Replogle R, Arcilla RA: Surgical correction of truncus arteriosus in infancy. Am J Cardiol 38:113, 1976

24. Marcelletti C, McGoon DC, Danielson GK, Wallace RB, Mair DD: Early and late results of surgical repair of truncus arteriosus. Circulation 55:636, 1977

25. Ebert PA, Robinson SJ, Stanger P, Engle MA: Pulmonary artery conduits in infants younger than six months of age. J Thorac Cardiovasc Surg 72:351, 1976

26. Stark J, Gandhi D, deLeval M, Macartney F, Taylor JFN: Surgical treatment of persistent truncus arteriosus in the first year of life. Br Heart J 40:1280, 1978

Complete Transposition of the Great Vessels

27. Campbell M: Incidence of cardiac malformations at birth and later, and neonatal mortality. Br Heart J 35:189, 1973

28. Nadas AS, Fyler DC: Pediatric Cardiology, 3rd ed. Philadelphia, Saunders, 1972, p 609

29. Keith JD, Rowe RD, Vlad P: Heart Disease in Infancy and Childhood. New York, Macmillan, 1958

30. Fanconi G: Die Transposition der grosseu Gefasse (das charakteristische Rontgenbild). Arch Kinderheilk 95:202, 1932

31. Taussig HB: Complete transposition of the great vessels. Clinical and pathologic features. Am Heart J 16:728, 1938

32. Mustard WT: Successful two-stage correction of transposition of the great vessels. Surgery 55:469, 1964

33. Keith A: The Hunterian lectures on malformations of the heart. Lancet 177:433, 1909

34. Lev M, Saphir O: A theory of transposition of the arterial trunks based on the phylogenetic and ontogenetic developments of the heart. Arch Pathol 39:172, 1945

35. Van Praagh R, Van Praagh S: Isolated ventricular inversion. A consideration of morphogenesis, definition and diagnosis of nontransposed and transposed great arteries. Am J Cardiol 17:395, 1966

36. Goor DA, Edwards JE: The spectrum of transposition of the great arteries. With specific reference to developmental anatomy of the conus. Circulation 48:406, 1973

37. Kidd BSL, Tyrell MJ, Pickering D: Transposition 1969. In Kidd BSL, Keith JD (eds): The Natural History and Progress in Treatment of Congenital Heart Defects. Springfield, Ill, Thomas, 1971, p 128

38. Rowe RD, Mehrizi A: The Neonate With Congenital Heart Disease. Philadelphia, Saunders, 1968, p 151

39. Liebman J, Cullum L, Belloc NB: Natural history of transposition of the great arteries. Anatomy and birth and death characteristics. Circulation 40:237, 1969

40. Mehrizi A, Drash A: Birth weight of infants with cyanotic and acyanotic congenital malformations of the heart. J Pediatr 59:715, 1961

41. Elliott LP, Anderson RC, Tuna N, Adams P Jr, Neufeld HN: Complete transposition of the great vessels. II. An electrocardiographic analysis. Circulation 27:1118, 1963

42. Solinger R, Elbl F, Minhas K: Deductive echocardiographic analysis in infants with congenital heart disease. Circulation 50:1072, 1974
43. Kidd BSL, Tyrell MJ, Pickering D: Transposition 1969. In Kidd BSL, Keith JD, (eds): The Natural History and Progress in Treatment of Congenital Heart Defects. Springfield, Ill, Thomas, 1971, p 130
44. Rashkind WJ, Miller WW: Creation of an atrial septal defect without thoracotomy. A palliative approach to complete transposition of the great arteries. JAMA 196:991, 1966
45. Rashkind WJ, Miller WW: Transposition of the great arteries. Results of palliation by balloon atrioseptostomy in thirty-one infants. Circulation 38:453, 1968
46. Baker F, Baker L, Zoltun R, Zuberbuhler JR: Effectiveness of the Rashkind procedure in transposition of the great arteries in infants. Circulation 43 [Suppl 1]:1, 1971
47. Gutgesell HP, McNamara DG: Transposition of the great arteries. Results of treatment with early palliation and late intracardiac repair. Circulation 51:32, 1975
48. Rashkind WJ: The complications of balloon atrioseptostomy. J Pediatr 76:649, 1970
49. Blalock A, Hanlon CR: The surgical treatment of complete transposition of the aorta and pulmonary artery. Surg Gynecol Obstet 90:1, 1950
50. Mustard WT, Chute AL, Keith JD, et al.: A surgical approach to transposition of the great vessels with extracorporeal circuit. Surgery 36:39, 1954
51. Blalock A: A consideration of some of the problems in cardiovascular surgery. J Thorac Cardiovasc Surg 21:543, 1951
52. Lillehei CW, Varco RL: Certain physiologic, pathologic, and surgical features of complete transposition of the great vessels. Surgery 34:376, 1953
53. Tynan M, Aberdeen E, Stark J: Tricuspid incompetence after the Mustard operation for transposition of the great arteries. Circulation 45 [Suppl 1]:111, 1972
54. Clarkson PM, Neutze JM, Barratt-Boyes BG, Brandt PWT: Late postoperative hemodynamic results and cineangiocardiographic findings after Mustard atrial baffle repair for transposition of the great arteries. Circulation 53:525, 1976
55. Park SC, Weiss FH, Siewers RD, et al.: Continuous murmur following Mustard operation for transposition of the great arteries. A sign of pulmonary venous obstruction. Circulation 54:684, 1976
56. Quaegebeur JM, Rohmer J, Brom AG: Revival of the Senning operation in the treatment of transposition of the great arteries. Preliminary report on recent experience. Thorax 32:517, 1977
57. Jarmakani JMM, Canent RV Jr: Preoperative and postoperative right ventricular function in children with transposition of the great vessels. Circulation 50 [Suppl 2]:39, 1974
58. Jatene AD, Fontes VF, Paulista PP, et al.: Anatomic correction of transposition of the vessels. J Thorac Cardiovasc Surg 72:364, 1976
59. Taussig HB, Bing RJ: Complete transposition of the aorta and a levoposition of the pulmonary artery. Am Heart J 37:551, 1949
60. Neufeld HN, Lucas RV Jr, Lester RG, et al.: Origin of both great vessels from the right ventricle without pulmonary stenosis. Br Heart J 24:393, 1962
61. Zamora R, Moller JH, Edwards JE: Double-outlet right ventricle. Anatomic types and associated anomalies. Chest 68:672, 1975
62 Tandon R, Moller JH, Edwards JE: Communication of mitral valve with both ventricles associated with double outlet right ventricle. Circulation 48:904, 1973
63. Kitamura N, Takaoi A, Ando M, Mai I, Konno S: Taussig-Bing heart with mitral valve straddling. Case reports and postmortem study. Circulation 49:761, 1974
64. Cameron AH, Acerete F, Quero M, Castro MC: Double outlet right ventricle. Study of 27 cases. Br Heart J 38,1124, 1976

65. Neufeld HN, DuShane JW, Wood EH, Kirklin JW, Edwards JE: Origin of both great vessels from the right ventricle. I. Without pulmonary stenosis. Circulation 23:399, 1961
66. Bharati S, Lev M: The conduction system in double outlet right ventricle with subpulmonic ventricular septal defect and related hearts (the Taussig-Bing group). Circulation 54:459, 1976

Tricuspid Atresia

67. Tandon R, Edwards JE: Tricuspid atresia. J Thorac Cardiovasc Surg 67:530, 1974
68. Kessler A, Adams P: Association of transposition of the great vessels and rudimentary right ventricle, with and without tricuspid atresia. Pediatrics 19:851, 1957
69. Marcano BA, Riemenschneider TA, Ruttenberg HD, Goldberg ST, Gyepes M: Tricuspid atresia with increased pulmonary blood flow. An analysis of 13 cases. Circulation 40:399, 1969
70. Williams WG, Rubis L, Fowler RS, et al.: Tricuspid atresia: Results of treatment in 160 children. Am J Cardiol 38:235, 1976
71. Davachi F, Lucas RV Jr., Moller JH: The electrocardiogram and vectorcardiogram in tricuspid atresia. Correlation with pathologic anatomy. Am J Cardiol 25:18, 1970
72. Dick M, Fyler DC, Nadas AS: Tricuspid atresia: Clinical course in 101 patients. Am J Cardiol 35:327, 1975
73. Folger GM Jr, Witham AC, Ellison RG: Tricuspid atresia with transposition of the great vessels. J Pediatr 74:946, 1969

Single Ventricle without Pulmonary Stenosis

74. Van Praagh R, Van Praagh S, Vlad P, Keith JD: Diagnosis of the anatomic types of single or common ventricle. Am J Cardiol 15:345, 1965
75. Van Praagh R, Ongley PA, Swan HJC: Anatomic types of single or common ventricle in man. Morphologic and geometric aspects of 60 necropsied cases. Am J Cardiol 13:367, 1964
76. Lev M, Liberthson RR, Kirkpatrick JR, Eckner FAO, Arcilla RA: Single (primitive) ventricle. Circulation 39:577, 1969
77. Marin-Garcia J, Tandon R, Moller JH, Edwards JE: Common (single) ventricle with normally related great vessels. Circulation 49:565, 1974
78. Marin-Garcia J, Tandon R, Moller JH, Edwards JE: Single ventricle with transposition. Circulation 49:994, 1974
79. Somerville J, Becu L, Ross D: Common ventricle with acquired subaortic obstruction. Am J Cardiol 34:206, 1974
80. Rahimtoola SH, Ongley PA, Swan HJC: The hemodynamics of common (or single) ventricle. Circulation 34:14, 1966
81. Morgan AD, Krovetz LJ, Schiebler GL: Electrovectorcardiographic analysis of nine cases of single ventricle with the great vessel arrangement of congenitally corrected transposition. In Hoffman I, Taymor RC (eds): Vectorcardiography. Philadelphia, Lippincott, 1966, pp 327–336
82. Gessner IH, Elliott LP, Schiebler GL, Van Mierop LHS, Miller BL: The vectorcardiogram in double inlet left ventricle, with and without ventricular inversion. In Hoffman I, Hamby RI, Glassman E (eds): Vectorcardiography 2. Philadelphia, Lippincott, 1971, pp 624–637
83. Davachi F, Moller JH: The electrocardiogram and vectorcardiogram in single ventricle. Anatomic correlations. Am J Cardiol 23:19, 1969

84. Guller B, Mair DD, Ritter DG, Smith RE: Frank vectorcardiogram in common ventricle: Correlation with anatomic findings. Am Heart J 90:290, 1975
85. Hallermann FJ, Davis GD, Ritter DG, Kincaid OW: Roentgenographic features of common ventricle. Radiology 87:109, 1966
86. Carey LS, Ruttenberg HD: Roentgenographic features of common ventricle with inversion of the infundibulum. Corrected transposition with rudimentary left ventricle. Am J Roentgenol Radium Ther Nucl Med 92:652, 1964
87. Seward JB, Tajik AJ, Hagler DJ, et al.: Echocardiogram in common (single) ventricle: Angiographic-anatomic correlation. Am J Cardiol 39:217, 1977
88. Seward JB, Tajik AJ, Hagler DJ, Ritter DG: Contrast echocardiography in single or common ventricle. Circulation 55:513, 1977
89. Bini RM, Bloom KR, Culham JAG, et al.: The reliability and practicality of single crystal echocardiography in the evaluation of single ventricle. Angiographic and pathological correlates. Circulation 57:269, 1978
90. Macartney FJ, Partridge JB, Scott O, Deverall PB: Common or single ventricle: An angiocardiographic and hemodynamic study of 42 patients. Circulation 53:543, 1976
91. Freedom RM, Sondheimer H, Dische R, Rowe RD: Development of "subaortic stenosis" after pulmonary arterial banding for common ventricle. Am J Cardiol 39:78, 1977
92. Edie RN, Ellis K, Gersony WM, et al.: Surgical repair of single ventricle. J Thorac Cardiovasc Surg 66:350, 1973
93. McGoon DC, Danielson GK, Ritter DG, et al.: Correction of the univentricular heart having two atrioventricular valves. J Thorac Cardiovasc Surg 74:218, 1977
94. Yacoub MH, Radley-Smith R: Use of a valved conduit from right atrium to pulmonary artery for "correction" of single ventricle. Circulation 54 [Suppl]:63, 1976

Total Anomalous Pulmonary Venous Connection

95. Delisle G, Ando M, Calder AL, et al.: Total anomalous pulmonary venous connection: Report of 93 autopsied cases with emphasis on diagnostic and surgical consideration. Am Heart J 91:99, 1976
96. Blake HA, Hall RJ, Manion WC: Anomalous pulmonary venous return. Circulation 32:406, 1965
97. Burroughs JT, Edwards JE: Total anomalous pulmonary venous connection. Am Heart J 59:913, 1960
98. Haworth SG, Reid L: Structural study of pulmonary circulation and of heart in total anomalous pulmonary venous return in early infancy. Br Heart J 39:80, 1977
99. Wilson A, Newfeld EA, Paul MH: The pulmonary vascular bed in total anomalous pulmonary venous drainage. Circulation 56 [Suppl 3]:193, 1977 (Abstr)
100. El-Said G, Mullins CE, McNamara DG: Management of total anomalous pulmonary venous return. Circulation 45:1240, 1972
101. Behrendt DM, Aberdeen E, Waterston DJ, Bonham-Carter RE: Total anomalous pulmonary venous drainage in infants. I. Clinical and hemodynamic findings, methods, and results of operation in 37 cases. Circulation 46:347, 1972
102. Bonham-Carter RE, Capriles M, Noe Y: Total anomalous pulmonary venous drainage. A clinical and anatomical study of 75 children. Br Heart J 31:45, 1969
103. Gathman GE, Nadas AS: Total anomalous pulmonary venous connection. Clinical and physiologic observations of 75 pediatric patients. Circulation 42:143, 1970
104. Gessner IH, Krovetz LJ, Wheat MW Jr, Shanklin DR, Schiebler GL: Total anomalous pulmonary venous connection. Electrovectorcardiographic, hemo-

dynamic, and anatomic correlations in 11 cases. Am Heart J 68:459, 1964

105. Tajik AJ, Gau GT, Schattenberg TT: Echocardiogram in total anomalous pulmonary venous drainage. Mayo Clin Proc 47:247, 1972

106. Bozio A, Davignon A: Interpreting the echocardiogram in TAPVC. Circulation 53:1041, 1976

107. Orsmond GS, Ruttenberg HD, Bessinger FB, Moller JH: Echocardiographic features of total anomalous pulmonary venous connection to the coronary sinus. Am J Cardiol 41:597, 1978

108. Gersony WM, Bowman FO Jr, Steeg CN, et al.: Management of total anomalous pulmonary venous drainage in early infancy. Circulation 43 [Suppl 1]:19, 1971

109. Mullins CE, El-Said GM, Neches WH et al.: Balloon atrial septostomy for total anomalous pulmonary venous return. Br Heart J 35:752, 1973

110. Serratto M, Bucheleres HG, Bicoff P, Miller RA, Hastreiter AR: Palliative balloon atrial septostomy for total anomalous pulmonary venous connection in infancy. J Pediatr 73:734, 1968

111. Miller WW, Rashkind WJ, Miller RA, et al.: Total anomalous pulmonary venous return: Effective palliation of critically ill infants by balloon atrial septostomy. Circulation 36 [Suppl 2]:189, 1967

112. Clarke DR, Stark J, deLeval M, Pincott JR, Taylor JFN: Total anomalous pulmonary venous drainage in infancy. Br Heart J 39:436, 1977

113. Wukasch DC, Deutsch M, Real GJ, Hallman GL, Cooley DA: Total anomalous pulmonary venous return. Review of 125 patients treated surgically. Ann Thorac Surg 19:622, 1975

114. Breckenridge IM, deLeval M, Stark J, Waterston DJ: Correction of total anomalous pulmonary venous drainage in infancy. J Thorac Cardiovasc Surg 66:447, 1973

115. Dillard DH, Mohri H, Hessel EA, et al.: Correction of total anomalous pulmonary venous drainage in infancy utilizing deep hypothermia with total circulatory arrest. Circulation 36 [Suppl 1]:105, 1967

116. Castaneda AR, Lamberti J, Sade RM, Williams RG, Nadas AS: Open-heart surgery during the first three months of life. J. Thorac Cardiovasc Surg 68:719, 1974

117. Parr GVS, Kirklin JW, Pacifico AD, Blackstone EH, Lauridsen P: Cardiac performance in infants after repair of total anomalous pulmonary venous connection. Ann Thorac Surg 17:561, 1974

118. Mathew R, Thilenius OG, Replogle RL, Arcilla RA: Cardiac function in total anomalous pulmonary venous return before and after surgery. Circulation 55:361, 1977

119. Silove ED, Behrendt DM, Aberdeen E, Bonham-Carter RE: Total anomalous pulmonary venous drainage. II. Spontaneous functional closure of interatrial communication after surgical correction in infancy. Circulation 46:357, 1972

120. Whight CM, Barratt-Boyes BG, Calder AL, Neutze JM, Brandt PWT: Total anomalous pulmonary venous connection. Long-term results following repair in infancy. J Thorac Cardiovasc Surg 75:52, 1978

12 Cyanosis and Decreased Pulmonary Blood Flow

The cardiac conditions leading to cyanosis and decreased pulmonary blood flow are associated with obstruction to pulmonary blood flow and an intracardiac defect. The intracardiac defect and the right-to-left shunt may be at either the ventricular or atrial level, and the hemodynamics and clinical features vary, depending upon the site of the right-to-left shunt.

In patients with obstruction to pulmonary blood flow and a defect at the ventricular level, the amount of right-to-left shunt is dependent upon the relative resistances to systemic and pulmonary blood flow imposed by the systemic arterioles and pulmonary stenosis, respectively. In these patients, hypoxemia is the major clinical feature, and congestive cardiac failure does not occur. The cardiac size is normal or near normal. The cardiac contour frequently shows right ventricular hypertrophy, and the latter is also reflected on the electrocardiogram.

In contrast, among patients in whom the shunt occurs at the atrial level, the flow is more dependent upon the relative ventricular compliances. In most of the conditions, filling of the right ventricle is severely limited, so that a shunt occurs at the atrial level. The roentgenogram usually shows cardiomegaly (from right atrial enlargement), and the cardiac contour may have a left ventricular contour. Because of the type of cardiac malformation, the electrocardiogram may show left ventricular hypertrophy. Hypoxemia is the major feature, but there may be hepatomegaly or other signs of increased venous pressure because of difficult egress of blood from the right atrium.

The lesions classified in this group include:

I. Ventricular septal communication
   A. Tetralogy of Fallot
   B. Variants of tetralogy of Fallot
      1. Double outlet right ventricle with pulmonary stenosis
      2. Tetralogy of Fallot and endocardial cushion defect

3. Single ventricle and pulmonary stenosis, with or without transposition of the great vessels
4. Complete transposition of the great vessels with ventricular septal defect and pulmonary stenosis
5. Congenitally corrected transposition of the great vessels with ventricular septal defect and pulmonary stenosis
6. Congenital cardiac anomalies associated with asplenia

II. Atrial septal communication
   A. Pulmonary valve atresia
   B. Tricuspid valve atresia
   C. Ebstein's malformation of the tricuspid valve
   D. Isolated hypoplasia of the right ventricle
   E. Endocardial fibroelastosis of the right ventricle
   F. Uhl's anomaly of the right ventricle
   G. Tricuspid insufficiency

VENTRICULAR SEPTAL COMMUNICATION

The classic and most frequent lesion with ventricular septal defect and obstruction to pulmonary blood flow is tetralogy of Fallot. There are a number of other cardiac conditions with a ventricular communication and pulmonary stenosis in which the hemodynamics resemble tetralogy of Fallot. These have been called "tetrad variants."

The obstruction to pulmonary blood flow is related usually to pulmonary stenosis (valvular or subvalvular) but may be caused by pulmonary atresia. In the latter instance, pulmonary blood flow is often derived from a patent ductus arteriosus, which may close during the neonatal period, leading to deterioration of the patient.

Tetralogy of Fallot

Initially described by Neels Stensen in the seventeenth century, this condition is named for Étienne Fallot, who made the clinical-pathologic correlation, stating that patients with (1) ventricular septal defect, (2) pulmonary stenosis, (3) right ventricular hypertrophy, and (4) overriding aorta show cyanosis. Tetralogy of Fallot is the most common condition occurring in the group of conditions with diminished pulmonary blood flow.

PATHOLOGY.   Three important anatomic features are present in patients with tetralogy of Fallot: ventricular septal defect, overriding aorta, and pulmonary stenosis. The developmental aspects of tetralogy of Fallot have been discussed by several authors, including Van Praagh et al.[1] and Becker et al.[2] The ventricular septal defect is large and situated posteriorly to the parietal band of the crista supraventricularis.[3] The defect includes part of the membranous septum and the adjacent myocardium and lies predominantly under the right aortic cusp. It is separated from the pulmonary valve by the crista supraventricularis. On the right ventricular side, it lies beneath the septal leaflet of the tricuspid valve.

The aorta may override the ventricular septal defect, but the degree to which it straddles the ventricular septum varies considerably, ranging from nearly the entire left ventricle to predominantly from the right ventricle. In the latter case, the term "dextroposition of the aorta" is applied. Regardless of the relationship of the aorta to the ventricular septum, continuity between the aorta and the mitral valve is preserved, and this anatomic relationship distinguishes tetralogy of Fallot from partial transposition of the great vessels, i.e., double outlet right ventricle.

In cyanotic forms of tetralogy of Fallot, the pulmonary stenosis is of sufficient severity to lead to a right-to-left shunt at the ventricular level. The site of obstruction may reside in the infundibular area, at the valve, in the supravalvular area, or, rarely, in the branch pulmonary arteries. Infundibular stenosis is almost always present and may occur as the only site of obstruction or be associated with valvular stenosis. The anatomic details vary according to the degree of stenosis and the amount of displacement of the structures of the crista supraventricularis by the ventricular septal defect. All portions of the crista supraventricularis may be hypertrophied, or the predominant narrowing may be caused by hypertrophy of the parietal band. The degree of infundibular stenosis increases with age.

Valvular stenosis occurs in most patients[4] and may be the sole site of obstruction. The degree of stenosis and the anatomic details of the valve vary considerably. It may be tricuspid, bicuspid, unicuspid, domed, or atretic. The pulmonary annulus and the pulmonary trunk are usually hypoplastic in direct relation to the degree of stenosis, and this also causes obstruction to right ventricular outflow. In patients with pulmonary valvular atresia, the pulmonary trunk may be atretic or patent to the level of the pulmonary valve.

The caliber of the pulmonary arteries reflects the caliber of the pulmonary trunk. In a few patients, the left pulmonary artery is absent, and the left lung is supplied by bronchial collateral arteries. In patients with pulmonary atresia, the lungs are supplied by a ductus arteriosus or by bronchial collateral vessels that communicate with the pulmonary arterial system at various sites within the pulmonary parenchyma.

In 25 percent of the patients, a right aortic arch is present and usually shows mirror-image branching, although, occasionally, the left subclavian artery may arise anomalously from the descending aorta.

In the review by Rao and associates,[4] a high incidence of atrial septal defect or valvular competent foramen ovale was found. In about 10 percent of patients, a persistent left superior vena cava was found.

From an operative viewpoint, anomalous origin of the anterior descending coronary artery from the right coronary artery is an important coexistent anomaly. In 5 percent of patients, the anterior descending coronary artery courses aberrantly across the outflow area of the right ventricle and could be accidentally interrupted at the time of operation and cause extensive myocardial damage.

HEMODYNAMICS.   In tetralogy of Fallot, the ventricular septal defect is large and offers little resistance to flow. The systolic pressures in the ventricles are equal. The direction and magnitude of blood flow through the defect are dependent upon the relation between resistances imposed by the pulmonary stenosis and the systemic vasculature. The overriding of the aorta is not an important determinant in the shunt or the direction of blood flow. Several of the symptoms of tetralogy of Fallot are believed to be related to alterations in the relative resistance to pulmonary and systemic blood flow. The degree of pulmonary stenosis can vary because of changes in the contractable state of the hypertrophied infundibular myocardium, and the systemic vascular resistance can vary because of the numerous factors that influence systemic arterioles.

Major symptoms in patients with tetralogy of Fallot result from the limitation of pulmonary blood flow and the resultant hypoxemia. Compensatory mechanisms for the hypoxemia include development of polycythemia and of bronchial collaterals, but these may be insufficient to meet the oxygen requirements.

CLINICAL FEATURES.   The age at onset and the severity of symptoms are related to the degree of stenosis. Patients with severe pulmonary stenosis or with pulmonary atresia may develop symptoms at 24 to 48 hours of age, presumably as the ductus arteriosus closes. If the ductus arteriosus remains patent and provides adequate pulmonary blood flow, the cyanosis may be slight, but usually the ductus closes eventually, and cyanosis increases.

Half of the neonates identified as having tetralogy of Fallot present with cyanosis, and the other half initially present with a cardiac murmur. The degree of cyanosis is variable, and factors, such as hot weather, meals, or exertion, lower systemic vascular resistance and are associated with increased cyanosis.

Attacks of paroxysmal dyspnea, also called "tetrad spells," are typical of tetralogy of Fallot and are characterized by the sudden onset of dyspnea, restlessness, and increasing cyanosis.[5] During the spell, the murmur decreases in intensity and length and may even disappear. The hypoxemia can become severe enough to lead to convulsions, coma, and death. The duration of the spell varies from minutes to hours and terminates usually in generalized weakness, lethargy, and sleepiness. These occur more commonly in the morning, during hot weather, and following exertion, such as passing a stool. These spells are uncommon in the first 1 to 2 months but can occur throughout the remainder of the first year of life. Their occurrence is not limited to patients with severe stenosis. Between episodes, the infant may be asymptomatic.

The genesis of the episodes is unknown but is believed to be related to sudden imbalance between the resistance to outflow, such as an increased degree of pulmonary stenosis by increased contractile state of the right ventricular outflow tract, or a decrease in systemic vascular resistance. Either change would favor an increase in right-to-left shunt and could be caused by endogenous release of catecholamines.

Morgan and associates[5] consider hyperpnea the initiating event, leading to an increased systemic venous return, while pulmonary blood flow remains fixed or decreased, so that the right-to-left shunt increases. As a consequence, the arterial Pco_2 increases, and the Po_2 falls, leading to further hyperpnea.

Signs and symptoms of congestive cardiac failure do not occur in tetralogy of Fallot. Regardless of the severity of the pulmonary stenosis, the right ventricle has free egress to the aorta, and right ventricular pressure is fixed by the systemic pressure and cannot rise. Furthermore, left ventricular volume is not increased and, in fact, may be smaller than normal.

Squatting, a symptom that occurs more commonly in children after they begin to walk, may be observed in infants as they sleep with their knees drawn up against their chest. This symptom, which is virtually diagnostic of tetralogy of Fallot, is believed to have two beneficial effects in these patients: (1) increase in systemic vascular resistance and (2) alteration in venous return from the legs. Guntheroth and co-workers[6] found that in patients with tetralogy of Fallot, on assuming the knee-chest position, inferior vena caval flow shows a transient increase and then a decrease. As a result, systemic venous return falls, and less desaturated blood returns to the heart and arterial saturation improves.

The infant may show retarded growth if the stenosis is severe and associated with moderate or severe cyanosis. The cardiac apex is located normally, and there may be a right ventricular heave. In tetralogy of Fallot, a pulmonary systolic ejection murmur is expected, and its loudness and duration are inversely related to the severity of stenosis. It may be associated with a thrill and is heard best in the third left intercostal spaces. Even in the same patient, the murmur varies from day to day, for example, decreasing during a tetrad spell. In patients with pulmonary atresia, a systolic murmur is not heard, but there may be a continuous murmur of a patent ductus arteriosus or enlarged bronchial collateral arteries, the latter frequently being higher pitched, more superficial, and heard more diffusely over the thorax.

The first heart sound is loud along the lower left sternal border. The second heart sound, which is loud along the upper left sternal border, appears single, since it represents the aortic valve closure. The pulmonary component is delayed, soft, and rarely audible. In patients with severe stenosis or pulmonary atresia, an aortic systolic ejection click is heard.

Hepatomegaly is not present, although the hepatic edge may be palpable 2 to 3 cm below the right costal margin because of hyperinflation of the lungs during a tetrad spell.

ELECTROCARDIOGRAM.   The electrocardiogram shows a QRS axis in the frontal plane, usually around $+120°$ (Fig. 12-1). A QRS axis greater than $+150°$ is rare. A pattern of right atrial enlargement is present in one fourth of the patients

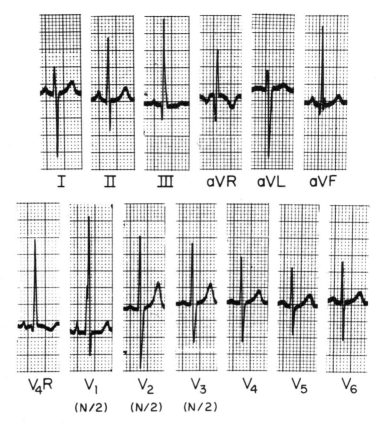

FIG. 12-1. Electrocardiogram of 4-month-old infant with tetralogy of Fallot. Right atrial enlargement. QRS axis is +110°. Right ventricular hypertrophy. N/2, half-standardization.

and is related to hypertrophy of the atrium from decreased right ventricular compliance. A pattern of right ventricular hypertrophy is found, and in lead V_1, the complex shows an rR' or Rs wave with slightly slurred upstroke of the R wave. The T waves in the right precordial leads may be either upright or inverted, and the specific pattern has no diagnostic significance. A pattern of right ventricular strain is not found.

THORACIC ROENTGENOGRAM. Cardiac size is normal. The cardiac contour has been described as "coeur en sabot." The cardiac apex is upturned, related to the right ventricular hypertrophy (Fig. 12-2). The pulmonary arterial segment is concave because the pulmonary trunk is small. The ascending aorta is enlarged, and in 25 percent of the patients, a right aortic arch is present. The pulmonary vasculature is diminished.

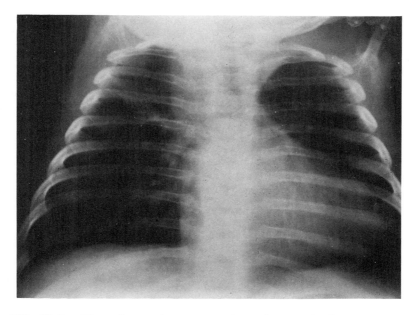

FIG. 12-2.   Thoracic roentgenogram of tetralogy of Fallot. Decreased pulmonary vascular markings. Normal cardiac size. Elevated cardiac apex. Concave pulmonary arterial segment. Right aortic arch.

In patients with coexistent pulmonary atresia and a large volume of bronchial collateral blood flow, the heart may be enlarged, and the left atrium may be prominent. The lung fields show no discrete hilar vessels, but there are diffuse tortuous vascular shadows, and pulmonary vasculature may appear increased.

ECHOCARDIOGRAM.   The echocardiogram of tetralogy of Fallot resembles that of persistent truncus arteriosus. In each condition, an enlarged arterial vessel is identified and overrides a thickened interventricular septum (Fig. 12-3). There is discontinuity between the anterior edge of this vessel and the interventricular septum. In both conditions, right ventricular hypertrophy is present, and the right ventricle may be enlarged. In tetralogy of Fallot, however, the pulmonary valve and the right ventricular outflow tract should be identifiable, whereas they would not be found in patients with truncus arteriosus. Because these structures are smaller than normal in tetralogy of Fallot,[7] they may not be demonstrated.

CARDIAC CATHETERIZATION AND ANGIOCARDIOGRAM.   Although the clinical and laboratory features are frequently diagnostic of tetralogy of Fallot, cardiac catheterization is necessary to obtain information on which to base operative decisions. The studies are needed (1) to confirm the diagnosis, (2) to visualize

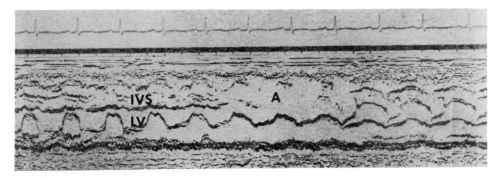

FIG. 12-3. Echocardiogram of tetralogy of Fallot. Sweep from left ventricle (LV) to aorta (A). Aorta overrides interventricular septum (IVS).

the anatomic details, and (3) to exclude cardiac conditions (tetrad variants) that may present a similar picture.

Particular care must be exercised in performance of the catheterization, for the infant can develop a tetrad spell during the procedure because of immobilization, sedation, or partial occlusion of the outflow tract by the catheter. We rarely sedate any infants with tetralogy of Fallot for cardiac catheterization. At the onset of the catheterization, the pH should be measured, and acidosis, if present, should be treated with bicarbonate. Continued observation of the infant and periodic determination of pH, Po_2, and Pco_2 are indicated. The blood samples can be obtained either through the venous catheter or from an arterial site. If the infant becomes irritable and restless, morphine 0.1 mg/kg should be administered.

The catheter is inserted into the saphenous vein and passed into the heart and should be initially placed in the right ventricle. At this site, the pressure and blood sample are obtained. The catheter should not be manipulated further, and a right ventriculogram should be performed. This study yields the greatest amount of diagnostic information, and if the infant's condition deteriorates, the necessary information will have been obtained. Following the angiogram, the catheter should be manipulated into the aorta for aortography. It is not necessary to catheterize the pulmonary artery, for the pressure is uniformly low, and manipulation of the catheter tip in the outflow tract of the right ventricle can produce arrhythmias or otherwise lead to a tetrad spell. Care should also be taken during manipulation of the catheter tip in the right atrium because a supraventricular tachycardia might be precipitated. This rhythm leads to a marked increase in right-to-left shunt and tetrad spells.[8,9]

During the procedure, oximetry data can be obtained but usually yield little additional information. Catheterization of the left side of the heart is rarely indicated in these infants. The entire catheterization procedure should be and can be performed expeditiously.

The oxygen saturation data show identical values throughout the right side of the heart, and these values are reduced and may be very low, particularly during a tetrad spell. Evidence of a right-to-left shunt at the atrial level may be found. Aortic oxygen saturation is low and can decrease considerably during the course of a cardiac catheterization or can vary, depending upon the status of the infant.

Right ventricular systolic pressures are elevated and equal to those of the left ventricle and the aorta. The pressure contour typically shows a square top. Pulmonary arterial pressure is low, and the site of pulmonary stenosis may be identified on careful withdrawal pressure recording. Right atrial pressure, particularly the a wave, may be increased slightly.

Right ventriculography is necessary to exclude other conditions that may mimic tetralogy of Fallot. The right ventriculogram shows simultaneous opacification of the aorta and the pulmonary artery (Fig. 12-4). The aorta is enlarged and shows a variable degree of overriding of the ventricular septum. There is continuity of the aorta and mitral valve, which can be seen on right ventriculogram.

Particular attention must be directed toward the details of the right ventricular outflow tract. The amount of infundibular narrowing should be noted, and this usually is caused by hypertrophy of the crista supraventricularis. The caliber of the pulmonary annulus, which is usually hypoplastic, must be assessed, and the details of the pulmonary valve must be observed. The caliber of the pulmonary trunk and major pulmonary arteries must also be measured.

The aortogram is performed to identify the course of the coronary arteries, looking for an anomalous course of the left coronary artery across the right ventricular outflow tract. Fellows and associates[10] have emphasized the need for preoperative aortography to outline abnormalities of the coronary arteries. In 5 percent of patients studied,[10] the coronary arterial pattern was abnor-

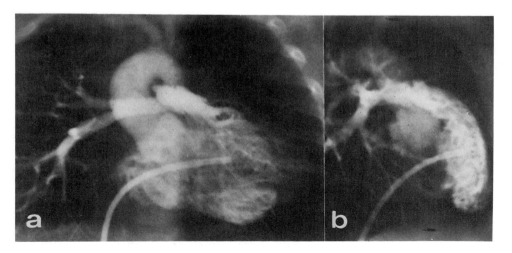

FIG. 12-4. Right ventriculogram of tetralogy of Fallot. **a.** Anteroposterior view. **b.** Lateral view. Opacification of both the aorta and pulmonary trunk. Hypoplasia of pulmonary annulus and trunk.

mal—either the anterior descending coronary artery arose from the right coronary artery, or a single left coronary artery was present. The incidence of coronary arterial anomalies in 195 autopsied patients was also 5 percent. In addition, aortography also identifies the location of the aortic arch and the origin of the brachiocephalic vessels, information which is useful if a Blalock-Taussig shunt is being considered. In patients with pulmonary atresia, the pulmonary arteries may be opacified on aortography by way of a patent ductus arteriosus or bronchial collateral arteries. In these patients, the pulmonary arteries are usually quite hypoplastic.

MANAGEMENT.   In infants with tetralogy of Fallot, cyanosis increases secondary to progressive pulmonary stenosis. Progression can be assessed by three clinical means: (1) history—with increasing severity of pulmonary stenosis, cyanosis and tetrad spells increase and exercise tolerance declines, (2) auscultation—with an increasing degree of pulmonary stenosis, the murmur becomes softer and shorter, and (3) red cell indices—with increasing hypoxemia, the hemoglobin and hematocrit increase, and this reflects more accurately the degree of hypoxia than does an arterial Po_2 determination. The latter measures the degree of hypoxemia at that particular moment, and it is well recognized that the Po_2 varies with crying, straining, time of day, and other factors. The electrocardiogram and roentgenogram show no changes to indicate increasing severity.

The infants must also be monitored to make certain they are not developing a relative anemia, that is, elevated hematocrit, without a corresponding rise of hemoglobin. Infants with relative anemia require treatment with iron, and if tetrad spells or other symptoms are present, these may improve considerably following therapy.

Treatment of tetrad spells includes placing the infant in a knee-chest position and administering oxygen. Oxygen, however, has little benefit because the volume of pulmonary blood flow is so low. Morphine 0.1 mg/kg should be given. The beneficial effect of morphine is unknown, but it decreases oxygen utilization by slowing the respiratory rate and sedating the infant. Acidosis, if present, should be treated, and as pH rises, the spell may ease. Propranolol may also be administered during the acute episode and results in relief of the symptoms.[11-13] This agent has also been used for long-term management, giving 1 mg/kg four times daily, for the prevention of further spells, but we have observed tachyphylaxis to this agent. Furthermore, the alternative of an operation, either palliative or corrective, must be seriously considered, since the spells may end fatally.

In patients with tetralogy of Fallot, Nudel and others[14] have described the effects of acutely increasing systemic vascular resistance by the infusion of phenylephrine and the resultant increased arterial oxygen saturation. These authors indicated that such therapy may be beneficial in treatment of protracted tetrad spells. This alpha adrenergic drug has no effect on the myocardium but does cause systemic vasoconstriction. Blood pressure elevation and reflex slowing of the heart rate are effects of the drug and revert following its discontinuance. Additional studies are needed before this becomes an acceptable adjunct to treatment of hypoxemic spells.

A palliative procedure is usually performed on the neonate with tetralogy of Fallot and severe pulmonary stenosis or atresia who shows severe hypoxemia and acidosis, that cannot be corrected or that recurs. Three types of palliative procedures are available:

1. Blalock-Taussig procedure—in which the subclavian artery usually opposite the side of the aortic arch, is divided and anastomosed to the pulmonary artery. The small size of the blood vessels in neonates and young infants makes it difficult to achieve an anastomosis of sufficient size which remains patent. This shunt, however, has the advantage in that the size of the communication is relatively constant and rarely leads to pulmonary hypertension or cardiac failure and can be easily ligated at the time of corrective operation.
2. Waterston procedure—in which a communication is made between the ascending aorta and the right pulmonary artery. Although technically easier to perform than a Blalock-Taussig, it is more difficult to control the size of the communication. Frequent complications include congestive cardiac failure,[15,16] kinking or narrowing of the pulmonary arteries,[16] and, less frequently, the development of pulmonary vascular disease. Although permitting the survival of the neonate, these complications are considerable and may make the ultimate repair difficult. Therefore, it is our policy to recatheterize all children with a Waterston shunt 1 year postoperatively.
3. Pott's procedure—in which the left pulmonary artery is anastomosed to the descending aorta. This is similar in concept and complications[17,18] to the Waterston procedure. The presence of pulmonary vascular disease leads to increased risk at the time of corrective operation. Corrective operation is more difficult because of its posterior location in the thorax. There is evidence that the size of the anastomosis may increase with age.

Miller and colleagues[19] reviewed 50 infants and children with tetralogy of Fallot and pulmonary atresia, 28 of whom underwent palliative procedures, and indicate an ascending aorta-right pulmonary artery shunt is the procedure of choice.

The primary purpose of the shunt is relief of hypoxemia by increasing the volume of pulmonary blood and allowing the infant to grow, so a corrective operation can be performed subsequently. Another consequence of the shunt procedure is that the augmented pulmonary blood flow may increase the caliber of hypoplastic pulmonary arteries and the size of the left atrium and left ventricle.

The indications for palliative operation in infants are progressive cyanosis, as indicated by increasing hemoglobin and hematocrit, or hypoxemic spells unassociated with anemia.

Formerly, corrective operation was delayed until the age of 3 to 4 years, but with the development of techniques of hypothermia and perfusion of small infants, it is possible to successfully perform corrective operations in infants.[20-23]

Bonchek and associates[24] described corrective operation in 28 patients with tetralogy of Fallot between the ages of 10 weeks and 2 years, 5 being under 6 months. They used cardiopulmonary bypass without circulatory arrest and had 2 operative and no late deaths. Furthermore, postoperative cardiac catheterization in 17 showed[25] a mean gradient of 19 mm between the right ventricle and the pulmonary artery, with a range of 6 to 55 mm Hg. Two had a small residual ventricular septal defect. Left ventricular performance was considered normal. The growth and development of the children were normal.

Castaneda and associates[21] operated upon 41 infants with tetralogy of Fallot, ranging from 12 days to 1 year (mean, 5.7 months), and used deep hypothermia and circulatory arrest. Thirty-eight required an outflow patch. There were 3 deaths (7 percent) and no late deaths. Postoperative cardiac catheterization showed relief of the gradient and successful closure of the defect in almost all infants.

Operation at an early age may prevent the progressive development of pulmonary stenosis and attendant fibrosis and the complications of reduced pulmonary blood flow and left ventricular size. Our surgeons have indicated that the relief of the stenosis is easier to accomplish in infants than in older children, but a patch must often be placed across the pulmonary annulus into the pulmonary trunk. Patients must be carefully selected for corrective operation because the size of the pulmonary arteries and the pulmonary trunk is a major limitation. If the branch pulmonary arteries are quite hypoplastic or if the pulmonary trunk is less than one third the size of the aorta, we perform a shunt, hoping to create a favorable increase in the size of these structures, so that corrective operation can be performed when the infant is older.

In the immediate postoperative period, the cardiac output may be low, and clinical evidence of poor perfusion may be found. Central venous pressure is elevated. Treatment consists of blood transfusion, increasing the central venous pressure even higher to improve right ventricular filling pressure, and systemic perfusion. Digitalis is given and respirator support is also often indicated.

About half of the patients develop congestive cardiac failure following correction, and they should be maintained on digitalis for 6 months postoperatively. While most patients no longer require this medication after 6 months, persistent cardiac failure indicates major residual anomalies that usually are operatively correctable.[26]

Jarmakani and associates[27] studied left ventricular function postoperatively in patients following operation for tetralogy of Fallot and indicate depressed left ventricular function in patients both prior to and following corrective operation. This was manifested by depressed left ventricular ejection function and lower left ventricular systolic pressure.

Graham and associates[28] found that right ventricular size and myocardial function are abnormal in patients whose operation includes a right ventricular outflow patch and may be compromised further by elevated right ventricular systolic pressure, pulmonary insufficiency or a large noncontractile outflow tract.

Tetralogy of Fallot with Absence of Pulmonary Valve

Tetralogy of Fallot with absence of the pulmonary valve is discussed in relation to tetralogy of Fallot because the anatomic details are similar. The clinical picture is, however, different, since congestive cardiac failure may occur, respiratory symptoms are prominent, and the thoracic roentgenogram has a characteristic appearance.

PATHOLOGY.   The basic anatomy is that of tetralogy of Fallot, except that the degree of infundibular stenosis is usually mild.[29,30] At the site of the pulmonary valve, a ring of nodular tissue is present that has no structural characteristics of the pulmonary valve. The histologic appearance of the valvular tissue is of large, pale-staining cells.[29] The pulmonary annulus is hypoplastic and causes stenosis. The pulmonary trunk and major pulmonary arteries, particularly the right, are dilated and may appear aneurysmal. The right ventricle is dilated because of the pulmonary regurgitation. The enlarged pulmonary arteries can compress major bronchi, particularly in the right lung, leading to emphysema or atelectasis.

HEMODYNAMICS.   At birth, because of the pulmonary stenosis and the elevated pulmonary vascular resistance, blood shunts right to left through the ventricular septal defect. As the pulmonary vascular resistance falls, a left-to-right shunt develops, the size depending upon the amount of pulmonary stenosis and the status of the pulmonary vasculature.[31] Usually there is a right-to-left shunt as well.

CLINICAL FEATURES.   Cyanosis, usually present in the neonatal period, disappears but may recur in infancy because of pulmonary complications. Cyanosis often escapes notice, and the infant presents with pulmonary symptoms of wheezing, dyspnea, and tachypnea related to bronchial compression.[32] Findings of congestive cardiac failure may be present.

A right ventricular heave is found. A loud, long pulmonary systolic ejection murmur is heard in the pulmonary area and is transmitted widely. The second heart sound is single and accentuated. It is followed by a grade 2–3/6 early diastolic murmur of pulmonary insufficiency, localized to the second and third left intercostal spaces. A pulmonary systolic ejection click may be present.

Auscultation of the lung fields may reveal signs of consolidation, emphysema, and pneumonia.

ELECTROCARDIOGRAM.   The electrocardiogram shows a pattern of right axis deviation and right ventricular hypertrophy, as in tetralogy of Fallot.

THORACIC ROENTGENOGRAM.   There is moderate cardiomegaly and prominence of the right ventricular outflow area and pulmonary trunk. The characteristic finding relates to the aneurysmal dilatation of the right pulmonary artery that forms a sausage-shaped mass projecting into the right hilus[29,30,32] (Fig. 12-5). On

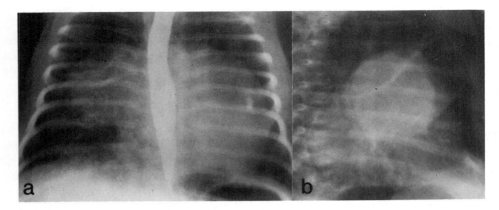

FIG. 12-5. Thoracic roentgenogram of tetralogy of Fallot with absent pulmonary valve. **a.** Posteroanterior view. **b.** Lateral view. Greatly enlarged right pulmonary artery. Moderate cardiomegaly.

lateral roentgenograms, the enlarged right pulmonary artery can be clearly seen. This enlarged right pulmonary artery may be misinterpreted as a tumor mass. The peripheral pulmonary vasculature is normal.

CARDIAC CATHETERIZATION AND ANGIOCARDIOGRAM.   The right ventricular and left ventricular pressures are equal. A pressure difference is found across the pulmonary valve, partially from the stenosis caused by the narrowed annulus and partially from the large volume of systolic flow across the valve. The pulmonary arterial pressures are usually normal. Bidirectional shunt is present at the ventricular level, but often the amount of right-to-left shunt is small.

Right ventriculography confirms the diagnosis (Fig. 12-6). There is simultaneous opacification of both great vessels. Infundibular stenosis may not be identified. The site of the pulmonary valvular annulus can be identified because of the nodular ring of tissue, but pulmonary valvular leaflets are not visualized. As in tetralogy of Fallot, the infundibulum is usually directed toward the right.[31] As a result, both the pulmonary trunk and the right pulmonary artery are greatly dilated and are very pulsatile. Because of the pulmonary regurgitation, contrast material slowly clears the right side of the heart.

MANAGEMENT.   Vigorous pulmonary therapy, including antibiotics, postural drainage, and humidity, is indicated for most patients who show a left-to-right shunt, cardiac failure, and pulmonary problems. The prognosis is poor for infants with these symptoms when medically managed, and operative treatment should be considered. Although several types of procedures have been tried, closure of the ventricular septal defect can be performed at relatively little risk, and usually nothing else is necessary in the infant.[31,33] This converts the condition to that of pulmonary valvular insufficiency with intact ventricular septum,

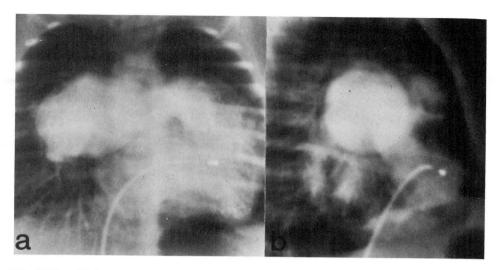

FIG. 12-6.   Right ventriculogram, anteroposterior view of tetralogy of Fallot with absent pulmonary valve. (Same infant as in Fig. 12-5.) Anteroposterior **(a)** and lateral **(b)** views of simultaneous opacification at aorta and pulmonary artery. Right pulmonary artery aneurysmally dilated.

which has a more favorable course in childhood. In infants, placement of a conduit or a pulmonary valve is not indicated, nor is resection or plication of the pulmonary arterial aneurysm.

Patients with minimal symptoms should be carefully followed and operation considered when they are older.

TETRAD VARIANTS

There are several cardiac conditions that can simulate tetralogy of Fallot and, while occurring much less frequently than tetralogy of Fallot, must be considered in the differential diagnosis. In each of these conditions,[34] there is a ventricular communication, pulmonary stenosis, and a right-to-left shunt at the ventricular level. Although there may be clinical and laboratory features that allow the suspicion of a variant of tetralogy of Fallot, definitive diagnosis depends upon angiography.

Like tetralogy of Fallot, the conditions discussed here have major symptoms related to hypoxemia, and congestive cardiac failure does not occur in uncomplicated cases. The major cardiac auscultatory finding is a pulmonary ejection systolic murmur, the loudness varying inversely with the severity of the stenosis. In most of the conditions discussed here, the electrocardiogram shows right ventricular hypertrophy. The thoracic roentgenogram shows decreased pulmonary blood flow and a cardiac size which is normal or slightly enlarged. There may be electrocardiographic or roentgenographic features that are characteristic of the underlying cardiac condition.

The conditions considered as tetrad variants are:

1. Double outlet right ventricle with pulmonary stenosis
2. Tetralogy of Fallot and endocardial cushion defect
3. Single ventricle and pulmonary stenosis, with or without transposition of the great vessels
4. Complete transposition of the great vessels, with ventricular septal defect and pulmonary stenosis
5. Congenitally corrected transposition of the great vessels, with ventricular septal defect and pulmonary stenosis
6. Congenital cardiac anomalies associated with asplenia

The anatomic details and the major clinical and laboratory features of these conditions are discussed elsewhere. In this section, only those relevant or unique features which must be considered in the differential diagnosis of tetralogy of Fallot will be discussed.

DOUBLE OUTLET RIGHT VENTRICLE WITH PULMONARY STENOSIS.   In virtually all patients with double outlet right ventricle coexisting with pulmonary stenosis, the ventricular septal defect is located below the crista supraventricularis, and the pulmonary stenosis is caused by valvular or infundibular narrowing or a combination of the two.[35] The distinguishing anatomic features of double outlet right ventricle, which closely resembles tetralogy of Fallot, are discontinuity of the aortic and mitral valves and a higher and more anterior position of the aortic valve.

Clinical and laboratory features resemble those of tetralogy of Fallot. Right ventriculography demonstrates the abnormal position of the aorta, and if a left ventriculogram is performed, the separation of the mitral and aortic valves can be verified. Echocardiography initially held promise in identifying discontinuity between the aortic and mitral valves, but unfortunately both false positives and false negatives occur.

The intracardiac operative procedure to correct double outlet right ventricle with pulmonary stenosis is similar to that for tetralogy of Fallot. The ventricular defect is closed, and a patch is placed so that left ventricular blood is delivered to the aorta and separated from right ventricular blood flow. The pulmonary stenosis is relieved as in tetralogy of Fallot.

TETRALOGY OF FALLOT AND ENDOCARDIAL CUSHION DEFECT.   Tetralogy of Fallot may coexist with endocardial cushion defect, either a partial or a complete atrioventricular canal.[36] Separate defects are present in the ventricular septum—one of tetralogy of Fallot and one of the ventricular component of the endocardial cushion defect.

On auscultation, the presence of an apical pansystolic murmur of mitral insufficiency should alert the physician to this diagnostic possibility. The electrocardiogram provides a more valuable clue. The QRS axis is superiorly directed and may be between $-90°$ and $-150°$, and leads I and aVL show a qR pattern. Left ventricular hypertrophy is usually not present. In a patient with clinical findings suggestive of tetralogy of Fallot and left QRS axis, a left ventriculogram should be performed. In patients with coexistent endocardial cushion defect, the typical gooseneck deformity of the left ventricular outflow tract will be found. Echocardiography is also helpful by showing characteristic findings of the mitral valve, described in Chapter 9.

The operative approach to this lesion in infancy depends upon the experience of the surgeon. If the infant develops hypoxic symptoms, an aorticopulmonary shunt can be performed at relatively low risk. Corrective operation can be performed by procedures to correct the endocardial cushion defect and to correct the tetralogy of Fallot. We have recently had experience with a successful correction of this condition in an infant,[37] and this has been reported by others.[38]

SINGLE VENTRICLE AND PULMONARY STENOSIS, WITH OR WITHOUT TRANSPOSITION OF THE GREAT VESSELS.   In single ventricle, the great vessels may be normally related or show either *l-* or *d-*transposition[39] and may occur with different morphologic types of single ventricle.[40] In each, pulmonary stenosis may coexist. Depending upon the severity of the pulmonary stenosis, the volume of pulmonary blood flow may be limited. In the patients discussed in this section, the pulmonary blood flow is less than normal. There are several anatomic forms of the pulmonary stenosis.[40,41] There may be valvular stenosis, either of the classic domed type or secondary to a dysplastic valve. Membranous subpulmonary stenosis can occur. In patients with normally related great vessels, stenosis may occur in the communication between the single ventricle and the subpulmonary infundibulum.

There are laboratory data that suggest single ventricle in some patients. While the electrocardiographic features may resemble those of tetralogy of Fallot, the QRS axis, particularly in patients with normally related vessels, may show left axis deviation. There may be a precordial lead pattern of left ventricular hypertrophy or posteriorly directed QRS forces or q waves in the right precordial leads.[40-42]

Although the thoracic roentgenogram may resemble that of tetralogy of Fallot, it may show a prominent bulge along the upper left cardiac border, as in corrected transposition of the great vessels.

Echocardiography provides the best noninvasive method of identifying single ventricle, and the features of the echocardiogram in single ventricle and the use of contrast echocardiography in this condition have been discussed in Chapter 11. Angiography provides the definitive diagnosis.

Most patients with single ventricle and pulmonary stenosis do not have severe symptoms in infancy, but an extracardiac shunt should be performed in symptomatic infants. We prefer a Blalock-Taussig shunt, since this procedure infrequently leads to pulmonary vascular disease or disturbs the continuity of the pulmonary arterial tree. Palliation allows the infant to grow until a corrective procedure can be performed at an older age. Preservation of the pulmonary vascular bed is important, for in one type of procedure, a valved conduit is placed between the right atrium and the pulmonary artery, and the tricuspid valve is sewn closed.[43] The experience of Edie and associates[44] has also indicated that single ventricle in older children can be corrected by division of the ventricle by placement of a septal patch.

COMPLETE TRANSPOSITION OF THE GREAT VESSELS WITH VENTRICULAR SEPTAL DEFECT AND PULMONARY STENOSIS. In less than 5 percent of patients with complete transposition of the great vessels, ventricular septal defect and pulmonary stenosis coexist. Usually, the ventricular septal defect underlies the pulmonary annulus, and the stenosis in these patients is valvular. Subpulmonary stenosis may be related to one of the following mechanisms: bulging of the interventricular septum, fibromuscular narrowing,[45] abnormalities of the structure of the mitral valve or its abnormal attachment to the ventricular septum[46] in the region of the ventricular septal defect, protrusion of redundant tricuspid valvular tissue,[47] or aneurysm of membranous septum.[48]

The clinical and laboratory features mimic tetralogy of Fallot, even the presence of a right aortic arch. When right aortic arch occurs in complete transposition of the great vessels, ventricular septal defect and pulmonary stenosis almost always coexist.[49] A stenotic murmur is heard and, in our experience, radiates well to the right back. Echocardiography can diagnose the transposed great vessels, especially when combined with a knowledge of the clinical status of the patient, and can identify the presence of subpulmonary obstruction.[50] Angiography is required to diagnose transposition of the great vessels by showing the anterior position of the aorta and the posterior portion of the pulmonary artery. The details of the pulmonary stenosis, particularly if subvalvular in location, may be difficult to identify, but with the concepts of axial cineangiography,[51,52] this area can be more clearly visualized.

For the symptomatic infant, a shunt procedure is performed. Many patients with moderate pulmonary stenosis are relatively asymptomatic, since the stenosis limits the volume of pulmonary blood flow. Congestive cardiac failure does not occur, and the ventricular communication allows sufficient mixing so that cyanosis is not severe.

Two corrective-type procedures are available for the older child with transposition of the great vessels and pulmonary stenosis. If the stenosis is valvular, a Mustard procedure can be combined with correction of the intracardiac anomalies. If, however, subpulmonary stenosis is present, a Rastelli-type operation can be performed by creating an intraventricular tunnel for left ventricular blood through the ventricular septal defect to the aorta and routing right ventricular blood to the pulmonary trunk through a valved conduit.[53]

CONGENITALLY CORRECTED TRANSPOSITION OF THE GREAT VESSELS WITH VENTRICULAR SEPTAL DEFECT AND PULMONARY STENOSIS. The basic anatomic details of congenitally corrected transposition of the great vessels have been discussed in Chapter 9. This condition may be associated with a ventricular septal defect and pulmonary stenosis of sufficient severity to lead to a right-to-left shunt at the ventricular level. The pulmonary stenosis may be either valvular or subvalvular. The latter can result from a membranous ring, muscular obstruction, accessory right atrioventricular valvular tissue[54] or aneurysm of membranous septum.[55]

Four features should lead to the suspicion of the presence of congenitally corrected transposition of the underlying anatomy for the variant of tetralogy of Fallot:

1. The second heart sound in the pulmonary area is extremely loud because the ascending aorta is located anteriorly and leftward.
2. The electrocardiogram characteristically shows a q wave in the right precordial leads and the absence of such a deflection in the left-sided leads.
3. Because of the location of the aorta on the thoracic roentgenogram, there is a prominent bulge along the left cardiac border. It should be mentioned that patients with corrected transposition, ventricular septal defect, and pulmonary stenosis frequently have mesocardia.
4. Finally, the echocardiogram, as indicated previously, can provide clues for the presence of congenitally corrected transposition of the great vessels.

The diagnosis is made angiographically, and the major differential point on these studies is to distinguish it from single ventricle with *l*-transposition. If symptomatic, a shunt should be performed.

CONGENITAL CARDIAC ANOMALIES ASSOCIATED WITH ASPLENIA.   Neonates or infants with asplenia usually present a picture of intense cyanosis, normal cardiac size, and diminished pulmonary blood flow. Despite the complexity of the form of cardiac anomalies with this syndrome, basically there is obstruction to pulmonary blood flow and a right-to-left shunt at the ventricular level.

The presence of asplenia can be suspected by identifying on the thoracic roentgenogram the findings of abnormal situs. Definite diagnosis depends upon identifying Howell-Jolly bodies and, at angiocardiography, finding other cardiac anomalies, such as abnormal relationship between the descending aorta and the inferior vena cava. The coexistence of total anomalous pulmonary venous connection in any patient with pulmonary stenosis and ventricular shunt suggests asplenia.

The diagnosis of asplenia as the underlying condition is important, for it signifies a poor prognosis.

SUMMARY

In neonates and infants with cyanosis, normal cardiac size, and diminished pulmonary vascular markings, a variety of anatomic conditions may be present in which there is a shunt at the ventricular level and pulmonary stenosis. Because of the availability of corrective procedures for several of these conditions in infancy, it is imperative that a correct diagnosis be made.

Physical examination and thoracic roentgenograms may yield data to indicate the presence of a tetrad variant, but the electrocardiogram and echocardiogram are much more valuable, as shown in Table 12-1.

ATRIAL COMMUNICATION

Among infants with the combination of cyanosis and decreased pulmonary blood flow, there are conditions in which the right-to-left shunt occurs at the atrial level. These conditions cause either marked decrease in right ventricular compliance or obstruction at the tricuspid valve. Unlike patients with tetralogy of Fallot or tetrad variants, cardiomegaly is usually present. Often, the electrocardiographic features are unique for a particular lesion and allow a definitive diagnosis of the underlying condition.

PULMONARY ATRESIA WITH INTACT VENTRICULAR SEPTUM

Pulmonary atresia with intact ventricular septum is an important congenital cardiac condition appearing in the neonatal period with cyanosis, decreased pulmonary vascularity, and cardiomegaly.

PATHOLOGY.   In pulmonary atresia, obstruction at the pulmonary valve is complete. The pulmonary valve is an imperforate membrane and shows three sinuses of Valsalva and three raphes radiating from the pulmonary annulus. The pulmonary annulus is hypoplastic. The pulmonary trunk, patent to the pulmonary valve, is funnel shaped. The pulmonary trunk arises from the pulmonary annulus and extends to normal-sized left and right pulmonary arteries. This is in marked contrast to the anatomy of the pulmonary trunk in patients with ventricular septal defect and pulmonary atresia, where the pulmonary trunk is markedly hypoplastic.

Pulmonary atresia with intact ventricular septum has been divided into two types on the basis of right ventricular size. In 80 to 85 percent of the patients, the right ventricle is hypoplastic, and in the remaining 15 to 20 percent, it is of normal size.

In the hypoplastic type, the right ventricle is diminutive, perhaps having a volume of 1 to 2 ml. The right ventricle is thick-walled and may be lined by endocardial fibroelastosis. It has been called "peachpit right ventricle" because of its size and internal appearance. The chamber consists of a conus and a markedly reduced sinus portion. The infundibular muscle is hypertrophied and narrows the subpulmonary area.[56]

The tricuspid valve is also hypoplastic and causes tricuspid stenosis. The structure of the tricuspid valve appears normal, although it is thickened.[57] It may be displaced into the right ventricle, as in Ebstein's malformation.[58]

The right ventricle may also be normal or near normal in size, and the wall is of normal thickness for a newborn. The conus portion of the right ventricle is narrowed, but the sinus portion is well formed. The tricuspid annulus is nor-

TABLE 12-1

Diagnostic Features of Tetrad Variants

CONDITION	PHYSICAL EXAMINATION	ELECTRO-CARDIOGRAM	X-RAY	ECHO-CARDIOGRAM
DORV	0	0	0	±
ECD	MI murmur	LAD ($-90°$ to $-150°$)	Increase in cardiac size	Typical for ECD
SV with PS	0	LAD (many cases), Abn Q waves, deep post-QRS loop	Prominent bulge left upper border	Typical for SV
d-TGV with VSD and PS	Ejection murmur over back	0	0	Typical for d-TGV
l-TGV with VSD and PS	Loud S_2	q V_1, no q V_6	Bulge upper left border	Typical for l-TGV
Asplenia	0	0	Abn situs	0

Abbreviations: Abn, abnormal; DORV, double outlet right ventricle; d-TGV, d-transposition of great vessels; ECD, endocardial cushion defect; LAD, left axis deviation; l-TGV, l-transposition of great vessels; MI, mitral insufficiency; PS, pulmonary stenosis; SV, single ventricle; VSD, ventricular septal defect; 0, no characteristic change.

mal, but abnormalities of the tricuspid valve are invariably present and lead to tricuspid insufficiency. These tricuspid valve abnormalities have been well described by Bharati and associates.[57] The anterior leaflet is large and nodular and has abnormal chordal and papillary muscle attachments. The medial leaflet is either absent or adherent to the ventricular wall. The inferior leaflet is often large and nodular. Histologically, the leaflets show disorganization of structure and alternate thick and thin areas.

The right atrium has a thickened wall and is enlarged, reaching marked degrees in patients with tricuspid regurgitation. The atrial septum shows a patent foramen ovale and, less frequently, an atrial septal defect. The left ventricle and aorta may be slightly dilated. The ductus arteriosus is patent but usually closes during the neonatal period.

The coronary circulation shows unique features. Intramyocardial sinusoid-coronary arterial communications are present.[59,60] These communications are evident as small openings in the endocardial surface of the right ventricle, and penetrate the myocardium to join the coronary arterial system. Over the surface of the right ventricle, particularly at the apex of the right ventricle, tortuous dilated coronary arterial branches arise and connect with the major coronary arteries.

HEMODYNAMICS. The primary hemodynamic abnormality results from the obstruction to blood flow from the right ventricle. Blood exits the right ventricle by either of two routes. One route is through the intramyocardial sinusoids.

Because of the obstruction to right ventricular outflow, the right ventricular systolic pressure rises to high levels, often exceeding aortic systolic pressure. Therefore, right ventricular blood flows through myocardial sinusoids into the coronary arterial system and, in fact, may flow retrograde into the aorta with systole. This has been well demonstrated angiographically.[60,61] The amount of flow through this pathway is small and occurs in patients with hypoplastic right ventricle. The volume of flow into the right ventricle is small, since it equals the amount exited through the sinusoids.

In patients with an abnormal tricuspid valve associated with tricuspid regurgitation, blood can exit the right ventricle retrograde through the tricuspid valve. In this situation, the degree of regurgitation varies greatly, but it can be massive and associated with a markedly pulsatile right ventricle and right atrium and with right ventricular dilatation.

Regardless of the details of the right ventricle, the basic pathway of the circulation is similar and depends upon a right-to-left shunt at the atrial level through the foramen ovale. If the atrial communication is small, flow to the left atrium is impeded, and right atrial pressure is elevated. In the neonate, a left-to-right shunt occurs through the ductus arteriosus and represents the sole source of pulmonary blood flow. As long as the ductus remains patent, pulmonary blood flow can be maintained, but as the ductus closes, pulmonary blood flow is reduced, leading to severe symptoms and death.

CLINICAL FEATURES.   The clinical features have been described by a number of authors.[62-66] The course is one of progressive neonatal cyanosis, respiratory distress, and early death. Cyanosis is almost always evident within the first 24 hours of life. The degree of cyanosis is inversely related to the size of the ductus, and as this closes, it becomes intense. In an occasional infant, the ductus remains patent, and cyanosis continues to be mild. Respiratory distress is related to the inadequacy of pulmonary blood flow. In most neonates, symptoms progress rapidly.

On physical examination, there is generalized cyanosis, and the neonate appears dyspneic. The jugular venous pulses may be engorged and show prominent a waves. Clinical evidence of cardiomegaly is present and most marked in the patients with tricuspid regurgitation. The second heart sound is single. Three types of murmurs have been described:

1. Ejection systolic murmur. This murmur is present in about half of the patients and is located along the mid to upper left sternal border. It is grade 1–2/6 and is believed to originate from the increased blood flow across the aortic valve.
2. Regurgitant systolic murmur. This is a high-pitched pansystolic murmur along the lower left sternal border. Although it may be grade 4/6, usually it is only grade 1–2/6. This murmur occurs more commonly in patients with a normal-sized right ventricle.
3. Continuous murmur. A continuous murmur may be heard early in the course of neonates but rarely persists.

In 20 percent of infants, no murmur is heard.

Hepatomegaly occurs in neonates with marked tricuspid regurgitation or a restrictive atrial communication. In the former, hepatic pulsations may be present.

ELECTROCARDIOGRAM.   The QRS axis in the frontal plane is usually between +60° and +120° (Fig. 12-7). In contrast to tricuspid atresia, left axis deviation is rare. Patients with a normal-sized right ventricle may have an axis directed slightly more to the right. Right atrial enlargement is usually present, invariably so after 1 month of age.

The precordial lead patterns are variable. A pattern of left ventricular hypertrophy or dominance is the most common and is believed to be related to hypoplasia of the right ventricle. It is manifested by an rS pattern and deep S wave in lead V_1 and a QRS or RS with R>S in lead V_6. The persistence of left ventricular hypertrophy beyond 1 month strongly suggests a hypoplastic right

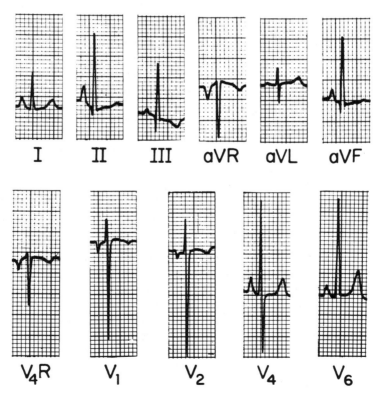

FIG. 12-7.   Electrocardiogram of pulmonary atresia with hypoplastic right ventricle in 6-month-old infant. Right atrial enlargement. QRS axis is +60°. Precordial leads show pattern of left ventricular hypertrophy. Small R wave in leads V_4R and V_1.

ventricle.[67] A few infants show a pattern of right ventricular hypertrophy, and this occurs most frequently in patients with a normal right ventricle.[67] A pattern of right ventricular hypertrophy, however, is not specific for a normal-sized right ventricle, because an occasional patient with a hypoplastic right ventricle may show right ventricular hypertrophy. Furthermore, it is more common in older patients.[62]

One report[63] describes serial observation of neonates whose initial electrocardiograms were normal or showed left ventricular hypertrophy and subsequently developed a pattern of right ventricular hypertrophy. Thus, the electrocardiographic findings have limitations in predicting right ventricular size.

THORACIC ROENTGENOGRAM.   The pulmonary vasculature is diminished. Cardiac size is increased because of right atrial and left ventricular enlargement (Fig. 12-8) and is larger in infants with tricuspid regurgitation. The cardiac contour usually is typical in showing a prominent right cardiac border (right atrial enlargement), a concave pulmonary artery, and a prominent convexity of cardiac apex (left ventricle).

ECHOCARDIOGRAM.   Pulmonary atresia is recognized by (1) a small right ventricular cavity (Fig. 12-9) and (2) an enlarged aorta. The identification of a tricuspid valve distinguishes pulmonary atresia from tricuspid atresia. It may be difficult to recognize this valve when the ventricle is hypoplastic. The pulmonary valve cannot be visualized.

CARDIAC CATHETERIZATION AND ANGIOCARDIOGRAM.   The diagnosis is confirmed by cardiac catheterization, and this study is necessary to determine right ventricular chamber size.

The oximetry data show no intracardiac left-to-right shunt. A right-to-left shunt is detected at the atrial level. Systemic arterial oxygen saturations vary considerably, primarily being determined by the volume of pulmonary blood flow, but most show marked reduction.

Pressure data show elevated right atrial pressure, especially a waves. Right atrial pressure exceeds left atrial pressure.[62] One report[63] indicates that pressure is higher in patients with a hypoplastic right ventricle than in those with a normal-sized right ventricle.

Right ventricular systolic pressure is increased, usually between 120 and 140 mm Hg, and significantly exceeds left ventricular systolic pressure. The pressure is greater in patients with hypoplastic right ventricle than in those with significant tricuspid regurgitation, where it may reach only 40 mm Hg. The pressure contour from the right ventricle typically shows symmetrical peaking.

Right atrial angiography shows a right-to-left shunt at the atrial level, but such a study is insufficient to diagnose pulmonary atresia. Right ventriculography must be performed. Once the catheter tip has been advanced into the right ventricle, a careful test injection must be performed, normally injecting

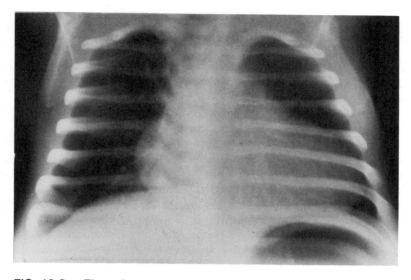

FIG. 12-8. Thoracic roentgenogram, posteroanterior view, of pulmonary atresia with hypoplastic right ventricle. Decreased pulmonary vasculature. Cardiomegaly. Right atrial border prominent. Broad, rounded contour of left cardiac border reflecting the left ventricle.

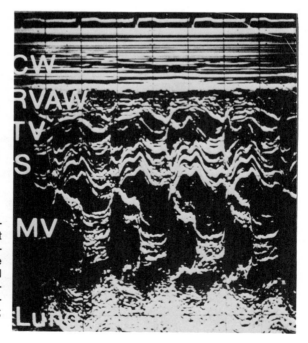

FIG. 12-9. Echocardiogram of pulmonary atresia with hypoplastic right ventricle. Small right ventricular cavity, containing small tricuspid valve (TV). The left ventricle and mitral valve (MV), by comparison, are enlarged. RVAW, right ventricular anterior wall; S, interventricular septum; CW, chest wall.

1/2 to 1 ml of contrast material to outline the right ventricle, for if it is hypo-plastic, this small volume may totally opacify the chamber.

In patients with a hypoplastic right ventricle, the small right ventricular cavity is opacified, and the chamber ends blindly at the pulmonary valve (Fig. 12-10). The chamber remains opacified as long as 10 sec. The myocardial sinu-soids are opacified and fill the coronary arteries.

If tricuspid regurgitation occurs, the right ventricle has an increased stroke volume, and the chamber is enlarged.

If the left ventricle or aorta is injected, a left-to-right shunt through the ductus arteriosus is seen, and the pulmonary arteries are opacified (Fig. 12-11). Characteristically, the pulmonary trunk is opacified to the level of the pulmo-nary valve. This observation led Freedom and associates[68] to use a double catheter technique to evaluate infants with pulmonary atresia, with simultane-ous ejection of contrast material into the right ventricle and into the aorta op-posite the ductus arteriosus. Both sides of the pulmonary valve are visualized simultaneously, and the valve thickness is outlined.

If the angiogram is technically satisfactory, right ventriculography can allow excellent estimation of right ventricular cavity size. Care must be taken not to misinterpret the sinusoids of a heavily trabeculated right ventricle.

MANAGEMENT.   Although the clinical findings of tachycardia, tachypnea, car-diomegaly, and hepatomegaly suggest congestive cardiac failure, these may be merely manifestations of the obstruction to blood flow from the right atrium. In patients with significant tricuspid insufficiency, there may be right-sided fail-ure, and digitalis may be helpful. It is not, however, the primary method of treatment.

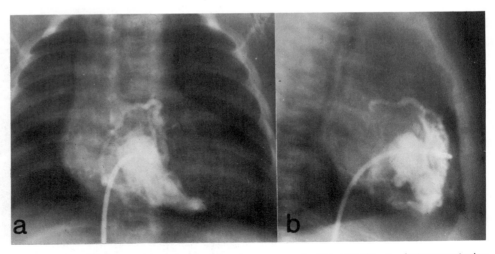

FIG. 12-10.   Right ventriculogram of pulmonary valvular atresia. **a.** Anteroposterior view. **b.** Lateral view. Hypoplastic right ventricle. No antegrade flow into pulmonary trunk. Through myocardial sinusoids, coronary arteries opacified in a retrograde direction.

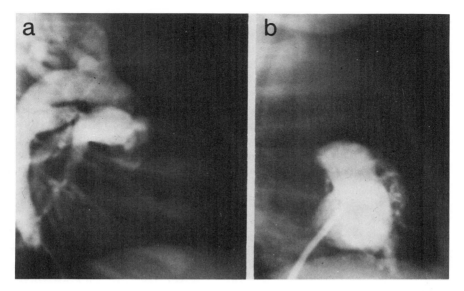

FIG. 12-11.   Lateral angiograms of pulmonary atresia. **a.** Aortogram. Opacification of pulmonary arteries through patent ductus arteriosus. Pulmonary trunk opacified to level of pulmonary valve. **b.** Right ventriculogram. Opacification of right ventricle and infundibulum to level of pulmonary valve.

The initial treatment should be directed toward hypoxemia and acidosis, using oxygen and bicarbonate. Following correction of acidosis, cardiac catheterization should be undertaken, and at that time, a Rashkind procedure should be performed to improve or make certain an adequate atrial communication exists.

At least half these infants die by 1 month of age, and virtually all patients die without operation. Even with operation, the mortality is high. In patients with pulmonary valvular atresia, the anatomy would seem extremely favorable for pulmonary valvotomy, since the pulmonary artery is patent to the level of the valve, and the right ventricle is patent beneath the valve. The hypoplasia of the pulmonary annulus, however, makes it difficult to relieve the obstruction, and the small right ventricle and tricuspid valve limit the inflow into the right ventricle. Pulmonary valvotomy alone has been performed in infants, but the operative mortality has been very high.[64,69–71] In patients with a normal-sized right ventricle, pulmonary valvotomy is, however, the preferred operation, but the risk is still high.

The preferred operation in infants with hypoplastic right ventricle is creation of both an aorticopulmonary shunt and an adequate atrial septal defect. The latter can be done by a Rashkind procedure, but our current policy is to perform a Waterston anastomosis and Blalock-Hanlon procedure at the same operation through a right thoracotomy. Other authors have reported favorable results from similar procedures. Trusler and Fowler[70] prefer a balloon atrial septostomy and a left aorticopulmonary anastomosis. Bowman[72] has described favorable results with a combination transventricular pulmonary valvotomy and Waterston shunt. Dhanavaravibul and associates[63] have described 11 of 15 survivors of an aorticopulmonary shunt, but 2 of the 11 survivors subsequently died, and another 5 survivors died at a second operation. This study indicates that although the patient may survive the palliative procedure, cyanosis usually persists and the unfavorable anatomy of a hypoplastic ventricle remains. Therefore, the ultimate hope of a normal circulation remains remote. A pulmonary valvotomy performed at or subsequent to the shunt has been advocated as a means of increasing right ventricular size, although long-term follow-up of such patients has not been reported. There is evidence, however, that a hypoplastic right ventricle can increase in size following pulmonary valvotomy.[69,73]

The ideal would be to allow the child to grow until a venous-pulmonary arterial conduit could be inserted. Unfortunately, the complications of pulmonary vascular disease and alterations of pulmonary arteries following a Waterston shunt or Potts operation could severely limit the potential for such procedures.

The infusion of prostaglandin E_1 during the initial management, catheterization, and in preparation for operation is extremely helpful in maintaining the infant and minimizing hypoxia and its complications.[74]

PULMONARY STENOSIS WITH HYPOPLASTIC RIGHT VENTRICLE

Severe pulmonary stenosis can occur with a diminutive right ventricle and present a clinical picture similar to pulmonary atresia, although the operative considerations and prognosis are different.

The pulmonary valve is thickened, deformed, and has a small central orifice. The pulmonary trunk may show slight dilatation. The right ventricular cavity is small and has an inflow portion and narrowed infundibulum, but the apical region is not developed.

In this condition, a right-to-left shunt is present at the atrial level because the right ventricular compliance is low on account of its small size and ventricular hypertrophy. Right ventricular output is reduced.

CLINICAL FEATURES.   Cyanosis is present from birth and can be severe. A murmur may be present at birth and is always discovered in the early neonatal period. The murmurs are of moderate intensity and may be from either pulmonary stenosis or tricuspid regurgitation. Systolic ejection clicks are rare. Hepatomegaly may be found.

ELECTROCARDIOGRAM.   The QRS axis is normal, and right atrial enlargement is present. The precordial leads almost always show left ventricular predominance. The rS ratio in lead V_1 is small, and this pattern is striking in comparison to the pattern expected for the age.

THORACIC ROENTGENOGRAM.   The pulmonary vasculature is diminished. Moderate cardiac enlargement is present, in part, because of right atrial dilatation. The pulmonary arterial segment is concave. The contour resembles a modern decanter.

CARDIAC CATHETERIZATION AND ANGIOCARDIOGRAM.   The important information derived from cardiac catheterization is the level of right ventricular pressure and size of the right ventricle.

A right-to-left shunt is present at the atrial level, and systemic arterial saturation may be very low (20 percent). Accordingly, saturations on the right side of the heart are also low.

Right ventricular systolic pressure may be as high as 175 mm Hg and the end-diastolic pressures also may be elevated.

After careful test injection, a small amount of contrast material should be injected. This shows antegrade flow into the pulmonary artery. The pulmonary valve may appear as a thick-domed valve or a thick immobile plate. A small amount of tricuspid regurgitation may be found that may be either real or artefactual. The right ventricular cavity is small. Right ventricular volumes were calculated by Freed and associates[75]: the mean right ventricular end-diastolic volume was 22 ml/m^2 (normal, 39 ± 8 ml/m^2), and right ventricular ejection fraction ranged from 50 to 88 percent. Nakazawa and associates[76] indicate that right ventricular function is reduced in patients with pulmonary stenosis and right-to-left atrial shunt.

MANAGEMENT.   These neonates should undergo prompt diagnostic studies, for the hypoxemia may lead to complications of acidosis. Efforts should be made to reduce oxygen utilization and to treat complications promptly.

The treatment of choice is pulmonary valvotomy, and we prefer to use inflow occlusion. Excellent results have been obtained with reduction in the degree of cyanosis. Some infants remain intensely cyanotic, probably from persistent problems in filling the right ventricle, and in these infants an aorticopulmonary shunt may need to be placed to provide a method for oxygenation.

Right ventricular volume increases postoperatively[69,73,75] but may never reach normal values, and in each of our survivors, a right-to-left shunt persists at the atrial level, even though right ventricular systolic pressures are near normal levels.

TRICUSPID ATRESIA WITH DIMINISHED PULMONARY BLOOD FLOW

Tricuspid atresia is associated with two cyanotic clinical pictures—one with diminished pulmonary blood flow which must be considered in the differential diagnosis of the other conditions discussed in this chapter, and the other associated with increased pulmonary blood flow (Chap. 11).

ANATOMY.   Tricuspid atresia is a complex of several separate anatomic anomalies, including (1) atresia of the tricuspid valve, (2) defect in the interatrial septum, (3) hypoplasia of the sinus portion of the right ventricle, and usually (4) a ventricular septal defect. Because the great vessels may be either normally related or transposed and the pulmonary valve may be normal, stenotic, or atretic, a classification of the forms of tricuspid atresia was developed by Edwards and Burchell in 1949.[77] Since that time, modifications of this classification have been made, including a recent one by Tandon and Edwards.[78]

For our purposes, the following classification is presented here and includes the number of patients we have catheterized in the first year of life (in parentheses):

Type I: Tricuspid atresia with normally related great vessels and:
     a. with coexistent pulmonary atresia (ventricular septum intact) (5)
     b. with pulmonary or subpulmonary stenosis and ventricular septal defect (24)
     c. normal pulmonary valve and large ventricular septal defect (3)
Type II: Tricuspid atresia with transposition of great vessels and:
     a. with coexistent pulmonary atresia (ventricular septum intact) (10)
     b. with pulmonary or subpulmonary stenosis and ventricular septal defect (2)
     c. normal pulmonary valve and large ventricular septal defect (1)

In this chapter, types Ia and Ib and IIa and IIb are discussed, since they are associated with decreased pulmonary blood flow, while types Ic and IIc were discussed in Chapter 11. Our distribution of anatomic types is similar to that of others, in which about 75 percent of patients with tricuspid atresia have normally related great vessels and 25 percent have transposition of the great vessels, and the distribution of cases between decreased and increased pulmonary blood flow is also about 75 percent to 25 percent.

The tricuspid valve is atretic, and its location is marked by a dimple.[79] In specimens, a tiny endocardial-lined blind pocket may be found in the floor of the right atrium in the location of the tricuspid valve. The right atrium is dilated, and its wall is hypertrophied. A communication is present in the atrial septum. The size of the communication varies, but often in infants, it is only a valvular competent foramen ovale. In a few infants, an atrial septal defect of fossa ovalis type is present.

The left atrium and the left ventricle are normally formed but are usually enlarged, the degree of enlargement being proportional to the volume of pulmonary blood flow.

In each patient other than those with coexistent pulmonary atresia, a ventricular septal defect is present and is located below the right and posterior aortic cusps[79] and includes the membranous septum. In infants with decreased pulmonary blood flow, the diameter of the ventricular septal defect is less than one-half the diameter of the aorta.

The right ventricle is composed primarily of the outflow area and does not contain papillary muscles. This chamber is small and may have hypertrophied infundibular muscles. The pulmonary valve is frequently stenotic, and the annulus is hypoplastic. The pulmonary artery is small. Obstruction to pulmonary blood flow can occur because of reduced size of the ventricular septal defect, infundibular stenosis, or coexistent valvular pulmonary stenosis.

If pulmonary atresia coexists, the ventricular septum is intact, and evidence of a right ventricle may be found only by identification of a minute blind endocardium-lined chamber. In these infants, pulmonary blood flow is dependent upon the ductus arteriosus.

Other than right aortic arch, associated cardiac malformations are rare in infants with tricuspid atresia and diminished pulmonary blood flow.

HEMODYNAMICS. Whether great vessels are normally related or transposed, the hemodynamics are similar. The systemic venous blood returns to the right atrium and has only one exit, the atrial communication. If the communication is narrowed, right atrial pressure is increased, and the right atrium becomes hypertrophied and dilated. This elevates systemic venous pressure and results in clinical features of hepatomegaly and distended neck veins.

A total right-to-left shunt occurs at the atrial level. The systemic venous and pulmonary venous returns enter the left atrium and mix completely in the left ventricle. The left ventricle ejects blood into both the aorta and the pulmonary artery. The volume of pulmonary blood flow is dependent upon the resistance to outflow, which is affected by the size of the ventricular septal defect and the degree of subpulmonary and valvular stenosis. In infants with coexistent pulmonary atresia, the volume of pulmonary blood flow depends upon the size of the patent ductus arteriosus.

Since there is mixing of both the pulmonary and systemic venous returns, tricuspid atresia is similar to an admixture lesion. As in all admixture lesions, an inverse relationship exists between the systemic arterial oxygen saturation and the magnitude of pulmonary blood flow. In the infants with tricuspid atresia discussed in this section, the volume of pulmonary blood flow is limited. Therefore, the volume of fully oxygenated pulmonary venous blood is small in relation to the amount of desaturated systemic venous return. The oxygen saturation of the aortic blood is quite reduced. When pulmonary stenosis is milder, pulmonary blood flow is larger, and systemic oxygen saturation is higher.

In infants with tricuspid atresia and diminished pulmonary blood flow, the volume of flow does not dilate the left ventricle sufficiently to cause congestive cardiac failure.

CLINICAL FEATURES. The major clinical finding is moderate generalized cyanosis, often being evident on the first day of life.[80,81] The degree of cyanosis reflects pulmonary blood flow and can become intense in patients with coexistent pulmonary atresia as the ductus arteriosus obliterates in the neonatal period. In some infants, congenital cardiac disease is discovered by finding a murmur. In neonates or infants with marked limitation of pulmonary blood flow, dyspnea may be present.

Rowe and Mehrizi[82] have indicated that the infant may have large a waves in the jugular venous pulse, but, in our experience, it has been difficult to identify these because of the rapid heart rate and short, chubby necks of infants. Hepatomegaly is not commonly found.

Although the murmur in tricuspid atresia is not diagnostic of that condition, it does reflect the volume of pulmonary blood flow. In patients with a patent pulmonary valve, the murmur originates from the blood flow through the ventricular septal defect and outflow area. The murmur is louder when there is a large pulmonary blood flow. It is usually pansystolic and located along the mid and upper left sternal border. In patients with coexistent pulmonary atresia, a continuous murmur may be present, but, occasionally, infants with severe pulmonary stenosis will have this type of murmur.

The second heart sound is single.

ELECTROCARDIOGRAM. The electrocardiogram, which has been the subject of many reports,[81,83-87] provides the major clinical diagnostic feature, left axis QRS complex.

Probably 85 percent of infants with tricuspid atresia and reduced pulmonary blood flow have left axis deviation, i.e., between 0 and $-90°$ (Fig. 12-12). In the remaining, the QRS axis may range to $+110°$ (Fig. 12-13). Patients with a normal QRS axis more commonly have coexistent pulmonary atresia or transposition of the great vessels. The QRS vector loop in the frontal plane is inscribed in a counterclockwise direction and helps in understanding that lead aVL almost invariably shows a qR pattern. This has been a helpful differential diagnostic point from pulmonary atresia, where a qR pattern is invariably found in lead aVF and no q in lead aVL.[88]

The precordial leads show the major QRS forces being directed posteriorly and leftward (Figs. 12-12 and 12-13). Thus, lead V_1 shows an rS pattern, and lead V_6 shows either a qR or an Rs pattern. The T waves may be inverted in the left precordial leads. The P waves are usually peaked and indicate right atrial enlargement. We[87] and others[81,86] have been unable to correlate the presence of right atrial enlargement with anatomic or hemodynamic factors. Although left atrial enlargement may coexist, this occurs primarily in older infants with increased pulmonary blood flow.

In our experience, about one half the patients have a short PR interval, despite having a normal P wave axis and no evidence of Wolff-Parkinson-White syndrome.

The reason for the left axis deviation has been studied by histologic analysis of the conduction system.[89,90] Guller and co-workers[89] identified the AV node adjacent to the central fibrous body and located by the dimple in the right atrium. They found early origin of the left bundle and elongation of the right

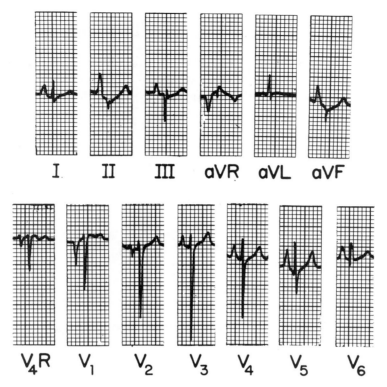

I   II   III   aVR   aVL   aVF

V_4R V_1 V_2 V_3 V_4 V_5 V_6

FIG. 12-12.   Electrocardiogram of 8-month-old infant with tricuspid atresia. Very large, peaked, pointed P waves of right atrial enlargement. QRS axis is $-60°$. Precordial leads show pattern of left ventricular hypertrophy. Small R wave in leads V_4R and V_1.

bundle, being located along the inferior aspect of the ventricular septal defect. This relation of the conduction system to the ventricular septal defect was also described by Bharati and Lev.[90]

THORACIC ROENTGENOGRAM.   The pulmonary vasculature is either normal or diminished. Cardiac size reflects the volume of pulmonary blood flow, being normal in patients with markedly limited flow. The cardiac contour, while not diagnostic, is often very suggestive of the diagnosis, perhaps more so in older patients. The right cardiac border may show a prominent convexity from the enlarged right atrium. The left cardiac border reveals a concave pulmonary arterial segment and a broad curvature of the left ventricle (Fig. 12-14). A right aortic arch may be present but, in our experience, is less frequent than the 5 to 10 percent reported elsewhere. The presence of cardiac enlargement and contour of left cardiac border help to distinguish tricuspid atresia from tetralogy of Fallot.

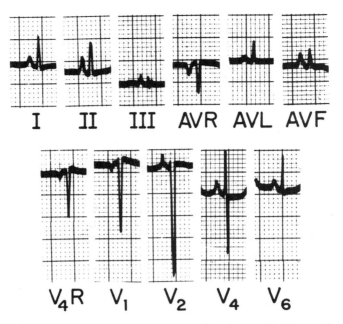

I II III AVR AVL AVF

V₄R V₁ V₂ V₄ V₆

FIG. 12-13. Electrocardiogram of patient with tricuspid atresia. Right atrial enlargement. QRS axis is +45°. Left ventricular hypertrophy.

ECHOCARDIOGRAM. The echocardiogram (Fig. 12-15) shows (1) absence of echoes from the tricuspid valve, (2) a hypoplastic anterior ventricle, and (3) an enlarged aorta. The left atrium and ventricle may be enlarged. If the pulmonary trunk is identified, it may be hypoplastic.

CARDIAC CATHETERIZATION AND ANGIOCARDIOGRAM. Cardiac catheterization is undertaken to distinguish tricuspid atresia from conditions with similar clinical and laboratory findings, although the electrocardiographic features permit a correct diagnosis in a high percentage of patients.

Despite numerous attempts, the catheter tip cannot be advanced into the right ventricle but can be passed from the right to the left atrium. There is evidence of a right-to-left shunt at the atrial level. The systemic arterial Po_2 in infants we have studied has ranged from 15 to 60 torr, with the lowest values usually being found in neonates.

Right atrial mean pressure and a wave are usually increased and higher than left atrial pressures,[81] the difference being particularly noted in a waves, as in one of our infants who had a 22 mm a wave in the right atrium and an 11 mm a wave in the left atrium. This pressure difference indicates obstruction at the level of the foramen ovale. Left-sided cardiac pressures are normal.

Right atrial injection of contrast material shows a dense right-to-left atrial shunt (Fig. 12-16a), subsequent opacification of the left ventricle (Fig. 12-16b),

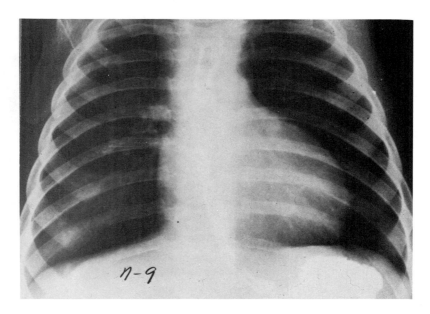

FIG. 12-14. Thoracic roentgenogram of tricuspid atresia. Diminished pulmonary vasculature. Concave pulmonary arterial segment. Broad round border of left cardiac contour reflecting the enlarged left ventricle.

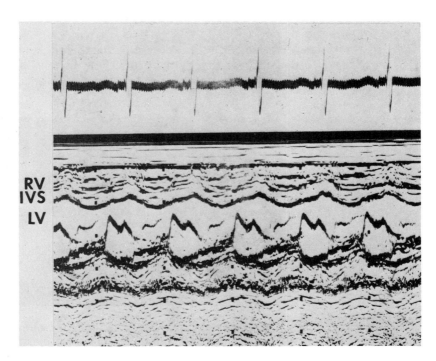

FIG. 12-15. Echocardiogram of tricuspid atresia. Enlarged left ventricle (LV) and minute right ventricle (RV). IVS, interventricular septum.

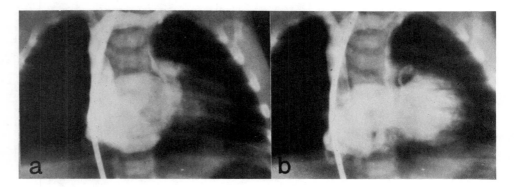

FIG. 12-16.   Anteroposterior venous angiogram of tricuspid atresia. **a.** Early exposure. **b.** Later exposure. Following opacification of right atrium, left atrium opacified and then left ventricle. Right ventricle not opacified.

and usually simultaneous opacification of both great vessels. Characteristically, there is a triangular filling defect between the medial aspect of the opacified right atrium and left ventricle.[91]

Left ventriculography (Fig. 12-17) is needed to identify the relationship of the great vessels, the presence and nature of obstruction to pulmonary blood flow, and the caliber of pulmonary arteries. These studies will help the planning for surgery.

At the time of cardiac catheterization, a balloon atrial septostomy should be performed to decompress the right atrium. The beneficial effects of this procedure in reducing elevated right atrial pressures have been described.[92,93]

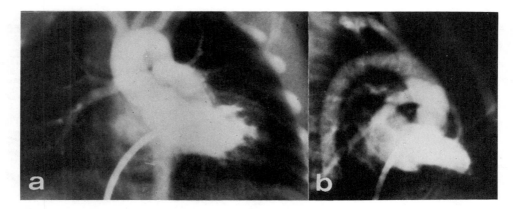

FIG. 12-17.   Left ventriculogram of tricuspid atresia. **a.** Anteroposterior view. **b.** Lateral view. From left ventricle, an enlarged aorta opacified. Minute column of opaque material passes through right ventricle (d) and opacifies pulmonary artery. Great vessels normally related.

Detailed studies of left ventricular function[94] have described an increased left ventricular diastolic volume and mildly depressed ejection fraction and have indicated that left ventricular function decreases with long-standing left ventricular volume overload.

MANAGEMENT.   Tricuspid atresia is a progressive condition because of the development of increased obstruction to pulmonary blood flow, usually by narrowing of the ventricular septal defect.[95,96] The major hemodynamic problems that lead to severe symptoms in infants are obstruction to right atrial emptying and reduced pulmonary blood flow. Most patients require operation.

The preferred operation is the combination of the creation of an atrial septal defect and an aorticopulmonary shunt.[92,97] Currently, we perform balloon atrioseptostomy during cardiac catheterization to improve the infant's status. At the time of operation, we combine the Blalock-Hanlon and Waterston procedures. Usually, we perform the operation soon after the cardiac catheterization.

Several reports have described the results of various types of aorticopulmonary shunts.[81,97-99] The results have not been encouraging, particularly in infants less than 1 month of age. Williams and co-workers[98] describe a 50 percent operative mortality in children of this age, using several types of shunts. They recommend the Potts procedure and stress the need to limit the volume of shunt.

Some infants may require a second operation to decrease the volume of pulmonary blood flow or to create a second shunt if the initial one occludes or becomes too narrow. A superior vena cava-pulmonary arterial shunt is not indicated in infants under 6 months of age. Dr. Taussig[100] has reported variable long-term results in patients with tricuspid atresia who underwent a Blalock-Taussig procedure in infancy.

The purpose of palliative procedures is the survival of infants to an age when a corrective procedure, using the Fontan approach, can be performed. Unfortunately, both the Waterston and Potts procedures are associated with the development of pulmonary vascular disease, which may make it impossible to perform such a corrective procedure. Thus, the Blalock-Taussig procedure has an advantage.

EBSTEIN'S ANOMALY OF THE TRICUSPID VALVE

Ebstein's malformation of the tricuspid valve is an infrequently occurring cardiac condition that may cause severe symptoms in the neonatal period.

ANATOMY.   In this condition, only a portion of the tricuspid valve is attached normally to the tricuspid annulus, while the remainder attaches from the right ventricular wall. This has led to the anomaly's also being called "downward displacement of the tricuspid valve." The anterior leaflet of the tricuspid valve is normal. In contrast, the posterior and septal leaflets originate abnormally, are thickened and deformed, and are only partially functional. The displaced leaflets adhere directly to the right ventricular wall or are attached by anomalous chordae tendineae and papillary muscles. The tricuspid valve often is insufficient.

The degree of tricuspid valvular displacement varies considerably, with the greatest degree of displacement being associated with the earliest onset and greatest severity of symptoms.

The size of the right ventricle distal to the tricuspid valve is reduced, but its wall has a normal thickness. The pulmonary orifice and pulmonary arteries may be small, depending upon the volume of pulmonary blood flow. The portion of the right ventricle between the tricuspid annulus and the location of the displaced tricuspid valve is thin walled and dilated. The right atrium is hypertrophied and dilated. The degree of dilatation depends on the amount of tricuspid insuffiency. A patent foramen ovale or atrial septal defect of the fossa ovalis type is present. The left side of the heart is normal.

In infants, Ebstein's malformation may coexist with pulmonary stenosis or atresia, and the clinical picture of these patients resembles that of the pulmonary valvular anomaly. Associated cardiac anomalies are uncommon.

HEMODYNAMICS. The severity of the hemodynamics varies considerably and depends principally on factors which influence right ventricular filling. Right ventricular filling is reduced and the volume of pulmonary blood flow is limited by several factors, one of which is the reduced volume of the right ventricular cavity. In the neonatal period, the right ventricular compliance is further reduced because of the increased pulmonary vascular resistance. Therefore, neonates with Ebstein's malformation may be severely symptomatic but improve within a week because the fall in pulmonary vascular resistance is associated with increase in ventricular compliance and improved pulmonary blood flow. Right ventricular filling may be further impeded because, as the atrium contracts, the atrialized portion of the right ventricle can expand so that flow into the right ventricle is decreased. Tricuspid regurgitation, which occurs in some patients, can further reduce pulmonary blood flow and cause dilatation of both the right atrium and right ventricle.

As a consequence of these factors altering right ventricular compliance, right atrial and systemic venous pressures are elevated.

Right atrial pressure can be further increased if the foramen ovale is small. A right-to-left shunt is present at the atrial level. The volume of shunt is inversely related to the amount of pulmonary blood flow.

CLINICAL FEATURES. Most patients with Ebstein's malformation are recognized in the neonatal period, and some of the infants may be critically ill. In neonates, cyanosis is the major feature leading to the initial recognition of cardiac disease and may be severe.[101-103] In one report,[104] 17 of 32 patients with Ebstein's malformation manifested cyanosis in the neonatal period, and in 11 of these, the cyanosis improved with age. Other authors have also indicated that cyanosis improves with age[102,103] because of the postnatal fall in pulmonary vascular resistance. The cyanosis in some infants improves to the point that they appear acyanotic. Cyanosis usually returns in later childhood.

Many neonates with severe Ebstein's malformation develop congestive cardiac failure, which may be present in utero.[105] Of 35 infants reported in an international cooperative study,[106] 72 percent had congestive cardiac failure. Although congestive cardiac failure may improve with age, the prognosis for such infants is poor.[106,107] Although it occurs more frequently in infants with tricuspid regurgitation, it is not limited to this group. One report states that following neonatal difficulties, survivors show normal growth and development after 2 months of age.[108]

The presence of a cardiac murmur or the development of supraventricular tachycardia are other features which lead to the suspicion of cardiac disease. Although we have emphasized that severely affected neonates have profound cyanosis, congestive cardiac failure, and respiratory distress, milder cases may have only mild cyanosis and no other symptoms.

Cardiomegaly is found clinically. The auscultatory findings may be very suggestive of the diagnosis, unlike many other cyanotic forms of congenital heart disease. A grade 2–3/6 systolic murmur is usually present along the left sternal border and is louder in patients with tricuspid regurgitation. A short, scratchy diastolic murmur is also present in many infants. The second heart sound is split,[109] and a fourth heart sound is often present, leading to a typical quadruple rhythm.

Hepatomegaly is present in patients with cardiac failure, but we have not observed a neonate with a pulsatile liver from the tricuspid regurgitation.

ELECTROCARDIOGRAM. The electrocardiogram provides valuable diagnostic clues (Fig. 12-18). Right atrial enlargement, evidenced by peaked P waves, is present in almost all patients and may reach 7 mm in height. The tallest P waves we have observed have occurred in infants with Ebstein's malformation or with tricuspid atresia.

Rowe and Mehrizi[110] indicate that the PR interval is prolonged in one half to two thirds of patients, but this has not been our experience.

The QRS axis is usually either normal or directed to the right, but it may occur in any quadrant because of the frequently associated intraventricular conduction defects. The precordial leads usually show right bundle-branch block,[102,104,107] but the QRS duration is less than 0.11 sec. With age, this interval prolongs. Others have emphasized that right bundle-branch block may develop following birth[108,111] and the QRS interval increases with age[107] Type B Wolff-Parkinson-White syndrome is found in other patients. The reasons for the association of these QRS abnormalities with Ebstein's anomaly are unknown. The R or R′ in lead V_1 does not exceed 11 mm.[102] Paroxysmal supraventricular tachycardia or atrial flutter may develop in these patients, perhaps because of the right atrial dilatation. These tachyarrhythmias occur in one fourth of patients.

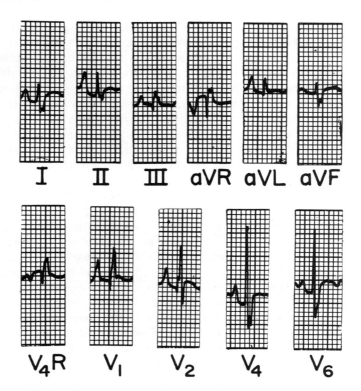

FIG. 12-18. Electrocardiogram of Ebstein's malformation of tricuspid valve in 6-day-old neonate. Right atrial enlargement. Complete right bundle branch block.

THORACIC ROENTGENOGRAM. The thoracic roentgenogram may show striking cardiomegaly. In fact, the largest cardiac silhouette we have seen occurred in a neonate with Ebstein's anomaly. Cardiac size tends to decrease with age. Milder forms of Ebstein's anomaly have normal cardiac size. The right cardiac border is prominent (Fig. 12-19). In older infants, the cardiac contour shows a more characteristic appearance, with a narrow base and a boxlike silhouette,[112] with a prominent upper portion of the left heart border from the enlarged right atrial appendage. The pulmonary vasculature is decreased.

ECHOCARDIOGRAM. The echocardiogram of Ebstein's malformation has been the subject of several reports.[113-117] The typical finding is delayed tricuspid valve closure, 60 msec or more following mitral valve closure, and the E-F slope of the tricuspid valve is reduced (Fig. 12-20). The excursion of the anterior leaflet of the tricuspid valve is increased. Paradoxical motion of the interventricular septum is present in most patients.

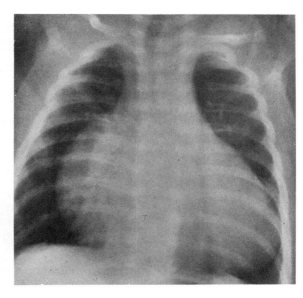

FIG. 12-19. Thoracic roentgenogram, posteroanterior view, of Ebstein's malformation of tricuspid valve in neonate. Cardiomegaly. Reduced pulmonary arterial markings. Prominent right cardiac border.

CARDIAC CATHETERIZATION AND ANGIOCARDIOGRAM. Cardiac catheterization is needed to confirm the diagnosis in sick infants, and in our view, the benefits derived from study outweigh the risks of catheterization in this particular condition. Cardiac arrhythmias, particularly supraventricular tachyarrhythmia, occur in these patients,[104,106,107] but these can usually be successfully controlled. In the cooperative study of 505 patients with Ebstein's malformation,[106] 363 underwent cardiac catheterization, and 90 of these developed paroxysmal atrial tachycardia. Thirteen deaths occurred during catheterization, including 5 of the 35 infants who were studied. Among 9 neonates less than 2 weeks of age we have studied, 1 developed atrial flutter and none died.

In neonates and infants, the right ventricular systolic pressure is usually normal and never greater than 40 mm Hg.[101,102] Right atrial pressure may be normal and the a wave larger than the v wave. In our symptomatic neonates, right atrial pressure was elevated, and the v waves predominated, reached 20 mm Hg, and was associated with tricuspid regurgitation. Oxygen saturation values are low on the right side of the heart and show a right-to-left atrial shunt.

Angiographic studies, particularly right ventriculograms, are usually diagnostic, but right atrial injections may be misleading because the right-to-left shunt and consequent opacification of left-sided chambers obscure the details of overlying cardiac structures.

Diagnosis rests on the identification of both the normal atrioventricular groove and a notch in the right ventricle that marks the location of the displaced tricuspid valve (Fig. 12-21). The distal part of the right ventricle is small. The right ventricle empties slowly. Paradoxical motion of the atrialized

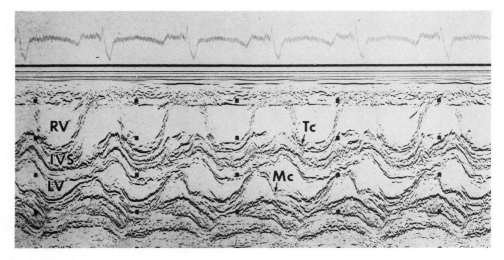

FIG. 12-20.   Echocardiogram of Ebstein's malformation of tricuspid valve. Wide excursion of tricuspid valve in right ventricle (RV). Delayed closure of tricuspid valve (Tc) compared to mitral closure (Mc). IVS, interventricular septum; LV, left ventricle.

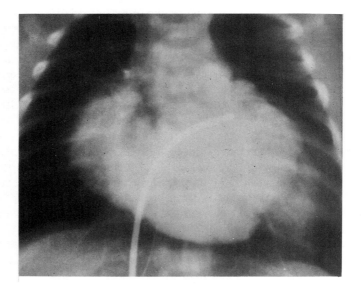

FIG. 12-21.   Right ventriculogram, anteroposterior view, of Ebstein's malformation of tricuspid valve. (Same patient as in Fig. 12-19.) Prompt opacification of right atrium, indicating tricuspid regurgitation. Scalloped border in the right ventricle indicates position of downward displacement of tricuspid valve.

portion of the right ventricle may be noted. Tricuspid regurgitation can also be identified.

MANAGEMENT.   The prognosis is poor for patients with severe symptoms in the neonatal period, particularly if they have tricuspid regurgitation, congestive cardiac failure, or paroxysmal supraventricular tachyarrhythmia. Of the 35 infants in the cooperative study,[106] 29 died, 15 from congestive cardiac failure, 8 others following cardiac operation, 5 others from cardiac catheterization, and 1 suddenly at 10 months of age. This incidence probably overestimates the severity of the condition, for mild degrees of Ebstein's may not be diagnosed in infancy, since it may cause few signs and symptoms. Other patients improve and may survive into childhood.

In symptomatic neonates, extensive treatment with digitalis and diuretics should be given, and operative treatment should be delayed while waiting for spontaneous improvement from changing pulmonary vascular resistance. Palliative procedures in infants have little to offer, and placement of a tricuspid valve or performance of a superior vena cava-pulmonary atrial shunt should be delayed until they are older, for the risk is high in early infancy.

ISOLATED HYPOPLASIA OF RIGHT VENTRICLE

Although a rare anomaly, isolated hypoplasia of the right ventricle must be considered in the differential diagnosis of pulmonary atresia. This anomaly has a strong familial tendency.[118-122]

PATHOLOGY.   In this anomaly, the left ventricle is enlarged when compared to the small right ventricle. Various degrees of hypoplasia of the right ventricle and the tricuspid valve are present, but in patients presenting in infancy,[118-121] the size is markedly reduced. Both the tricuspid and pulmonary valves are structurally normal. The underdevelopment usually involves the sinus portion of the right ventricle. The right ventricular endocardium may be thickened by fibroelastosis. The right atrium is dilated and hypertrophied. An atrial communication, either patent foramen ovale or atrial septal defect, is present.

HEMODYNAMICS.   The diminutive right ventricle and narrowed tricuspid valve limit right ventricular filling and reduce pulmonary blood flow. Blood flows predominantly from the right atrium into the left atrium, leading to reduced oxygen saturations in the left side of the heart and cyanosis. Right atrial pressure is elevated, but right ventricular systolic pressure is normal.

CLINICAL FEATURES.   Patients show significant cyanosis in the neonatal period. There may be hepatomegaly. Our infants initially appeared vigorous,[118,119] but without treatment, they developed progressive hypoxemia. The apex impulse is displaced laterally. The first and second heart sounds are normal, and we have not heard a fourth heart sound, although this has been described in older patients.[123] There may be no murmur, a soft systolic murmur along the left sternal border, or a continuous murmur of patent ductus arteriosus.

ELECTROCARDIOGRAM. In our patients, the electrocardiogram resembled that of pulmonary valvular atresia[118,119]: right atrial enlargement, left ventricular hypertrophy, a normal QRS axis, and q waves in leads aVF and III. The T waves were normal.

THORACIC ROENTGENOGRAM. The pulmonary vascular markings are diminished. Cardiac size is usually increased, with a prominent convexity of the right cardiac border (right atrial enlargement) and concave pulmonary arterial segment.

ECHOCARDIOGRAM. The echocardiogram resembles pulmonary atresia with hypoplastic right ventricle.

CARDIAC CATHETERIZATION AND ANGIOCARDIOGRAM. The catheter can be passed into the right ventricle, indicating patency of the tricuspid valve. The right ventricular and pulmonary arterial pressures are normal. Right atrial pressure, particularly a waves, is increased.

Angiography from the right atrium reveals a dense right-to-left shunt at the atrial level. It may be difficult to identify the right ventricle on an anteroposterior view because of the opacification of the overlying left atria. Careful selective injection of the right ventricle shows the reduced size of the right ventricle and the normal appearance of the pulmonary valve (Fig. 12-22).

At the time of cardiac catheterization, balloon atrial septostomy should be performed.

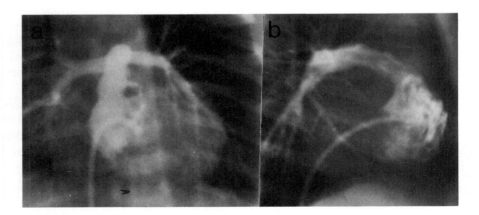

FIG. 12-22.   Right ventriculogram of hypoplastic right ventricle. **a.** Anteroposterior projection. **b.** Lateral projection. Hypoplastic right ventricle. Normal pulmonary valve.

MANAGEMENT. Although the patient has features of congestive cardiac failure, digitalis has little effect, since the congested features are related to limited egress from the right atrium and can only be effectively treated by creating an enlarged exit from the right atrium, either by the Rashkind procedure or the Blalock-Hanlon operation. In infants, an aorticopulmonary shunt is also needed to improve the hypoxemia.

PROGNOSIS. The prognosis for infants with cyanosis in the neonatal period is poor. A few cases of hypoplasia of the right ventricle have been reported in adulthood, but these have had lesser degrees of hypoplasia and no symptoms in infancy.[122]

ENDOCARDIAL FIBROELASTOSIS OF THE RIGHT VENTRICLE

A single neonate has been reported with extensive endocardial fibroelastosis of the right ventricle.[124] At autopsy, the right ventricular volume was normal, but the right ventricular endocardium was thickened and white. The left ventricle was dilated.

The clinical picture of this neonate was similar to that of hypoplastic right ventricle. Cyanosis and rapid respirations were present within 12 hours of birth. There was no murmur. The electrocardiogram showed a QRS axis of $+25°$, right atrial enlargement, and left ventricular hypertrophy and strain. Thoracic roentgenogram showed cardiomegaly, decreased pulmonary vasculature, and concave pulmonary arterial segment.

The circulating pattern of this neonate was considered similar to that of one with hypoplastic right ventricle. Decreased right ventricular compliance limits pulmonary blood flow, and a right-to-left shunt occurs at the atrial level. This condition must be considered in the differential diagnosis of the other conditions discussed in this section, but the clinical features alone would not allow differentiation. Treatment, however, would be a systemic-pulmonary arterial shunt and creation of an atrial septal defect.

UHL'S ANOMALY OF THE HEART

This is an uncommon cardiac anomaly, initially described by Uhl[125] and the subject of two additional reports.[126,127] It must be considered in the differential diagnosis of Ebstein's malformation and of tricuspid regurgitation. In this anomaly, there is marked hypoplasia or aplasia of the right ventricular myocardium. The right ventricular myocardium, over virtually the entire free wall, is absent, and the endocardium and epicardium are adjacent without intervening myocardium. The tricuspid valve is structurally normal, but the annulus is dilated. Both the right atrium and the right ventricle are greatly dilated. The left side of the heart is normal, including the left ventricular myocardium. The foramen ovale is intact.

Because the myocardium is absent, the right ventricle empties poorly, becomes dilated, and offers resistance to filling. The right ventricle contracts forcefully to fill the pulmonary artery, but this is not fully effective, and the cardiac output is reduced. Right atrial pressure is elevated.

The history and physical examination show findings of congestive cardiac failure, including the development of peripheral pitting edema and a puffy face. Marked cardiomegaly, weak heart sounds, and absence of a murmur are other features. Cyanosis is not present except in a terminal state. Hepatomegaly is found.

The electrocardiogram shows right atrial enlargement and low voltage QRS complex and may have ST and T wave changes. The axis may be normal, or there may be marked right axis deviation.

On roentgenography, there is striking cardiomegaly and normal pulmonary vascular markings. Cardiac catheterization in one infant[127] showed tall a waves in the right atrium which were transmitted to the right ventricle and pulmonary artery. At angiography, the right ventricle is enlarged and noncontractile, and its wall is thin and has no trabeculation. The right atrium is dilated, and emptying of the right side of the heart is delayed.

Treatment consists of digitalis and diuretics, but these only provide symptomatic relief and are only partially effective. One operative approach would be a Fontan-type operation, although we know of no patients who have been operated upon.

TRICUSPID INSUFFICIENCY

Tricuspid insufficiency may be related to a variety of cardiac problems and should not in itself be considered a primary diagnosis until various etiologic factors have been excluded. A number of the conditions that lead to tricuspid insufficiency are discussed in other portions of this chapter. A classification is given below:

I. Involvement of tricuspid valve as part of another cardiac condition directly involving the tricuspid valve.
   A. Ebstein's malformation (Chap. 12)
   B. Endocardial cushion defect (Chap. 11)
   C. Endocarditis
II. Tricuspid insufficiency secondary to a condition affecting the right ventricle
   A. Associated with increased right ventricular systolic pressure
      1. Pulmonary stenosis or atresia with intact ventricular septum (Chaps. 10, 12)
      2. Pulmonary hypertension (Chap. 14)
   B. Right ventricular dilatation
      1. Cardiomegaly (Chap. 12)
      2. Premature closure of foramen ovale
      3. Obstructive pulmonary disease (Chap. 14)
      4. Endocardial fibroelastosis (Chap. 10)

III. Primary abnormalities of the tricuspid valve
   A. Dysplastic tricuspid valve
   B. Papillary muscle dysfunction secondary to asphyxia or metabolic insult (can be transient)

In each of the conditions associated with significant tricuspid insufficiency, the neonate has cyanosis, a greatly enlarged heart, and congestive cardiac failure. The clinical and laboratory findings often permit the diagnosis of the condition underlying the tricuspid insufficiency. The diagnosis can be be assisted by finding elevated right ventricular systolic pressure at cardiac catheterization or by demonstrating a diagnostic angiographic appearance of the right ventricle.

In this section, only isolated tricuspid regurgitation from primary abnormalities of the tricuspid valve is considered, since most of the other conditions are discussed elsewhere in the text.

PATHOLOGY.   The amount of autopsy material in isolated tricuspid insufficiency is limited.[128] The right atrium and right ventricle are dilated, and the right atrial wall is thickened. The foramen ovale is patent. The tricuspid valve may be normal but usually shows thickening of the valve cusps, shortened or absent chordae tendineae, and small papillary muscles. The valve originates from the annulus or is slightly displaced into the right ventricle.

Recently, studies[129,130] have indicated that even massive tricuspid insufficiency of neonates may undergo spontaneous resolution, and they have suggested that dysfunction of the tricuspid valve occurs from myocardial abnormalities. Bucciarelli and associates[129] described necropsy findings of two neonates with tricuspid regurgitation and showed necrosis of the anterior papillary muscle of the tricuspid valve. Neonates who have transient tricuspid insufficiency often have a history of neonatal distress, manifested by a low Apgar score at birth and hypoxemia and hypoglycemia. Furthermore, Nelson and colleagues[131] have shown elevation of serum creatine phosphokinase fraction 2 in neonates with tricuspid regurgitation, providing supporting evidence for myocardial damage. These authors believe that hypoxemia and the associated depletion of limited myocardial glycogen stores lead to damage of the particularly vulnerable papillary muscles. With restoration of glycogen stores and improvement of oxygenation, the papillary muscle function returns.

HEMODYNAMICS.   Regardless of its etiology, tricuspid insufficiency in the neonatal period can be associated with congestive cardiac failure because the normally elevated pulmonary vascular resistance of the neonatal period elevates right ventricular preload and magnifies the degree of regurgitation. As pulmonary vascular resistance falls postnatally, the load on the right ventricle lessens. The degree of tricuspid regurgitation depends upon the extent of the tricuspid valvular abnormality and the level of pulmonary vascular resistance, which in itself may be raised by hypoxemia or acidosis.

With major tricuspid regurgitation, right ventricular end-diastolic and right atrial pressures are elevated. The foramen ovale can be stretched open, allowing a right-to-left atrial shunt and resultant cyanosis.

CLINICAL FEATURES. The clinical features have been described in several reports.[132-141] This is a neonatal condition presenting symptoms in the first week of life, often on the first day. Cyanosis is the initial symptom and may be combined with features of congestive cardiac failure.

The degree of cyanosis is variable but can be severe. Tachypnea and tachycardia are present. A grade 1-4/6 systolic murmur is found along the lower left sternal border, and its presence may lead to the recognition of cardiac disease. The murmur is often of high frequency and radiates to the right sternal border. The first heart sound has usually been described as normal and the second heart sound as single. This latter finding may result from the reduced volume of flow across the pulmonary valve. The presence of a single second heart sound makes it difficult to distinguish isolated tricuspid regurgitation from the tricuspid insufficiency associated with pulmonary stenosis or atresia. Systolic pulsations of the liver may have been reported.[137]

ELECTROCARDIOGRAM. There are no characteristic electrocardiographic features of this condition. The QRS axis in the frontal plane is normal for the age, but in two of our neonates, left axis deviation ($-105°$ and $-60°$) was present. Right atrial enlargement is the most consistent finding (Fig. 12-23). The precordial leads may be normal for the age or show right ventricular hypertrophy. Occasionally, complete right bundle-branch block is present.[139] Bucciarelli and associates[129] described ST segment depression in the midprecordial leads and T wave inversion in the left precordial leads and believe these findings indicated myocardial ischemia.

THORACIC ROENTGENOGRAM. Massive cardiomegaly is present (Fig. 12-24), and the right cardiac border is prominent and rounded, presumably from right atrial enlargement. The cardiac contour resembles that of Ebstein's malformation or that of severe pulmonary stenosis. The pulmonary vasculature appears normal or diminished.

ECHOCARDIOGRAM. We performed echocardiograms in three neonates,[141] and in each a normal M-mode tracing was obtained, showing neither abnormal tricuspid valve motion nor paradoxical septal motion. The tricuspid valve opening was normal, helping to distinguish it from Ebstein's malformation.

CARDIAC CATHETERIZATION AND ANGIOCARDIOGRAM. The cardiac catheterization in these neonates is usually performed to determine the underlying cardiac condition, and usually the differential diagnosis is among the conditions that obstruct the pulmonary blood flow and have a right-to-left atrial shunt.

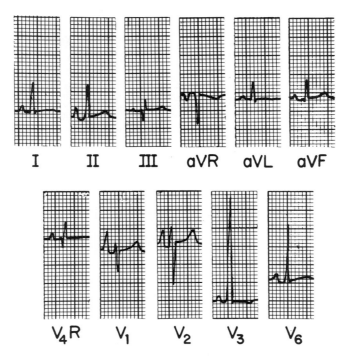

FIG. 12-23. Electrocardiogram of 4-day-old neonate with tricuspid insufficiency. Right atrial enlargement. QRS axis is +30°. Small QRS voltages right precordial leads.

The catheter tip can be advanced into the right ventricle, eliminating tricuspid atresia, and the ease with which this can be accomplished would tend to exclude cases of pulmonary atresia or stenosis with hypoplastic right ventricle.

The right ventricular systolic pressure is usually less than the systemic arterial pressure[130,136,139-141] but may equal[137] or exceed the left ventricular systolic pressure.[129,130] The highest right ventricular systolic pressure reported is 90 mm Hg, but usually the value is less than 55 mm Hg. If pulmonary arterial pressure is measured, it is similar to right ventricular systolic pressure, tending to exclude pulmonary stenosis. Right atrial pressures are normal or show slight elevation of a and v waves, but the a wave is taller.

Oximetry data show a right-to-left shunt at the atrial level.[129,130,137,141] Right ventriculography shows a large degree of tricuspid regurgitation, a markedly enlarged right atrium, and an extremely contractile right ventricle (Fig. 12-25). Occasionally, there may be no forward flow of contrast material into the pulmonary artery, giving the false impression of pulmonary atresia.[137,141] The tricuspid valve appears at the normal site. Passage of contrast material occurs from the right to the left atrium.

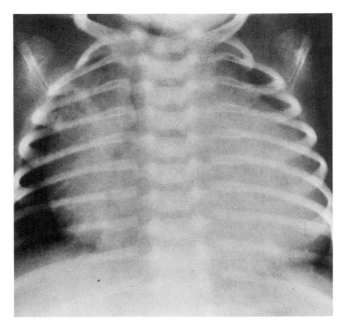

FIG. 12-24. Thoracic roentgenogram, posteroanterior view, of congenital tricuspid insufficiency. Massive cardiomegaly. Reduced pulmonary arterial markings.

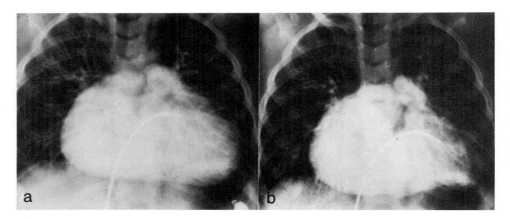

FIG. 12-25. Right ventriculogram, anteroposterior view, of congenital tricuspid insufficiency. **a.** Diastolic film. **b.** Systolic film. Massive tricuspid regurgitation.

Boucek and associates[130] have measured the volumes of the right-sided chambers angiographically and found: (1) right atrium of 225 to 759 percent of normal, (2) right ventricular end-diastolic of 121 to 357 percent of normal, and (3) right ventricular ejection fraction normal.

MANAGEMENT.   Prior to the reports of Boucek et al.[130] and Bucciarelli et al.,[129] nearly every patient with this condition died. However, these studies have provided new insight into the therapy and prognosis.

Digitalis and diuretics should be given and prompt attention directed toward correction of acidosis, hypoglycemia, or other metabolic abnormalities. Cardiac catheterization is undertaken to exclude operative conditions. The neonate is managed medically. With a fall in pulmonary arteriolar resistance or improvement of papillary muscle dysfunction, the infant's condition improves.

In Bucciarelli's experience,[129] in each survivor there was resolution of cardiomegaly, cyanosis, and the murmur by 2 weeks of age, while electrocardiographic changes persisted for 2 months. Follow-up examination of their patients at 8 months to 5 years was normal. Boucek and associates[130] report residual abnormalities of auscultation and electrocardiographic or thoracic roentgenograms in some patients, but the severity of the abnormalities was less. Cardiac volume measurements determined at follow-up cardiac catheterization also improved.

REFERENCES

Tetralogy of Fallot

1. Van Praagh R, Van Praagh S, Nebesar RA, et al.: Tetralogy of Fallot: Underdevelopment of the pulmonary infundibulum and its sequelae. Am J Cardiol 26:25, 1970
2. Becker AE, Connor M, Anderson RH: Tetralogy of Fallot: A morphometric and geometric study. Am J Cardiol 35:402, 1975
3. Rosenquist GC, Sweeney LJ, Stemple DR, Christianson SD, Rowe RD: Ventricular septal defect in tetralogy of Fallot. Am J Cardiol 31:749, 1973
4. Rao BNS, Anderson RC, Edwards JE: Anatomic variations in the tetralogy of Fallot. Am Heart J 81:361, 1971
5. Morgan BC, Guntheroth WG, Bloom RS, Fyler DC: A clinical profile of paroxysmal hyperpnea in cyanotic congenital heart disease. Circulation 31:66, 1965
6. Guntheroth WG, Morgan BC, Mullins GL, Baum D: Venous return with knee-chest position and squatting in tetralogy of Fallot. Am Heart J 75:313, 1968
7. Morris DG, Felner JM, Schlant RC, Franch RH: Echocardiographic diagnosis of tetralogy of Fallot. Am J Cardiol 36:908, 1975
8. King SB, Franch RH: Production of increased right-to-left shunting by rapid heart rates in patients with tetralogy of Fallot, Circulation 46:265, 1971
9. Young D, Elbl F: Supraventricular tachycardia as cause of cyanotic syncopal attacks in tetralogy of Fallot. N Engl J Med 284:1359, 1971
10. Fellows KE, Freed MD, Keane JF, et al.: Results of routine preoperative coronary angiography in tetralogy of Fallot. Circulation 51:561, 1975

11. Ponce FE, Williams LC, Webb HM, Riopel DA, Hohn AR: Propranolol palliation of tetralogy of Fallot: Experience with long-term drug treatment in pediatric patients. Pediatrics 52:100, 1973

12. Cummings GR, Carr W: Relief of dyspnoeic attacks in Fallot's tetralogy with
propranolol. Lancet 1:519, 1966

13. Cummings GR: Propranolol in tetralogy of Fallot (Editorial). Circulation 41:13,
1970

14. Nudel DB, Berman MA, Talner NS: Effects of acutely increasing systemic vascular resistance on oxygen tension in tetralogy of Fallot. Pediatrics 58:248, 1976

15. Bernhard WF, Jones JE, Friedberg DZ, Litwin SB: Ascending aorta-right pulmonary artery shunt in infants and older patients with certain types of cyanotic
congenital heart disease. Circulation 43:580, 1971

16. Norberg WJ, Tadavarthy M, Knight L, Nicoloff DM, Moller JH: Late hemodynamic and angiographic findings after ascending aorta-pulmonary artery anastomosis. J Thorac Cardiovasc Surg 76:345, 1978

17. Cole RB, Muster AJ, Fixler DE, Paul MH: Long-term results of aortopulmonary
anastomosis for tetralogy of Fallot. Morbidity and mortality, 1946–1969. Circulation 43:263, 1971

18. von Bernuth G, Ritter DG, Frye RL, et al.: Evaluation of patients with tetralogy
of Fallot and Potts anastomosis. Am J Cardiol 27:259, 1971

19. Miller WW, Nadas AS, Bernhard WF, Gross RE: Congenital pulmonary atresia
with ventricular septal defect. Review of the clinical course of fifty patients with
assessment of the results of palliative surgery. Am J Cardiol 21:673, 1968

20. Starr A, Bonchek LI, Sunderland CO: Total correction of tetralogy of Fallot in
infancy. J Thorac Cardiovasc Surg 65:45, 1973

21. Castaneda AR, Freed MD, Williams RG, Norwood WI: Repair of tetralogy of
Fallot in infancy. Early and late results. J Thorac Cardiovasc Surg 74:372, 1977

22. Pacifico AD, Bargeron LM Jr, Kirklin JW: Primary total correction of Fallot in
children less than four years of age. Circulation 48:1085, 1973

23. Kerr AR, Barratt-Boyes BG: Surgery of tetralogy of Fallot in infancy: Compari-
son of shunt palliation and primary intracardiac repair. In Barratt-Boyes BG,
Neutze JM, Harris EA (eds): Heart Disease in Infancy. Diagnosis and Surgical
Treatment. Edinburgh and London, Churchill Livingstone, 1973, pp 197–203

24. Bonchek LI, Starr A, Sunderland CO, Menashe VD: Natural history of tetralogy
of Fallot in infancy. Clinical classification and therapeutic implications. Circulation 48:392, 1973

25. Sunderland CO, Matarazzo RG, Lees MH, et al.: Total correction of tetralogy of
Fallot in infancy. Postoperative hemodynamic evaluation. Circulation 48:398,
1973

26. Rocchini AP, Rosenthal A, Freed M, Castaneda AR, Nadas AS: Chronic congestive heart failure after repair of tetralogy of Fallot. Circulation 56:305, 1977

27. Jarmakani JMM, Graham TP Jr, Canent RV, Jewett PH: Left heart function in
children with tetralogy of Fallot before and after palliative or corrective surgery.
Circulation 46:478, 1972

28. Graham TP Jr, Cordell D, Atwood GF, et al.: Right ventricular volume characteristics before and after palliative and reparative operation in tetralogy of Fallot. Circulation 54:417, 1976

Tetralogy of Fallot with Absence of Pulmonary Valve

29. Ruttenberg HD, Carey LS, Adams P Jr, Edwards JE: Absence of the pulmonary
valve in the tetralogy of Fallot. Am J Roentgenol Radium Ther Nucl Med
91:500, 1964

30. Miller RA, Lev M, Paul MH: Congenital absence of the pulmonary valve. The

clinical syndrome of tetralogy of Fallot with pulmonary regurgitation. Circulation 26:266, 1962

31. Lakier JB, Stanger P, Heymann MA, Hoffman JIE, Rudolph AM: Tetralogy of Fallot with absent pulmonary valve. Natural history and hemodynamic considerations. Circulation 50:167, 1974
32. Bove EL, Shaher RM, Alley R, McKneally M: Tetralogy of Fallot with absent pulmonary valve and aneurysm of the pulmonary artery: Report of two cases presenting as obstructive lung disease. J Pediatr 81:339, 1972
33. Stafford EG, Mair DD, McGoon DC, Danielson GK: Tetralogy of Fallot with absent pulmonary valve. Surgical considerations and results. Circulation 47, 48[Suppl 3]:24, 1973

Tetrad Variants

34. Rao BN, Edwards JE: Conditions simulating the tetralogy of Fallot. Circulation 49:173, 1974
35. Zamora R, Moller JH, Edwards JE: Double-outlet right ventricle. Anatomic types and associated anomalies. Chest 68:672, 1975
36. Tandon R, Moller JH, Edwards JE; Tetralogy of Fallot associated with persistent common atrioventricular canal (endocardial cushion defect). Br Heart J 36:197, 1974
37. Lindsay WG: Personal communication
38. Zavanella C, Matsuda H, Subramanian S: Successful correction of a complete form of atrioventricular canal associated with tetralogy of Fallot: Case report. J Thorac Cardiovasc Surg 74:195, 1977
39. Rahimtoola SH, Ongley PA, Swan HJC: The hemodynamics of common (or single) ventricle. Circulation 34:14, 1966
40. Marin-Garcia J, Tandon R, Moller JH, Edwards JE: Single ventricle with transposition. Circulation 49:994, 1974
41. Marin-Garcia J, Tandon R, Moller JH, Edwards JE; Common (single) ventricle with normally related great vessels. Circulation 49:565, 1974
42. Davachi F, Moller JH: The electrocardiogram and vectorcardiogram in single ventricle. Anatomic correlations. Am J Cardiol 23:19, 1969
43. Yacoub MH, Radley-Smith R: Use of a valved conduit from right atrium to pulmonary artery for "correction" of single ventricle. Circulation 54 [Suppl 3]:63, 1976
44. Edie RN, Ellis K, Gersony WM, et al.: Surgical repair of single ventricle. J Thorac Cardiovasc Surg 66:350, 1973
45. Shaher RM, Puddu GC, Khoury G, Moës CAF, Mustard WT: Complete transposition of the great vessels with anatomic obstruction of the outflow tract of the left ventricle. Surgical implications of anatomic findings. Am J Cardiol 19:658, 1967
46. Layman TE, Edwards JE: Anomalies of the cardiac valves associated with complete transposition of the great vessels. Am J Cardiol 19:247, 1967
47. Riemenschneider TA, Goldberg SJ, Ruttenberg HD, Gyepes MT: Subpulmonic obstruction in complete d-transposition produced by redundant tricuspid tissue. Circulation 39:603, 1969
48. Vidine BA, Subramanian S, Wagner HR: Aneurysm of the membranous ventricular septum in transposition of the great arteries. Circulation 53:157, 1976
49. Mathew R, Rosenthal A, Fellows K: The significance of right aortic arch in d-transposition of the great arteries. Am Heart J 87:314, 1974
50. Nanda NC, Gramiak R, Manning JA, Lipchik EO: Echocardiographic features of subpulmonic obstruction in dextrotransposition of the great vessels. Circulation 51:515, 1975

51. Bargeron LM Jr, Elliott LP, Soto B, Bream RP, Curry GC: Axial cineangiography in congenital heart disease. Section I. Concept, technical, and anatomic considerations. Circulation 56:1075, 1977
52. Elliott LP, Bargeron LM Jr, Bream PR, Soto B, Curry GC: Axial cineangiography in congenital heart disease. Section II. Specific lesions. Circulation 56:1084, 1977
53. Rastelli GC, Wallace RB, Ongley PA: Complete repair of transposition of the great arteries with pulmonary stenosis. A review and report of a case corrected by using a new surgical technique. Circulation 39:83, 1969
54. Levy MJ, Lillehei CW, Elliott LP, et al.: Accessory valvular tissue causing subpulmonary stenosis in corrected transposition of the great vessels. Circulation 27:494, 1963
55. Krongrad E, Ellis K, Steeg CN, et al.: Subpulmonary obstruction in congenitally corrected transposition of the great arteries due to ventricular membranous septal aneurysms. Circulation 54:679, 1976

Pulmonary Atresia

56. Arom KV, Edwards JE; Relationship between right ventricular muscle bundles and pulmonary valve. Significance in pulmonary atresia with intact ventricular septum. Circulation 54 [Suppl 3]:79, 1976
57. Bharati S, McAllister HA Jr, Chiemmongkoltip P, Lev M: Congenital pulmonary atresia with tricuspid insufficiency. Morphologic study. Am J Cardiol 40:70, 1977
58. Elliott LP, Adams P Jr, Edwards JE: Pulmonary atresia with intact ventricular septum. Br Heart J 25:489, 1963
59. Grant RT: An unusual anomaly of coronary vessels in the malformed heart of a child. Heart 13:273, 1926
60. Freedom RM, Harrington DP: Contributions of intramyocardial sinusoids in pulmonary atresia and intact ventricular septum to a right-sided circular shunt. Br Heart J 36:1061, 1974
61. Lauer RM, Fink HP, Petry EL, Dann MI, Diehl AM: Angiographic demonstration of intramyocardial sinusoids in pulmonary-valve atresia with intact ventricular septum and hypoplastic right ventricle. N Engl J Med 271:68, 1964
62. Cole RB, Muster AJ, Lev M, Paul MH: Pulmonary atresia with intact ventricular septum. Am J Cardiol 21:23, 1968
63. Dhanavaravibul S, Nora JJ, McNamara DG: Pulmonary valvular atresia with intact ventricular septum: Problems in diagnosis and results of treatment. J Pediatr 77:1010, 1970
64. Shams A, Fowler RS, Trusler GA, Keith JD, Mustard WT: Pulmonary atresia with intact ventricular septum: Report of 50 cases. Pediatrics 47:370, 1971
65. Celermajer JM, Bowdler JD, Gengos DC, Cohen DH, Stuckey DS: Pulmonary valve fusion with intact ventricular septum. Am Heart J 76:452, 1968
66. Benton JW Jr, Elliott LP, Adams P Jr, et al.: Pulmonary atresia and stenosis with intact ventricular septum. Am J Dis Child 104:161, 1962
67. Davignon AL, Greenwold WE, DuShane JW, Edwards JE: Congenital pulmonary atresia with intact ventricular septum. Clinicopathologic correlation of two anatomic types. Am Heart J 62:591, 1961
68. Freedom RM, White RI Jr, Ho CS, et al.: Evaluation of patients with pulmonary atresia and intact ventricular septum by double catheter technique. Am J Cardiol 33:892, 1974
69. Moller JH, Girod DA, Amplatz K, Varco RL: Pulmonary valvotomy in pulmonary atresia with hypoplastic right ventricle. Surgery 68:630, 1970
70. Trusler GA, Fowler RS: The surgical management of pulmonary atresia with

intact ventricular septum and hypoplastic right ventricle. J Thorac Cardiovasc Surg 59:740, 1970
71. Gersony WM, Bernhard WF, Nadas AS, Gross RE: Diagnosis and surgical treatment of infants with critical pulmonary outflow obstruction. Study of thirty-four infants with critical pulmonary stenosis or atresia, and intact ventricular septum. Circulation 35:765, 1967
72. Bowman FO Jr, Malm JR, Hayes CJ, Gersony WM, Ellis K: Pulmonary atresia with intact ventricular septum. J Thorac Cardiovasc Surg 61:85, 1971
73. Rao PS, Liebman J, Borkat G: Right ventricular growth in a case of pulmonic stenosis with intact ventricular septum and hypoplastic right ventricle. Circulation 53:389, 1976
74. Heymann MA, Rudolph AM: Ductus arteriosus dilatation by prostaglandin E$_1$ in infants with pulmonary atresia. Pediatrics 59:325, 1977

Pulmonary Stenosis

75. Freed MD, Rosenthal A, Bernhard WF, Litwin SB, Nadas AS: Critical pulmonary stenosis with a diminutive right ventricle in neonates. Circulation 48:875, 1973
76. Nakazawa M, Marks RA, Isabel-Jones J, Jarmakani JM: Right and left ventricular volume characteristics in children with pulmonary stenosis and intact ventricular septum. Circulation 53:884, 1976

Tricuspid Atresia

77. Edwards JE, Burchell HB: Congenital tricuspid atresia: A classification. Med Clin North Am 33:1177, 1949
78. Tandon R, Edwards JE: Tricuspid atresia. J Thorac Cardiovasc Surg 67:530, 1974
79. Guller B, Titus JL: Morphological studies in tricuspid atresia. Circulation 38:977, 1968
80. Gasul BM, Fell EH, Mavrelis W, Casas R: Diagnosis of tricuspid atresia or stenosis in infants. Based upon a study of 10 cases. Pediatrics 6:862, 1950
81. Dick M, Fyler DC, Nadas AS: Tricuspid atresia: Clinical course in 101 patients. Am J Cardiol 36:327, 1975
82. Rowe RD, Mehrizi A: The Neonate with Congenital Heart Disease. Philadelphia, Saunders, 1968, p 288
83. Gamboa R, Gersony WM, Nadas AS: The electrocardiogram in tricuspid atresia and pulmonary atresia with intact ventricular septum. Circulation 34:24, 1966
84. Somlyo AP, Halloran KH: Tricuspid atresia. An electrocardiographic study. Am Heart J 63:171, 1962
85. Guller B, Titus JL, DuShane JW: Electrocardiographic diagnosis of malformations associated with tricuspid atresia: Correlation with morphologic features. Am Heart J 78:180, 1969
86. Neill CA, Brink AJ: Left axis deviation in tricuspid atresia and single ventricle. The electrocardiogram in 36 autopsied cases. Circulation 12:612, 1955
87. Davachi F, Lucas RV Jr, Moller JH: The electrocardiogram and vectorcardiogram in tricuspid atresia. Correlation with pathologic anatomy. Am J Cardiol 25:18, 1970
88. Keith JD, Rowe RD, Vlad P: Heart Disease in Infancy and Childhood, 2nd ed. New York, Macmillan, 1967, pp 644–681
89. Guller B, DuShane JW, Titus JL: The atrioventricular conduction system in two cases of tricuspid atresia. Circulation 40:217, 1969
90. Bharati S, Lev M: The conduction system in tricuspid atresia with and without regular (d−) transposition. Circulation 56:423, 1977

91. Baron MG: Hypoplasia of the inflow portion of the right ventricle: An angiocardiographic sign of tricuspid atresia. Circulation 44:746, 1971

92. Rashkind W, Waldhausen J, Miller W, Friedman S: Palliative treatment in tricuspid atresia. Combined balloon atrioseptostomy and surgical alteration of pulmonary blood flow. J Thorac Cardiovasc Surg 57:812, 1969

93. Singh SP, Astley R, Parson CG: Haemodynamic effects of balloon septostomy in tricuspid atresia. Br Med J 1:225, 1968

94. LaCorte MA, Dick M, Scheer G, LaFarge CG, Fyler DC: Left ventricular function in tricuspid atresia. Angiographic analysis in 28 patients. Circulation 52:996, 1975

95. Gallaher ME, Fyler DC: Observations on changing hemodynamics in tricuspid atresia without associated transposition of the great vessels. Circulation 35:381, 1967

96. Rao PS: Natural history of the ventricular septal defect in tricuspid atresia and its surgical implications. Br Heart J 39:276, 1977

97. Kyger ER III, Reul GJ Jr, Sandiford FM, et al.: Surgical palliation of tricuspid atresia. Circulation 52:685, 1975

98. Williams WG, Rubis L, Fowler RS, et al.: Tricuspid atresia: Results of treatment in 160 children. Am J Cardiol 38:235, 1976

99. Subramanian S, Carr I, Waterston DJ, Bonham-Carter RE: Palliative surgery in tricuspid atresia. Forty-two cases. Circulation 32:977, 1965

100. Taussig HB, Keinonen R, Momberger N, Kirk H: Long-time observations on the Blalock-Taussig operation. IV. Tricuspid atresia. Johns Hopkins Med J 132:135, 1973

Ebstein's Anomaly

101. Newfeld EA, Cole RB, Paul MH: Ebstein's malformation of the tricuspid valve in the neonate. Functional and anatomic pulmonary outflow tract obstruction. Am J Cardiol 19:727, 1967

102. Schiebler GL, Adams P Jr, Anderson RC, Amplatz K, Lester RG: Clinical study of twenty-three cases of Ebstein's anomaly of the tricuspid valve. Circulation 19:165, 1959

103. Engle MA, Payne TPB, Bruins C, Taussig HB: Ebstein's anomaly of the tricuspid valve. Report of three cases and analysis of clinical syndrome. Circulation 1:1246, 1950

104. Simcha A, Bonham-Carter RE: Ebstein's anomaly. Clinical study of 32 patients in childhood. Br Heart J 33:46, 1971

105. Moller JH, Lynch RP, Edwards JE: Fetal cardiac failure resulting from congenital anomalies of the heart. J Pediatr 68:699, 1966

106. Watson H: Natural history of Ebstein's anomaly of tricuspid valve in children and adolescence. An international co-operative study of 505 cases. Br Heart J 36:417, 1974

107. Kumar AE, Fyler DC, Miettinen OS, Nadas AS: Ebstein's anomaly. Clinical profile and natural history. Am J Cardiol 28:84, 1971

108. Yamauchi T, Cayler GG: Ebstein's anomaly in the neonate. A clinical study of three cases observed from birth through infancy. Am J Dis Child 107:165, 1964

109. Crews TL, Pridie RB, Benham R, Leatham A: Auscultatory and phonocardiographic findings in Ebstein's anomaly. Correlation of first heart sound with ultrasonic records of tricuspid valve movement. Br Heart J 34:681, 1972

110. Rowe RD, Mehrizi A: The Neonate with Congenital Heart Disease. Philadelphia, Saunders, 1968, pp 307–315

111. Lowe KG, Emslie-Smith D, Roberston PGC, Watson H: Scalar, vector, and intracardiac electrocardiograms in Ebstein's anomaly. Br Heart J 30:617, 1968

112. Amplatz K, Lester RG, Schiebler GL, Adams P Jr, Anderson RC: The roentgenologic features of Ebstein's anomaly of the tricuspid valve. Am J Roentgenol Radium Ther Nucl Med 81:788, 1959
113. Tajik AJ, Gau GT, Giuliani ER, Ritter DG, Schattenberg TT: Echocardiogram in Ebstein's anomaly with Wolff-Parkinson-White preexcitation syndrome, type B. Circulation 47:813, 1973
114. Farooki ZQ, Henry JG, Green EW: Echocardiographic spectrum of Ebstein's anomaly of the tricuspid valve. Circulation 53:63, 1976
115. Lundström NR: Echocardiography in the diagnosis of Ebstein's anomaly of the tricuspid valve. Circulation 47:597, 1973
116. Matsumoto M, Matsuo H, Nagata S, et al.: Visualization of Ebstein's anomaly of the tricuspid valve by two-dimensional and standard echocardiography. Circulation 53:69, 1976
117. Hirschklau MJ, Sahn DJ, Hagan AD, Williams DE, Friedman WF: Cross-sectional echocardiographic features of Ebstein's anomaly of the tricuspid valve. Am J Cardiol 40:400, 1977

Isolated Hypoplasia

118. Raghib G, Amplatz K, Moller JH, Jue KL, Edwards JE: CPC. Hypoplasia of right ventricle and of tricuspid valve. Am Heart J 70:806, 1965
119. Davachi F, McLean RH, Moller JH, Edwards JE: Hypoplasia of the right ventricle and tricuspid valve in siblings. J Pediatr 71:869, 1967
120. Becker AE, Becker MJ, Moller JH, Edwards JE: Hypoplasia of right ventricle and tricuspid valve in three siblings. Chest 60:273, 1971
121. Medd WE, Neufeld HN, Weidman, WH, Edwards JE: Isolated hypoplasia of the right ventricle and tricuspid valve in siblings. Br Heart J 23:25, 1961
122. Sackner MA, Robinson MJ, Jamison WL, Lewis DH: Isolated right ventricular hypoplasia with atrial septal defect or patent foramen ovale. Circulation 24:1388, 1961
123. Gasul BM, Arcilla RA, Lev M: Heart Disease in Children—Diagnosis and Treatment. Philadelphia, Lippincott, 1966, p 706

Endocardial Fibroelastosis

124. Morgan AD, McLoughlin TG, Bartley TD, Shanklin DR: Endocardial fibroelastosis of the right ventricle in the newborn. Presenting the clinical picture of the hypoplastic right heart syndrome. Am J Cardiol 18:933, 1966

Uhl's Anomaly

125. Uhl HSM: A previously undescribed congenital malformation of the heart: Almost total absence of the myocardium of the right ventricle. Bull Johns Hopkins Hosp. 91:197, 1952
126. Perrin EV, Mehrizi A: Isolated free-wall hypoplasia of the right ventricle. Am J Dis Child 109:558, 1965
127. Arcilla RA, Gasul BM: Congenital aplasia or marked hypoplasia of the myocardium of the right ventricle (Uhl's anomaly). J Pediatr 58:381, 1961

Tricuspid Insufficiency

128. Becker AE, Becker MJ, Edwards JE: Pathologic spectrum of dysplasia of the tricusid valve. Features in common with Ebstein's malformation. Arch Pathol 91:167, 1971

129. Bucciarelli RL, Nelson RM, Egan EA II, Eitzman DV, Gessner IH: Transient tricuspid insufficiency of the newborn: A form of myocardial dysfunction in stressed newborns. Pediatrics 59:330, 1977
130. Boucek RJ Jr, Graham TP Jr, Morgan JP, Atwood GF, Boerth RC: Spontaneous resolution of massive congenital tricuspid insufficiency. Circulation 54:795, 1976
131. Nelson RM, Bucciarelli RL, Eitzman DV, Egan EA II, Gessner IH: Serum creatine phosphokinase MB fraction in newborns with transient tricuspid insufficiency. N Engl J Med 298:146, 1978
132. Ariel MB. Ein seltener Fall von angeborenem Herzfehler bei einem neugeborenen. Virchows Arch [Pathol Anat] 277:501, 1930
133. Abbott ME; Atlas of Congenital Cardiac Disease. New York, American Heart Association, 1936, p 24
134. Dubin IN, Hollinshead WH: Congenitally insufficient tricuspid valve accompanied by an anomalous septum in the right atrium. Arch Pathol 38:225, 1944
135. Palladino VS, Kenney TD: Cardiac hypertrophy and congenital tricuspid insufficiency. Bull Int Assoc Med Mus 28:23, 1948
136. Kincaid OW, Swan HJC, Ongley PA, Titus JL: Congenital tricuspid insufficiency: Report of two cases. Proc Staff Meet Mayo Clin 37:640, 1962
137. Reisman M, Hipona FA, Bloor CM, Talner NS: Congenital tricuspid insufficiency. A cause of massive cardiomegaly and heart failure in the neonate. J Pediatr 66:869, 1965
138. Sanayl SK, Bhargava SK, Saxena HMK, Ghosh S: Congenital insufficiency of the tricuspid valve. A rare cause of massive cardiomegaly and congestive cardiac failure in neonate. Indian Heart J 20:214, 1968
139. Barr PA, Celermajer JM, Bowdler JD, Cartmill TB: Severe congenital tricuspid incompetence in the neonate. Circulation 49:962, 1974
140. Freymann R, Kallfelz HC: Transient tricuspid incompetence in a newborn. Eur J Cardiol 2:467, 1975
141. Shrivastava S, Moller JH: Severe isolated tricuspid regurgitation in the neonate. Unpublished observations

13 Pulmonary Venous Obstruction

A variety of different forms of congenital cardiac anomalies obstruct blood flow into the left ventricle. Although the anatomic form of the anomalies differs, each elevates pulmonary venous pressure and the pressure in each portion of the vascular system proximal to the obstruction. In fact, many of the clinical and laboratory features of the malformations reflect the changes in the pulmonary vessels and parenchyma rather than those in the malformation itself.

The cardiac anomalies leading to pulmonary venous obstruction can be divided into two groups[1]: (1) conditions located distal to the mitral valve and (2) conditions located at or proximal to the mitral valve. The former consists of many conditions, such as aortic stenosis or endocardial fibroelastosis, discussed in Chapter 10. These conditions decrease left ventricular compliance and increase left ventricular end-diastolic pressure. Thus, left atrial and, therefore, pulmonary venous pressures are elevated. The second group causing pulmonary venous obstruction consists of conditions discussed in this chapter, in which cardiac abnormality occurs at the mitral valve, in the left atrium, or in the pulmonary veins.

The consequences of the condition upon the heart and pulmonary circulation depend upon the site and severity of obstruction. Usually, those conditions occurring distal to the mitral valve (Chap. 10) show electrocardiographic evidence of left ventricular hypertrophy and cardiomegaly on thoracic roentgenograms, while those in the second group usually show only right ventricular hypertrophy and normal cardiac size.

In most patients with pulmonary venous obstruction related to the second category, the cardiac septae are intact, and no shunt is present. In a few patients, however, defects in the cardiac septae may coexist, and a shunt occurs in addition to pulmonary venous obstruction. On the basis of the location of obstruction and the presence of a shunt, the anomalies leading to left ventricular inflow obstruction are classified (Table 13-1).

TABLE 13-1

Left Ventricular Inflow Obstruction at or Proximal to Mitral Valve

I. With intact atrial septum
  A. Involving mitral valve mechanism
    1. Excessive papillary muscle
    2. Parachute mitral valve
    3. Commissural fusion
    4. Accessory mitral valvular tissue
  B. Occurring within the left atrium
    1. Supravalvular stenosing ring
    2. Cor triatriatum
  C. Occurring in pulmonary veins
    1. Pulmonary vein stenosis
    2. Pulmonary vein hypoplasia

II. With atrial septal communication
  A. With anomalously connecting pulmonary connection
    1. Total anomalous pulmonary venous connection
      a. With obstruction
        (1) To infradiaphragmatic site
        (2) Supradiaphragmatic, with narrowing of connecting vein
      b. With atresia
        (1) Atresia of the common pulmonary vein
  B. With normally connecting pulmonary veins
    1. Associated with hypoplastic left ventricle
      a. Aortic atresia
      b. Severe aortic stenosis
      c. Mitral atresia
      d. Coexistent mitral and aortic atresia
    2. Associated with normal sized left ventricle. Any cardiac anomaly associated with a shunt may coexist with any form of left ventricular inflow obstruction

PATHOLOGY. Several pathologic changes occur as a result of elevated left atrial pressure or pulmonary venous pressure, regardless of the underlying cardiac condition. These pathologic abnormalities have direct implications in understanding the clinical and laboratory findings common to all infants with pulmonary venous obstruction.[2]

In infants whose level of obstruction resides within the left ventricle or at the level of the mitral valve, left atrial pressure is elevated. The pressure elevation in the left atrium leads to myocardial hypertrophy, and the endocardial surface becomes thickened by a proliferation of fibrous and elastic tissue, giving it a whitish appearance. The left atrium is dilated.

The pressure elevation leads to dilatation of the pulmonary veins, particularly those in the upper lobes. The media of the pulmonary veins thickens, and the intima proliferates. Because of communications normally present between the pulmonary and the bronchial veins, elevation of pulmonary venous pressure leads to a marked pressure differential between the pulmonary and the bronchial venous systems. This causes enlargement of these communications, so that blood flows from pulmonary to bronchial veins. As a consequence, the bronchial veins dilate and become tortuous.

The pulmonary capillary pressure is also elevated and leads to pulmonary edema and alveolar hemorrhage. Pulmonary edema is partially removed from the lungs by the pulmonary lymphatic system, which is located in the intralobar septae and subpleural areas.

Pulmonary arterial pressure is elevated, not only passively because of the elevated pulmonary venous pressure, but also from reflex pulmonary vasoconstriction. The pulmonary arteries show medial hypertrophy and, at times, intimal proliferation.

The major pulmonary arterial branches and the pulmonary trunk are dilated and may compress the major bronchi and cause atelectasis, pneumonia, or emphysema distal to the obstruction. This most frequently involves the right middle and left lower lobes. In patients with left atrial enlargement, particularly in conditions with left ventricular dilatation, the left main stem bronchus may be compressed between the enlarged left atrium and hypertensive left pulmonary artery, causing changes in the left lower lobe.

Right ventricular hypertrophy results from elevated pulmonary arterial pressure. The hypertrophy decreases ventricular compliance and affects ventricular filling.

CLINICAL CORRELATIONS.   Various clinical and laboratory findings correlate with these pathologic changes and are outlined in Table 13-2. The findings are present in any infant with pulmonary venous obstruction. The major clinical features resemble pulmonary disease. Dyspnea and tachypnea are described in the history and found on physical examination. These reflect decreased pulmonary compliance from pulmonary edema and pulmonary hypertension. Rales of the pulmonary edema may be present on auscultation of the lungs.

The electrocardiogram shows right ventricular hypertrophy, reflecting that pulmonary hypertension and right atrial enlargement may be present also.

The thoracic roentgenogram can be easily confused with pulmonary parenchymal disease, particularly in the neonatal period, because the pulmonary edema shows diffuse stippling of lung fields (Fig. 13-1). The lungs appear congested, the upper lobe pulmonary veins are dilated, and later in infancy, Kerley's B lines appear, representing dilated pulmonary lymphatics. Cardiac size is normal or only slightly enlarged.

Pulmonary venous obstruction occurring at or proximal to the mitral valve can occur from several types of cardiac anomalies. Each condition leading to pulmonary venous obstruction in infancy will be discussed separately.

LEFT VENTRICULAR INFLOW OBSTRUCTION WITH INTACT ATRIAL SEPTUM

Anomalies causing left ventricular inflow obstruction with an intact atrial septum can occur at the mitral valve, within the left atrium, or within the pulmonary veins. In these anomalies, the pulmonary veins connect normally to the

TABLE 13-2

Physiologic Changes and Related Clinical Manifestations in Pulmonary Venous Obstruction.

PHYSIOLOGIC CHANGE	CLINICAL MANIFESTATION
Elevated left atrial pressure	Left atrial enlargement (x-ray)
Elevated pulmonary venous pressure	Dilated upper lobe pulmonary veins (x-ray)
Elevated pulmonary capillary pressure	Pulmonary edema (x-ray), dyspnea, rales
Dilated lymphatics	Kerley's B lines
Elevated pulmonary arterial pressure	Increased P2, dilated pulmonary artery
Elevated right ventricular pressure	Right ventricular hypertrophy (EKG)

left atrium. There may be cyanosis because of pulmonary edema but not from an intracardiac right-to-left shunt.

MITRAL STENOSIS

Among the causes of pulmonary venous obstruction, mitral stenosis is common, being second in frequency only to total anomalous pulmonary venous connection with obstruction.

PATHOLOGY.   Mitral stenosis results in infancy from several different anatomic states,[3] the most frequent being parachute mitral valve.[4] In this form, only a single left ventricular papillary muscle is present. The chordae tendineae from

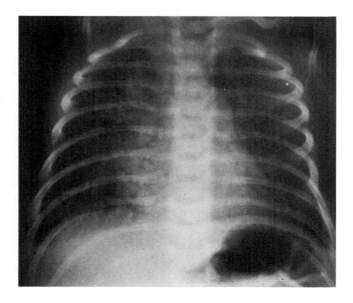

FIG. 13-1.   Thoracic roentgenogram of atresia of common pulmonary vein. Pulmonary venous obstruction and edema. Normal cardiac size.

both mitral valve leaflets insert into this single papillary muscle. The chordae tendineae are short and thickened, so movement of the leaflets is restricted. The mitral valvular leaflets and commissures are normal. Mitral stenosis results from convergence of the chordae tendineae and narrowing of the interchordae spaces by thickening and fusion of chordae tendineae.

Parachute mitral valve is frequently a portion of a developmental complex that includes supravalvular mitral stenosis, subaortic stenosis, and coarctation of the aorta. It also occurs in patients with ventricular septal defect or origin of both great vessels from the right ventricle and supracristal ventricular septal defect.[5]

Mitral stenosis also occurs from abnormally large papillary muscles.[3,6] In this condition, the mitral valvular leaflets are normal. Large bulky papillary muscles are situated immediately beneath the mitral valve and attach to the valvular leaflets by shortened chordae tendineae. The obstruction is basically related to subvalvular mitral stenosis.

Another anatomic cause of mitral stenosis is congenital commissural fusion, and this resembles rheumatic mitral stenosis.[3] The leaflets are thickened and fused.[7] The chordae tendineae are also distorted, and the papillary muscles may be poorly developed.

Mitral stenosis, regardless of anatomic detail, can occur as an isolated lesion or coexist with other conditions.[3,4,8] In this chapter, the isolated form is considered, and associated conditions will be referred to only in specific instances. When mitral stenosis coexists with another lesion, the major clinical features usually resemble those of the associated condition.

CLINICAL FEATURES. Several articles describe the clinical and laboratory findings of mitral stenosis.[7-10] Respiratory symptoms are prominent and include frequent respiratory infections and pneumonia. The symptoms, signs, and laboratory findings suggesting pneumonia may actually be caused by pulmonary edema. The infants are often treated for pneumonia and respond poorly. In our experience, weight gain is slow, and the infants appear irritable and fretful. Signs of congestive cardiac failure are common and respond only partially to digitalization.

Infants with major coexistent conditions develop signs and symptoms earlier than do those with isolated mitral stenosis. Infants with isolated mitral stenosis rarely develop symptoms within the first month of life, but more often between the ages of 4 and 8 months.

On physical examination, the infant may appear generally normal or scrawny. Dyspnea and tachypnea are present. Mild to moderate cardiomegaly may be evident clinically. A left precordial bulge and right ventricular precordial heave are common. The first heart sound is often accentuated at the apex,[9] and the pulmonary component of the second heart sound is accentuated. An opening snap is rarely identified in infants.[8]

A murmur is present in almost every infant with mitral stenosis and may be initially heard in the neonatal period. The murmur is a grade 1-3/6, low-pitched, long, mid to late diastolic murmur and may, but not always, have presystolic accentuation (Fig. 13-2). In most forms of congenital cardiac anomalies, cardiac murmurs are systolic in timing. Physicians may not concentrate carefully on the timing of the murmur, so that in infants with mitral stenosis, the murmur may be falsely interpreted as being systolic in timing. In some infants with mitral stenosis, a soft pansystolic murmur may, however, also be present and related to either mitral regurgitation from an abnormality of the valve or to tricuspid regurgitation from the effects of pulmonary hypertension upon the right ventricle.

Hepatomegaly is found. Rales occur, but infrequently.

ELECTROCARDIOGRAM.   The QRS axis lies between $+90°$ and $+150°$.[8] The precordial leads usually show isolated right ventricular hypertrophy, with an Rs pattern usually present in lead V_1. The T waves may be upright in the right precordial leads. Although left ventricular hypertrophy rarely occurs, we have seen two infants with mitral stenosis who had large q waves in lead V_6. The P waves may be normal or show right atrial or left atrial enlargement (Fig. 13-3).

THORACIC ROENTGENOGRAM.   Cardiac enlargement of a variable degree is present but is usually not significant. Cardiac enlargement is accounted for by the right ventricle and right atrium. The pulmonary arterial segment is prominent (Fig. 13-4). Left atrial enlargement is present and is a valuable finding in locating the site of the pulmonary venous obstruction because conditions proximal to the mitral valve often do not show left atrial enlargement. The lung fields, of course, show pulmonary edema and prominent upper lobe pulmonary veins.

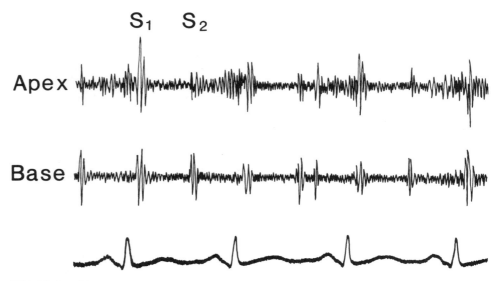

FIG. 13-2.   Phonocardiogram of mitral stenosis in 16-month-old infant. Diastolic murmur with presystolic accentuation. S_1, first heart sound; S_2, second heart sound.

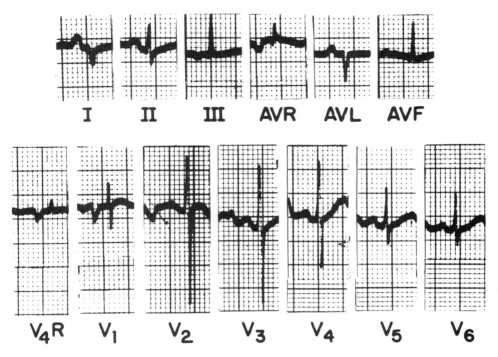

FIG. 13-3. Electrocardiogram of congenital mitral stenosis. Broad P waves indicate left atrial enlargement.

ECHOCARDIOGRAM. Echocardiography can help identify mitral stenosis. The E-F slope of the anterior valvular leaflet is reduced, the mitral valvular excursions during diastole are reduced, and the A wave may be absent (Fig. 13-5). These findings are not diagnostic of mitral stenosis because left ventricular failure or other causes of pulmonary venous obstruction may reduce flow from the left atrium to the left ventricle to such an extent as to cause decreased mitral valvular excursion. Multiple echoes may be recorded from the stenotic mitral valve, but this finding is also not specific.

CARDIAC CATHETERIZATION AND ANGIOCARDIOGRAM. In infants with a clinical picture of pulmonary venous obstruction, cardiac catheterization and angiocardiography are needed to define (1) the level of the obstruction, (2) the anatomic details of the lesion, and (3) the severity of the obstruction. Measurement of the pulmonary arterial wedge or left atrial pressure must be done, for elevation of this pressure is the hallmark of mitral stenosis, provided left ventricular end-diastolic pressure is normal. Attempts should be made to measure the latter simultaneously, if possible, to make certain that the elevation is not caused by elevated left ventricular end-diastolic pressure. The left atrial or pulmonary arterial wedge pressure in infants may be elevated to 30 or 35 mm Hg, and the a

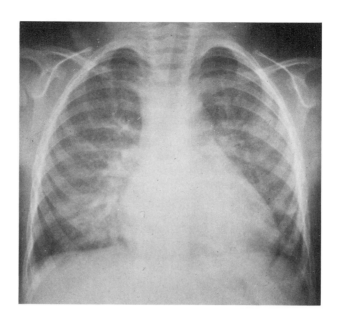

FIG. 13-4. Thoracic roentgenogram, posteroanterior view, of congenital mitral stenosis. Slightly enlarged heart. Prominent pulmonary arterial segment. Pulmonary venous obstruction.

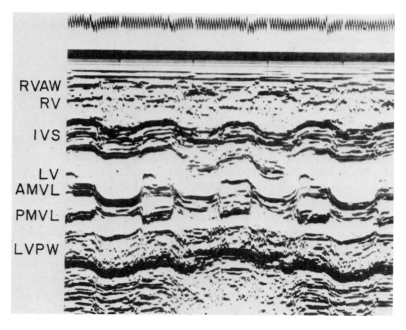

FIG. 13-5. Echocardiogram of congenital mitral stenosis. Thickened mitral valve leaflets (AMVL, PMVL) within left ventricle (LV). Flat E-F slope. RVAW, right ventricular anterior wall; RV, right ventricle; IVS, interventricular septum; LVPW, left ventricular posterior wall.

wave is greater than the v wave. Pulmonary arterial systolic pressure is also increased, often to 75 to 100 mm Hg.[6,8,10-12]

In infants, systemic arterial desaturation may be present,[10] presumably from pulmonary edema and not from an intracardiac right-to-left shunt. The cardiac output has been normal in infants, but pulmonary vascular resistance is elevated and frequently between 10 and 15 units.

The usual angiographic studies performed in patients with isolated mitral stenosis are pulmonary arteriography or left ventriculography because the foramen ovale is usually sealed by the elevated left atrial pressure, making it nearly impossible to pass the catheter from the right to the left atrium.

Pulmonary arteriograms show dilatation of the pulmonary trunk and major pulmonary arteries. Flow through the lungs is slow. The left atrium remains opacified a long time, is dilated, and fails to show the normal pattern of contraction.

On left ventriculography, the left ventricle is normal or slightly reduced in volume. In an occasional case, the occurrence of mitral regurgitation allows visualization of the superior aspect of the mitral valve, but frequently the mitral valve is not clearly visualized. The left ventricle may show a filling defect in infants with parachute mitral valve[13,14] or with enlarged bulky papillary muscles.[6] One report[14] describes the ventricular filling defect as having an egg-timer appearance during diastole, the posterior-superior portion of the egg-timer formed from the coned mitral valvular leaflets and chordae tendineae and the anteroinferior portion of the papillary muscle.

Mitral stenosis and the next two conditions to be discussed, supravalvular stenosing ring and cor triatriatum, may be difficult to distinguish angiographically because it is difficult to delineate clearly anatomic structures about the mitral valve. Each condition causes an enlarged, slowly emptying, poorly contracting left atrium, and a normal appearing left ventricle. These features indicate the general location of obstruction to the vicinity of the mitral valve. Often, operation is undertaken which, in part, is exploratory—and the surgeon inspects the left atrium and identifies and corrects the obstructive lesion.

MANAGEMENT. Management includes aggressive treatment of congestive cardiac failure and pulmonary edema and prompt performance of a cardiac catheterization. Although mitral commissurotomy has been successfully performed,[11,15] the anatomic features of the mitral valve preclude commissurotomy in most infants. Mitral valvular replacement is the treatment of choice in symptomatic infants and has been performed successfully.[6,12,15,16] The operative risk is high in infants with mitral stenosis because of the frequent association of other cardiac malformations that also require repair.

SUPRAVALVULAR STENOSING RING OF THE LEFT ATRIUM

In this condition, a circumferential ridge of connective tissue is located in the left atrium, attached to the base of the mitral valve leaflets, and protrudes into the mitral valve orifice (Fig. 13-6). Depending upon the diameter of the ring,

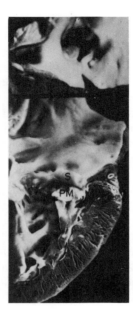

FIG. 13-6.   Supravalvular stenosing ring of left atrium. **Top.** View of membrane from left atrium. **Bottom.** View of left side of heart above posterior mitral (PM) valve leaflet. Supravalvular stenosing ring (S) is present.

various degrees of obstruction are present, but it can act as a significant stenotic lesion. When it causes obstruction, the left atrium shows dilatation and a thickened endocardium.

This is a rare condition and is usually associated with other cardiac conditions.[1,3,17-20] The association with parachute mitral valve and other left-sided obstructive lesions has been well described,[4] but it also occurs with ventricular septal defect, tetralogy of Fallot, and corrected transposition of the great vessels. In these latter conditions, the stenosing ring can lead to pulmonary venous obstruction, but in patients with conditions with reduced pulmonary blood flow, such as tetralogy of Fallot, the presence of the stenosing ring may not be evident until after a corrective or palliative procedure has been performed and pulmonary blood flow becomes normal.

The hemodynamics resemble the hemodynamics of mitral stenosis. It is difficult to develop a clinical picture of this condition, since it usually coexists with other cardiac anomalies. The symptoms are related to congestive cardiac failure and pulmonary congestion. Usually, no murmur originates from the membrane, although we have heard a middiastolic murmur in one patient. If murmurs are present, they are usually related to the associated malformation. The pulmonary component of the second heart sound is accentuated.

On the electrocardiogram, right axis deviation and right ventricular hypertrophy are present. Thoracic roentgenograms may show cardiac enlargement, depending upon the type of coexistent cardiac malformation. The left atrium and pulmonary trunk are enlarged. The pulmonary venous markings are accentuated.

We have had no experience with this condition on echocardiography but would believe a membrane may be found and the mitral valvular movements reduced.

The pulmonary arterial wedge pressure is elevated. Angiography may demonstrate a ledge in the left atrium,[21] but usually it is difficult to distinguish angiographically from mitral stenosis, since details of the mitral valvular area are difficult to visualize. As in mitral stenosis, the left atrium is dilated and empties slowly if the left ventricular cavity is normal. If contrast material refluxes across the mitral valve, the undersurface of the membrane may be delineated.

Management consists of resecting the membrane. At operation, the mitral valve should also be explored, for it may also be stenotic and require operation.

COR TRIATRIATUM

This is a rare cardiac anomaly in which the pulmonary veins enter a chamber that communicates with the left atrium through a small orifice. It must be considered in the differential diagnosis of pulmonary venous obstruction, since it can be operatively corrected, and the results are excellent.

PATHOLOGY.   Several reviews[22-24] have described the anatomy of cor triatriatum. This anomaly is generally considered to result from faulty incorporation of the common pulmonary vein into the left atrium, so that the pulmonary veins do not directly join the left atrium. Rather, they enter an accessory atrial chamber that communicates through an opening or, occasionally, through several openings into the left atrium proper. The size of the orifice varies but may be only 2 mm in diameter. Marin-Garcia and co-workers[24] classified cor triatriatum into three types: (1) diaphragmatic type—in which a fibromuscular diaphragm divides the left atrium from the accessory chamber, and there is no external evidence of two distinct chambers, (2) hourglass type—in which a constriction is observed externally between the two chambers, and (3) tubular type—which is apparent externally, with a tubular channel joining the chambers receiving the pulmonary veins with the left atrium.

The left atrial appendage arises from the left atrium below the cor triatriatum. This is an important anatomic feature which distinguishes cor triatriatum from mitral stenosis and supravalvular stenosing ring. The fossa ovalis almost always connects between the right atrium and the true left atria.

Partial anomalous pulmonary venous connection can coexist with cor triatriatum.[25-28] In the experience of Marin-Garcia and co-workers,[24] associated anomalies were common.

HEMODYNAMICS.   The hemodynamics of this condition resemble those of mitral stenosis, with elevated pulmonary venous pressure resulting from the narrowed orifice in the channel separating the anomalous chamber from the left atria. This leads to the previously described changes in pulmonary parenchyma and vasculature.

CLINICAL FEATURES.   The age at which symptoms appear is related to the size of the orifice. Infants with cor triatriatum show irritability, slow growth, and respiratory symptoms usually starting after 1 month of age.[23,29] The respiratory symptoms are tachypnea and persistent respiratory infections. There may be episodes of acute pulmonary edema and congestive cardiac failure.

The infants appear scrawny and may be in respiratory distress. A left precordial bulge is common, and the pulmonary component of the second heart sound is accentuated. Murmurs are not consistently found and, if present, are nonspecific, soft, and variable in timing and location. Perhaps this variability is related to the size of the communication and the volume of flow. Both systolic and diastolic murmurs have been described. The systolic murmur may be related to tricuspid insufficiency occurring secondary to pulmonary hypertension.

ELECTROCARDIOGRAM.   As in other conditions with pulmonary venous obstruction, right axis deviation (usually between $+100°$ and $+150°$), right atrial enlargement, and right ventricular hypertrophy are found.

THORACIC ROENTGENOGRAM.   The roentgenographic picture of pulmonary edema is observed as in other conditions in this group. Mild to moderate cardiac enlargement is found. The cardiac contour is not characteristic. The pulmonary trunk is prominent. Displacement of the barium-filled esophagus, suggesting mild left atrial enlargement, has been described,[30-32] although others[24] have not found it. Thus, the presence of left atrial enlargement on thoracic roentgenogram does not uniformly distinguish mitral stenosis and supravalvular mitral stenosis from cor triatriatum.

ECHOCARDIOGRAM.   Reports[33-35] have described dense linear echoes in the left atrium or behind the mitral valve of patients with cor triatriatum (Fig. 13-7). Care must be taken in interpreting such echoes because artifacts may occur.

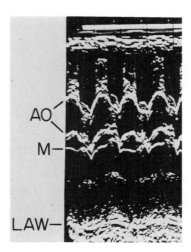

FIG. 13-7.   Echocardiogram of cor triatriatum. A linear echo (M) visualized within the left atrium behind the aorta (AO). LAW, left atrial wall.

The mitral valvular motions may be normal[34] or abnormal.[33] There are, in addition, findings of right ventricular hypertrophy and pulmonary hypertension. Left atrial enlargement has been described.[33]

CARDIAC CATHETERIZATION AND ANGIOCARDIOGRAM.   The pulmonary arterial wedge and pulmonary arterial pressures are elevated, the wedge pressure being in the area of 30 to 35 mm Hg and the pulmonary arterial systolic pressure 70 to 100 mm Hg.[24,30,31,36] There is no intracardiac shunt.

As in all cases of pulmonary venous obstruction, pulmonary arteriography shows slow passage of contrast through the lung and left atrium (Fig. 13-8). A membrane may be identified within the left atrium, but in many patients, the exact site of obstruction is not clearly defined.

MANAGEMENT.   Management consists of treatment with digitalis and diuretics and prompt diagnostic studies. The diaphragm of the cor triatriatum should be resected, and this can be done successfully.[30,32,36]

The success of operation depends upon the age of the child and the status of pulmonary parenchyma and vasculature. The elevated pulmonary vascular resistance falls to normal following relief of the obstruction.

STENOSIS OF INDIVIDUAL PULMONARY VEINS

In a few infants, pulmonary venous obstruction results from stenosis of individual pulmonary veins.[37-41] The pulmonary veins are either stenotic or atretic at the venoatrial junction (Fig. 13-9). The stenosis is usually less than 5 mm long,

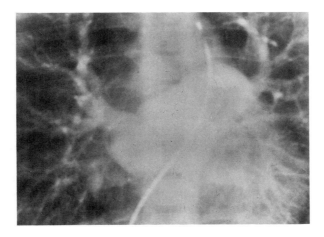

FIG. 13-8.   Pulmonary arteriogram, late phase, of cor triatriatum. Opacification of pulmonary veins entering small chamber (to right of spine). Separated from left atrium by curvilunar membrane.

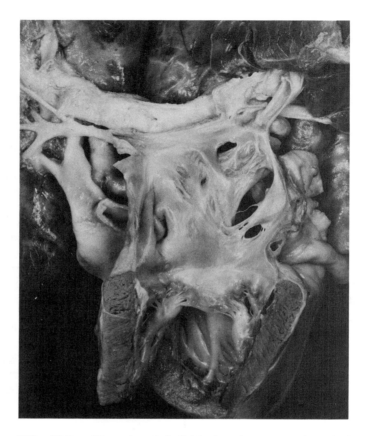

FIG. 13-9. Stenosis of individual pulmonary veins. Left atrium (above) and left ventricle (below). Fibrous thickening of pulmonary veins at entrance to left atrium.

and although the external appearance of the pulmonary veins is normal, there is intrinsic thickening of the walls. In one case, the pulmonary veins were diffusely hypoplastic throughout the lung fields.[39]

The major clinical features are failure to gain weight, dyspnea, and recurrent respiratory infections. There may be episodes of acute pulmonary edema. The only abnormal ausculatory finding is an accentuated pulmonary component of the second heart sound. Electrocardiogram shows right axis deviation, right atrial enlargement, and right ventricular hypertrophy. On thoracic roentgenogram, cardiac size is usually normal. A pattern of pulmonary edema is found, but left atrial enlargement is absent. Echocardiograms should show no abnormalities in the left side of the heart, but in one infant, we found a decreased E-F slope and reduced mitral valve excursion. The right side of the heart is dilated and hypertrophied.

Cardiac catheterization shows elevated wedge pressure and pulmonary arterial hypertension, which, in the case reported by Shone,[37] was 170/80 mm Hg. Left atrial pressure is normal. Pulmonary angiography may show passage of contrast material through the lungs and only faint opacification of the left atrium. The stenotic lesions of the pulmonary veins may, however, be demonstrated. Treatment is supportive, and no operative procedure is available.

PULMONARY VENOUS OBSTRUCTION WITH AN ATRIAL SEPTAL COMMUNICATION

Pulmonary venous obstruction can be associated also with a variety of anomalies in which there is an atrial septal defect and cardiac shunt. In each, bidirectional shunting and cyanosis are present.

Among the anomalies in this category, there are two groups of conditions. In the first form, the pulmonary veins connect abnormally, and there is a right-to-left atrial shunt. In the second, the pulmonary veins connect normally to the left atrium, and there is either left ventricular inflow or outflow obstruction.

Compared to the causes of pulmonary venous obstruction with an intact atrial septum, those with an atrial communication usually lead to symptoms in the neonatal period. Neonates with total anomalous pulmonary venous connection and obstruction resemble those with pulmonary parenchymal disease, and those with a hypoplastic left ventricle present a picture of profound circulatory shock.

TOTAL ANOMALOUS PULMONARY VENOUS CONNECTIONS WITH OBSTRUCTION

As indicated in Chapter 11, total anomalous pulmonary venous connection may cause two clinical pictures—one form shows minimal cyanosis and greatly increased pulmonary blood flow, and the other form, discussed here, is associated with obstruction to pulmonary venous return. The infants discussed here have the clinical and laboratory features of pulmonary venous obstruction and moderate or marked cyanosis.

PATHOLOGY. The developmental aspects and anatomic variations of total anomalous pulmonary venous connection were presented in Chapter 11.

Although most forms of total anomalous pulmonary venous connection can be associated with pulmonary venous obstruction, connection to an infradiaphragmatic site is always associated with this physiologic state. In the infradiaphragmatic form, the connecting vein joins a tributary of the portal vein, usually at the junction of the splenic and superior mesenteric veins. Less commonly, it connects to the ductus venosus.[42] Rarely, it connects to the hepatic vein or inferior vena cava. Four sites lead to pulmonary venous obstruction: (1) the pulmonary venous blood must pass through the hepatic capillary bed, (2) narrowing at the junction of anomalous venous channel and portal vein or ductus venosus, (3) extrinsic compression of the venous channel at the level of the diaphragm, and (4) perhaps the length of the venous channel.[43,44]

Supradiaphragmatic sites of anomalous connection can also be associated with pulmonary venous obstruction. This occurs more frequently than previously recognized. Gathman and Nadas[45] reviewed 75 patients with total anomalous pulmonary venous connection, and 40 had pulmonary venous obstruction, including 24 of their 59 cases (41 percent) with supradiaphragmatic connection. In two other series,[44,46] pulmonary venous obstruction also occurred frequently. In an anatomic study,[47] of 93 patients, 58 patients had no major associated cardiac anomaly, and 30 of these were found to have pulmonary venous obstruction. Among 28 patients in this study[47] with supracardiac connection, 14 had pulmonary venous obstruction. Obstruction can occur at one of several sites. In total anomalous pulmonary venous connection to the left superior vena cava, obstruction can result if the venous channel passes between the left pulmonary artery and left main stem bronchus,[28,48] forming the hemodynamic vise. Less commonly, there may be an intrinsic stenotic area in the vertical vein or at its junction with the innominate vein.[1,44,47,49] In total anomalous pulmonary venous connection to right superior vena cava, stenosis can occur from similar mechanisms.

In patients with total anomalous pulmonary venous connection to the azygous vein, obstruction can occur from hypoplasia or stenosis of the connecting vein.[47]

In patients with obstruction, the right ventricle is hypertrophied, but not dilated, since the volume of blood flow through the right side of the heart is limited. The ductus arteriosus may be patent.

HEMODYNAMICS. The central circulatory pattern is governed by the same factors controlling total anomalous pulmonary venous connection without pulmonary venous obstruction. Blood flow into the ventricles is dependent upon the relative ventricular compliances. Because of the pulmonary venous obstruction, the pulmonary arterial pressure is elevated and does not fall postnatally. As a result, the right ventricle remains thick walled, and its compliance is low. Therefore, the volume of flow into the right ventricle and so into the lungs is limited. Since total anomalous pulmonary venous connection is an admixture lesion, the degree of cyanosis is inversely related to the volume of pulmonary blood flow, and these patients with pulmonary venous obstruction show considerable cyanosis.

CLINICAL FEATURES. Severe symptoms develop in the neonatal period, and most patients die in the first or second month of life. In the series of Delisle and co-workers,[47] the median age of death in the patients with pulmonary venous obstruction was 3 weeks, but patients may survive for several months. Several reports[44,45,50–57] give information about the clinical features, and these are perhaps best defined in neonates with infradiaphragmatic connection. There is a marked tendency for infradiaphragmatic connection to occur in males.[50,51,54]

The principal symptoms are tachypnea, dyspnea, cyanosis, and difficulty with feeding. The symptoms are progressive, and the cyanosis and respiratory distress may intensify on feeding or straining in patients with an infradiaphragmatic form because of pressure upon the connecting venous channel.

The presence of a cardiac cause for these symptoms may be overlooked initially because the auscultatory findings are normal. On clinical examination, cardiac size is normal, and in about half the patients, no murmur is present. In the others, a soft pulmonary flow murmur may be present. The pulmonary component of the second heart sound is accentuated. There may be rales and hepatomegaly. Duff and co-workers[50] described two patients in whom a soft systolic murmur was heard over the liver.

ELECTROCARDIOGRAM.   The QRS axis is located between +110° and +160° and is considered normal for the age. Right atrial enlargement is uncommon.[50,52] As expected, right ventricular hypertrophy is found, and lead V_1 may show a qR pattern.[50] Lead V_6 shows an rS pattern.

THORACIC ROENTGENOGRAM.   Cardiac size is almost always normal.[50,51] There is no left atrial enlargement. The pulmonary trunk is prominent. The lung fields show a diffuse reticular pattern of pulmonary edema[1,58] (Fig. 13-10).

ECHOCARDIOGRAM.   The echocardiogram may be difficult to distinguish from normal. The left atrium and left ventricle may be slightly smaller than normal. Recordings of the pulmonary valve show changes of pulmonary hypertension, but this is by no means specific. Occasionally, an echo-free space may be found behind the left atrium.

CARDIAC CATHETERIZATION AND ANGIOCARDIOGRAM.   Several authors present cardiac catheterization data of patients with total anomalous pulmonary venous connection and pulmonary venous obstruction.[45,50,57,59,60] The oxygen satura-

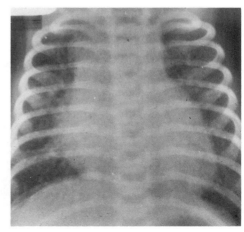

FIG. 13-10.   Thoracic roentgenogram, posteroanterior view, of total anomalous pulmonary venous connection with pulmonary venous obstruction. Slightly enlarged heart. Increased pulmonary venous markings.

tion values in each cardiac chamber and both great vessels are nearly identical. Systemic arterial desaturation is present and can vary considerably from 20 percent to 90 percent. In most infants, systemic arterial oxygen saturations range from 50 to 70 percent. Duff[50] indicates that oxygen saturation was higher in patients with an atrial septal defect than in those with a patent foramen ovale.

Pulmonary hypertension is present, and in most infants, pulmonary arterial pressure exceeds systemic arterial pressure. The pulmonary arterial wedge pressure is elevated. In most infants, atrial pressures are equal.

Pulmonary angiography is required to identify the site of the anomalous pulmonary venous connection and may reveal the cause of obstruction (Fig. 13-11). Because of pulmonary venous obstruction, blood flow through the lungs is slow, and delayed films (up to 10 sec) may be necessary to outline the pulmonary veins and connecting venous channels. Tynan and associates[61] describe two infants with infradiaphragmatic total anomalous pulmonary venous connection in whom portal venous system catheterization was performed through the umbilical vein. Contrast material was injected, and excellent visualization of the pulmonary veins and connecting venous channel was accomplished. In their infants, a pressure gradient was demonstrated at the junction of the connecting venous channel with the portal vein in one and with the inferior vena cava in the other. Injection of contrast material into the right atrium shows a

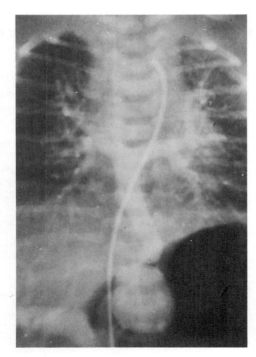

FIG. 13-11. Pulmonary arteriogram, anteroposterior view, late phase, of total anomalous pulmonary venous connection to infradiaphragmatic site. Opacification of pulmonary vein, which forms a venous channel that passes through diaphragm and enters portal vein.

right-to-left atrial shunt and denser opacification of aorta than of pulmonary artery.

Mathew and co-workers[59] present cardiac chamber volume studies in four neonates. The right ventricular end-diastolic volume was increased, while the left ventricular end-diastolic volume was abnormally small (75 percent of predicted normal) in three of four infants studied. The maximum left atrial volume was smaller than normal.

Balloon atrial septostomy has been recommended,[62,63] at the time of catheterization, for patients with total anomalous pulmonary venous connection (Chap. 11). In patients with pulmonary venous obstruction, this is unlikely to be beneficial.

MANAGEMENT.   The outlook for infants with total anomalous pulmonary venous connection with pulmonary venous obstruction is poor, particularly for those with infradiaphragmatic connection. Engle[64] summarized the history of developments related to total anomalous pulmonary venous connection and described the 1970s as the era of definitive treatment for this anomaly. During this period, operative techniques and perioperative support have improved, but the mortality for infradiaphragmatic connection remains high. Cases of total anomalous pulmonary venous connection with pulmonary venous obstruction have been successfully corrected and reported as individual cases[65-67] or included in larger series of patients.[46,50,68-71] Since medical management nearly always fails, operative therapy is indicated and should be performed as an emergency procedure, as the condition of a neonate can rapidly deteriorate. The high mortality is related to several factors—the critical status of the neonate, pulmonary hypertension and status of the lungs, and, in some, the small left atrial size.

Several survivors have been reported who have shown resolution of pulmonary hypertension and have become asymptomatic.[50,59,65]

At the time of operation, the common pulmonary vein is anastomosed to the left atrium, and the connecting vein is ligated. There are questions about whether the atrial defect should be closed at the time of operation, since this might compromise the left atrial size. Silove and associates[72] have reported spontaneous closure of the interatrial communication following correction in infancy.

ATRESIA OF COMMON PULMONARY VEIN

Although it is a rare condition, several neonates have been described with atresia of the common pulmonary vein.[73-77] In this anomaly, there is no functional connection between the pulmonary veins and the left atrium or other cardiac or venous structures. The pulmonary veins converge behind the left atrium, forming a confluence, but there is no exit for pulmonary venous blood (Fig. 13-12). The confluence may be attached to the left atrium by a fibrous strand.[74, 76] Small venous channels may lead from the confluence to the eso-

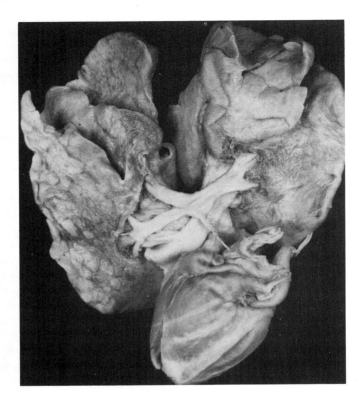

FIG. 13-12.   Atresia of common pulmonary vein. Posterior view of the heart, with lungs retracted superiorly. Pulmonary veins connected to left atrium by fibrous band.

phageal or other mediastinal veins. The lungs show gross and histologic findings of pulmonary venous congestion, particularly dilated lymphatics.[77]

Atresia of the common pulmonary vein is developmentally similar to total anomalous pulmonary venous obstruction. In this condition, the common pulmonary vein is believed to become obliterated after the communications to the splanchnic or cardinal venous systems have disappeared.

Pulmonary blood flow is minimal, since blood can exit the lungs only through minute connections to systemic veins in the mediastinum. An obligatory shunt is present at the atrial level, and cyanosis is marked.

CLINICAL FEATURES.   The patients present in the neonatal period, usually in the first 24 hours, with respiratory distress and cyanosis unresponsive to oxygen. Congestive cardiac failure may develop in patients who live for several days. Most patients died in the first 1 to 2 days, but some may survive until 1 month of age. Aside from an accentuated pulmonary component of the second heart sound, the cardiac findings are not diagnostic. No murmur is present, although occasionally a soft nonspecific murmur has been described.[73,74,76]

ELECTROCARDIOGRAM.   The electrocardiogram may be normal for the age or show right axis deviation and right ventricular hypertrophy.

THORACIC ROENTGENOGRAM.   Thoracic roentgenograms show a normal cardiac size and a striking reticular pattern of pulmonary venous obstruction. In most patients, the thymus is not evident, and the pulmonary trunk is enlarged.

CARDIAC CATHETERIZATION AND ANGIOCARDIOGRAM.   Pulmonary angiography shows slow passage of contrast material through the lungs. The pulmonary veins may be opacified and course toward the hila,[74,75] but no venous confluence is visualized, nor is the left atrium or a venous channel opacified. The failure to opacify the left atrium or systemic veins helps to distinguish this from other conditions causing pulmonary venous obstruction. A reversing patent ductus arteriosus may be seen, and the opaque material may flow retrograde in the arch toward the aortic valve, indicating low left ventricular output.[75] Systemic venous angiography shows a dense right-to-left shunt at the atrial level.

Three angiographic findings are nearly diagnostic of this condition: (1) visualization of pulmonary veins but neither the left atrium nor other veins, (2) right-to-left atrial shunt, and (3) evidence of reduced left ventricular output.

Attempts to anastomose the pulmonary venous confluence to the left atrium have been unsuccessful.[73-75] Atresia of the common pulmonary vein is theoretically correctable, but perhaps because of the small size of the child and delay in diagnosis, success has not been achieved. The clinical and laboratory features strongly suggest pulmonary parenchymal disease, and, undoubtedly, cases of atresia of the common pulmonary vein are missed because of failure to consider a cardiac condition.

AORTIC VALVULAR ATRESIA

Aortic atresia was one of the conditions classified by Lev[78] into the term "hypoplasia of the aortic tract complexes." Subsequently, Noonan and Nadas[79] used the term "hypoplastic left heart syndrome" to include all patients with a small left ventricle and ascending aorta, regardless of associated conditions. Because of its clinical course, poor prognosis, and lack of an operative approach, aortic atresia is considered separately from other conditions with a hypoplastic left ventricle.

PATHOLOGY.   In aortic valvular atresia, the aortic valve is an imperforate membrane, usually showing three raphes. The aortic annulus is narrowed. The ascending aorta is markedly hypoplastic, although the aortic arch is usually of normal caliber. The left ventricle is diminutive and lined by a thickened whitish endocardium. There may be prominent myocardial sinusoids connecting with the coronary arterial system. In about 25 percent of patients, the mitral valve is also atretic, and in these patients, the left ventricle can only be identified as a minute blind endocardium-lined crevice.[80] If the mitral valve is patent, it is hypoplastic, and the left atrium is also small. The foramen ovale usually shows communication with the right atrium, frequently because of herniation and prolapse of the valve of the foramen ovale. Less frequently, an atrial septal defect of the primum type may be present. In a few cases, premature closure of the foramen ovale occurs,[81,82] and in these patients, egress from the left side of the heart may be through a levoatrial cardinal vein or through myocardial sinusoids.

The right atrium, ventricle, and pulmonary trunk are enlarged, since they carry both the systemic and the pulmonary venous return. A patent ductus arteriosus is present.

Coarctation of the aorta commonly coexists.[83] The pulmonary arterioles show an increased amount of medial tissue. The thickened media is presumably present before birth and occurs in response to elevated pulmonary venous pressure.[81,84,85]

In perhaps 5 percent of patients, the left ventricle may be normal or near normal in size.[86–88]

HEMODYNAMICS. Because of the aortic atresia, the obstruction of the blood flow from the left ventricle is absolute. The pulmonary venous blood flows from the left to the right atrium, where it mixes with the systemic venous return. The blood passes into the right ventricle and is ejected into the pulmonary trunk. Blood then flows both into the lungs and right to left through the ductus arteriosus. The volume of blood flow into the two vascular systems is dependent upon the resistances of the two circuits. The entire systemic output passes through the ductus and flows both into the descending aorta and in a retrograde direction around the arch to supply blood to the brachiocephalic vessels and, finally, the coronary arteries. The hypoplastic ascending aorta acts essentially as a common coronary artery.

The systemic circulation is thus maintained by the right ventricle and is dependent upon elevation of pulmonary vascular resistances. Likewise, patency of the ductus arteriosus is mandatory. Although the ductus may be found widely patent at postmortem examination, catheterization data may show a pressure gradient between the pulmonary trunk and aorta, suggesting that it is narrowed.[85, 89] The increased arterial oxygen saturation postnatally can cause constriction of the ductus. Resistance to pulmonary blood flow is accentuated in the patients with a narrowed foramen ovale and no exit from the left atrium.

Aortic atresia is an admixture lesion, since both the systemic and pulmonary venous returns mix in the right atrium and ventricle. The right-sided cardiac chambers and pulmonary trunk are dilated. In most patients, pulmonary blood flow is increased, so that the degree of cyanosis is initially minimal in neonates. The fetal circulation is severely disturbed in this cardiac anomaly.

The condition of these neonates deteriorates rapidly, and peripheral perfusion is decreased. The roles of the ductus arteriosus and coarctation of the aorta are unknown, and more detailed studies are needed to understand the decreased peripheral perfusion. In fact, one study[90] showed that the patients had normal mean systemic arterial pressures, although in some, the pulse pressure was narrow. Yet, at postmortem examination, the liver and other organs show changes of hypoperfusion.

Systemic blood flow is adversely affected by the fall in pulmonary vascular resistance and by constriction of the patent ductus arteriosus. It is likely that cerebral and myocardial blood flow is preserved at the expense of visceral and cutaneous perfusion. Indeed, these neonates have azotemia and a mottled appearance.

CLINICAL FEATURES.   Several authors[81,83,85,88] have indicated the high incidence of aortic atresia in males. In our experience,[83] of 31 patients with aortic atresia and patent mitral valve, 27 were males, while of 10 patients with coexistent aortic and mitral atresia, 5 were males.

Although neonates with aortic atresia appear normal at birth, they deteriorate rapidly, the average age of death being 4.5 days.[81] Ninety percent are dead by 2 weeks of age.

Several authors have described the classic features of aortic atresia.[81,85,88,91] The initial symptoms, tachypnea and dyspnea, develop within hours of birth and suggest the presence of pulmonary disease. Cyanosis appears but is not marked, and early systemic arterial saturation may be 85 to 90 percent.[90] With the administration of 100 percent oxygen, the Po_2 may rise to 250 torr. Congestive cardiac failure usually develops by 24 hours of age, and the liver quickly descends to the level of the umbilicus or further.

Subsequently, the neonate develops poor peripheral perfusion and shows a mottled, cool skin, but still cyanosis is not marked. The skin may also show jaundice, in part related to decreased hepatic perfusion. The status of peripheral perfusion varies.

Early in the course, the peripheral arterial pulses are normal, but they become weak or impalpable.

The auscultatory findings are not diagnostic. Early in the course, a grade 2/6 murmur may be heard along the left sternal border, but it subsequently may disappear as the condition deteriorates. We have noted a soft systolic murmur in the left paraspinal area in many of these infants. The second heart sound is loud and single. A prominent gallop may be heard. A middiastolic murmur, presumably from increased tricuspid blood flow, has been described.[81]

ELECTROCARDIOGRAM.   In most instances, the electrocardiogram may be normal for the age or show a pattern of right axis deviation and right ventricular hypertrophy.[81,92] This pattern results from hypertrophy of the right ventricle and hypoplasia of the left ventricle (Fig. 13-13). Right atrial enlargement is usually present. We have seen no patient with a q wave in lead V_6,[92] and this has been commented upon by others.[85,91] Flat or inverted T waves may be present in the left precordial leads.

Occasionally, left axis deviation may be present and, rarely, left ventricular hypertrophy. We have found patients with Wolff-Parkinson-White syndrome or other types of ventricular conduction abnormalities.[92]

THORACIC ROENTGENOGRAM. Thoracic roentgenograms show moderate or marked cardiomegaly (Fig. 13-14). Aortic atresia is the leading cause of gross cardiomegaly in the first week of life. Left atrial enlargement is not present. The pulmonary vascularity shows increased venous and arterial markings. Although the contour is not considered diagnostic, one report[91] noted in the frontal plane an acute angulation between the shadow of the superior vena cava

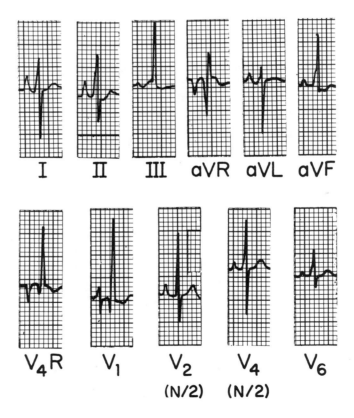

FIG. 13-13. Electrocardiogram of 1-month-old infant with aortic atresia. Right atrial enlargement. QRS axis is +120°. Right ventricular hypertrophy. No q wave in lead V_6. N_2, half-standardization.

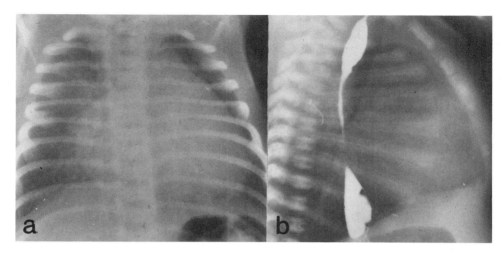

FIG. 13-14.   Thoracic roentgenogram of aortic atresia. **a.** Posteroanterior view. **b.** Lateral view. Marked cardiomegaly. Increased pulmonary vascular markings. No left atrial enlargement.

and the right atrium. This is probably related to the enlargement of the right atrium.

ECHOCARDIOGRAM.   Four echocardiographic features (Fig. 13-15) in combination are strongly suggestive of aortic atresia: (1) small aortic root, (2) small left ventricular cavity, (3) enlarged right ventricular cavity, and (4) abnormal form and

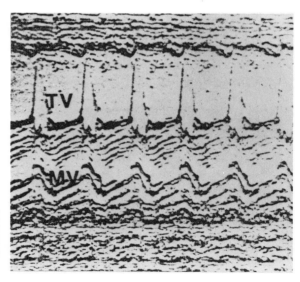

FIG. 13-15.   Echocardiogram of aortic atresia. Small left ventricle and reduced movement of mitral valve (MV). Tricuspid valve (TV) within enlarged right ventricle.

excursion of mitral valve. We have found some neonates with aortic atresia in whom the aortic root and left ventricle had measurements within the normal range.

CARDIAC CATHETERIZATION AND ANGIOCARDIOGRAM. It is only recently that cardiac catheterization data have been reported. Although catheterization data assist in the diagnosis, angiography provides the important information. Usually this diagnosis can be made clinically, and cardiac catheterization and angiography are performed to exclude cardiac conditions that are operatively treatable.

The pressure data show elevated pulmonary venous and left atrial pressure, although it may be difficult to advance the catheter into the left atrium. Right atrial pressures are also elevated, frequently the mean pressure being 10 mm Hg or greater.[85,90,91] Right atrial a waves are predominant and reach 20 mm Hg. Right ventricular and pulmonary arterial systolic pressures are usually greater than 65 mm Hg, and a pressure difference may be recorded between the aorta and the pulmonary artery.[85,90] The aortic systolic pressure may range from 30 to 45 mm Hg in a critically ill neonate.

Oximetry data show a left-to-right shunt at the atrial level in most patients, except in those with premature closure of the atrial septum. Some streaming may occur in the atria, but oxygen saturations are similar in the right ventricle, pulmonary artery, and aorta. The oxygen saturations in the systemic arteries may reach 90 percent, but as systemic perfusion decreases, oxygen saturations fall in the vena cava and the aorta.

Angiography is paramount in the diagnosis. In our experience, injection into the right ventricle, pulmonary artery, or aorta is sufficient to make the diagnosis. A right-to-left shunt occurs at the ductus, and both the descending and the ascending aorta are opacified. The ascending aorta is opacified as contrast material flows in a retrograde direction around the aortic arch. The ascending aorta, which is usually quite hypoplastic, is opacified to the level of the aortic valve, and then the coronary arteries opacify. There is no other condition we know of that gives this appearance. On occasion, the ascending aorta is nearly normal in caliber. If the catheter is advanced into the left atrium, injection should be made at that site, but we do not consider this necessary for the diagnosis.

Retrograde aortography may demonstrate the aortic atresia very well[93] (Figure. 13-16).

Care must be taken during the procedure to limit the amount of contrast material used because the systemic pressure is low, and renal damage can result or be accentuated, leading to oliguria or anuria. These neonates are usually severely ill at the time of catheterization, and bradycardia and cardiac arrest may occur. The infants must be carefully monitored and the known complications aggressively treated.

MANAGEMENT. Early treatment should include a digitalis preparation and diuretics. As systemic perfusion decreases, the complications of hypoglycemia,

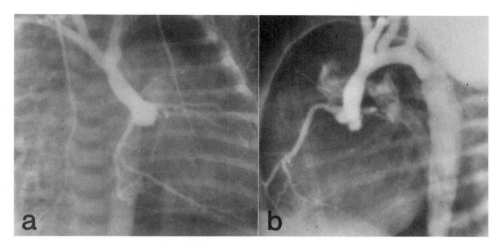

FIG. 13-16. Aortogram of aortic atresia. **a.** Anteroposterior view. **b.** Lateral view. Opacification to level of aortic valve. Dense opacification of coronary arteries. Ascending aorta small in comparison to size of descending aorta. On lateral view, slight opacification of pulmonary arteries through patent ductus arteriosus.

azotemia, and acidosis develop and require management. Disseminated intravascular coagulation ultimately develops. Therefore, blood sugar, BUN, pH, and coagulation factors must be monitored. Usually, sick neonates are placed in an oxygen-enriched environment. This may have deleterious effects in aortic atresia by (1) constricting the ductus arteriosus, causing decreased systemic perfusion, and (2) causing pulmonary vasodilatation. Rudolph[89] did not administer high oxygen concentrations and found that the infants survived longer.

Recently, a technique was described[94] in which a single roentgen exposure was made following injection of contrast material through an umbilical arterial catheter placed at the level of the ductus. Such films can be diagnostic of aortic atresia. This can save the risks and cost of cardiac catheterization or the transfer of patients to other hospitals. It is imperative, however, that the films be interpreted by experienced physicians so that correctable lesions are not missed.

Aortic atresia is usually rapidly fatal in the neonatal period, and there is no corrective procedure available. A palliative procedure has been described[95] that requires (1) enlargement of the atrial septal defect to reduce pulmonary venous obstruction, (2) protection of the lungs from elevated pulmonary arterial pressure, and (3) a means of increasing systemic arterial perfusion because of a constricting patent ductus arteriosus. This operation requires creation of an atrial septal defect, banding of both pulmonary arteries, and a Waterston-type shunt between the pulmonary artery and the aorta. This is an extensive procedure for an infant for whom no corrective procedure is currently available. Until a corrective operation becomes available, we believe little is gained by undertaking the palliative procedure. We have not encouraged the parents of our patients to undertake such a procedure. Once we make the diagnosis, we discuss the prognosis with the parents and conservatively manage the infant.

AORTIC STENOSIS WITH HYPOPLASTIC LEFT VENTRICLE

The pathology, hemodynamics, and clinical features of aortic stenosis with hypoplastic left ventricle resemble those of aortic atresia.[79, 96]

PATHOLOGY.   Unlike the valve in aortic atresia, the aortic valve is patent but severely stenotic. The aortic valve is unicommissural. Both the aortic annulus and the ascending aorta are smaller than normal but not to the same degree as with aortic atresia. The mitral valve and left ventricle are hypoplastic, and the left ventricle shows marked endocardial fibroelastosis (Fig. 13-17). The left atrium, which is not enlarged, shows endocardial fibroelastosis. The foramen ovale may be sealed or herniated into the right atrium. The right atrium and ventricle are dilated and hypertrophied. There is a patent ductus.

HEMODYNAMICS.   The major difference from aortic atresia is that forward flow occurs through the aortic valve, but the volume is limited by the degree of stenosis and the impediment of left ventricular inflow by the mitral valve hypoplasia and decreased left ventricular compliance.

There may be a left-to-right shunt at the atrial level, but this is usually small. Left atrial pressure is elevated and causes pulmonary venous obstruction. There is a right-to-left shunt at the ductal level, and this is the major source of systemic blood flow.

CLINICAL FEATURES.   This condition occurs more frequently in males. Symptoms generally develop in the first 2 days of life. The major symptoms are those of dyspnea, cyanosis, and congestive cardiac failure. Decreased systemic perfusion and its complications develop.

On physical examination, initially the neonates are acyanotic, show normal perfusion, and have normal peripheral pulses, but they quickly become mottled and cyanotic and have impalpable pulses. A systolic murmur is present over the precordium, presumably from the aortic stenosis. The second sound is single. Hepatomegaly is prominent.

ELECTROCARDIOGRAM.   The electrocardiogram shows a QRS axis which is normal for the age. Right atrial enlargement and right ventricular hypertrophy are present (Fig. 13-18). T waves may be inverted in the left precordial leads.

THORACIC ROENTGENOGRAM.   Cardiomegaly is present, and the right atrium and ventricle are prominent. Slight left atrial enlargement may be found. The pulmonary vascular markings show a mixed pattern of increased arterial and venous vessels.

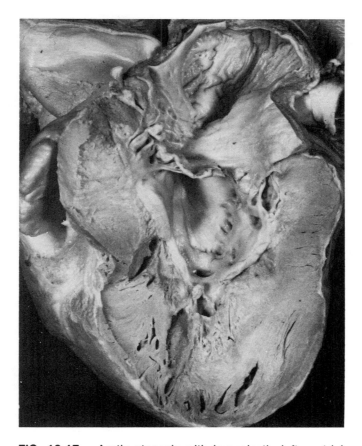

FIG. 13-17. Aortic stenosis with hypoplastic left ventricle. Left atrium (above) and left ventricle (below) are hypoplastic. Endocardial surface of left ventricle white and thickened by endocardial fibroelastosis. Small dimples on left ventricular endocardial surface represents the lumina of intramyocardial sinusoid-coronary arterial communications.

ECHOCARDIOGRAM. The echocardiogram resembles that of aortic atresia, although in aortic atresia, there is a range in the size of the left ventricular cavity and the caliber of the ascending aorta. In aortic stenosis and hypoplastic left ventricle, the size of the left-sided structures may be at the lower limits of normal. In contrast to aortic atresia, opening of the aortic valve can be observed. Multiple echoes may be recorded from the aortic valve, perhaps because the leaflets are thick. Aortic valvular closure is asymmetrical.

CARDIAC CATHETERIZATION AND ANGIOCARDIOGRAM. Generally, because the features of these neonates resemble those of infants with aortic atresia, the diag-

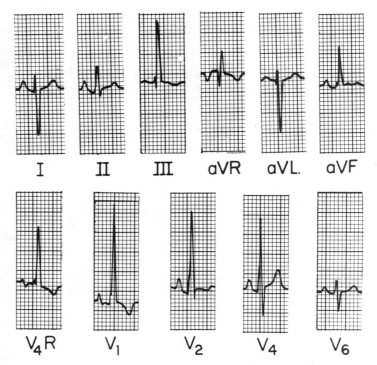

FIG. 13-18. Electrocardiogram of aortic stenosis and hypoplastic left ventricle. Right atrial enlargement. QRS axis is +120°. Right ventricular hypertrophy.

nosis is initially suspected on angiography. Whether the approach is through the umbilical artery, pulmonary angiography, or other, a right-to-left shunt occurs at the ductal level, and there may be retrograde flow about the aortic arch. In contrast to angiography in aortic atresia, the contrast material in the ascending aorta is washed out, indicating antegrade flow through that valve. The aortic valve may dome. If antegrade flow occurs in the ascending aorta, the size of the left ventricular cavity must be determined. The left ventricle may be visualized by passing a catheter across the atrial septum into the left ventricle (Fig. 13-19). If it is impossible to pass the catheter across the atrial septum, a pulmonary arteriogram is an alternative to visualizing the left ventricle.

Pressure data show pulmonary hypertension and, at times, a pressure difference between the pulmonary artery and the descending aorta. Pulmonary venous left atrial and left ventricular pressures are also elevated.

MANAGEMENT. Infants with aortic stenosis and hypoplastic left ventricle show progressive congestive cardiac failure and hypoperfusion. Most die by 2 weeks of age. Aortic valvotomy is rarely indicated because the left ventricle is so hypoplastic, but there may be an occasional infant whose left ventricular cavity

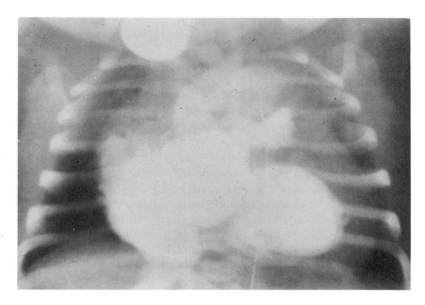

FIG. 13-19.   Left atriogram, anteroposterior view, of aortic stenosis with hypoplastic left ventricle. Left ventricle reduced in size. Ventricular wall thickened. Left-to-right shunt at atrial level.

size approaches normal, in whom an operation should be performed, but the risk is extremely high.

MITRAL ATRESIA WITH NORMAL AORTIC VALVE

Mitral atresia with normal aortic valve can mimic aortic atresia but shows a more variable clinical picture. It occurs less frequently than aortic atresia and must be considered in the differential diagnosis of that condition and other causes of pulmonary venous obstruction.

PATHOLOGY.   The mitral valve is absent, and its position is marked by a dimple on the floor of the left atrium. The left atrium is small, and its wall is hypertrophied and may show endocardial fibroelastosis. The left atrium usually communicates with the right atrium through a patent foramen ovale and less frequently through an atrial septal defect. Premature closure of the foramen ovale may occur, and in these situations, the pulmonary venous return passes through a levoatriocardinal vein[97] or other anomalous pulmonary venous connection.[98] The right atrium and right ventricle are enlarged. Usually a ventricular septal defect is present, which communicates with a diminutive left ventricle that serves as the aortic outflow tract. The great vessels may be normally related and transposed, or there may be varying degrees of dextroposition of the aorta.[99]

Pulmonary stenosis or coarctation of the aorta may coexist. Mitral atresia may also occur in patients with the syndromes associated with asplenia or polysplenia.[100,101]

HEMODYNAMICS.   There is total obstruction of blood flow from the left atrium to the left ventricle. Blood leaves the left atrium through either an atrial communication or a levoatriocardinal vein. If the atrial communication is small or nonexistent, pulmonary venous obstruction results, causing the typical clinical and laboratory features of that physiologic state. In addition, pulmonary blood flow is limited, so a severe degree of arterial desaturation occurs. The entire systemic and pulmonary venous returns enter the right atrium and are ejected by the right ventricle into the aorta and pulmonary artery, the amount of flow going to each vascular system depending upon the volume of blood flow. Resistance to pulmonary blood flow can occur, as indicated by pulmonary venous obstruction or by coexistent pulmonary stenosis. If a coarctation of the aorta coexists, pulmonary blood flow is increased.

Although many infants show pulmonary venous obstruction and severe cyanosis, if the atrial communication is sufficient, pulmonary blood flow is greatly increased, and the degree of desaturation is minimal.

CLINICAL FEATURES.   Although many patients present with symptoms in the neonatal period, survival is much more variable than in aortic atresia.[100,101] One report[101] finds the average age of death is 6 months, with longer survival in patients with atrial septal defect or pulmonary stenosis. There is an equal sex distribution.[101,102]

Most patients develop cyanosis, tachypnea, or respiratory distress in the first week of life and often in the first 24 hours of life.[102,103] In our experience, congestive cardiac failure and the development of cyanosis occurred after the onset of a murmur. As indicated, the degree of cyanosis is inversely related to the volume of pulmonary blood flow. Murmurs have been described in infants and were present in most of our patients. They were usually ejection type and generally loud (grade 3/6). We were unable to relate the murmur to specific associated defects. In other infants, no murmur or an unimpressive systolic murmur is found. Unless pulmonary stenosis is present, the pulmonic component of the second heart sound is loud.

The liver is enlarged. In patients with severe pulmonary venous obstruction, systemic blood flow is limited, and the infant shows signs of inadequate peripheral perfusion.

ELECTROCARDIOGRAM.   The electrocardiogram is not diagnostic. The QRS axis is usually normal or right, but a few patients have left axis deviation.[100,101] We found a QRS axis between 0 and $-120°$ in 6 of our 26 patients.[102] Right ventricular hypertrophy is found, as expected, and lead V_1 frequently shows a qR pattern. Some of our patients with coexistent single ventricle have a pattern of biventricular hypertrophy.

THORACIC ROENTGENOGRAM. Unlike many conditions described in this chapter, mitral atresia is usually associated with cardiomegaly. There is no specific cardiac contour. The left atrium is not enlarged. The pulmonary vascular markings may show one of four patterns, depending upon the associated hemodynamics: (1) decreased, (2) increased pulmonary arterial, (3) increased pulmonary venous, or (4) mixed pulmonary arterial and venous.

CARDIAC CATHETERIZATION AND ANGIOCARDIOGRAM. There is little information reported about cardiac catheterization. A left-to-right shunt is present at the atrial level, and pulmonary arterial and aortic oxygen saturations are equal. Right ventricular systolic pressure is elevated to systemic levels. Usually, left atrial pressure is elevated and may reach mean values of 40 mm Hg.[101] The a wave is the prominent atrial wave. Pulmonary arterial pressure equals aortic pressure unless pulmonary stenosis coexists.

Left atrial injection of contrast material would ideally demonstrate the mitral atresia, but it is frequently impossible to pass the catheter tip into that chamber. As a substitute, pulmonary arterial injection can show the hemodynamics of mitral atresia, but because of the slow pulmonary blood flow, the details of the left atrium are not clearly visualized. In patients with a levoatriocardinal vein or other pulmonary venous connection, the pulmonary arteriogram may be confused with total anomalous pulmonary venous connection. However, the latter has a right-to-left atrial shunt, and mitral atresia has a left-to-right shunt at this level. Right ventriculography shows simultaneous opacification of both great vessels and antegrade flow across the aortic valve, thus excluding the diagnosis of aortic atresia. This study also shows other details of ventricular and great vessel anatomy.

Balloon atrial septostomy should be attempted but is usually unsatisfactory because the atrial septum is thickened and tough.

MANAGEMENT. Decongestive measures are indicated in most patients. Although no corrective type of operation is available, palliative procedures may help some patients. In those with pulmonary venous obstruction, operative creation of an atrial septal defect relieves the left atrial obstruction. In those with large atrial septal defect, pulmonary arterial banding decreases the shunt. Patients with pulmonary stenosis may be assisted by a systemic-pulmonary arterial shunt, provided there is an adequate atrial communication. In patients with pulmonary stenosis, the coexistent mitral atresia may first be recognized postoperatively following a shunt when the patient develops pulmonary edema, as described by Friedman.[104]

LEFT VENTRICULAR INFLOW OBSTRUCTION WITH NORMAL-SIZED LEFT VENTRICLE

Any cardiac anomaly associated with a shunt may coexist with any form of left ventricular inflow obstruction. In conditions associated with a left-to-right shunt, the magnitude of the shunt is increased. It the shunt occurs at the atrial level, the coexistent stenotic lesion at the mitral valve is difficult to visualize angiographically because of the atrial shunt. Likewise, because of the shunt, pressure data do not reveal the obstruction. Echocardiography is helpful in outlining the mitral valve and adjacent structures.

In those with left-to-right shunt distal to the mitral valve, the elevated left atrial and pulmonary venous pressures increase pulmonary vascular resistance and limit pulmonary blood flow.

Among patients with cyanotic conditions associated with decreased pulmonary blood flow, the obstructing condition may not be recognized because of the small volume of pulmonary blood flow. If it increases because of corrective or palliative procedures, signs of pulmonary venous obstruction may appear.

In those with cyanosis and increased pulmonary blood flow, the hemodynamics resemble those with left-to-right shunts.

REFERENCES

Mitral Stenosis

1. Lucas RV Jr, Anderson RC, Amplatz K, Adams P Jr, Edwards JE: Congenital causes of pulmonary venous obstruction. Pediatr Clin North Am 10:781, 1963
2. Moller JH: Congenital causes of left ventricular inflow obstruction. In Edwards JE, Lev M (eds): The Heart. Baltimore, Williams & Wilkins, 1974, pp 271–296
3. Davachi F, Moller JH, Edwards JE: Diseases of the mitral valve in infancy. An anatomic analysis of 55 cases. Circulation 43:565, 1971
4. Shone JD, Sellers RD, Anderson RC, et al.: The developmental complex of "parachute mitral valve," supravalvular ring of left atrium, subaortic stenosis, and coarctation of aorta. Am J Cardiol 11:714, 1963
5. Zamora R, Moller JH, Edwards JE: Double-outlet right ventricle. Anatomic types and associated anomalies. Chest 68:672, 1975
6. Castaneda AR, Anderson RC, Edwards JE: Congenital mitral stenosis resulting from anomalous arcade and obstructing papillary muscles. Report of correction by use of ball valve prosthesis. Am J Cardiol 24:237, 1969
7. Ferencz C, Johnson AL, Wiglesworth FW: Congenital mitral stenosis. Circulation 9:161, 1954
8. van der Horst RL, Hastreiter AR: Congenital mitral stenosis. Am J Cardiol 20:773, 1967
9. Dauod G, Kaplan S, Perrin EV, Dorst JP, Edwards FK: Congenital mitral stenosis. Circulation 27:185, 1963
10. Elliott LP, Anderson RC, Amplatz K, Lillehei CW, Edwards JE: Congenital mitral stenosis. Pediatrics 30:552, 1962
11. Braudo JL, Javett SN, Adler DI, Kessel I: Isolated congenital mitral stenosis. Report of two cases with mitral valvotomy in one. Circulation 15:358, 1957
12. Young D, Robinson G: Successful valve replacement in an infant with congenital mitral stenosis. N Engl J Med 270:660, 1964
13. Glancy DL, Chang MY, Dorney ER, Robert WC: Parachute mitral valve: Further observations and associated lesions. Am J Cardiol 27:309, 1971
14. Macartney FJ, Scott O, Ionescu MI, Deverall PB: Diagnosis and management of

parachute mitral valve and supravalvar mitral ring. Br Heart J 36:641, 1974

15. Khalil KG, Shapiro I, Kilman JW: Congenital mitral stenosis. J Thorac Cardiovasc Surg 70:40, 1975

16. Blieden LC, Castaneda AR, Nicoloff DM, Lillehei CW, Moller JH: Prosthetic valve replacement in children. Results in 44 patients. Ann Thorac Surg 14:545, 1972

Supravalvular Stenosing Ring of Left Atrium

17. Rao S, Anderson RC, Lucas RV Jr, et al.: Clinical pathologic conference. Am Heart J 77:538, 1969

18. Hohn AR, Jain KK, Tamer DM: Supravalvular mitral stenosis in a patient with tetralogy of Fallot. Am J Cardiol 22:733, 1968

19. Chesler E, Beck W, Barnard CN, Schrire V: Supravalvular stenosing ring of the left atrium associated with corrected transposition of the great vessels. Am J Cardiol 31:84, 1973

20. Benrey J, Leachman RD, Cooley DA, Klima T, Lufschanowski R: Supravalvular mitral stenosis associated with tetralogy of Fallot. Am J Cardiol 37:111, 1976

21. Mehrizi A, Hutchins GM, Wilson EF, Breckinridge JC, Rowe RD: Supravalvular mitral stenosis. J Pediatr 67:1141, 1965

Cor Triatriatum

22. Van Praagh R, Corsini I: Cor triatriatum: Pathologic anatomy and a consideration of morphogenesis based on 13 postmortem cases and a study of normal development of the pulmonary vein and atrial septum in 83 human embryos. Am Heart J 78:379, 1969

23. Niwayama G: Cor triatriatum. Am Heart J 59:291, 1960

24. Marin-Garcia J, Tandon R, Lucas RV Jr, Edwards JE: Cor triatriatum: Study of 20 cases. Am J Cardiol 35:59, 1975

25. Jennings RB Jr, Innes BJ: Subtotal cor triatriatum with left partial anomalous pulmonary venous return. Successful surgical repair in an infant. J Thorac Cardiovasc Surg 74:461, 1977

26. Wilson JW, Graham TP, Gehweiler JA, Canent RV: Cor triatriatum with intact subdividing diaphragm and partial anomalous pulmonary venous connection to the proximal left atrial chamber (an unreported type). Pediatrics 47:745, 1971

27. Shone JD, Anderson RC, Amplatz K, et al.: Pulmonary venous obstruction from two separate coexistent anomalies. Subtotal pulmonary venous connection to cor triatriatum and subtotal pulmonary venous connection to left innominate vein. Am J Cardiol 11:525, 1963

28. Nakib A, Moller JH, Kanjuh VI, Edwards JE: Anomalies of the pulmonary veins. Am J Cardiol 20:77, 1967

29. Grondin C, Leonard AS, Anderson RC, Amplatz KA, Edwards JE: Cor triatriatum: A diagnostic surgical enigma. J Thorac Cardiovasc Surg 48:527, 1964

30. Jegier W, Gibbons JE, Wiglesworth FW: Cor triatriatum: Clinical, hemodynamic and pathological studies: Surgical correction in early life. Pediatrics 31:255, 1963

31. Miller GAH, Ongley PA, Anderson MW, Kincaid OW, Swan HJC: Cor triatriatum. Hemodynamic and angiocardiographic diagnosis. Am Heart J 68:298, 1964

32. Anderson RC, Varco RL: Cor triatriatum: Successful diagnosis and surgical correction in a three year old girl. Am J Cardiol 7:436, 1961

33. Moodie DS, Hagler DJ, Ritter DG: Cor triatriatum. Echocardiographic findings. Mayo Clin Proc 51:289, 1976

34. LaCorte M, Harada K, Williams RG: Echocardiographic features of congenital left ventricular inflow obstruction. Circulation 54:562, 1976

35. Canedo MI, Stefadouros MA, Frank MJ, Moore HV, Cundey DW: Echocardiographic features of cor triatriatum. Am J Cardiol 40:615, 1977

36. Perry LW, Scott LP, McClenathan JE: Cor triatriatum: Preoperative diagnosis and successful surgical repair in a small infant. J Pediatr 71:840, 1967

Stenosis of Individual Pulmonary Veins

37. Shone JD, Amplatz K, Anderson RC, Adams P Jr, Edwards JE: Congenital stenosis of individual pulmonary veins. Circulation 26:574, 1962

38. Sherman FE, Stengel WF, Bauersfeld SR: Congenital stenosis of pulmonary veins at their atrial junction. Am Heart J 56:908, 1958

39. Moller JH, Noren GR, David PR, et al.: Clinical pathologic conference. Am Heart J 72:530, 1966

40. Mortensson W, Lundstrom NR: Congenital obstruction of the pulmonary veins at their atrial junction. Review of the literature and a case report. Am Heart J 87:359, 1974

41. Contis G, Fung RH, Vawter GF, Nadas AS: Stenosis and obstruction of the pulmonary veins associated with pulmonary artery hypertension. Am J Cardiol 20:718, 1967

Anomalous Pulmonary Venous Connection

42. Lucas RV Jr, Schmidt RE: Anomalous venous connections, pulmonary and systemic. In Moss AJ, Adams FH, Emmanouilides GC (eds): Heart Disease in Infants, Children and Adolescents. Baltimore, Williams & Wilkins, 1977, pp 437–470

43. Burroughs JT, Edwards JE: Total anomalous pulmonary venous connection. Am Heart J 59:913, 1960

44. Bonham-Carter RE, Capriles M, Noe Y: Total anomalous pulmonary venous drainage. A clinical and anatomical study of 75 children. Br Heart J 31:45, 1969

45. Gatham GE, Nadas AS: Total anomalous pulmonary venous connection. Clinical and physiologic observations of 75 pediatric patients. Circulation 42:143, 1970

46. Gomes MMR, Feldt RH, McGoon DC, Danielson GK: Total anomalous pulmonary venous connection. Surgical considerations and results of operation. J Thorac Cardiovasc Surg 60:116, 1970

47. Delisle G, Ando M, Calder AL, et al.: Total anomalous pulmonary venous connection: Report of 93 autopsied cases with emphasis on diagnostic and surgical considerations. Am Heart J 91:99, 1976

48. Elliott LP, Edwards JE: The problem of pulmonary venous obstruction in total anomalous pulmonary venous connection to left innominate vein. Circulation 25:913, 1962

49. Carey LS, Edwards JE: Severe pulmonary venous obstruction in total anomalous pulmonary venous connection to the left innominate vein. Am J Roentgenol Radium Ther Nucl Med 90:593, 1963

50. Duff DF, Nihill MR, McNamara DG: Infradiaphragmatic total anomalous pulmonary venous return. Review of clinical and pathological findings and results of operation in 28 cases. Br Heart J 39:619, 1977

51. Lucas RV Jr, Adams P Jr, Anderson RC, et al.: Total anomalous pulmonary venous connection to the portal venous system: A cause of pulmonary venous obstruction. Am J Roentgenol Radium Ther Nucl Med 86:561, 1961

52. Hastreiter AR, Paul MH, Molthan ME, Miller RE: Total anomalous pulmonary

venous connection with severe pulmonary venous obstruction. A clinical entity. Circulation 25:916, 1962

53. Kauffman SL, Ores CN, Anderson DH: Two cases of total anomalous pulmonary venous return of the supracardiac type with stenosis simulating infradiaphragmatic drainage. Circulation 25:376, 1962

54. Johnson AL, Wiglesworth FW, Dunbar JS, Siddoo S, Grajo M: Infradiaphragmatic total anomalous pulmonary venous connection. Circulation 17:340, 1958

55. Gott VL, Lester RG, Lillehei CW, Varco RL: Total anomalous pulmonary return. An analysis of thirty cases. Circulation 13:543, 1956

56. Guntheroth WG, Nadas AS, Gross RE: Transposition of the pulmonary veins. Circulation 18:117, 1958

57. Higashino SM, Shaw GG, May IA, Ecker RR: Total anomalous pulmonary venous drainage below the diaphragm. Clinical presentation, hemodynamic findings, and surgical results. J Thorac Cardiovasc Surg 68:711, 1974

58. Robinson AE, Chen JTT, Bradford WD, Lester RG: Kerley B lines in total anomalous pulmonary venous connection below the diaphragm (Type III). Am J Cardiol 24:436, 1969

59. Mathew R, Thilenius OG, Replogle RL, Arcilla RA: Cardiac function in total anomalous pulmonary venous return before and after surgery. Circulation 55:361, 1977

60. Behrendt DM, Aberdeen E, Waterston DJ, Bonham-Carter RE: Total anomalous pulmonary venous drainage in infants. I. Clinical and hemodynamic findings, methods, and results of operation in 37 cases. Circulation 46:347, 1972

61. Tynan M, Behrendt D, Urquhart W, Graham GR: Portal vein catheterization and selective angiography in diagnosis of total anomalous pulmonary venous connexion. Br Heart J 36:1155, 1974

62. Serratto M, Bucheleres HG, Bicoff P, Miller RA, Hastreiter AR: Palliative balloon atrial septostomy for total anomalous pulmonary venous connection in infancy. J Pediatr 73:734, 1968

63. Mullins CE, El-Said GM, Neches WH, et al.: Balloon atrial septostomy for total anomalous pulmonary venous return. Br Heart J 35:752, 1973

64. Engle MA: Total anomalous pulmonary venous drainage. Success story at last. Circulation 46:209, 1972

65. Jegier W, Charrette E, Dobell ARC: Infradiaphragmatic anomalous pulmonary venous drainage. Normal hemodynamics following operation in infancy. Circulation 35:396, 1967

66. Mody MR, Gallen WJ, Lepley D: Total anomalous pulmonary venous drainage below the diaphragm. Successful surgical correction in an infant. Am J Cardiol 24:575, 1969

67. Joffe HS, O'Donovan TG, Glaun BP, Chesler E, Schrire V: Subdiaphragmatic total anomalous pulmonary venous drainage: Report of a successful surgical correction. Am Heart J 81:250, 1971

68. Buckley MJ, Behrendt DM, Goldblatt A, Laver MB, Austen WG: Correction of total anomalous pulmonary venous drainage in the first month of life. J Thorac Cardiovasc Surg 63:269, 1972

69. Breckenridge IM, de Leval M, Stark J, Waterston DJ: Correction of total anomalous pulmonary venous drainage in infancy. J Thorac Cardiovasc Surg 66:447, 1973

70. Gersony WM, Bowman FO Jr, Steeg CN, et al.: Management of total anomalous pulmonary venous drainage in early infancy. Circulation 43 [Suppl 1]:19, 1971

71. El-Said G, Mullins CE, McNamara DG: Management of total anomalous pulmonary venous return. Circulation 45:1240, 1972

72. Silove ED, Behrendt DM, Aberdeen E, Bonham-Carter RE: Total anomalous pulmonary venous drainage: II. Spontaneous functional closure of interatrial communication after surgical correction in infancy. Circulation 46:357, 1972

Atresia of Common Pulmonary Vein

73. Hawker RE, Celermajer JM, Gengos DC, Cartmill TB, Bowdler JD: Common pulmonary vein atresia. Premortem diagnosis in two infants. Circulation 46:368, 1972
74. Levine MA, Moller JH, Amplatz K, Edwards JE: Atresia of the common pulmonary vein; case report and differential diagnosis. Am J Roentgenol Radium Ther Nucl Med 100:322, 1967
75. Mody GT, Folger GM Jr: Atresia of the common pulmonary vein: Report of one case. Pediatrics 54:62, 1974
76. Lucas RV Jr, Woolfrey BF, Anderson RC, Lester RG, Edwards JE: Atresia of the common pulmonary vein. Pediatrics 29:729, 1962
77. Rywlin AM, Fojaco RM: Congenital pulmonary lymphangiectasis associated with a blind common pulmonary vein. Pediatrics 41:931, 1968

Aortic Valvular Atresia

78. Lev M: Pathologic anatomy and interrelationship of hypoplasia of the aortic tract complexes. Lab Invest 1:61, 1952
79. Noonan JA, Nadas AS: The hypoplastic left heart syndrome. An analysis of 101 cases. Pediatr Clin North Am 5:1029, 1958
80. Kanjuh VI, Eliot RS, Edwards JE: Coexistent mitral and aortic valvular atresia. A pathologic study of 14 cases. Am J Cardiol 15:611, 1965
81. Watson DG, Rowe RD: Aortic-valve atresia. Report of 43 cases. JAMA 179:14, 1962
82. Raghib G, Bloemendaal RD, Kanjuh VI, Edwards JE: Aortic atresia and premature closure of foramen ovale. Myocardial sinusoids and coronary arteriovenous fistula serving as outflow channel. Am Heart J 70:476, 1965
83. Von Rueden TJ, Knight L, Moller JH, Edwards JE: Coarctation of the aorta associated with aortic valvular atresia. Circulation 52:951, 1975
84. Wagenvoort CA, Edwards JE: The pulmonary arterial tree in aortic atresia with intact ventricular septum. Lab Invest 10:924, 1961
85. Sinha SN, Rusnak SL, Sommers HM, et al.: Hypoplastic left ventricle syndrome. Analysis of thirty autopsy cases in infants with surgical considerations. Am J Cardiol 21:166, 1968
86. Freedom RM, Williams WG, Dische MR, Rowe RD: Anatomical variants in aortic atresia. Potential candidates for ventriculoaortic reconstruction. Br Heart J 38:821, 1976
87. Pellegrino PA, Thiene G: Aortic valve atresia with a normally developed left ventricle. Chest 69:121, 1976
88. Roberts WC, Perry LW, Chandra RS, et al.: Aortic valve atresia: A new classification based on necropsy study of 73 cases. Am J Cardiol 37:753, 1976
89. Rudolph AM: Congenital Diseases of the Heart. Chicago, Year Book, 1974, p 569
90. Krovetz LJ, Rowe RD, Schiebler GL: Hemodynamics of aortic valve atresia. Circulation 42:953, 1970
91. Saied A, Folger GM Jr: Hypoplastic left heart syndrome. Clinicopathologic and hemodynamic correlation. Am J Cardiol 29:190, 1972
92. Von Rueden TJ, Moller JH: The electrocardiogram in aortic valvular atresia. Chest 73:66, 1978
93. Neufeld HN, Adams P Jr, Edwards JE, Lester RG: Diagnosis of aortic atresia by retrograde aortography. Circulation 25:278, 1962
94. Rosengart R, Jarmakani JM, Emmanouilides GC: Single film retrograde umbilical aortography in the diagnosis of hypoplastic left heart syndrome with aortic atresia. Circulation 54:345, 1976
95. Cayler GG, Smeloff EA, Miller GE Jr: Surgical palliation of hypoplastic left side of the heart. N Engl J Med 282:780, 1970

Aortic Stenosis

96. Moller JH, Lucas RV Jr, Adams P Jr, et al.: Endocardial fibroelastosis. A clinical and anatomic study of 47 patients with emphasis on its relationship to mitral insufficiency. Circulation 30:759, 1964

Mitral Atresia

97. Lucas RV Jr, Lester RG, Lillehei CW, Edwards JE: Mitral atresia with levoatriocardinal vein. A form of congenital pulmonary venous obstruction. Am J Cardiol 9:607, 1962
98. Shone JD, Edwards JE: Mitral atresia associated with pulmonary venous anomalies. Br Heart J 26:241, 1964
99. Eliot RS, Shone JD, Kanjuh VI, et al.: Mitral atresia. A study of 32 cases. Am Heart J 70:6, 1965
100. Watson DG, Rowe RD, Conen PE, Duckworth JWA: Mitral atresia with normal aortic valve. Report of 11 cases and review of the literature. Pediatrics 25:450, 1960
101. Moreno F, Quero M, Diaz LP: Mitral atresia with normal aortic valve. A study of eighteen cases and a review of the literature. Circulation 53:1004, 1976
102. Seidel FG, Edwards JE, Moller JH: Unpublished observations
103. Summerell J, Miller C, Persaud V, Talerman A: Congenital mitral atresia. Br Heart J 30:249, 1968
104. Friedman S, Edmunds LH, Saraclar M, Weinstein EM: Mitral atresia with premature closure of foramen ovale. A rare hemodynamic cause for failure of Blalock-Taussig anastomosis to relieve inadequate pulmonary blood flow. J Thorac Cardiovasc Surg 71:118, 1976

14 Specific Cardiopulmonary Problems of the Neonate and Their Management

The diagnosis and treatment of infants with cardiac disease is often rewarding, sometimes heart rending, but always a formidable challenge. This chapter addresses the management of complications related to cardiac disease in infants. Treatment of the specific cardiac lesions has been presented in previous chapters of the book. Here, management of the problems of congestive cardiac failure, profound hypoxemia, persistence of fetal vasculature, sepsis, and shock will be discussed in a general way.

Since infants with cardiac disease frequently have one of these complications, the pediatrician hopefully will approach these problems with confidence built upon experience and knowledge. It is not necessary to be a cardiologist to recognize and begin treatment of the critically ill infant with cardiac disease. Indeed, if treatment was not started promptly at the referring hospital, too few infants would survive long enough to benefit from the tertiary level of cardiac care. The sixth sense of the experienced pediatrician will often provide the correct diagnostic possibilities, and confidence in one's judgment allows decisive initiation of appropriate therapy.

CONGESTIVE CARDIAC FAILURE

Defined simply, congestive cardiac failure means that the heart is not performing adequately as a pump commensurate with normal metabolic activity.[1] When certain adaptive physiologic mechanisms are effective in maintaining normal cardiac output, cardiac failure is said to be "compensated." Low cardiac output despite maximal interplay of cardiocirculatory protective mechanisms implies a noncompensated state.

PATHOPHYSIOLOGY. Congestive cardiac failure in infants is usually caused by structural anomalies of the heart, though, less commonly, primary myocardial disease may be the precipitating cause (Chap. 10). Structural anomalies can be

This chapter was prepared with the assistance of Bradley P. Fuhrman, M.D.

divided into (1) those which cause volume overload of the heart, as from left-to-right shunt or valvular insufficiency, and (2) those which cause pressure overload, as from obstructive lesions, such as aortic or pulmonic stenosis and coarctation of the aorta. The morphologic patterns resulting from pressure and volume stress of the heart are distinctly different and affect performance characteristics.[2]

The four major determinants of myocardial performance are preload (estimated by end-diastolic volume), afterload (resistance to fiber shortening), contractility, and heart rate.[3,4] Prolonged hemodynamic stress can alter any of these factors and affect the others. The fundamental indicator of depressed myocardial performance, however, is diminished cardiac contractility.[5,6] Recent data suggest that impaired contractility is related to suboptimal calcium transport within the sarcoplasmic reticulum.[7-9]

A number of important adaptive mechanisms come into play in congestive cardiac failure. Chronic volume overload results in ventricular dilatation, which, according to the Frank-Starling mechanism,[10] enhances stroke volume and contractility to a certain point. The development of myocardial hypertrophy in response to pressure overload results in decreased contractility of each sarcomere, the basic unit of contraction, but there is a beneficial effect because of the increase in overall contractile mass.[11] During congestive cardiac failure, an increase in circulating catecholamines, especially the neurotransmitter norepinephrine, increases cardiac rate and the velocity of ejection.[12] In advanced cardiac failure, decreased cardiac output is accompanied by peripheral vasoconstriction and redistribution of blood flow to areas of greatest metabolic need.[13] Renal blood flow is decreased, and, therefore, glomerular filtration rate is reduced. This, in turn, stimulates the release of aldosterone and renin, resulting in fluid retention.[14] Tissue oxygenation, which may be suboptimal in congestive cardiac failure, is improved by an increase in red blood cell 2,3-diphosphoglycerate, shifting the oxygen dissociation curve to the right.[15]

CLINICAL FEATURES.   The diagnosis of congestive cardiac failure is facilitated by information provided by the parents or primary physician (Chap. 2) and is confirmed by physical examination (Chap. 3).

Young parents caring for their first child may not be aware of abnormal patterns of feeding, respiration, and growth. It is sometimes helpful to question grandparents, babysitters, or close friends who have participated in the care of the infant.

The most consistent feature of congestive cardiac failure during infancy is tiring during feedings, a manifestation of dyspnea upon exertion. A normal infant will generally take 15 to 20 min to consume a volume of formula or breast milk appropriate for its age and size. A 6-week-old infant with easy fatigability due to congestive cardiac failure may require 45 to 60 min to consume 1 or 2 ounces of formula.

Diaphoresis may be noted by parents, but this symptom is more difficult to evaluate reliably, since some infants are simply dressed too warmly.[16]

A history of chronic cough is sometimes obtained and can suggest pulmonary infection or edema. Frequently, the infant is irritable because sleep and feeding patterns are interfered with.

Physical examination should confirm the presence of congestive cardiac failure. Plotting the infant's height, weight, and head circumference on a standard growth chart allows accurate determination if the infant is falling below his expected growth curve. Infants with congestive cardiac failure show slow weight gain, and if cardiac failure is severe, protracted, or accompanied by cyanosis, they show slow growth in length. Head circumference is normal unless there is either a coexistent central nervous system disease or a chromosomal abnormality which affects brain growth.

The hallmarks of congestive cardiac failure are tachypnea, tachycardia, hepatomegaly, and cardiomegaly, and each must be present before the diagnosis is made. In order to obtain meaningful information, cardiac and respiratory rates should be counted while the infant is resting quietly or sleeping. Physical examination is more reliable than x-ray in determining hepatic enlargement, but hepatomegaly may be incorrectly diagnosed by palpating the hepatic edge more than 2 cm below the right costal margin in conditions, such as bronchiolitis, which cause air trapping. Cardiomegaly is most accurately determined by thoracic roentgenogram. A posteroanterior film taken during deep inspiration is essential for reliable interpretation of the contour and size of the heart.

Additional physical signs of congestive cardiac failure include pale, clammy skin, rales, and gallop rhythm. Rales are an uncommon finding in congestive cardiac failure, though diffuse expiratory wheezes are sometimes audible. Neck vein distention and peripheral edema are rarely present, even in fulminant failure.

TREATMENT.   The basic goals of treatment of congestive cardiac failure are to lessen the workload of the heart and to improve its efficiency. Obviously, definitive correction of the cause of the cardiac failure is most desirable but not always possible. Even when operative palliation or correction is feasible, the risk is less when cardiac function has improved from medical management and supportive care.

Digitalis remains the drug of choice in the treatment of congestive cardiac failure.[17-19] It most likely acts by augmenting calcium transport to the contractile proteins,[20,21] causing greater force of contraction and increasing cardiac output.[22,23]

Digoxin, the cardiac glycoside most commonly used in the treatment of congestive cardiac failure in infants, is absorbed, metabolized, and excreted as in adults.[24] Infants, however, seem to require larger doses of digoxin per unit of body mass than is required in adults.[25,26] It is unclear if this is related to differences in distribution or receptor site saturation. In neonates and infants, the usual therapeutic dose of digoxin is 0.04 to 0.06 mg/kg administered either orally or intravenously in three divided doses over 12 to 24 hours. Once digitalization is complete, maintenance is continued by administering one eighth of the total digitalizing dose twice a day. In critically ill infants with severe congestive cardiac failure, digitalization should be completed within 8 hours provided urinary output is satisfactory.

Hospitalization is usually indicated when a diagnosis of congestive cardiac failure is made. Digitalization can then be safely carried out while diagnostic studies are in progress. If congenital cardiac disease is suspected as the underlying cause of cardiac failure, cardiac catheterization should be performed to establish the cardiac diagnosis and determine cardiac function. In the rare event that one elects not to hospitalize the infant, digitalization is best managed by starting the maintenance dosage, realizing that the full therapeutic benefit will not be obtained for approximately 5 days.

Diuretic agents are valuable adjuncts in the treatment of congestive cardiac failure. Furosemide is commonly used when congestive cardiac failure is severe, and when given in a dose of 1 mg/kg, causes a vigorous diuresis within 15 to 20 min. Once the infant is stable, oral chlorothiazide, 10 mg/kg, may be started in combination with an aldosterone antagonist to prevent hypokalemia. There is evidence to suggest that some infants will remain refractory to a thiazide diuretic alone because of secondary hyperaldosteronism.[27]

Afterload reduction has been used recently in severe refractory cardiac failure, but the results have been variable.[28,29] Theoretically, peripheral vasodilatation should improve performance characteristics of the heart by unloading the left ventricle, thereby increasing cardiac output, reducing ventricular diastolic pressure and volume, and enhancing subendocardial perfusion. Nitroprusside has been used as an acute measure, and this will be discussed in greater detail later in this chapter. Data are inconclusive regarding the efficacy of oral vasodilator therapy in infants with congestive cardiac failure.[30] Prazosin and hydralazine are currently being used but, in our limited experience, have had little demonstrable effect.

Finally, ventilatory assistance should be used when cardiac failure is fulminant and uncontrolled. Placing such an infant on a ventilator often results in dramatic improvement within minutes, thus providing additional time for more definitive therapy. Respiratory assistance improves cardiac failure by diminishing the work of breathing and, thereby, reducing oxygen consumption. Diffusion defects secondary to pulmonary edema are partially overcome by ventilation, but systemic venous return to the heart is impeded to some degree.

Management of congestive cardiac failure is a four-step process: (1) recognition of cardiac failure, (2) treatment of cardiac failure, (3) diagnosis of underlying conditions, and (4) treatment of underlying conditions.

Once the cardiac failure has been treated, the infant should be referred to a cardiac center where appropriate diagnostic studies, which usually include cardiac catheterization, can be performed. Based upon knowledge of the underlying cardiac conditions, decisions can be made about further management, including cardiac operation.

HYPOXEMIA

Profound hypoxemia leading to metabolic acidosis is a frequent complication of cyanotic congenital cardiac disease in infants. Medical management provides short-term support at best, but optimizing this important aspect of supportive care can spell the difference between success or failure in the operating suite. Once maximal care has been expediently instituted and the patient has improved as much as possible, further delay in providing operative palliation or correction is counterproductive.

OXYGEN. The first supportive measure readily available to the hypoxemic infant is oxygen. A primary function of the cardiovascular system is the delivery of oxygen to tissues. Three major factors affect oxygen transport: (1) the amount of oxygen in the blood, (2) hemoglobin content, and (3) cardiac output.

The amount of oxygen in blood may be variously measured and expressed as oxygen tension(P_{O_2}), percent hemoglobin saturation (%sat), and oxygen content (vol%).

The total amount of oxygen present in blood is primarily dependent upon the hemoglobin level. One gram of hemoglobin can combine with 1.36 ml of oxygen. Thus, a patient with 10 g% hemoglobin has an *oxygen-carrying capacity* of 13.6 vol%, while a patient with a hemoglobin of 15 g% has a capacity of 20.4 vol%. Oxygen bound to hemoglobin plus that which is dissolved in plasma represents the *oxygen content* of the blood. The amount of oxygen dissolved is dependent upon the P_{O_2}; 1 mm P_{O_2} will dissolve 0.003 vol% of oxygen in blood. Oxygen content can be determined by the Van Slyke method, but this method is rarely used today except to calibrate other methods of oxygen determination.

More commonly, oxygen saturation is determined spectrophotometrically and represents the amount of oxyhemoglobin present as a percentage of total hemoglobin. The relationship between oxygen saturation, oxygen-carrying capacity, and oxygen content may be expressed as follows:

$$\text{Oxygen saturation (\%)} = \frac{\text{oxygen content} - P_{O_2} \times 0.003}{\text{oxygen capacity}} \times 100$$

Oxygen saturation is routinely measured during cardiac catheterization to calculate shunts. By measuring oxygen consumption, pulmonary and systemic blood flow can be calculated using the Fick method (Chap. 7).

Hemoglobin, oxygen saturation, and P_{O_2} are related through the familiar S-shaped hemoglobin-oxygen saturation curve (Fig. 14-1). This relationship indicates that, depending upon the partial pressure of oxygen in the blood (P_{O_2}), hemoglobin binds a certain amount of oxygen (percent saturation). The curve has a steep midportion, favoring oxygen release to tissues.

A family of oxygen dissociation curves exists, depending upon the following factors: hydrogen ion concentration (H^+), carbon dioxide tension (P_{CO_2}), temperature, and the amount of the organic phosphate, 2,3-diphosphoglycerate (2,-

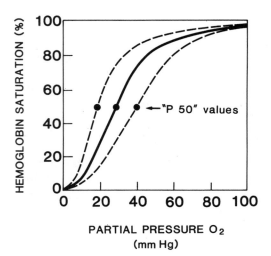

FIG. 14-1. Diagram of hemoglobin-oxygen dissociation curves. *P50* values indicate partial pressure of O_2 at which hemoglobin is 50 percent saturated.

3-DPG), present in the red blood cell. A decrease in any of these factors shifts the oxygen dissociation curve to the left, meaning that at any level of Po_2 more oxygen is combined with hemoglobin. Though hemoglobin affinity for oxygen is increased, release of oxygen to tissues is impaired. A rightward shift of the curve, produced by acidosis, hyperthemia, or increased 2,3-DPG, results in weaker oxygen binding to hemoglobin and enhanced release of oxygen at the tissue level. This shift is sometimes expressed by measurement of P50, i.e., the Po_2 at which hemoglobin is 50 percent saturated with oxygen. When the P50 is raised, the curve is shifted to the right, and hemoglobin has less affinity for oxygen. A lowered P50 has the opposite meaning.

2,3-DPG exerts its influence on the oxygen dissociation curve by competing with hemoglobin for oxygen. This organic phosphate is present in increased amounts in cyanotic congenital cardiac disease, chronic pulmonary disease, and anemia. Levels of 2,3-DPG are decreased in septic shock, severe acidosis, and after transfusion of stored blood. In the normal neonate, the oxygen dissociation curve is shifted to the left because fetal hemoglobin has poor affinity for 2,3-DPG.

The effect of changes of hemoglobin-oxygen dissociation curves is particularly critical in neonates with cyanotic congenital cardiac disease. In hypoxemic neonates, such factors as fetal hemoglobin and hypothermia limit oxygen release by shifting the curve to the left. During cardiac catheterization, the shift can be accentuated by the injection of contrast material.

When hypoxemia is caused by cyanotic congenital cardiac disease, administration of high ambient oxygen concentration in the inspired air is of limited but definite value. Assuming pulmonary function is normal (i.e., no diffusion defect), the hemoglobin molecules in the red blood cells perfusing the lungs are nearly fully saturated, and there is no appreciable increase in the oxyhemoglobin content. At normal body temperature, 37C, 0.00003 ml of oxygen is dissolved in 1 ml of plasma for each mm Hg partial pressure of oxygen. Thus, when breathing room air, arterial blood has an oxygen partial pressure of approximately 100 mm Hg and a dissolved oxygen content of 0.3 ml/100 ml blood, representing only about 1.5 percent total blood oxygen. Administration of high concentrations of oxygen can increase the arterial partial pressure to 600 mm Hg, causing 1.8 ml/100 ml blood to be dissolved in plasma. This represents about a 10 percent increase in total oxygen available to body tissues.

This is a small but potentially significant increase in the available oxygen supply. By correction of such factors as hypothermia, frequently present in hypoxic infants, which tend to shift the oxygen dissociation curve to the left, oxygen bound to hemoglobin is more readily released to tissues.

The level of hemoglobin is also important in oxygen delivery to tissues and can present a major problem in patients with anemia. At the capillary level, oxygen is transported from blood to tissue because of an oxygen gradient. The capillary Po_2 necessary for tissue oxygenation is at least 20 torr and varies among different tissues and their metabolic rates. For a range of 20 to 30 torr, the corresponding hemoglobin oxygen saturation would be 35 to 55 percent. In neonates and infants with severe cyanotic cardiac conditions, blood perfusing capillaries may have an extremely low Po_2. Therefore, oxygen transfer to tissues may be extremely limited because the blood-tissue oxygen gradient is small. As a consequence, cellular function is maintained by anaerobic metabolism, which leads to H^+ production and the possibility of acidosis if renal and pulmonary mechanisms cannot compensate.

OTHER SUPPORTIVE MEASURES.   Metabolic acidosis is corrected by intravenous administration of sodium bicarbonate in a dose of 1 to 3 mEq/kg, depending upon the severity of the acidosis. Sodium bicarbonate, diluted 1:1 with sterile water to avoid rapid changes in blood osmolarity, should be given slowly over several minutes. Correction of acidosis to a pH of at least 7.25 (1) shifts the oxygen dissociation curve to the right, (2) improves cardiac contractility and, indirectly, peripheral vascular perfusion, and (3) decreases pulmonary vascular resistance to a variable degree, augmenting pulmonary blood flow and improving oxygenation.

Respiratory assistance with a ventilator is an additional supportive measure in the extremely hypoxemic, acidotic infant with congenital cardiac disease. Although a ventilator will not appreciably increase oxygenation unless pulmonary edema is present, it reduces oxygen consumption by eliminating the work of breathing, which may cause a significant requirement for oxygen in the hyperventilating infant attempting to compensate for hypoxemia and acidosis. Mechanical hyperventilation effectively blows off CO_2 and contributes to increases in pH.

The seriously ill infant with cardiac disease should be provided maintenance fluids, glucose, and electrolytes intravenously until his condition is stabilized and definitive operative palliation or correction is accomplished. Oral feedings increase the work of digestion, require greater oxygen consumption, and increase the risk of aspiration.

PROSTAGLANDIN E.   Prostaglandin E_1 has revolutionized the care of the neonate who is extremely hypoxemic because of a ductus-dependent congenital cardiac condition. The pharmacologic agent, currently undergoing clinical trials in selected centers around the country, is a potent dilator of the ductus arteriosus.

Elliott[31] was the first to demonstrate this effect in vitro in fetal calves, and its effect was confirmed upon human ductus tissue by Starling and Elliott in 1974.[32] Elliott and co-workers[33] reported the first successful infusion of PGE_1 into two infants with cyanotic congenital cardiac disease who depended upon patency of the ductus arteriosus to maintain arterial oxygen saturation. These results have been repeatedly confirmed by other investigators, and there is little doubt as to the efficacy of PGE_1 in this situation.[34-37]

Muscle tone of the fetal ductus arteriosus appears to be controlled by the endogenous production of prostaglandin compounds.[38] These 20-carbon hydroxy fatty acids are present in many tissues, including brain, lung, kidney, liver, intestine, uterus, heart, placenta, and ductus arteriosus. Though in vitro studies suggest that PGE_1 has a limited relaxant effect upon the ductus after exposure to oxygen, clinical responsiveness has been noted in nonhypoxemic infants with left-sided obstructive lesions.[39]

PGE_1 appears to be most beneficial when administered to infants less than 2 weeks of age. It should be given in a dose of 0.1 μg/kg/min. Frequently within minutes, it doubles the arterial Po_2 values of neonates. Relief of profound hypoxemia results in improved acid-base balance, more effective cardiopulmonary function, and greatly enhanced potential for surviving operative intervention. Once complete anatomic closure of the ductus arteriosus has occurred, the effectiveness of prostaglandin is limited.

Side effects of PGE_1 infusion include pyrexia, focal seizures, and tremors,[40] minor electroencephalographic changes,[41] apnea, and mild hypotension, the latter presumably due to peripheral vasodilatation.

SURGICAL PALLIATION.   Total correction of complex cyanotic congenital cardiac lesions often is not feasible during early infancy, and one must resort to palliative procedures to insure survival until correction can be safely performed. Palliative procedures generally are designed to either improve pulmonary blood flow in ductus-dependent lesions (pulmonary or tricuspid atresia) or improve mixing of pulmonary and systemic venous return in admixture lesions (transposition of the great vessels).

Pulmonary blood flow can be augmented by any one of several systemic artery-pulmonary artery anastomoses (Fig. 14-2). Most commonly in young infants, a Waterston-Cooley anastomosis of the ascending aorta to the pulmonary artery (usually right) is employed, whereas a Blalock-Taussig anastomosis of the subclavian artery to the pulmonary artery is performed in older

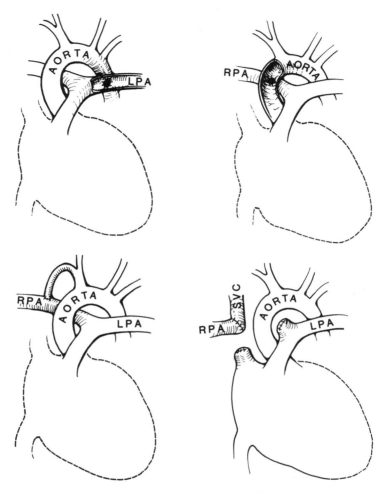

FIG. 14-2.   Diagram of various types of palliative procedures for neonates and infants with reduced volume of pulmonary blood flow. **Upper left.** Potts anastomosis: descending aorta to left pulmonary artery (LPA). **Upper right.** Waterston-Cooley anastomosis: ascending aorta to right pulmonary artery (RPA). **Lower left.** Blalock-Taussig anastomosis: subclavian artery to ipsilateral pulmonary artery. **Lower right.** Glenn procedure: anastomosis of superior vena cava (SVC) to right pulmonary artery (RPA).

infants and children. Additional shunts less often performed today include the Potts anastomosis (descending aorta to left pulmonary artery) and Glenn procedure (superior vena cava to right pulmonary artery). Finally, some institutions are using Gortex tube grafts sewn between a systemic and a pulmonary artery to effect the same purpose.

The most practical way to improve intracardiac mixing of blood is to create an atrial septal defect or enlarge the fossa ovalis sufficiently to allow nonrestrictive flow between the two atria. The Rashkind procedure (balloon atrial septostomy), described in the section dealing with transposition of the great vessels, is often a successful means of enlarging the fossa ovalis in newborns. Alternatively, surgical creation of an atrial septal defect can be accomplished without cardiopulmonary bypass by excision of the posterior portion of the atrial septum (Blalock-Hanlon procedure). This should not be confused with a shunt procedure, since its purpose and method are entirely different from a systemic artery-pulmonary artery anastomosis.

PERSISTENCE OF THE FETAL CIRCULATION

Adequate oxygenation of the tissues is an essential role of the circulation. In the neonate, this function may be impaired in spite of a morphologically normal heart by circulatory disturbances, which either mimic or physiologically resemble congenital cardiac defects. Specific therapy depends upon both proper identification of the homeostatic derangement and an understanding of the underlying pathophysiology.

PATHOPHYSIOLOGY. There is an increasing capacity for pulmonary vasoconstriction with advancing gestational age.[42] After birth, the vascular bed of the lung normally becomes less muscular and less reactive with increasing postpartum age.[43] The capacity to develop acute pulmonary hypertension secondary to pulmonary vasoconstriction is, therefore, a function of both gestational and postpartum age. Whereas normal adults with acute pulmonary vasoconstriction develop only moderately elevated pulmonary arterial pressures,[44] term infants are acutely capable of achieving suprasystemic resistance.[45] The potential for reestablishment of a fetal pattern of circulation, that is, right-to-left shunting across the ductus arteriosus and foramen ovale, should be readily apparent. With ductus closure, pulmonary vasoconstriction may potentially cause right heart decompensation or a low cardiac output state.

Factors that can initiate or sustain pulmonary vasoconstriction[46] include inadequate pulmonary expansion,[47,48] parenchymal pulmonary disease,[45] hypoxia,[49,50] acidosis,[49] hypercarbia,[51] shock,[52] left heart failure or obstruction,[53] and hyperviscosity secondary to polycythemia.[54-57]

Adequate pulmonary inflation is critical to the establishment of adequate pulmonary blood flow at birth. Inflation with air facilitates the fall in pulmonary vascular resistance, independent of changes in arterial oxygen tension.[58]

Various respiratory diseases which impair ventilation induce pulmonary arterial constriction in the neonate. High pulmonary vascular resistance has been a particular problem in the management of infants with diaphragmatic hernia[59,60] and aspiration syndromes.[56] These conditions are frequently associated with significant right-to-left shunting. The use of oxygen to treat hypoxia in these conditions may be disadvantageous. The higher the inspired oxygen tension, the lower the alveolar nitrogen tension. When a lung segment is plugged by secretions or by aspirated materials, oxygen distal to the obstruction is absorbed. If the nitrogen content of these alveoli is insufficient to maintain a residual volume greater than the critical collapsing column of the alveoli, collapse occurs. The bellows action necessary for removal of the obstruction is then lost, and reexpansion is impaired. The use of oxygen to treat hypoxia unresponsive to an enriched oxygen atmosphere, therefore, carries with it the risk of progressive atelectasis, pulmonary vasoconstriction, and progressively increasing right-to-left shunting.

Acidosis from any cause can raise pulmonary vascular resistance[49] and promote right-to-left shunting of the blood.

In asphyxia, the combination of severe hypoxemia and acidosis may cause profound pulmonary vasoconstriction. Whereas at normal pH, hypoxemia may have little effect on pulmonary vascular resistance,[49] in the presence of acidosis, hypoxemia is a potent pulmonary vasoconstrictor.

Some newborns have an extremely elevated hemoglobin level and consequent hyperviscosity. These neonates show cardiorespiratory symptoms, including tachypnea and right-to-left shunting.[61-63] Hyperviscosity raises both pulmonary and systemic vascular resistance[54-57] and has complex effects on the circulation.

Neonatal right-to-left shunting may occur within the lung, across the ductus arteriosus, across the foramen ovale, or at each site. An intrapulmonary right-to-left shunting occurs when pulmonary blood flow bypasses alveoli and arrives desaturated in the pulmonary veins. Bypass of alveoli results from atelectasis, consolidation, or perfusion of underventilated lung. Airway obstruction secondary to aspiration may prevent ventilation of areas of the lung, which are nonetheless perfused, and lead to cyanosis.[64]

Flow of blood across the widely patent ductus arteriosus is determined by the relationship between the pulmonary and systemic vascular resistances. Elevated pulmonary vascular resistance plays a major role in the genesis or right-to-left shunting. Reduced systemic vascular resistance can have a similar effect.

Elevation of right ventricular end-diastolic pressure, as occurs in right heart failure, or reduction of left atrial pressure, such as may occur when pulmonary venous return is diminished by ductal right-to-left shunting, causes persistently higher right atrial than left atrial pressures. The foramen ovale will then permit right-to-left shunting at the atrial level.

These three forms of right-to-left shunt, intrapulmonary, ductal, and atrial, have similar effects. In the presence of such shunts, aortic blood is desaturated. In the case of isolated right-to-left shunting at the ductal level, differential cyanosis may be expected, but such an isolated shunt is not the general rule in the newborn. Left ventricular blood which perfuses the ascending aorta is often also desaturated because of associated atrial or pulmonary level shunting.

Whatever the etiology of right-to-left shunting, the greater the magnitude of right-to-left shunt or the lower the pulmonary blood flow, the lower the value of systemic arterial Po_2.

Furthermore, tissue oxygen extraction (which markedly affects mixed venous oxygen saturation) has a pronounced effect on arterial oxygen saturation in the presence of right-to-left shunting. Factors which cause a major increase in oxygen consumption and further lower arterial Po_2 include cold stress, respiratory distress, the work of feeding, and agitation.

A right-to-left shunt is a significant disturbance of neonatal homeostasis because the reduction in pulmonary blood flow which accompanies a right-to-left shunt potentiates pulmonary vasoconstriction.

CLINICAL FEATURES. Persistence of the fetal circulation (PFC) is a disturbance of the normal transition from a fetal to an adult circulatory pattern, characterized predominantly by evidence of right-to-left shunting. While it has been associated with various conditions which promote right-to-left shunting in the neonate,[65] it may occur without etiologic explanation. In the latter patients, there is often a history of perinatal hypoxia suggestive of antepartum depression.[66] Most descriptions of PFC exclude patients with coexistent pulmonary or structural cardiac disease, although similar hemodynamic mechanisms may underlie the right-to-left shunting seen in such instances. PFC occurs often in term or postmature infants, with a tendency toward greater severity in more mature infants.

Symptoms of cyanosis, tachypnea, tachycardia, and often mild respiratory distress begin generally in the first day or two of life. Cardiac examination is generally unremarkable, although the pulmonary component of the second sound may be prominent. Breath sounds are normal. Slight hepatomegaly may be present.

The electrocardiogram is normal, and a thoracic roentgenogram does not show parenchymal disease. Vascular markings may be diminished, and mild cardiomegaly may be present. Because the heart is structurally normal, echocardiography is only of value in excluding anatomic cardiac disease. Right ventricular systolic time intervals may be abnormal, with an increased preejection period to systolic ejection period ratio. However, this is not diagnostic, for normal infants may have similar right and left ventricular systolic time intervals during the first 2 days of life.[67]

Confirmation of right-to-left shunting of blood can be made by simultaneously measuring Po_2 from the right radial artery and descending aorta (via an umbilical arterial catheter). A right radial artery Po_2 10 torr or more than the value obtained from the umbilical catheter is significant and indicates a reversing ductus arteriosus. Acidosis is usually present. Cardiac catheterization is rarely necessary to exclude the presence of structural cyanotic cardiac disease.

TREATMENT. The treatment of infants with PFC should focus on the management of identifiable causes of elevated pulmonary resistance. Correction of acidosis, hyperviscosity, metabolic disorders, myocardial dysfunction, shock, atelectasis, or hypoventilation is essential to altering the circulatory disorder.

Attention has recently been focused on various pharmacologic pulmonary vasodilators, most importantly tolazoline,[68] on persistent fetal circulation. Tolazoline is a potent pulmonary and systemic vasodilator.[69] It, therefore, should be used with caution after other supportive measures, such as correction of acidosis with sodium bicarbonate and hyperventilation, have failed. Intraarterial blood pressure should be followed closely before and during administration of the drug so that volume expansion and/or ionotropic drugs can be given if systemic hypotension develops. Tolazoline is generally administered by scalp vein or central venous pressure catheter, though some of the drug will still be delivered to the systemic circulation because of atrial and ductal right-to-left shunting.

Tolazoline is very effective in some neonates but has little benefit in others. When the desired rise in Po_2 does not occur within several hours, continued use of the drug is unwarranted and may be considered contraindicated. The focus of therapy in neonates with PFC should remain directed at possible underlying causes.

BACTERIAL INFECTION AND CARDIAC DISEASE DURING INFANCY

Not infrequently, the pediatric cardiologist or consulting pediatrician is asked to substantiate the presence or absence of structural cardiac disease in an infant who is subsequently found to be septic. Neonatal sepsis with the group B streptococcus warrants special comment because there has been a striking increase in the incidence of this infection in recent years[70,71] and because it may clinically suggest the presence of either left ventricular outflow obstruction or severe cyanotic congenital cardiac disease.

GROUP B STREPTOCOCCAL DISEASE. Two forms of infantile group B streptococcal sepsis have been described.[72] Early onset infection has been attributed to colonization in the immediate perinatal period[73] and is generally manifest in the first day of life. It is a fulminant infection that characteristically appears as pneumonia and overwhelming septicemia. Shock is a prominent manifestation,[74] and apnea is common.[75] Thoracic roentgenograms are often indistinguishable from those of respiratory distress syndrome.[76-78] There may be cardiomegaly and increased pulmonary vascular markings. Meningitis may occur but is not a regular feature of disease in neonates. Late onset infection may occur up to 2 months after birth and is unassociated with maternal colonization. Meningitis is a regular feature of late onset infection.[71] Other soft tissue involvement may include arthritis, cerebritis, cellulitis, conjunctivitis, ethmoiditis, impetigo, pneumonia, osteomyelitis, and otitis media. Late onset disease is seldom confused with cardiac disease.

Two aspects of early onset group B streptococcal sepsis make differentiation from cardiac disease challenging. First, there is a very marked tendency to develop profound shock in this disease. Shock from any cause may injure the myocardium and produce secondary myocardial depression. Differentiation of primary from secondary cardiac decompensation can be difficult. Secondly, group B sepsis is often associated with right-to-left shunting.[74] This may merely reflect the severity of lung disease or its impact on pulmonary vascular resistance. Nonetheless, it produces cyanosis that may be minimally responsive to oxygen therapy. Ventilatory support and positive end-expiratory pressure ventilation may dramatically reduce the degree of right-to-left shunting and improve arterial oxygen tension.

COEXISTENT PNEUMONIA AND CONGESTIVE CARDIAC FAILURE.   In general, the infant with heart disease is no more or less likely than any other child to acquire a severe infection or septicemia. With few exceptions (asplenia syndrome, DiGeorge syndrome), the infant's immune system is intact and fully capable of responding to invading organisms. Nevertheless, we still occasionally see a child who is placed on continuous antibiotic therapy "because of the heart problem," but this practice is neither necessary nor desirable.

There are several exceptions that should be considered. These are the infant with congestive cardiac failure in whom pneumonia cannot be excluded by clinical laboratory evaluations, the infant or child with asplenia syndrome, and the infant who has DiGeorge syndrome.

The first of these, the infant with congestive cardiac failure and possible pneumonia, is perhaps the most nebulous and least clear-cut situation, and the physician may be inclined to treat with antibiotics more readily than usual. Substantiating data are scarce, but it appears that infants who have chronic pulmonary edema secondary to cardiac disease experience lower respiratory tract infection more commonly than do healthy children. Whether this is because of the presence of interstitial and alveolar fluid which enhance bacterial growth or because altered pulmonary dynamics somehow predispose the infant to become infected is uncertain. Diagnosis is more difficult due to the similarity of presenting signs and symptoms. The critically ill infant who may have pneumonia as a complicating feature of congestive cardiac failure should be treated with antibiotics, in addition to anticongestive drugs, until infection can be excluded.

ASPLENIA SYNDROME, DIGEORGE SYNDROME.   Asplenia syndrome is associated with complex cyanotic congenital cardiac disease, malrotation of the gut, and dysrhythmias. The majority of babies with this syndrome die during early infancy, primarily because of the severity of their cardiac defect. Those who survive, however, are at considerable risk of succumbing to overwhelming infection with a gram-negative or encapsulated organism by the time they reach 1 year of age. Waldman and co-workers[79] reviewed the course of 59 children with congenital asplenia and found 16 instances of documented sepsis (27 percent). Thus, daily prophylaxis with an antibiotic effective against both gram-negative and gram-positive organisms is advised prior to 6 months of age. Thereafter, gram-positive coverage alone should be provided. Immunization with pneumococcal vaccine would seem a reasonable precaution, but this has not been documented in infants with asplenia syndrome.

The coexistence of thymic aplasia or hypoplasia, absent parathyroid glands, aortic arch anomalies, and distinctive facial features makes up the DiGeorge anomalad.[80] These infants are more susceptible to severe infections because of deficient cellular immunity.

SHOCK

The basic principles of treatment of an infant in shock are no different from those followed in any other patient. The term "shock" implies inadequate perfusion of body tissue sufficient to maintain normal metabolic function.[81,82] It may result from hypovolemia, myocardial failure, or causes which directly or indirectly affect cellular integrity, such as bacterial toxins, hypoxemia, or hypoglycemia.

Infants with congenital cardiac disease may develop shock as a terminal event secondary to profound hypoxemia and acidosis, as a consequence of severe left-sided obstructive lesions, or following cardiac surgery. The underlying cause of shock must be sought and therapy directed appropriately. Several general supportive measures are discussed, since they can be applied regardless of the cause of the shocklike state.

PHYSIOLOGIC MONITORING. Supportive therapy is based upon knowledge of important physiologic variables,[83] such as cardiac rate, arterial blood pressure, central venous pressure, urine output, and capillary filling. Management of postoperative shock, in particular, is facilitated by measurement of cardiac index and left atrial pressure.

The umbilical vessels of neonates are routinely used for catheter insertion, allowing ready access to the umbilical artery for blood gas sampling, fluid administration, and measurement of central arterial blood pressure. Frequently, a catheter can be advanced from the umbilical vein through the ductus venosus into the right or left atrium. This is a safer position for an umbilical venous line than below the diaphragm (within the portal venous system).

In older infants, it is usually possible to insert percutaneously a 22 gauge Teflon-coated polyvinyl catheter into the radial artery and external jugular vein for continuous pressure measurements. The jugular vein is also a site for fluid administration. Indwelling catheters in the brachial artery should be avoided because of the danger of ischemic necrosis of the arm. A thermodilution catheter should be inserted into the pulmonary artery of infants undergoing major cardiac surgery so that cardiac output can be monitored by saline injection. Left ventricular end-diastolic pressure can be assessed by measurement of pulmonary artery wedge pressure with a balloon catheter or of left atrial pressure by a catheter.

Shock is almost always accompanied by intense peripheral vasoconstriction and inadequate peripheral perfusion. Peripheral perfusion cannot be assessed objectively, so we must depend on clinical judgment of the adequacy of capillary filling and warmth of the extremities. Further experience with the transcutaneous Po_2 monitor may prove a useful means of quantitating peripheral perfusion, since the relationship between capillary Po_2 and intraarterial Po_2 is largely dependent upon peripheral perfusion.

FLUID AND ELECTROLYTE ADMINISTRATION. The rate of fluid administration in the treatment of shock is determined by the cause of peripheral vascular collapse, the rapidity with which it developed, changes in weight over an 8- to 12-hour period, urine output, arterial and central venous pressures, and left atrial pressure if available. Acute blood loss, though uncommon in a hospitalized infant, must be treated by rapid infusion of whole blood or colloid. Other causes of shock, such as myocardial failure following cardiac surgery, require sufficient fluids to raise the central venous pressure to 5 to 10 cm of water pressure and left atrial pressure to a maximum of 15 cm of water. Further fluid administration beyond measured and insensible losses may precipitate pulmonary edema.

Maintenance fluids should consist of 5 percent dextrose in a balanced electrolyte solution containing 30 to 40 meq of NaCl and approximately 20 meq/l KCl, assuming urine output is normal ($\simeq$ 1 ml/kg/hour). Postoperative patients may not require sodium-containing solutions for a day or two after surgery because of sodium retention secondary to hyperaldosteronism. Serum potassium must be followed closely and must be judiciously replaced in patients who have been on cardiopulmonary bypass. These patients, including infants, experience an incompletely understood potassium wasting which may result in severe hypokalemia. This effect is not present in infants with shock and low or absent urine output. In the postoperative patient, chest tube drainage is replaced volume for volume with plasminate or salt-poor albumin.

Anuria associated with shock is an extremely difficult management problem. Administration of 5 percent dextrose sufficient to replace insensible losses (approximately 500 ml/m^2/day) plus measured gastrointestinal and chest tube drainage should satisfy fluid requirements. Sodium bicarbonate may be indicated to counteract metabolic acidosis secondary to inadequate peripheral perfusion. The end result often is hypernatremia, hyperkalemia, and sometimes hypervolemia. These may be treated by peritoneal or hemodialysis or by Kayexalate and sorbitol via a nasogastric tube and by enema, providing intestinal function and motility are satisfactory.

IONOTROPIC AGENTS. Appropriate fluid therapy maximizes the ability of the heart to augment systemic output by achieving optimal stroke volume. Unless there is acquired or congenital heart block, manipulation of heart rate is not necessary. Further increase in cardiac output can frequently be attained by improving cardiac contractility. Digitalis and certain catecholamines, such as isoproterenol, dopamine, and dobutamine, are routinely used for this purpose.[84]

Isoproterenol infused at a rate of 0.25 µg/kg/min increases cardiac output and causes mild peripheral vasodilatation.[85] Its disadvantages include tachycardia, ventricular arrhythmias, and markedly increased myocardial oxygen consumption, shifting myocardial metabolism to anaerobic.[86]

Dopamine and dobutamine are more desirable beta-adrenergic stimulants, in that their ionotropic effect on the heart is comparable to isoproterenol without a marked chronotropic effect and increased myocardial oxygen consumption.[87] Dopamine produces significant redistribution of systemic blood flow, especially enhanced renal blood flow, when used in a dosage of 10 µg/kg/min or greater. Dobutamine, synthesized by modifying the sidechain of dopamine, effectively increases left ventricular performance in a dose of 5 to 10 µg/kg/min without significant alteration of peripheral vascular resistance.[88]

PERIPHERAL VASODILATORS. The concept of decreasing the impedence of left ventricular ejection by afterload reduction has been increasingly employed in acute and chronic low cardiac output states,[89] especially following cardiac surgery. Low cardiac output is invariably accompanied by intense peripheral vasoconstriction due to excessive circulating endogenous catecholamines. Central blood pressure may be normal or even slightly elevated and urine output may be satisfactory, yet the patient has cool extremities and poor capillary filling. Metabolic acidosis ensues, thereby further decreasing cardiac contractility and output. Left ventricular filling pressure is elevated, interfering with myocardial perfusion during diastole. Reversal of peripheral vasoconstriction substantially improves myocardial performance. Intravenous nitroprusside or phentolamine are the most potent peripheral vasodilator drugs available for this purpose. In order to avoid a precipitous fall in blood pressure, a relatively high preload and normal or slightly increased vascular volume are required. The pulmonary wedge or left atrial pressures must be monitored during use of these drugs. Glucocorticoids and phenothiazines have been suggested because of their mild vasodilating properties, but we have not been impressed with their clinical efficacy.

With physiologic monitoring as a guide to therapy, appropriate administration of fluids, ionotropic drugs, and afterload reduction can reverse shock in many infants with cardiac disease. As always, early recognition is a prerequisite to expedient successful therapy.

REFERENCES

Congestive Cardiac Failure

1. Goldring D, Hernandez A, Hartmann AF Jr: The critically ill child: Care of the infant in cardiac failure. Pediatrics 47:1056, 1971
2. Linzbach AJ: Heart failure from the point of view of quantitative anatomy. Am J Cardiol 5:370, 1960
3. Braunwald E, Ross J Jr, Sonnenblick EH: Mechanisms of Coarctation of the

Normal and Failing Heart. Boston, Little, Brown, 1968, p 77

4. Mason DT, Spann JF Jr, Zelis R, Amsterdam EA: Alterations of hemodynamics and myocardial mechanics in patients with congestive heart failure: Pathophysiologic mechanisms and assessment of cardiac function and ventricular contractility. Prog Cardiovasc Dis 12:507, 1970
5. Spann JF Jr, Mason DT, Zelis RF: Recent advances in the understanding of congestive heart failure. I. Mod Concepts Cardiovasc Dis 39:73, 1970
6. Spann JF Jr, Mason DT, Zelis RF: Recent advances in the understanding of congestive heart failure. II. Mod Concepts Cardiovasc Dis 39:79, 1970
7. Gertz EW, Hess ML, Lain RF, Briggs FN: Activity of the vesicular calcium pump in the spontaneously failing heart-lung preparation. Circ Res 20:477, 1967
8. Muir JR, Dhalla NS, Orteza JM, Olson RE: Energy-linked calcium transport in subcellular fractions of the failing rat heart. Circ Res 26:429, 1970
9. Entman ML, Bornet EP, Schwartz A: Phasic components of calcium binding and release by canine cardiac relaxing system (sarcoplasmic reticulum fragments). J Mol Cell Cardiol 4:155, 1972
10. Miller GAH, Swan HJC: Effect of chronic pressure and volume overload on left heart volumes in subjects with congenital heart disease. Circulation 30:205, 1964
11. Spann JF Jr, Buccino RA, Sonnenblick EH, Braunwald E: Contractile state of cardiac muscle obtained from cats with experimentally produced ventricular hypertrophy and heart failure. Circ Res 21:341, 1967
12. Chidsey CA, Braunwald E, Morrow AG: Catecholamine excretion and cardiac stores of norepinephrine in congestive heart failure. Am J Med 39:442, 1965
13. Zelis R, Mason DT: Compensatory mechanisms in congestive heart failure—the role of the peripheral resistance vessels. N Engl J Med 282:962, 1970
14. Davis JO, Hartroft PM, Titus EO, et al.: The role of the renin-angiotensin system in the control of aldosterone secretion. J Clin Invest 41:378, 1962
15. Miller WW, Oski FA, Delivoria-Papadopoulas M: Increased oxygen release in hypoxemia and heart failure. Pediatr Res 4:444, 1970 (Abstr)
16. Morgan CL, Nadas AS: Sweating and congestive heart failure. N Engl J Med 268:580, 1963
17. Kreidberg MB, Chernoff HL, Lopez WL: Treatment of cardiac failure in infancy and childhood. N Engl J Med 268:23, 1963
18. Lees MH: Heart failure in the newborn infant. Recognition and management. J Pediatr 75:139, 1969
19. Neill CA: The use of digitalis in infants and children. Prog Cardiovasc Dis 7:399, 1965
20. Nayler WG: Calcium exchange in cardiac muscle: A basic mechanism of drug action. Am Heart J 73:379, 1967
21. Langer GA: Effects of digitalis on myocardial ionic exchange. Circulation 46:180, 1972
22. Ferrer MI, Conroy RJ, Harvery RM: Some effects of digoxin upon the heart and circulation in man. Digoxin in combined (left and right) ventricular failure. Circulation 21:372, 1960
23. Mason DT, Spann JF Jr, Zelis R: New developments in the understanding of the actions of the digitalis glycosides. Prog Cardiovasc Dis 11:443, 1969
24. Hernandez A, Burton RM, Pagtakhan RD, Goldring D: Pharmacodynamics of ^{3}H-digoxin in infants. Pediatrics 44:418, 1969
25. Nadas AS, Rudolph AM, Reinhold JDL: The use of digitalis in infants and children. A clinical study of patients in congestive heart failure. N Engl J Med 248:98, 1953
26. Hauck AJ, Ongley PA, Nadas AS: The use of digoxin in infants and children. Am Heart J 56:443, 1958
27. Baylen BG, Johnson G, Tsang RC, Srivastava L, Kaplan S: Hyperaldosteronism

and aldosterone antagonists in congestive heart failure (CHF) and cor pulmonale (CP) in infancy. Pediatr Res 10:310, 1976 (Abstr)

28. Bolen JL, Alderman EL: Hemodynamic consequences of afterload reduction in patients with chronic aortic regurgitation. Circulation 53:879, 1976
29. Chatterjee K, Parmley WW: The role of vasodilator therapy in heart failure. Prog Cardiovasc Dis 19:301, 1977
30. Kaplan S, Gaum WE, Benzing G III, Meyer RA, Schwartz DC: Therapeutic advances in pediatric cardiology. Pediatr Clin North Am 25:891, 1978

Hypoxemia

31. Elliott RB, Starling MB: The effect of prostaglandin $F_{2\alpha}$ in the closure of the ductus arteriosus. Prostaglandins 2:399, 1972
32. Starling MB, Elliott RB: The effects of prostaglandins, prostaglandin inhibitors in oxygen on the closure of the ductus arteriosus, pulmonary arteries and umbilical vessels in vitro. Prostaglandins 8:187, 1974
33. Elliott RB, Starling MB, Neutze JM: Medical manipulation of the ductus arteriosus. Lancet 1:140, 1975
34. Olley PM, Coceani F, Bodach E: E-type prostaglandins. A new emergency therapy for certain cyanotic congenital heart malformations. Circulation 53:728, 1976
35. Neutze JM, Starling MB, Elliott RB, Barratt-Boyes BG: Palliation of cyanotic congenital heart disease in infancy with E-type prostaglandins. Circulation 55:238, 1977
36. Lewis AB, Takahashi M, Lurie PR: Administration of prostaglandin E_1 in neonates with critical congenital cardiac defects. J Pediatr 93:481, 1978
37. Heymann MR, Rudolph AM: Ductus arteriosus dilatation by prostaglandin E_1 in infants with pulmonary atresia. Pediatrics 59:325, 1977
38. Coceani F, Olley PM: The response of the ductus arteriosus to prostaglandins. Can J Physiol Pharmacol 51:220, 1973
39. Lang P, Freed MD, Rosenthal A, Castaneda AR, Nadas AS: The use of prostaglandin E_1 in an infant with interruption of the aortic arch. J Pediatr 91:805, 1977
40. Coceani F: Prostaglandins and the central nervous system. Arch Intern Med 133:119, 1974
41. Fariello R, Olley PM, Coceani F: Neurological and electroencephalographic changes in newborns treated with prostaglandin E_1 and E_2. Prostaglandin 13:901, 1977

Persistence of the Fetal Circulation

42. Rudolph AM, Heymann MA: Pulmonary circulation in fetal lambs. Pediatr Res 6:341, 1972 (Abstr)
43. Rosen L, Bowden DH, Uchida I: Structural changes in pulmonary arteries in the first year of life. Arch Pathol 63:316, 1957
44. Doyle JT, Wilson JS, Warren JV: The pulmonary vascular responses to short-term hypoxia in human subjects. Circulation 5:263, 1952
45. Fox WW, Gewitz MH, Dinwiddie R, Drummond WH, Peckham GJ: Pulmonary hypertension in the perinatal aspiration syndromes. Pediatrics 59:205, 1977
46. Assali NS, Brinkman CR III: Control of systemic and pulmonary vasomotor tone before and after birth. Adv Exp Med Biol 22:13, 1972
47. Cussin S, Dawes GS, Mott JC, Ross BB, Strang LB: The vascular resistance of the foetal and newly ventilated lung of the lamb. J Physiol 171:61, 1964
48. Colebatch HJH, Dawes GS, Goodwin JW, Nadeau RA: The nervous control of the circulation in the foetal and newly expanded lungs of the lamb. J Physiol 178:544, 1965

49. Rudolph AM, Yuan S: Response of the pulmonary vasculature to hypoxia and H^+ ion concentration changes. J Clin Invest 45:399, 1966

50. Dawes GS, Mott JC, Widdicombe JG, Wyatt DG: Changes in the lungs of the new-born lamb. J Physiol 121:141, 1953

51. Malik AB, Kidd BSL: Independent effects of changes in H^+ and CO_2 concentrations on hypoxic pulmonary vasoconstriction. J Appl Physiol 34:318, 1973

52. Sugg WL, Craver WD, Webb WR, Ecker RR: Pressure changes in the dog lung secondary to hemorrhagic shock: Protective effect of pulmonary reimplantation. Am Surg 169:592, 1969

53. Ferencz C, Dammann JF Jr: Significance of the pulmonary vascular bed in congenital heart disease. V. Lesions of the left side of the heart causing obstruction of the pulmonary venous return. Circulation 16:1045, 1957

54. Tyson KRT, Sciarrotta N, Fender HR, McNeel LA: Effect of blood viscosity on pulmonary vascular resistance. J Pediatr Surg 6:559, 1971

55. Fouron JC, Hébert F: The circulatory effects of hematocrit variations in normovolemic newborn lambs. J Pediatr 82:995, 1973

56. Tyson KRT, Ferder HR: Direct influence of blood viscosity on pulmonary vascular resistance. J Pediatr Surg 10:779, 1975

57. Mair DD: Effect of markedly elevated hematocrit level on blood viscosity and assessment of pulmonary vascular resistance. J Thorac Cardiovasc Surg 77:682, 1979

58. Lauer RM, Evans JA, Aoki H, Kittle CF: Factors controlling pulmonary vascular resistance in fetal lambs. J Pediatr 67:568, 1965

59. Naeye RL, Shochat SJ, Whitman V, Maisels MJ: Unsuspected pulmonary vascular abnormalities associated with diaphragmatic hernia. Pediatrics 58:902, 1976

60. Levin DL: Morphologic analysis of the pulmonary vascular bed in congenital left-sided diaphragmatic hernia. J Pediatr 92:805, 1978

61. Gatti RA, Muster AJ, Cole RB, Paul MH: Neonatal polycythemia with transient cyanosis and cardiorespiratory abnormalities. J Pediatr 69:1063, 1966

62. Gross GP, Hathaway WE, McGaughey HR: Hyperviscosity in the neonate. J Pediatr 82:1004, 1973

63. Kontras SB: Polycythemia and hyperviscosity syndromes in infants and children. Pediatr Clin North Am 19:919, 1972

64. Avery ME: Lung development. In Avery ME, Fletcher BD (eds): The Lung and Its Disorders in the Newborn Infant, 3rd ed. Philadelphia, Saunders, 1974, pp 3–21

65. Gersony WM: Persistence of the fetal circulation: A commentary. J Pediatr 82:1103, 1973

66. Gersony WM, Morishima HO, Daniels S, et al.: The hemodynamic effects of intrauterine hypoxia: An experimental model in newborn lambs. J Pediatr 89:631, 1976

67. Riggs T, Hirschfeld S, Bormuth C, Fanaroff A, Liebman J: Neonatal circulatory changes: An echocardiographic study. Pediatrics 59:338, 1977

68. Goetzman BW, Sunshine P, Johnson JD, et al.: Neonatal hypoxia and pulmonary vasospasm: Response to tolazoline. J Pediatr 89:617, 1976

69. Grover RF, Reeves JT, Blount S Jr: Tolazoline hydrochloride (Priscoline). An effective pulmonary vasodilator. Am Heart J 61:5, 1961

Bacterial Infection and Cardiac Disease

70. McCracken GH Jr: Group B streptococci: The new challenge in neonatal infections. J Pediatr 82:703, 1973

71. Howard JB, McCracken GH Jr: The spectrum of group B streptococcal infections in infancy. Am J Dis Child 128:815, 1974

72. Gotoff SP: Emergence of group B streptococci as major perinatal pathogens. Hosp Pract 12:85, 1977
73. Baker CJ: Early onset group B streptococcal disease. J Pediatr 93:124, 1978
74. Ablow RC, Driscoll SG, Effmann EL, et al.: A comparison of early-onset group B streptococcal neonatal infection and the respiratory-distress syndrome of the newborn. N Engl J Med 294:65, 1976
75. Quirante J, Ceballos R, Cassady G: Group B β-hemolytic streptococcal infection in the newborn. Am J Dis Child 128:659, 1974
76. Leonidas JC, Hall RT, Beatty EC, Fellows RA: Radiographic findings in early onset neonatal group B streptococcal septicemia. Pediatrics 59[Suppl]:1006, 1977
77. Ablow RC, Gross I, Effmann EL, Uauy R, Driscoll S: The radiographic features of early onset group B streptococcal neonatal sepsis. Radiology 124:771, 1977
78. Weller MH, Katzenstein AA: Radiological findings in group B streptococcal sepsis. Radiology 118:385, 1976
79. Waldman JD, Rosenthal A, Smith AL, Shurin S, Nadas AS: Sepsis and congenital asplenia. J Pediatr 90:555, 1977
80. Kretschmer R, Say B, Brown D, Rosen FS: Congenital aplasia of the thymus gland (DiGeorge's syndrome). N Engl J Med 279:1295, 1968

Shock

81. MacLean LD: Shock and metabolism. Surg Gynecol Obstet 126:299, 1968
82. Thal AP, Wilson RF, Kalfuss L, Andre J: The role of metabolic and humoral doctors in irreversible shock. In Mills LC, Moyer JH (eds): Shock and Hypotension. New York, Grune & Stratton, 1965
83. Rapaport E, Scheinman M: Rationale and limitations of hemodynamic measurements in patients with acute myocardial infarction. Mod Concepts Cardiovasc Dis 38:55, 1969
84. Harrison DC, Kerber RE, Alderman EL: Pharmacodynamics and clinical use of cardiovascular drugs after cardiac surgery. Am J Cardiol 26:385, 1970
85. Rosenblum R, Berkowitz WD, Lawson D: Effect of acute intravenous administration of isoproterenol on cardiorenal hemodynamics in man. Circulation 38:158, 1968
86. Braunwald E, Covell JW, Maroko PR, Ross J Jr: The effect of drugs and of counterpulsation on myocardial oxygen consumption. Observations on the ischemic heart. Circulation 40[Suppl 4]:220, 1969
87. Goldberg LI: Cardiovascular and renal actions of dopamine: Potential clinical applications. Pharmacol Rev 24:1, 1972
88. Loeb HS, Bredakis J, Gunner R: Superiority of dobutamine over dopamine for augmentation of cardiac output in patients with chronic low output cardiac failure. Circulation 55:375, 1977
89. Miller RR, Vismara LA, Williams DO, Amsterdam EA, Mason DT: Pharmacological mechanisms for left ventricular unloading in clinical congestive heart failure. Differential effects of nitroprusside, phentolamine, and nitroglycerin on cardiac function and peripheral circulation. Circ Res 39:127, 1976

INDEX

Abdomen, examination of, 36
Acidosis
  in angiography, 154
  in aortic atresia, 448
  in catheterization, 155
  in corrective therapy, 469
  in persistence of fetal circulation, 472–474
  in pulmonary vascular disorders, 163–164,
    391, 393, 472
Acrocyanosis, in severe pulmonary stenosis,
  239
Acyanosis
  in congenital cardiac anomalies, 166–167
  increased pulmonary blood flow with,
    171–234
  normal pulmonary blood flow with, 235–318
Admixture lesion(s), 167, 319, 340
  aortic atresia as, 444
  cyanosis in, 349
  differential diagnosis of, 347
  oxygen saturation in, 319, 355
Afterload reduction, 466, 479
Age
  in blood pressure changes, 146–149
  in cardiac dysrhythmia, 57–58
  in complete transposition of the great ves-
    sels, 328
  in congestive cardiac failure diagnosis, 3,
    11, 15
  in electrocardiogram changes, 40–47
  in heart rate of neonates, 40–41
  in infant death due to congenital cardiac
    anomalies, 2–3
  in vectocardiogram changes, 54–57
Aminophylline, in apnea and bradycardia, 59

Anastamoses. *See also* Surgical shunts; *specific procedures*
  in pulmonary blood flow palliation, 470–471
Anemia
  at birth, 11
  iron deficiency, 121–122
  relative, in tetralogy of Fallot, 374
Angiocatheter, NIH, 140
Angiography, 149–151. *See also* Aortography;
  Catheterization
  acidosis during, 155
  in anomalous left coronary artery, 289–290
  in aortic arch interruption, 264
  in aortic atresia, 448
  in aortic stenosis, 452
  in arteriovenous fistulas, 223
  brachial artery approach in, 138
  catheters used in, 140
  in coarctation of the aorta, 257
  diagnostic role and techniques, 149–151
  in glycogen storage disease, 298
  in great vessel transposition, 196
  in Kawasaki disease, 293–294
  in mitral stenosis, 431
  in pericardial effusion, 307
  in pulmonary valvular dysplasia, 243
  in pulmonary vein atresia, 443
  in rhabdomyomas, 302–303
  in single ventricle, 346
  in Taussig-Bing malformation, 335–336
  in tetralogy of Fallot, 372–373; in variants
    of, 379–383
  in total anomalous pulmonary venous con-
    nection, 354, 356; with pulmonary venous
    obstruction, 440
  in tricuspid insufficiency, 415

Auscultation. *See also* Heart sounds; Murmurs
  in atrial septal defects, 215–216, 219
  in endocardial cushion defect, 206
  technique of, 33–36

Bacterial infection, in infant cardiac disease, 475–477
Balloon, with flow directed catheters, 140–141
Balloon atrial septostomy, 156, 472. *See also* Rashkind procedure
  in pulmonary atresia, 391
  in right ventricle hypoplasia, 408
  in tricuspid atresia, 400–401
Behrman angio catheter, 140
Blalock-Hanlon procedure
  in atrial septum excision, 472
  in pulmonary atresia, 391
  in right ventricle hypoplasia, 408
  in transposition of the great vessels, 333
Blalock-Taussig procedure, 470–471
  in tetralogy of Fallot, 374, 375
  in tricuspid atresia, 401
Blood chemistry determinations, 133
Blood flow/Circulation
  in anomalous left coronary artery, 287
  in aortic arch interrupted, 262
  in aortic isthmus narrowing, 258–259
  in atrial communications, 168–170
  in complete transposition of the great vessels, 327–328, 331
  in congenital cardiac anomaly classification, 166–170
  in endocardial fibroelastosis, 281–282
  in glycogen storage disease, 298
  neonatal and later changes in, 161–165
  in pericardial effusion, 304
  in peripheral pulmonary arterial stenosis, 247
  in pulmonary atresia, 385–386
  in pulmonary stenosis, 237–238
  via pulmonary veins, 168. *See also* Pulmonary blood flow
  in pulmonary venous obstruction, 438
  in single ventricle anomaly, 341–346
  in tricuspid atresia with diminished pulmonary flow, 395
  in truncus arteriosus, 321
Blood gas monitoring. *See also* Oximetry; Oxygen saturation
  calculations in, 129–130, 143–146, 467–469
  in cardiac catheterization, 132
  in defect diagnosis, 143–144
  via umbilical catheter, 137

Blood loss
  due to catheterization, 153
  monitoring by catheterization, 132
Blood pressure
  age changes in ventricular, 164–165
  calculation of vascular, 148–149
  infant examination for, 24–26
  infant values for, 25
  intravascular measurement of, 132
  left ventricular, 148
  in lesion diagnosis, 146–149
  measurement of, in catheterization, 132, 140, 143, 146–149
Brachial artery, in catheterization, 138–139
Bradycardia, sinus, 59
Bundle of HIS
  electrocardiography of, 54
  endocardial cushion defect displacement of, 206
  endocardial fibroelastosis in interruption of, 280
  inversion of, 195

Cardiac. *See* Heart
Cardiac anomalies/malformations
  age of onset of, 2–3, 11, 15, 17, 19
  case history in diagnosis of, 15–19
  congenital. *See* Congenital cardiac anomalies/malformations
  diagnostic considerations in, 15–19. *See also specific symptoms*
Cardiac apex, in physical examination, 26
Cardiac catheterization. *See* Catheterization
Cardiac chamber enlargement. *See* Cardiomegaly
Cardiac contour, diagnostic aspects of, 77, 84–86. *See also specific disorders*
Cardiac contractility
  iotronic agents in improvement of, 478–479
  measurement of, 117–118
  in myocardial function, 464
  neonatal changes in, 165
Cardiac failure. *See* Congestive cardiac failure
Cardiac murmurs. See Murmur(s), cardiac
Cardiac output. *See also* Blood flow/Circulation
  measurement of, 130, 145, 146
Cardiac sounds, 28–31. *See also* Heart sounds
Cardiac size
  diagnostic aspects of, 84–85
  evaluation of, 77–78

Pulmonary arteries
absent, 6
aortic origin of, 199–200
peripheral stenosis of, 249–250
in truncus arteriosus, 321
Pulmonary atresia
in catheterization, 5
of common pulmonary vein, 441–443
Ebstein's malformation with, 402
incidence of, 3–8
right ventricle isolated hypoplasia vs.,
407–409
tetralogy of Fallot with, 275, 377–379
treatment of, 390–391
tricuspid atresia vs., 388
ventricular septum intact with, 384–392
Pulmonary blood flow. *See also* Blood
flow/Circulation
at birth, initiation of, 161–162, 472–473
in congenital cardiac anomaly classification, 166–167
decreased, with cyanosis, 365
effective (QEP), calculation of, 331
in fetal circulation, 159–162
increased, with acyanosis, 171
increased, with cyanosis, 319–320
obstructed. *See* Pulmonary stenosis; Pulmonary venous obstruction
operative augmentation of, 470–471
vascular resistance vs., 167, 174, 175,
366–384
Pulmonary edema, 425
in cor triatriatum, 434
in mitral stenosis, 428, 434
in pulmonary individual vein stenosis, 436
roentgenography of, 434
Pulmonary hypertension
in aortic stenosis, 452
in endocardial cushion defect, 205
fetal development of, 472
in operative mortality for total anomalous
pulmonary venous connection, 357–358
in total anomalous pulmonary venous connection with venous obstruction, 440
ventricular, 147. *See also* Pulmonary arterial pressure
Pulmonary parenchymal disorder
cyanosis and, 16
pulmonary vasoconstriction and, 472
pulmonary venous obstruction and, 437
roentgenographic indications of, 82–83
Pulmonary valvular area (PVA), calculation
of, 237–238, 243
Pulmonary valvular dysplasia, 236, 243

Pulmonary valvular stenosis, 236–243
anatomy of valve formations in, 236–237
asymptomatic, 244
atrial septal defects in, 236–237
dome shaped valve in, 236
double outlet right ventricle with, 239
dyplastic, 236, 243
Ebstein's malformation and, 402
with hypoplastic right ventricle, 392–401
incidence of, 3–8
mild to moderate type, 444–445
severe type, 239–243
single ventricle and, 381–382
in tetralogy of Fallot, 366, 367, 375
in tetralogy of Fallot variants, 379, 382
Pulmonary vascularity. *See also* Pulmonary
vasculature
diagnostic role of, 77
patterns and roentgenography of, 81–82
Pulmonary vascular resistance. *See also* Systemic vascular resistance
at birth, 161–163
blood flow volume vs., 168
disorders affecting, in neonate, 472–473
echocardiography of, 116
fetal, 161
at higher elevations, 164
hypoxemia and, 163–164, 473
pulmonary blood flow vs., 167, 174, 175
Pulmonary vasculature. *See also* Pulmonary
vascularity
changes in, at birth, 161–162
in congenital cardiac anomaly classification, 165–166
fetal development of, 162–163
ventricular septal defects and, 174
Pulmonary veins
atresia of common, 441–443
congenital transposition of, 194
oxygen saturation in, 145
stenosis of individual, 435–437
Pulmonary venous obstruction, 423–456
Pulse, examination of, 25–26
Pulse monitoring, in cardiac catheterization,
131–132
Pulsus paradoxus, in pericardial effusion, 304
Pulse rate
in arteriovenous fistulas, 221, 223
in infant examination, 24–26
in purulent pericarditis, 305
Purulent pericarditis, 304–308
P waves
abnormality indications in, 48
age change characteristics of, 42
in premature infants, 45–46